欧阳德方　编著

计算药剂学
——制药4.0中的人工智能和建模

Computational Pharmaceutics

AI and Modeling in Pharma 4.0

化学工业出版社

·北京·

内容简介

《计算药剂学：制药4.0中的人工智能和建模》全书共17章，主要内容包括：计算药剂学简介（第1章）、人工智能在药物递送领域的机遇与挑战（第2章）、药剂学计算资源（第3章）、干粉吸入给药方式的计算机数值模拟技术（第4章）、药物递送中的分子模拟（第5章）、固体制剂3D结构研究（第6章）、基于非平衡热力学模型研究药物及制剂的溶解机制（第7章）、PBPK建模在制剂开发中的应用（第8章）、药物递送中的分子建模（第9章）、基于树枝状聚合物的递送技术与计算药剂学的结合及其在纳米医学时代的潜力（第10章）、人工智能与计算建模在经口吸入药物研发中的应用（第11章）、使用3D打印技术的数字处方开发（第12章）、专家系统在药物处方工艺设计中的研究与应用（第13章）、固体片剂药物生产工艺研发及其多尺度模型（第14章）、药物开发中的机器学习（第15章）、生物医药专利大数据分析及应用（第16章）以及模型引导的药物研发监管要求与思考（第17章）。

《计算药剂学：制药4.0中的人工智能和建模》可为制药领域研究人员、高等院校相关专业研究生和本科生提供将人工智能和多尺度模拟技术应用于药物制剂研究的一个全景概貌。

图书在版编目（CIP）数据

计算药剂学：制药4.0中的人工智能和建模/欧阳德方编著．－－北京：化学工业出版社，2025.3．
ISBN 978-7-122-46862-8

Ⅰ. R94-39

中国国家版本馆CIP数据核字第2024TV9094号

责任编辑：褚红喜	装帧设计：关 飞
责任校对：李露洁	

出版发行：化学工业出版社
　　　　（北京市东城区青年湖南街13号　邮政编码100011）
印　　装：河北京平诚乾印刷有限公司
787mm×1092mm　1/16　印张 29¾　字数 699 千字
2025年3月北京第1版第1次印刷

购书咨询：010-64518888　　　售后服务：010-64518899
网　　址：http://www.cip.com.cn

凡购买本书，如有缺损质量问题，本社销售中心负责调换。

定　　价：298.00元　　　　　　　　　版权所有　违者必究

《计算药剂学：制药 4.0 中的人工智能和建模》编写人员

（排名不分先后）

王南男 （澳门大学）
王 维 （澳门大学）
钟 豪 （澳门大学）
欧阳德方 （澳门大学）
叶祝一帆 （澳门理工大学）
董 界 （中南大学）
胡驾纬 （萨里大学）
张 凌 （萨里大学）
邬传宇 （萨里大学）
亚历克斯·邦克（Alex Bunker）（赫尔辛基大学）
约瑟夫·克赖因（Josef Kehrein）（赫尔辛基大学）
殷宪振 （中国科学院上海药物研究所；临港实验室）
黄晨夕 （临港实验室）
曹泽颖 （中国科学院上海药物研究所）
伍 丽 （中国科学院上海药物研究所）
肖体乔 （中国科学院上海应用物理所）
彼得·约克（Peter York）（布拉德福德大学）
张继稳 （中国科学院上海药物研究所）
吉远辉 （东南大学）
张 政 （东南大学）

葛 凯 （东南大学）
拉斐尔·波斯（Raphael Paus）（多特蒙德工业大学）
加布里埃莱·萨多夫斯基（Gabriele Sadowski）（多特蒙德工业大学）
刘 波 （武汉工程大学）
李 学 （英翰医药科技（上海）有限公司）
王佳文 （澳门科技大学；苏州大学）
于 怡 （苏州大学）
李有勇 （澳门科技大学；苏州大学）
卡纳克·R. 图帕利 （Karnaker R. Tupally）（昆士兰大学）
普拉桑吉特·西尔 （Prasenjit Seal）（坦佩雷大学）
普里蒂·潘迪 （Preeti Pandey）（昆士兰大学）
林克-扬·洛曼 （Rink-Jan Lohman）（昆士兰大学）
肖恩·史密斯 （Sean Smith）（澳大利亚国立大学）
哈伦德拉·帕雷克 （Harendra Parekh）（昆士兰大学）
李韧杰 （莫纳什大学）
缪 浩 （莫纳什大学）

周旭东 （莫纳什大学）
邹瑞萍 （莫纳什大学）
佟振博 （东南大学；东南大学-莫纳什大学联合研究院）
蒂莫西·特雷西（Timothy Tracy）（南京三迭纪医药科技有限公司）
吴　磊 （南京三迭纪医药科技有限公司）
成森平 （南京三迭纪医药科技有限公司）
李霄凌 （南京三迭纪医药科技有限公司；太平洋大学）
杜若飞 （上海中医药大学；中药现代制剂技术教育部工程研究中心）
张　裕 （上海中医药大学；中药现代制剂技术教育部工程研究中心）
陈锡忠 （上海交通大学；谢菲尔德大学）
刘　锴 （谢菲尔德大学）

王利戈 （山东大学）
李　亮 （上海交通大学）
罗正鸿 （上海交通大学）
约翰·伯特克（Johan Bøtker）（哥本哈根大学）
尤卡·兰塔宁（Jukka Rantanen）（哥本哈根大学）
安德斯·马德森（Anders Madsen）（哥本哈根大学）
徐佳琪 （澳门大学）
袁嘉璐 （澳门大学）
蔡　鸿 （澳门大学）
胡元佳 （澳门大学）
王玉珠 （国家药品监督管理局药品审评中心）

前言

当前药物开发高成本、长周期、低成功率的问题驱使制药科学家们思考如何提高药物开发效率。过去十年间制药行业的数字化转型浪潮为提高药物开发效率带来了新的机会。自2011年起，我们将人工智能和多尺度模拟技术用于药物制剂研究，开拓了"计算药剂学"这一新的研究领域。

2015年，我们编写了本领域第一部专著《Computational Pharmaceutics》，得到了广泛关注和好评。近十年来，计算药剂学领域迅猛发展并广泛应用于制药产业界。为了回应国内外广大读者的期待，我们自2021年起着手编著英文版《Exploring Computational Pharmaceutics: AI and Modeling in Pharma 4.0》，并于2024年8月正式出版，与此同时，我们进行了中文版《计算药剂学：制药4.0中的人工智能和建模》编写工作，相较于第一部专著，本书在广度和深度上有明显的提升。

在本书中，我们探讨了计算药剂学的最新进展，包括人工智能和机器学习在药物制剂中的应用、多尺度建模在药物递送中的应用，以及这些技术在药物开发全生命周期的整合。在此，我们要向为本书作出贡献的合作者表示诚挚的感谢，并感谢化学工业出版社长期以来的支持和帮助。我们希望本书能成为制药领域科学家、学生和专业人士的宝贵资源，并期待本书能激励国内计算药剂学领域的进一步发展。

计算药剂学是一个全新且迅速发展的领域，因作者水平和经验的限制，书中难免存在疏漏，恳请读者给予批评和指正，并希望在未来的再版中进行修正。

欧阳德方
2024年10月

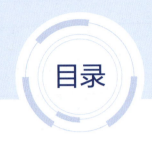

目录

第 1 章
计算药剂学简介 —— 001

- 1.1 药剂学研究现状 / 002
- 1.2 什么是计算药剂学？ / 004
- 1.3 关于本书 / 006
- 参考文献 / 007

第 2 章
人工智能在药物递送领域的机遇与挑战 —— 009

- 2.1 引言 / 010
- 2.2 机器学习算法 / 012
  - 2.2.1 线性模型 / 014
  - 2.2.2 人工神经网络 / 014
  - 2.2.3 深度学习 / 014
  - 2.2.4 遗传算法 / 015
  - 2.2.5 模糊神经网络 / 016
  - 2.2.6 支持向量机 / 016
  - 2.2.7 决策树 / 016
  - 2.2.8 集成学习 / 017
- 2.3 机器学习在药剂学中的应用 / 017
  - 2.3.1 速释片剂 / 022
  - 2.3.2 硬明胶胶囊 / 023
  - 2.3.3 口服缓释制剂 / 023
  - 2.3.4 乳液、微乳液和纳米乳液药物递送系统 / 024
  - 2.3.5 水凝胶经皮给药系统 / 025
  - 2.3.6 纳米药物递送系统 / 025
  - 2.3.7 固体分散体 / 028
  - 2.3.8 环糊精 / 028
- 2.4 大模型在药物发现和药物开发领域的应用 / 029
  - 2.4.1 下游药物发现与开发任务的语言模型预训练 / 029
  - 2.4.2 多任务学习和多性质预测的预训练在药物发现与开发领域的应用 / 030
- 2.5 人工智能在临床与精准医学领域的应用 / 032
- 2.6 机遇与挑战 / 033
- 2.7 总结 / 035
- 参考文献 / 035

第 3 章
药剂学计算资源 —————————————— 043

- 3.1 计算药剂学的概念 / 044
- 3.2 计算药剂学数据库 / 045
  - 3.2.1 数据库技术推动药物制剂领域快速发展 / 045
  - 3.2.2 药剂学数据库资源 / 046
- 3.3 药物制剂计算平台资源 / 050
  - 3.3.1 人工智能推动药物剂型快速研发和评价 / 050
  - 3.3.2 计算药剂学中的人工智能模型 / 051
  - 3.3.3 计算平台/网络服务器 / 055
- 3.4 数据库和计算平台的实现方法 / 058
- 3.5 总结 / 060
- 参考文献 / 061

第 4 章
干粉吸入给药方式的计算机数值模拟技术 —————————————— 063

- 4.1 引言 / 064
- 4.2 离散元法 / 065
- 4.3 颗粒团聚模拟 / 066
  - 4.3.1 仅药物颗粒团聚体的形成 / 066
  - 4.3.2 基于载体的团聚体的形成 / 067
- 4.4 颗粒团聚体解聚模拟 / 068
  - 4.4.1 空气动力学力引起的解聚 / 068
  - 4.4.2 机械冲击引起的解聚 / 069
- 4.5 DPI 中颗粒沉积模拟 / 071
  - 4.5.1 装置尺度上的 DEM-CFD 模拟 / 071
  - 4.5.2 CFD-DPM 雾化建模 / 072
- 4.6 总结 / 073
- 参考文献 / 074

第 5 章
药物递送中的分子模拟：一项聚合物保护修饰的案例研究 —————————————— 079

- 5.1 引言 / 080
  - 5.1.1 前药和纳米医学：缓解药物递送中的平衡作用 / 080
  - 5.1.2 药物递送中的聚合物 / 082
  - 5.1.3 机制阐释：制药学中的生物物理学范式 / 087
  - 5.1.4 分子动力学模拟：一种机制阐释的工具 / 088
- 5.2 聚合物在药物递送中的分子动力学模拟 / 094
  - 5.2.1 基于脂质的体系 / 094
  - 5.2.2 基于聚合物的体系 / 099
  - 5.2.3 基于蛋白质的体系 / 114
  - 5.2.4 无机纳米颗粒 / 119
- 5.3 结论 / 124
- 参考文献 / 125

第 6 章
固体制剂 3D 结构研究　　　　　　　　151

- 6.1　引言　／152
- 6.2　固体制剂的结构与研究方法概述　／152
  - 6.2.1　固体制剂的结构　／152
  - 6.2.2　固体制剂结构的研究方法　／153
- 6.3　同步辐射 X 射线显微断层扫描成像技术　／154
- 6.4　基于 SR-μCT 的三维结构重建　／155
  - 6.4.1　样品的制备　／155
  - 6.4.2　图像采集和三维重建　／157
  - 6.4.3　模型构建与分析　／158
- 6.5　三维可视化和定量表征　／159
  - 6.5.1　颗粒和颗粒系统的微观结构　／159
  - 6.5.2　固体剂型的静态结构和材料分布　／162
  - 6.5.3　亲水性基质片的动态结构　／164
  - 6.5.4　渗透泵片的动态结构　／166
- 6.6　展望　／174
- 参考文献　／174

第 7 章
基于非平衡热力学模型研究药物及制剂的溶解机制　　　　　　　　179

- 7.1　引言　／180
- 7.2　理论基础和模型　／182
  - 7.2.1　相平衡和化学势　／182
  - 7.2.2　化学势梯度模型　／183
  - 7.2.3　统计速率理论　／184
  - 7.2.4　微扰-统计缔合流体理论（PC-SAFT）　／185
  - 7.2.5　用 PC-SAFT 计算活度系数　／185
  - 7.2.6　溶解动力学的计算　／186
- 7.3　实验方法　／186
  - 7.3.1　API 溶解度的测定　／186
  - 7.3.2　量热性质的测定　／186
  - 7.3.3　API/聚合物制剂的制备　／187
  - 7.3.4　DSC、XRD 和 SEM 表征　／187
  - 7.3.5　体外本征溶解动力学测定　／187
  - 7.3.6　紫外-可见分光光度分析　／188
- 7.4　机制分析与模型预测　／188
  - 7.4.1　晶体 API 的溶解动力学与溶解机制　／188
  - 7.4.2　API/聚合物制剂的溶解动力学　／193
- 7.5　总结　／202
- 参考文献　／202

第 8 章
PBPK 建模在制剂开发中的应用　　　　　　　　209

- 8.1　引言　／210
- 8.2　用于建模的药代动力学软件　／210
  - 8.2.1　定量构效/构性关系（QSAR/QSPR）建模　／210
  - 8.2.2　药物从头设计（*de novo*）和合成计划　／211

8.2.3	使用分子动力学模拟进行药物制剂设计 / 212	8.3.2	针对吸入制剂的模型 / 215
8.2.4	基于生理的药代动力学模型的制剂开发设计 / 212	8.3.3	皮肤模型 / 216
		8.3.4	长效注射剂模型 / 217
8.3	不同类型制剂的建模机制 / 213	8.3.5	不足与改进 / 220
8.3.1	针对口服固体制剂的模型 / 214	8.4	总结 / 220
		参考文献	/ 221

第 9 章
药物递送中的分子建模 _____ 225

- 9.1 引言 / 226
- 9.2 分子动力学模拟的基本原理和分子建模方法 / 230
  - 9.2.1 分子动力学模拟的基本原理 / 231
  - 9.2.2 分子建模 / 232
  - 9.2.3 分子动力学模拟 / 232
- 9.3 纳米颗粒给药策略中的分子动力学模拟 / 233
  - 9.3.1 碳基纳米材料 / 233
  - 9.3.2 硅基纳米材料 / 238
  - 9.3.3 金属基纳米材料 / 239
  - 9.3.4 其他纳米材料 / 243
  - 9.3.5 分子动力学在药物递送系统中的其他应用 / 245
- 9.4 总结 / 246
- 参考文献 / 247

第 10 章
基于树枝状聚合物的递送技术与计算药剂学的结合及其在纳米医学时代的潜力 _____ 253

- 10.1 引言 / 254
- 10.2 树枝状聚合物作为药物/基因递送系统及其制药应用 / 256
  - 10.2.1 多功能载体系统 / 256
  - 10.2.2 增溶剂 / 262
  - 10.2.3 渗透促进剂 / 266
  - 10.2.4 药物递送系统 / 271
  - 10.2.5 治疗剂 / 275
  - 10.2.6 基因递送系统 / 277
  - 10.2.7 树枝状大分子在新型冠状病毒感染中的应用 / 281
- 10.3 树枝状聚合物给药的计算问题与挑战 / 282
- 10.4 总结 / 286
- 参考文献 / 287

第 11 章
人工智能与计算建模在经口吸入药物研发中的应用 —————— 295

11.1	引言		/296
11.2	慢性呼吸系统疾病与吸入治疗		/296
11.2.1	慢性呼吸系统疾病		/296
11.2.2	吸入治疗		/296
11.2.3	吸入给药装置		/297
11.3	计算建模简介		/298
11.3.1	计算流体力学模型		/298
11.3.2	生理药代动力学模型		/298
11.3.3	人工智能模型		/299
11.3.4	计算模型的验证与确认		/300
11.4	计算模型在吸入装置与制剂研发过程中的应用		/301
11.4.1	计算模型在雾化器研发过程中的应用		/301
11.4.2	计算模型在 pMDI 研发过程中的应用		/301
11.4.3	计算模型在 SMI 研发过程中的应用		/302
11.4.4	计算模型在 DPI 研发过程中的应用		/302
11.4.5	计算模型在吸入药物制剂研发过程中的应用		/303
11.5	计算模型在吸入药物药效评价中的应用		/304
11.5.1	药物沉积的预测模型		/304
11.5.2	吸入药物吸收与溶出的 PBPK 建模		/306
11.6	计算模型在慢性呼吸系统疾病管理中的应用		/308
11.6.1	基于吸入药物装置的电子检测设备		/308
11.6.2	患者依从性的改善		/309
11.6.3	吸入参数的测量		/309
11.6.4	急性加重的预测模型		/310
11.7	当前挑战与未来		/310
11.8	总结		/312
参考文献			/312

第 12 章
使用 3D 打印技术的数字处方开发：人工智能与建模 —————— 319

12.1	引言		/320
12.2	药物制剂处方中的 3D 打印方法		/321
12.2.1	挤出法		/322
12.2.2	粉末法		/322
12.2.3	液体法		/323
12.2.4	板材层压法		/323
12.3	使用 3D 打印技术实现新颖的片剂结构		/323
12.3.1	使用 3D 打印技术构建独特的片剂外部几何结构		/323
12.3.2	使用 3D 打印技术构建独特的片剂内部几何结构		/324
12.4	使用 3D 打印进行处方开发的人工智能		/325
12.4.1	辅料选择		/325
12.4.2	使用 3D 打印的制剂开发		/325

12.5 使用3D打印进行处方开发中的		12.6.1 3D打印处方源于设计（3DFbD®）	
数学建模	/329	的方法	/335
12.5.1 预测可打印性	/329	12.6.2 3DFbD®对质量源于设计的贡献	/336
12.5.2 溶出曲线预测	/330	12.7 总结	/337
12.6 3D打印处方源于设计	/335	参考文献	/338

第13章
专家系统在药物处方工艺设计中的研究与应用 　　　341

13.1 引言	/342	13.3 应用	/350
13.2 专家系统的结构	/343	13.3.1 SeDeM专家系统	/353
13.2.1 数据库	/343	13.3.2 中药质量控制专家系统	/356
13.2.2 规则库	/346	13.4 总结	/362
13.2.3 推理引擎	/347	参考文献	/363
13.2.4 用户界面	/349		

第14章
固体片剂药物生产工艺研发及其多尺度模型 　　　369

14.1 引言	/370	14.4.1 谢菲尔德大学的中型试验工厂	/379
14.2 片剂的药物制造过程	/371	14.4.2 连续直接压片过程的模拟	/380
14.3 计算模型	/373	14.5 总结	/383
14.4 研究案例	/379	参考文献	/384

第15章
药物开发中的机器学习 　　　387

15.1 引言	/388	15.4.2 作为数据源的过程分析	/395
15.2 制药材料科学	/389	15.4.3 与个性化药品生产系统有关的	
15.2.1 与制药相关的数据库实例	/389	方面	/396
15.2.2 模拟	/391	15.5 制药环境中的分析化学	/397
15.3 产品设计	/392	15.6 总结	/397
15.4 药品制造	/394	参考文献	/398
15.4.1 过程数据和预测模型	/394		

第 16 章
生物医药专利大数据分析及应用 　　　　　　　　　　401

- 16.1　引言　　/ 402
  - 16.1.1　专利数据的应用现状　　/ 402
  - 16.1.2　专利数据在生物医药研究中的应用　　/ 402
  - 16.1.3　概念框架　　/ 403
- 16.2　专利格局分析　　/ 403
  - 16.2.1　数据收集和标准化处理　　/ 404
  - 16.2.2　文献计量分析　　/ 404
  - 16.2.3　专利格局分析标准　　/ 404
  - 16.2.4　专利检索数据库　　/ 406
- 16.3　从专利数据中挖掘化学信息　　/ 407
  - 16.3.1　专利中的化学信息　　/ 407
  - 16.3.2　化学信息数据挖掘方法　　/ 408
  - 16.3.3　专利化学信息数据库　　/ 410
  - 16.3.4　常用 OCSR 工具比较　　/ 411
- 16.4　从专利数据中挖掘生物信息　　/ 411
  - 16.4.1　专利中的生物信息　　/ 411
  - 16.4.2　生物序列专利挖掘方法　　/ 412
  - 16.4.3　专利生物信息数据库　　/ 414
  - 16.4.4　专利中抗体序列数据挖掘—案例介绍　　/ 417
- 16.5　药剂学专利数据挖掘　　/ 418
  - 16.5.1　药剂学专利分析　　/ 418
  - 16.5.2　药剂学专利数据挖掘　　/ 419
- 16.6　实际操作及相关问题　　/ 420
  - 16.6.1　专利检索数据库　　/ 421
  - 16.6.2　化学信息数据库　　/ 423
  - 16.6.3　生物信息数据库　　/ 424
  - 16.6.4　现有专利数据库面临的挑战　　/ 428
  - 16.6.5　生物医药专利分析流程　　/ 429
- 16.7　总结　　/ 430
- 参考文献　　/ 430

第 17 章
模型引导的药物研发（MIDD）监管要求与思考 　　　　　　　　　　435

- 17.1　MIDD 发展的驱动力　　/ 436
- 17.2　建模方法的监管指南　　/ 438
  - 17.2.1　E-R 模型或 PK/PD 模型　　/ 438
  - 17.2.2　Pop-PK 模型　　/ 438
  - 17.2.3　PBPK 模型　　/ 439
  - 17.2.4　计算流体动力学建模和其他建模技术　　/ 440
- 17.3　关于 MIDD 的一些新思考　　/ 440
  - 17.3.1　PBPK 模拟用于体内试验的豁免　　/ 440
  - 17.3.2　通过 PK 相关的模拟以减轻 BE 研究的负担　　/ 442
  - 17.3.3　机器学习及其统计方法的应用　　/ 444
  - 17.3.4　监管部门正努力促进 MIDD 的应用　　/ 444
- 17.4　我国在定量药理学方面的进展　　/ 445
- 17.5　总结　　/ 446
- 参考文献　　/ 446

本书缩略词一览表

缩略词	英文全称	中文全称
0D	Zero-dimensional	零维
1D	One-dimensional	一维
2D	Two-dimensional	二维
3D	Three-dimensional	三维
4LANN	Four-layer artificial neural network	四层人工神经网络
AA	All-atom	全原子
AAD	Average absolute deviation	平均绝对偏差
ABC	Accelerated blood clearance	加速血清清除
ABS	Polymers acrylonitrile butadiene styrene	丙烯腈丁二烯苯乙烯
ACAT	Compartmental distribution and transit	隔室分布和转运模型
ACC	Accuracy	准确率
ACI	Anderson cascade impactor	安德森级联撞击器
ADME	Absorption, distribution, metabolism, and excretion	吸收、分布、代谢和排泄
ADMET	Absorption, distribution, metabolism, excretion, and toxicity	吸收、分布、代谢、排泄以及毒性
AFM	Atomic force microscope	原子力显微镜
AG	Berberine	穿心莲内酯
AgNP	Silver nanoparticle	银纳米颗粒
AI	Artificial intelligence	人工智能
AIDD	Artificial intelligence drug design	人工智能辅助药物设计
AIT	Artificial intelligence tool	人工智能工具
AMP	Antimicrobial peptide	抗菌肽
ANDA	Abbreviated new drug application	简化新药申请
ANN	Artificial neural network	人工神经网络
API	Active pharmaceutical ingredient	活性药物成分
AR	Augmented reality	增强现实技术
ARA	Acid-reducing agent	抗酸药

缩略词	英文全称	中文全称
ARD	Average relative deviation	平均相对偏差
ARLA	Aerosol Research Laboratory of Alberta	加拿大阿尔伯塔大学气溶胶研究实验室
ASD	Amorphous solid dispersions	无定形固体分散体
ASGPR	Asialoglycoprotein receptor	非糖基化蛋白受体
ASTM	American Society for Testing and Materials	美国材料试验协会
ATTR	Transthyretin-mediated amyloidosis	转甲状腺激素蛋白淀粉样变性
AUC	Area under curve	曲线下面积
AuNP	Au nanoparticle	金纳米颗粒
Aβ	β-amyloid protein	β 淀粉样蛋白
BA	Bioavailability	生物利用度
BCS	Biopharmaceutical classification system	生物药剂学分类系统
BE	Bioequivalence	生物等效性
BERT	Bidirectional encoder representations from Transformer	基于 Transformer 的双向编码器
BLA	Biologic License Application	生物制品许可申请
BP	Back propagation	反向传播
BPNN	Back propagation neural network	多层前馈神经网络
BSA	Bovine serum albumin	牛血清白蛋白
CAD	Computer-aided design	计算机辅助设计
CADD	Computer-aided drug design	计算辅助药物设计
CADFD	Computer-aided drug formulation design	计算机辅助药物制剂设计
CAESAR	Chemical substances according to regulations	符合规定的化学物质
CAS	Chemical Abstracts Service	化学文摘
CCD	Charge coupled device	电荷耦合器件
CD	Cyclodextrin	环糊精
CDE	Center for Drug Evaluation	中国药品审评中心
CEMP	Chemical entity mention in patents	化学实体标注识别
CFC	Chlorofluorocarbon	氯氟烃
CFD	Computational fluid dynamics	计算流体动力学
CG	Coarse-grained	粗粒化
CHEMDNER	Chemical compound and drug name recognition	化合物和药物名称识别
CHS	Chitosan	壳聚糖
CIF	Crystallographic information file	晶体学信息文件

缩略词	英文全称	中文全称
CLSM	Confocal laser scanning microscope	激光共聚焦扫描显微镜
CM	Continuous manufacturing	连续制造
CMA	Critical material attribute	关键物料属性
C_{max}	Maximum concentration	最大浓度
CMD	Carboxymethyl dextran	羧甲基葡聚糖
cMolGPT	Conditional molecular generative pre-trained Transformer model	有条件的分子生成预训练Transformer模型
CNER	Chemical named entity recognition	化学命名实体识别
CNN	Convolutional neural network	卷积神经网络
CNT	Carbon nanotube	碳纳米管
COD	Crystallography Open Database	晶体学开放数据库
COPD	Chronic obstructive pulmonary disease	慢性阻塞性肺疾病
CPP	Critical process parameter	关键工艺参数
CQA	Critical quality attribute	关键质量属性
CRCG	Center for Research on Complex Generics	复杂仿制药研究中心
CRF	Conditional random field	条件随机场
CRITIKAL	CRITical Inhaler mistaKes and Asthma control (*clinical trial*)	关于哮喘控制以及吸入装置错误使用的临床试验
cryo-EM	Cryo-electron microscopy	冷冻电子显微镜
CSD	Cambridge Structural Database	剑桥结构数据库
C_{ss}	Steady state concentration	稳态浓度
CHS-λ-CG	Chitosan-λ-carrageenan	壳聚糖-λ-卡拉胶
CT	Computed tomography	计算机断层扫描
CV	Computer vision	计算机视觉
CYP	Cytochrome P450	细胞色素 P450
DC	Diclofenac	双氯芬酸
DDBJ	DNA Data Bank of Japan	日本 DNA 数据库
DDI	Drug-drug interaction	药物相互作用
DDL	Drug delivery liposome	药物递送脂质体
DDPM	Dense discrete particle model	密集离散颗粒模型
DDS	Drug delivery system	药物递送系统
DEM	Discrete element method	离散元法
D_f	Dimension of fractal	分形维数
DF	Dispersion fraction	分散度分数
DFTB	Tight-binding density functional theory	紧束缚密度泛函理论

缩略词	英文全称	中文全称
DHA	Docosahexanoic acid	二十二碳六烯酸
DL	Deep learning	深度学习
DLLA	D, L-lactic acid	羟基乙酸，乳酸
DLP	Digital light processing	数字光处理
DNN	Deep neural network	深度神经网络
DOC	Docetaxel	多西他赛
DoE	Design of experiments	实验设计
DOPA	3, 4-dihydroxy-l-phenylalanine	3, 4-二羟基-L-苯丙氨酸
DOX	Doxorubicin	多柔比星
DPD	Dissipative particle dynamics	耗散粒子动力学
DPI	Dry powder inhaler	干粉吸入器
DPM	Discrete particle model	离散颗粒模型
DS	Distearyl	二硬脂酰
DSC	Differential scanning calorimeter	差示扫描量热仪
DSD	Distance between sample and detector	样品与检测器之间的距离
dsDNA	Double stranded DNA	双链 DNA
DSS	Decision support system	决策支持系统
DTI	Drug-target interaction	药物-靶标相互作用
DUSA	Dose unite sampling apparatus	剂量单位取样装置
DWPI	Derwent World Patents Index	德温特世界专利索引
DXT	Dextran	葡聚糖
EC	Ethylcellulose	乙基纤维素
ED	Emitted dose	释放剂量
ELF	Epithelia lining fluid	支气管上皮衬液
EMA	European Medicines Agency	欧洲药品管理局
E-MATIC	E-Monitoring of Asthma Therapy to Improve Compliance in Children Trial（clinical trial）	关于使用电子监控设备来改善儿童依从性的临床试验
EMBL-EBI	EMBL's European Bioinformatics Institute	欧洲生物信息研究所
ENA	European Nucleotide Archive	欧洲核酸数据库
EPI	Estimation programs interface	评估程序接口
EPO	European Patent Office	欧洲专利局
EPR	Enhanced permeability and retention	增强渗透和滞留
ER	Extended-release	缓释
E-R	Exposure-response	暴露-反应

缩略词	英文全称	中文全称
ESO	Esomeprazole magnesium enteric coated microsphere	艾司奥美拉唑镁肠溶微丸
FAIR	Findable, accessible, interoperable, and reusable	可查找，可访问，可互操作，可重复
FbD	Formulation by design	处方源于设计
FDA	Food and Drug Administration	美国食品药品管理局
FDM	Fused deposition modeling	熔融沉积建模
FEM	Finite element method	有限元法
FG	Fluorinated graphene	氟化石墨烯
FGO	Fluorinated graphene oxide	氟化氧化石墨烯
FN	False negative	假阴性
FNN	Feedforward neural network	前馈神经网络
FP	False positive	假阳性
FPF	Fine particle fraction	细颗粒分数
FTO	Free to operate	自由实施
GA	Genetic algorithm	遗传算法
GAN	Generative adversarial network	生成对抗网络
GBRT	Gradient boost regression tree	梯度增强回归树
G-CSF	Granulocyte colony-stimulating factor	嗜中性粒细胞集落刺激因子
GDUFA	Generic Drug User Fee Amendments	仿制药使用者费用法案
GLIB	Glibenclamide	格列本脲
GLP-1	Glucagon-like peptide-1	胰高血糖素样肽-1
GMP	Good manufacturing practice for drugs	药物生产质量管理规范
GNR	Gold nanorod	金纳米棒
GOF	Goodness of fit	拟合度
GOQD	Graphene oxide quantum dot	氧化石墨烯量子点
GPT	Generative pre-trained Transformer	生成式预训练 Transformer
GQD	Graphene quantum dot	石墨烯量子点
GRM	Graphene related material	石墨烯相关材料
GRNN	General regression neural network	广义回归神经网络
GSA	Global sensitive analysis	全局敏感度分析
GSD	Geometric standard deviation	几何标准偏差
GWO	Gray wolf optimization	灰狼优化

续表

缩略词	英文全称	中文全称
HCT	Hydrochlorothiazide	氢氯噻嗪
HES	Hydroxyethyl starch	羟乙基淀粉
HFA	Hydrofluoroalkane	氢氟烷
HFM	Homogeneous frozen model	均质冻结模型
hGH	Human growth hormone	人生长激素
HIPS	High-impact polystyrene	高冲击聚苯乙烯
HMA	Heads of Medicines Agencies	药品监管机构负责人组织
HME	Hot-melt extrusion	热熔挤出
HPG	Hyperbranched poly（glycerol）	高支化聚甘油
HPMC	Hydroxyl propyl methylcellulose	羟丙甲纤维素
HRP	Horseradish peroxidase	辣根过氧化物酶
IAPP	Human islet amyloid polypeptide	人胰岛淀粉样多肽
IB	Ipratropium bromide	异丙托溴铵
IBU	Ibuprofen	布洛芬
ICH	International Conference on Harmonization	国际协调会议
ICRP	International Commission on Radiological Protection	国际辐射防护委员会
ICSD	Inorganic Structural Database	无机结构数据库
IEMD	Inhaler-based electronic monitoring devices	基于吸入装置的电子监测设备
IFM	Internal flow model	内部流动模型
IFN	Interferon	干扰素
INCA	Inhaler compliance assessment device	吸入装置依从性评估设备
IND	Investigational New Drug Application	新药研究申请
INPADOC	International Patent Documentation	国际专利文献索引
INSDC	International Nucleotide Sequence Database Collaboration	国际核苷酸序列协作数据库
IONP	Iron oxide nanoparticle	铁氧化物纳米颗粒
IR	Immediate-release	速释
IR	Infrared radiation	红外线
ISE	Iterative stochastic elimination	迭代随机消除
ISPE	The International Society for Pharmaceutical Engineering	国际制药工程学会
IUPAC	International Union of Pure and Applied Chemistry	国际纯粹与应用化学联合会
IVIVC	*In vitro-in vivo* correlation	体内-体外相关性
JKR	Johnson-Kendal-Roberts	约翰逊-肯德尔-罗伯茨

续表

缩略词	英文全称	中文全称
JPO	Japan Patent Office	日本专利局
K-CV	K-fold cross-validation	K 折交叉验证
KNN	K-nearest neighbors	K 最近邻
L/S	Liquid/Solid	液固比
LAI	Long-acting injectable	长效注射剂
LAP	Locally acting product	局部作用产品
LBM	Lattice Boltzmann method	格子玻尔兹曼方法
LC	Liquid crystalline	液晶
LC-ELSD	Liquid chromatography-evaporative light scattering detector	液相色谱-蒸发光散射检测器
LC-MS	Liquid chromatography-mass spectrometry	液相色谱-质谱联用
LDS	Liposome-based delivery system	基于脂质体的递送系统
LightGBM	Light gradient boosting machine	光梯度提升机
LLE	Liquid-liquid equilibrium	液-液平衡
LLM	Large language model	大型语言模型
LNP	Lipid nanoparticle	脂质纳米颗粒
LOD	Loss on drying	干燥失重
logBB	Barrier permeabilities（logarithmic）	屏障渗透性（对数值）
log$P$	Partition coefficient（logarithmic）	油水分配系数（对数值）
LOO	Leave-one-out cross-validation	留一法交叉验证
LPG	Linear poly（glycerol）	线性聚（甘油）
LR	Logistic regression	逻辑回归
LSTM	Long short term memory	长短期记忆
MBDD	Model-based drug development	基于模型的药物研发
MBP	Monolayer black phosphorus	单层黑磷
MC	Monte Carlo	蒙特卡洛
MCC	Microcrystalline cellulose	微晶纤维素
MCC	Mucociliary clearance	黏膜睫状清除
MCC	Matthews correlation coefficient	马修斯相关系数
MCMG	Multi-constraint molecular generation	多重约束分子生成
MD	Molecular dynamics	分子动力学
MDI	Metered dose inhaler	定量吸入器
ME	Microemulsion	微乳剂
MED	Melt extrusion deposition	熔融挤出沉积
MIDD	Model-informed drug development	模型引导的药物研发

续表

缩略词	英文全称	中文全称
MIE	Model-integrated evidence	模型整合实证
ML	Machine learning	机器学习
ML	Matrix layer	基质层
MLP	Multilayer perceptron	多层感知机
MLR	Multivariate linear regression	多元线性回归
MLR	Mixed logistic regression	混合逻辑回归
MM	Molecular mechanics	分子力学
MMAD	Mass median aerodynamic diameter	质量中值气动直径
MMF	Model master file	模型主文件
MM-GBSA	Molecular mechanics generalized-Born surface area	分子力学广义玻恩表面积
MM-PBSA	Molecular mechanics Poisson-Boltzmann surface area	分子力学泊松-玻尔兹曼表面积
MOPT	Monolithic osmotic pump tablet	单室渗透泵片
MP	Melting point	熔点
MPS	Mononuclear phagocyte system	单核吞噬细胞系统
MRI	Magnetic resonance imaging	磁共振成像
MSD	Mean-square displacement	均方位移
MSPC	Multivariate statistical process control	多变量统计过程控制
MTR	Mixer torque rheometer	混合扭矩流变仪
MVC	Model-controller-view	模型-控制-视图
MWCNT	Multi-walled carbon nanotube	多壁碳纳米管
Nano-CT	Nano-computed tomography	纳米计算机断层扫描
NAP	Naproxen	萘普生
NAS	Network architecture search algorithm	网络架构搜索算法
NCBI	National Center for Biotechnology Information	美国国家生物技术信息中心
NCI	National Cancer Institute	美国国家癌症研究所
NCRP	National Council on Radiation Protection and Measurement	美国辐射防护与测量委员会
NDA	New drug application	新药申请
NER	Named entity recognition	命名实体识别
NGI	Next generation impactor	下一代撞击器
NGO	Nano graphene oxide	纳米氧化石墨烯
NIH	National Institutes of Health	美国国立卫生研究院
NiONP	Nickel oxide nanoparticle	氧化镍纳米颗粒

缩略词	英文全称	中文全称
NIR	Near-infrared spectroscopy	近红外光谱
NLP	Natural language processing	自然语言处理
NME	New molecular entity	新分子实体
NMPA	National Medical Products Administration	国家药品监督管理局
NMR	Nuclear magnetic resonance	核磁共振
NN	Neural network	神经网络
NP	Nanoparticle	纳米颗粒
OCR	Optical character recognition	光学字符识别
OCSR	Optical chemical structure recognition	光学化学结构识别
ODDS	Osmosis drug delivery system	渗透药物递送系统
OECD	Organization for Economic Cooperation and Development	经济合作与发展组织
OFDF	Oral fast disintegrating film	口服快速崩解膜
OME	Omeprazole magnesium microsphere	奥美拉唑镁微丸
PAA	Poly（acrylic acid）	聚丙烯酸
PAC	Paclitaxel	紫杉醇
PAcM	Poly（N-acryloylmorpholine）	聚（N-丙烯酰吗啉）
PAE	Poly（β-amino ester）	聚（β-氨基酯）
PAEMA	Poly（aminoethyl methacrylate）	聚（氨乙基甲基丙烯酸酯）
PaLM	Pathways language model	路径语言模型
PAMAM	Poly amidoamine	聚酰胺-胺
PARA	Paracetamol	对乙酰氨基酚
PASP	Poly（aspartic acid）	聚（天冬氨酸）
PASS	Prediction of activity spectra for substance	物质活性谱预测
PAT	Process analytical technology	过程分析技术
PBBM	Physiologically based biopharmaceutics modeling	基于生理的生物药剂学模型
PBCA	Poly（n-butylcyanoacrylate）	聚正丁基氰基丙烯酸酯
PBCMA	Poly（carboxybetaine methacrylate）	聚（羧基甲基丙烯酸酯）
PBLG	Poly（γ-benzyl-L-glutamate）	聚（γ-苯基-L-谷氨酸）
PBM	Population balance model	种群平衡模型
PBPK	Physiologically-based pharmacokinetic	基于生理的药代动力学
PC	Phosphatidyl choline	磷脂酰胆碱
PCA	Principle component analysis	主成分分析

缩略词	英文全称	中文全称
PCAT	Pulmonary compartmental absorption & transit model	肺部分区吸收和转运模型
PCC	Preclinical candidate	临床前候选药物
PCL	Protective layer	保护层
PCL	Polycaprolactone	聚己内酯
PCS	Physicalpharmaceutics classification system	中药提取物粉体物理药剂学分类系统
PC-SAFT	Perturbed-chain statistical associating fluid theory	微扰-统计缔合流体理论
PCT	Patent cooperation treaty	国际专利申请
PD	Pharmacodynamics	药效动力学
PDB	Protein Data Bank	蛋白质数据库
PDEAEMA	Poly（N,N-diethylaminoethyl methacrylate）	聚（N,N-二乙基氨基乙基甲基丙烯酸酯）
PDF	Pair distribution function	成对分布函数
PDI	Polydispersity index	多分散指数
PDLA	Poly（D-lactic acid）	聚（D-乳酸）
PDLLA	Poly（D, L-lactic acid）	聚（D, L-乳酸）
PDMA	Poly（N, N-dimethylacrylamide）	聚（N, N-二甲基丙烯酰胺）
PdNP	Palladium nanoparticle	钯纳米颗粒
PDUFA Ⅵ	Prescription Drug User Fee Act Ⅵ	第六次处方药使用者费用法案
PEG	Polyethylene glycol	聚乙二醇
PEGMA	Poly（ethylene glycol methacrylate）	聚乙二醇甲基丙烯酸酯
PEOZ	Poly（2-ethyl-2-oxazoline）	聚（2-乙基-2-噁唑啉）
PE-PEG	Phosphatidyl ethanolamine-poly（ethylene glycol）	磷脂酰乙醇胺-聚乙二醇
PES	Polyethersulfone	聚醚砜
PGLU	Poly（glutamic acid）	聚谷氨酸
PHBV	Poly（3-hydroxybutyrate-co-3-hydroxyvalerate）	聚（3-羟基丁酸-co-3-羟基戊酸酯）
PHEMA	Poly（2-hydroxyethyl methacrylate）	聚（2-羟乙基甲基丙烯酸酯）
PHPMA	Poly[N-(2-hydroxypropyl)methacrylamide]	聚[N-（2-羟丙基）甲基丙烯酰胺]
PIF	Peak inspiratory flow rate	峰值吸入流速
PK	Pharmacokinetics	药代动力学
PK/PD	Pharmacokinetic/parmacodynamics	药代动力学/药效动力学
pK_a	Dissociation constant	解离常数
PL	Particle layer	颗粒层

缩略词	英文全称	中文全称
PLA	Polylactic acid	聚乳酸
PLA-PEG-PLA	Poly(lactide)-poly(ethylene glycol)-poly(lactide)	三嵌段聚乳酸-聚乙二醇-聚乳酸
PLGA	Poly（lactic-co-glycolic acid）	聚乳酸-羟基乙酸共聚物
PLLA	Poly（L-lactic acid）	聚L-乳酸
PLS	Partial least squares	偏最小二乘法
PLSR	Partial least squared regression	偏最小二乘回归
pMDI	Pressurized metered-dose inhaler	压力定量吸入器
PMF	Potential of mean force	平均力势
PMMA	Poly（methyl methacrylate）	聚甲基丙烯酸甲酯
PMOZ	Poly（2-methyl-2-oxazoline）	聚（2-甲基-2-噁唑啉）
PNIPAAm	Poly（N-isopropylacrylamide）	聚（N-异丙基丙烯酰胺）
POEGMA	Poly[oligo(ethylene glycol)methacrylate]	聚寡聚乙二醇甲基丙烯酸酯
POPC	1-palmitoyl-2-oleoyl-sn-glycero-3-phospho-choline	1-棕榈酰-2-油酰-sn-甘油-3-磷酸胆碱
POPE	1-palmitoyl-2-oleoyl-sn-glycero-3-phospho-ethanolamine	1-棕榈酰-2-油酰-sn-甘油-3-磷酸乙醇胺
popPK	Population pharmacokinetic	群体药代动力学
POX	Poly（oxazoline）	聚（2-噁唑啉）
PPEGMA	Poly（poly(ethylene glycol)methyl ether methacrylate）	聚（聚乙二醇甲基醚甲基丙烯酸酯）
PPI	Poly（propylene imine）	聚丙烯亚胺
PPO	Poly（propylene oxide）	聚丙烯醚
PPOP	Push pull osmosis pump	推拉渗透泵片
PR	Percent of release	释放百分比
PRISMA	Preferred Reporting Items for Systematic reviews and Meta-Analyses	系统评价和荟萃分析的首选报告项目
PSA	Poly（sarcosine）	聚肌氨酸
PSA	Polar surface area	极性表面积
PSBMA	Poly（sulfobetaine methacrylate）	聚甲基丙烯酸磺基甜菜碱
PSD	Particle size distribution	粒径分布
PSG	Product-specific guidance	特定药品指导原则
PSIPS	The USPTO publication site for issued and published sequences	USPTO已授权和已公开序列
PSO	Particle swarm algorithm	粒子群优化算法
PVA	Polyvinyl alcohol	聚乙烯醇

续表

缩略词	英文全称	中文全称
PVAc	Poly（vinyl acetate）	聚乙酸乙烯酯
PVI	Poly（4-vinyl imidazole）	聚（4-乙烯基咪唑）
PVP	Polyvinylpyrrolidone	聚乙烯吡咯烷酮；聚（N-乙烯基-2-吡咯烷酮）
PVP K25	Polyvinylpyrrolidone K25	聚乙烯吡咯烷酮 K25
PVPVA	Polyvinylpyrrolidone/vinyl acetate	聚乙烯吡咯烷酮/乙酸乙烯酯
PVPVA 64	Polyvinylpyrrolidone/vinyl acetate 64	聚乙烯吡咯烷酮/乙酸乙烯酯 64
Q3D	Quasi 3D	准三维
QbD	Quality by Design	质量源于设计
QM	Quantum mechanics	量子力学
QSAR	Quantitative structure-activity relationship	定量结构-活性关系（构效关系）
QSP	Quantitative systems pharmacology	定量系统药理学
QSPR	Quantitative structure-property relationship	定量结构-性质关系（构性关系）
QTPP	Quality target product profile	目标产品质量概况
R&D	Research and development	研究和开发
R^2	Coefficient of determination	决定系数
RBD	Receptor binding domain	受体结合域
RDF	Radial distribution function	径向分布函数
ReaxFF	Reaction force field	反应力场
RES	Reticulo-endothelial system	网状内皮系统
RF	Random forest	随机森林
RFE	Recursive feature elimination	递归特征消除
RGD	Arginylglycylaspartic acid	精氨酰甘氨酰天冬氨酸
RGO	Reduced graphene oxide	还原氧化石墨烯
RH	Relative humidity	相对湿度
RIPL	Reporting items for patent landscapes	专利格局分析的报告项目
RMSD	Root mean square deviation	均方根偏差
RMSE	Root mean square error	均方根误差
RMSEP	Relative mean square error percentage	相对均方误差百分比
RMSF	Root-mean-square fluctuation	均方根波动
RNN	Recurrent neural network	循环神经网络
ROC	Receiver operating characteristic curve	受试者工作特征曲线
ROR	Receptor-related orphan receptor	受体相关孤儿受体
RSC	Royal Society of Chemistry	英国皇家化学会

缩略词	英文全称	中文全称
RSM	Response surface methodology	响应面法
RTD	Residence time distribution	停留时间分布
RTRT	Real-time release testing	实时释放测试
SA	Surface area	表面积
SAM	Segment anything model	分割模型
SAMN	Naked surface active maghemite nanoparticle	裸露表面活性磁赤铁矿纳米颗粒
SAR	Structure-activity relationship	构效关系
SASA	Solvent-accessible surface area	溶剂可及表面积
SBIA	Small Business and Industry Assistance	小企业和行业援助
SCID	Severe combined immunodeficiency disorder	重症联合免疫缺陷病
SD	Solid dispersion	固体分散体
SE	Sensitivity	灵敏度
SEDDS	Self-emulsifying drug delivery system	自乳化给药系统
SEM	Scanning electron microscope	扫描电子显微镜
SGF	Simulated gastric fluid	模拟胃液
SLE	Solid-liquid equilibrium	固-液平衡
SLS	Selective laser sintering	选择性激光烧结
SMI	Soft mist inhaler	软雾吸入器
SNS	Single cell sequencing	单细胞测序
SOM	Self-organizing map	自组织映射
SP	Specificity	特异性
SPECT	Single photon emission computed tomography	单光子发射计算断层扫描
SPH	Smoothed particle hydrodynamics	平滑粒子流体动力学
SR-FTIR	Synchrotron radiation fourier transform infrared	同步辐射傅里叶变换红外光谱
SRMT	Sustained release matrix tablet	缓释基质片
SR-μCT	Synchrotron radiation X-ray microcomputed tomography	同步辐射 X 射线显微断层扫描成像
ssDNA	Single stranded DNA	单链 DNA
SSE	Semi-solid extrusion	半固态挤出
suPAR	Soluble urokinase plasminogen activator receptor	可溶性尿激酶纤溶酶原激活剂受体
SVM	Support vector machine	支持向量机
TB	Tracheobronchial region	气管支气管
TCA	Triamcinolone acetonide	曲安奈德

续表

缩略词	英文全称	中文全称
TFF	Thin film freezing	薄膜冷冻
TSH	Tamsulosin hydrochloride sustained release capsule	盐酸坦索罗辛缓释胶囊
TLR	Toll-like receptor	Toll 样受体
TMC	Trimethylchitosane	三甲基壳聚糖
TN	True negative	真阴性
TP	True positive	真阳性
TR	Time of rotation	旋转时间
TRAP	Tartrate-resistant acid phosphatase	抗酒石酸磷酸酶
TTC	Thresholds of toxicological concern	毒理学相关阈值
TV	Time of vibration	振动时间
US EPA	United States Environmental Protection Agency	美国环境保护署
USP	United States Pharmacopeia	美国药典
USPTO	United States Patent and Trademark Office	美国专利商标局
UV	Ultraviolet	紫外线
UV-Vis	Ultraviolet-visible	紫外线-可见光
VBE	Virtual bioequivalence	虚拟生物等效性
VDW	Van der Waals	范德华力
vGNP	Virtual gold nanoparticle	虚拟金纳米颗粒
VIP	Vasoactive intestinal peptide	血管活性肠肽
ViT	Vision Transformer	视觉 Transformer
VR	Virtual reality	虚拟现实
WIPO	World Intellectual Property Organization	世界知识产权组织
XGBoost	Extreme gradient boosting	极限梯度提升
XRD	X-ray diffraction	X 射线衍射
α-PC	α-phase phosphorus carbide	α 相磷碳化合物
αS	α-synaptic nucleoprotein	α-突触核蛋白
μCT	Microcomputed tomography	显微计算机断层扫描成像

第1章

计算药剂学简介

王南男　　澳门大学，澳门，中国
王　维　　澳门大学，澳门，中国
钟　豪　　澳门大学，澳门，中国
欧阳德方　澳门大学，澳门，中国

当前药物开发高成本、长周期、低成功率的问题驱使制药科学家们思考如何才能提高药物制剂开发的效率。过去十年间制药行业的数字化转型浪潮催生了名为"计算药剂学"的药物开发新范式,为提高制剂开发效率带来了新的机会。本章初步介绍了计算药剂学的概念和常用工具。此外,本章还阐述了《计算药剂学》出版的初衷,内容框架和优势。

1.1 药剂学研究现状

现代药剂学与新型药物递送系统(drug delivery system,DDS)的发展密切相关,在过去70多年间历经了巨大的变革。1952年,Smith Kline & French公司使用Spansule®技术开发了第一个12小时缓释制剂,被认为开创了现代药剂学的历史新时期[1]。现代药剂学在过去70年间的进展可分为两个时期[2, 3]。第一代现代药剂学(1950年至1980年)通过将物理化学的基本原理与药剂学相结合,逐渐发展了物理药剂学,它主要侧重于控释制剂的开发。在此期间,药物递送技术快速发展,并在临床应用中取得了巨大成功,包括口服缓释制剂、透皮贴剂(Scop®)[4]和压力定量吸入剂(pMDI)[5]。第二代现代药剂学(1980年至2010年)致力于开发先进的给药系统,包括基于纳米技术的给药系统、自我调节给药系统和长效制剂等先进药物递送技术。然而,由于存在人体生物屏障,新型制剂进入临床的阻碍大,临床成功率低[6]。

当前的新分子实体(new molecular entity,NME)产出与研发投入与之间存在明显的鸿沟。NME的研发成本正以平均每年13.4%的速度增长[7]。然而,NME在临床试验中的成功率仅为10%左右。2007年对68种已获批准的药物进行研究显示,将一个NME推向市场平均需要花费15年[8]和2.558亿美元[9]。如图1-1所示,2022年美国食品药品管理局(Food and Drug Administration,FDA)仅批准了37个NME。在过去30年中,尽管投入的资源呈指数级增长,FDA每年批准的NME数量却一直在20到50个之间徘徊,这种现象被称为"Eroom's law"[10]。此外,由于溶解度低、稳定性差、靶向效果差等问题,当前的一些药品在临床实践中远未达到最佳效果。从理论上讲,开发一种新制剂的成本总体上只是开发一个NME的数十亿美元成本的一小部分,耗时仅需3至4年,这促使许多制药公司转向新型药物制剂的开发。

近40年来,药剂学学术研究取得了令人瞩目的进展。如图1-2(A)所示,1980—2022年间,影响因子在1以上的药剂学领域SCI期刊共发表论文141523篇,呈稳定增长趋势。2022年的药剂学领域论文发表数量高达8420篇,几乎是1980年(1523篇)的5.5倍。然而,新型给药系统的临床成功率(已上市药物产品与临床试验数量的比率)甚至低于NME开发的成功率(10%)[11]。主要原因是传统的药物制剂研发仍依赖于低效的试错模式,缺乏对药物递送系统与生物系统之间多尺度相互作用的关注和理解。

药物开发高成本、长周期、低成功率的挑战为我们提出了一个问题,即如何提高药物制剂开发的效率?当前影响药物制剂开发效率的问题应当归咎于药剂学原理与传统药物开发范式之间的冲突。药剂学研究从本质上讲是在材料特性和工艺参数组成的高维空间中进行多目标优化。据估算[12],制剂开发的空间维度可高达10^{25}~10^{30}。在如此高维的空间中试错是极为

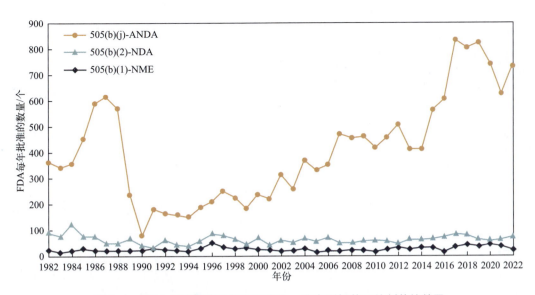

图1-1　FDA年度批准的新分子实体、改良型新药和仿制药的数量

505（b）（1）-NME：505（b）（1）审评通道下的新分子实体的批准数量；505（b）（2）-NDA：505（b）（2）审评通道下的改良型新药的批准数量，包括新的活性药物成分、新剂型、新组合、新制剂以及新适应证；505（b）（j）-ANDA：505（b）（j）审评通道下的仿制药批准数量

低效的。一个直截了当的想法是，在生产和检验之前应该对药物递送的基本原理有深入的认识，这显然比依靠幸运女神的眷顾进行无休止的试错试验更高效，正如FDA提倡的"质量源于设计（quality by design，QbD）"理念，鼓励将对产品和工艺的理解融入药品设计中，以提高药品质量。

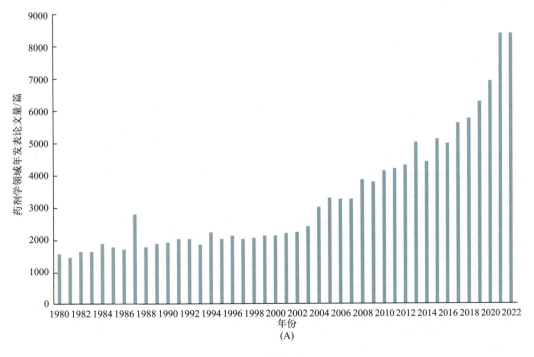

(A)

图1-2

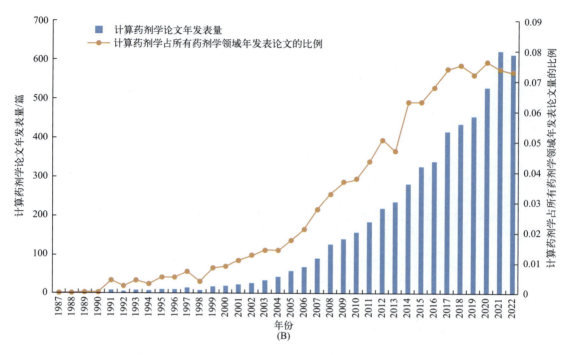

图1-2　从1980年到2022年药剂学领域发表论文情况

（A）从1980年到2022年，药剂学领域年发表论文量；（B）计算药剂学论文年发表量及其在当年所有药剂学领域年发表论文中所占的比例，其中1987年至1990年计算药剂学的发表论文数量分别为1、0、1和1

1.2 什么是计算药剂学？

过去10年间，计算能力的飞跃发展推动了各行各业的数字化转型，制药行业也不例外。人工智能（artificial intelligence，AI）和多尺度建模与药剂学的深度融合，催生了"计算药剂学"新领域[12]。如图1-3所示，与传统的"筛选-验证-再筛选"药物制剂开发流程不同，计算药剂学强调计算机驱动的"理解-设计-验证-优化"的药物制剂设计新范式[13]。利用建模和模拟工具来全面理解药物递送机理，结合人工智能的高效设计和优化算法，QbD理念正在计算药剂学中得到很好的践行。由此推断，计算药剂学新范式不仅能提高药物制剂开发的效率，还有望促进目标导向的个性化药物开发。

计算药剂学的常用工具包括机器学习或人工智能、量子力学（quantum mechanics，QM）模拟、分子动力学（molecular dynamics，MD）模拟、数学建模、过程模拟和基于生理的药代动力学（physiologically-based pharmacokinetics，PBPK）建模。通过在现有数据上训练模型，机器学习或人工智能算法可以发现潜在的关联，并对新场景进行预测。QM模拟使用分子的空间电子密度和量子化学函数精确计算分子特性和化学反应的变化。MD模拟是基于分子内部和分子之间的势能和牛顿运动定律，模拟和分析分子结构和所构成系统的动态变化。数学建模是用数学方程来描述宏观过程，其中数学方程是多种模拟的基础，但在药剂学中，数学建模一词通常用于溶解或沉淀过程的模拟。过程模拟指模拟药物在生产线上的工艺过程中材料的变化，涉及的技术包括计算流体动力学（CFD）、离散元法（DEM）以及利用统计算法从数据中训练的自动监测系统。PBPK是一种利用一组涉及药物和生理参数的微分方程来模拟给药后药物代谢动力学的方法。此外，如果已知药代动力学/药效动力学（PK/PD）关系，也可以建立PBPK/PD模型。

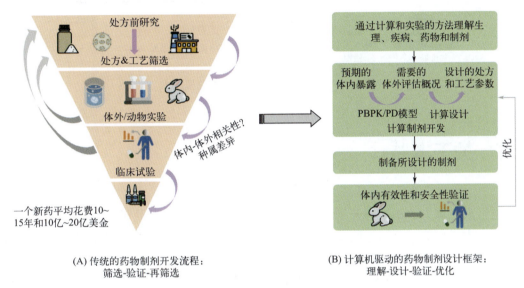

图1-3 计算药剂学驱动的药物制剂开发范式转变

如今，计算药剂学的相关研究越来越受欢迎。在Web of Science中搜索截至2022年计算药剂学领域的出版物[12]，共找到5547篇论文。在这些论文中，85.2%（4724篇）为研究文章，10.6%（590篇）为综述论文，其他类型约占4.2%。图1-2（B）展示了论文发表情况，在过去几十年中，尤其是2000年后，计算药剂学领域每年发表论文的数量及其在所有药剂学领域发表论文中所占比例均呈现快速增长。仅2022年计算药剂学领域的论文发表数量已超过600篇。

图1-4展示了计算药剂学的应用前景，从图中可以看出，药物开发的各个阶段都可能涉及建模技术。在数据收集得当的情况下，几乎所有情况下都可以使用人工智能或机器学习来挖掘数据背后的关联。QM模拟和MD模拟可用于研究生物分子、药物分子、辅料及其相互作用的微观机制。当遇到更大尺度的问题时，QM模拟和MD模拟就不适用了，因为它们的计算精度太高，而目前的计算能力不支持模拟太大的体系。在这种情况下，必须使用基于数学建模的方法。现有的数学公式涵盖了固体溶解、分子扩散、流体或粉末流动、颗粒碰撞以及药物的吸收、分布、代谢、排泄（ADME）等过程。这些过程与处方设计、工艺开发和临床阶段的特定问题相对应。

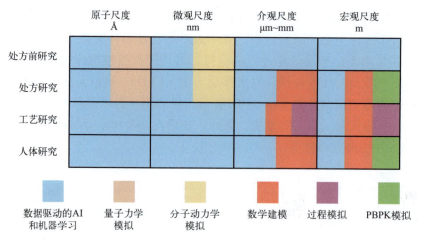

图1-4 计算药剂学中的多尺度建模技术

1.3 关于本书

近些年来，算力的不断提升为药剂学中的分子模拟开辟了新的场景，定量药理学研究也为以临床为导向的计算药物制剂开发提供了新的思路，尤其是人工智能的飞速发展为计算药剂学注入了新的动力。此外，计算药剂学不仅仅是一个学术概念，近年来，越来越多的工业界头部制药公司和监管机构引进和实施了计算药剂学[14, 15]。计算药剂学正在为药物开发的范式转变提供源源不断的驱动力。2017年，国际制药工程学会（International Society for Pharmaceutical Engineering，ISPE）提出了制药4.0的倡议，旨在将数字化、智能化和自动化技术融入药物开发的整个生命周期。FDA鼓励模型引导的药物开发（model-informed drug development，MIDD）[16]并提倡在药物开发和制造过程中使用AI技术。在制药4.0时代，计算药剂学驶入了发展的快车道，各个研究分支都积累了诸多宝贵的研究成果。

在本章中，我们首先对药剂学和计算药剂学的研究成果进行了回顾和大数据分析，并简要阐述计算药剂学的内涵。计算药剂学的系统介绍可以从最近的两篇综述文章[12, 13]中获得。本书其余章节的内容按以下几个部分组织编写。

（1）方法学

第2章至第8章详细介绍了药剂学中主要应用的计算技术和资源，包括人工智能、分子模拟、过程模拟、PK/PD建模以及药物开发中的数据库资源等。本部分还介绍了物理药剂学基础理论的计算研究方法（如药物三维固态结构计算、药物制剂的溶出理论计算）。方法学部分将帮助读者构建计算药剂学的理论基础和思维模式。

（2）工业应用和纳米药物

计算药剂学在制药4.0产业升级计划中的潜力和价值正在得到验证。在第9章至第15章中，我们邀请了具有工业和学术背景的专家讨论计算药剂学在制药工业界以及纳米药物研究中的应用、挑战和前景。涉及的主题包括人工智能、多尺度建模和数字孪生在片剂、吸入制剂、3D打印制剂和中药制剂等的设计、制造和临床应用中的作用。此外，纳米药物一直是药剂学研究的热点之一，因此本部分还将讨论计算药剂学在纳米药物结构和性质研究、药物负载和释放机制探索、纳米药物与生物系统相互作用理解的计算研究等，所涉及的纳米药物包括无机纳米颗粒和树枝状聚合物。

（3）监管科学

在制药4.0时代，计算药剂学领域的健全离不开监管科学的同步发展。第16章将介绍专利分析研究，计算药剂学可以为监管科学提供有关技术创新和市场动态的情报。第17章分析了全球药物监管机构对模型引导的药物开发（MIDD）以及人工智能用于药物开发的积极态度和监管要求。

总的来说，本书由来自全球计算药剂学领域学术界、工业界和药品监管机构的顶尖专家合力撰写完成，系统地介绍了制药4.0时代计算药剂学的前沿发展、其在新兴制药技术中的应用和计算药剂学相关的监管科学。

参考文献

[1] Park H, Otte A, Park K. Evolution of drug delivery systems: From 1950 to 2020 and beyond[J]. Journal of Controlled Release, 2022, 342: 53-65.
[2] Park K. Controlled drug delivery systems: Past forward and future back[J]. Journal of Controlled Release, 2014, 190: 3-8.
[3] Park K. Drug delivery of the future: Chasing the invisible gorilla[J]. Journal of Controlled Release, 2016, 240: 2-8.
[4] Pastore M N, Kalia Y N. Transdermal patches: History, development and pharmacology[J]. British Journal of Pharmacology, 2015, 172: 2179-2209.
[5] Clark A R. Medical aerosol inhalers: Past, present, and future[J]. Aerosol Science and Technology, 1995, 22(4): 374-391.
[6] Park K. The beginning of the end of the nanomedicine hype[J]. Journal of Controlled Release, 2019, 305: 221-222.
[7] Munos B. Lessons from 60 years of pharmaceutical innovation[J]. Nature Reviews Drug Discovery, 2009, 8(12): 959-968.
[8] Chong C R, Sullivan D J.New uses for old drugs[J]. Nature, 2007, 448(7154): 645-646.
[9] DiMasi J A, Grabowski H G, Hansen R W. Innovation in the pharmaceutical industry: New estimates of R&D costs[J]. Journal of Health Economics, 2016, 47: 20-33.
[10] Scannell J W, Blanckley A, Boldon H, et al. Diagnosing the decline in pharmaceutical R&D efficiency[J]. Nature Reviews Drug Discovery, 2012, 11(3): 191-200.
[11] Zhong H, Chan G, Hu Y, et al. A comprehensive map of FDA-approved pharmaceutical products[J]. Pharmaceutics, 2018, 10(4): 19.
[12] Wang W, Ye Z, Gao H, et al. Computational pharmaceutics: A new paradigm of drug delivery[J]. Journal of Controlled Release, 2021, 338: 119-136.
[13] Wang N N, Zhang Y S, Wang W, et al. How can machine learning and multiscale modeling benefit ocular drug development？[J]. Advanced Drug Delivery Reviews, 2023, 196: 114772.
[14] Schuhmacher A, Gatto A, Hinder M, et al.The upside of being a digital pharma player[J]. Drug Discov Today, 2020, 25(9): 1569-1574.
[15] Schuhmacher A, Gassmann O, Hinder M, et al. The art of virtualizing pharma R&D[J]. Drug Discov Today, 2019, 24(11): 2105-2107.
[16] Madabushi R, Seo P, Zhao L, et al. Role of model-informed drug development approaches in the lifecycle of drug development and regulatory decision-making[J]. Pharmaceutical Research, 2022, 39(8): 1669-1680.

第2章

人工智能在药物递送领域的机遇与挑战

叶祝一帆　澳门理工大学，澳门，中国
欧阳德方　澳门大学，澳门，中国

随着新分子实体（NME）开发成本急剧上升，以药物递送系统研究为主的现代药剂学正逐渐成为制药行业的核心领域。目前，传统的药品开发仍然主要依赖基于经验的试错方法。然而，先进的人工智能（AI）和机器学习技术在促进药物递送系统的发展方面具有巨大潜力。AI可以处理海量数据，发现潜在关联，提供准确预测，并在高维度空间中导航，为改变药物递送研究的范式提供了巨大机遇。数据驱动方法可应用于药剂学领域的各个环节，包括处方前研究、处方筛选以及临床精准医学。特别是在开发复杂剂型，如纳米粒子和蛋白质药物方面，AI具有显著优势。本文全面详细地审视了药剂学领域中AI应用的各个方面，包括统计优化方法、质量源于设计、机器学习算法、AI在药剂学领域的应用以及精准医学。此外，我们还探讨了AI在制药工业当前面临的挑战和未来前景。

2.1 引言

目前人们已经普遍认识到，药物的疗效受到其化学特性和制剂特征的双重影响。近年来，开发新分子实体（NME）变得愈发困难。40%~70%的药物候选分子存在溶解度和生物利用度不佳的问题[1, 2]。每年批准的NME数量一直在20~50个之间徘徊。随着NME的开发效率下降，创新的和复杂的剂型逐渐引起关注，并进入制药行业的主要关注领域，目的是提升药物性能[3]。尽管目前市场上的大多数药品都是安全有效的，但许多药物并未被设计成具有最佳的递送系统。

传统上，制剂科学家通过反复的实验室试验、多年的经验和领域知识积累来回答制剂问题，一直通过试错的方法模糊地理解各种参数对临床治疗效果的作用。然而，以传统方法筛选多种制剂处方需要消耗大量时间和样品，因此在控制、预测和优化制剂性能方面仍然面临复杂性和挑战性的考验[4]。

药物递送系统的开发是一个高维空间的优化问题，药物制剂处方设计空间估计在10^{25}到10^{30}之间[5]。影响药物的药代动力学（PK）和药效动力学（PD）特征的因素有很多，包括处方中活性药物成分（API）和辅料的理化特性与比例、工艺参数以及包装材料。药物递送系统的开发涉及许多不同领域的研究内容，如化合物的理化特性、给药途径、剂型、工艺放大和临床用药方案的确定。

质量源于设计（quality by design，QbD）最初是由Joseph M. Juran博士首次提出的概念[6]。2009年，人用药品注册技术国际协调会议（The International Council for Harmonisation of Technical Requirements for Pharmaceuticals for Human Use，ICH）发布了一份指南，明确了QbD的原则[7]。QbD侧重于理解关键物料属性（critical material attributes，CMA）和关键工艺参数（critical process parameter，CPP），以确保药品质量。通过确定CMA、CPP与质量之间的关系，优化这些关键因素来保证质量，这对于开发新的制剂至关重要。对于制药行业来说，QbD既是一次机遇，也是一项挑战[8]。QbD可以缩短研发时间、减少原材料消耗，并提高药品质量。

20世纪80年代，统计优化方法首次引入药剂学领域，用于量化制剂处方因素的影响。这些优化方法如响应面法（response surface methodology，RSM）等已成为药剂学的标准方法。此外，制剂科学家也引入了统计理论支持的实验设计（design of experiment，DoE）方法，以提高试验效率[9]。从那时起，科学家们有时可以通过使用这些统计分析方法来确定关键的制剂处方因素[10]。然而，处方因素与处方目标性质之间的相互关系非常复杂且尚未得到完全理解，因此这些统计分析方法不足以揭示它们真正的关系。

近年来，人工智能（AI）技术取得了显著进展，并取得了许多令人印象深刻的成就[11-14]。AI擅长处理大数据、揭示潜在关联、提供准确的预测，并在高维空间中导航。它已成功应用于许多领域，包括零售和安全，以解决实际问题[15]。

在药学领域，人工智能首先被用于药物研发，包括预测靶标活性、蛋白质结构和药物毒性等方面。例如，在蛋白质折叠预测竞赛中，机器学习方法明显优于传统方法[16]。药学是一门多学科交叉科学，几十年来积累了大量数据。随着算法的持续发展和计算能力的指数级增长，数据驱动的方法可以识别潜在的模式并近似非常复杂的函数，这有助于创新药物的研发，并且数据驱动的方法还能帮助药学家探索新的研究问题。

早期的研究使用了浅层人工神经网络（artificial neural network，ANN），这是一种传统的人工智能技术，用于预测体外药物释放参数，如溶出度，其准确性明显优于响应面分析法[17]，这表明ANN在药物开发中有广泛的应用潜力。近年来，人工智能在药剂学领域的应用呈上升趋势[18, 19]。如图2-1所示，自2001年以来，相关出版物的年度公开发表数量逐渐增加，并在过去七年中急剧上升，到2021年已经超过100篇。

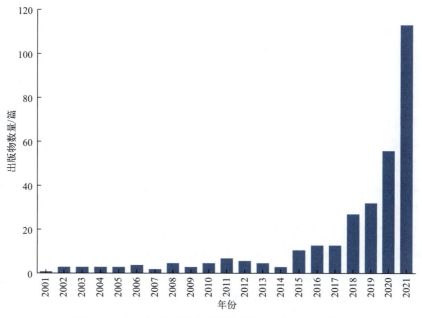

图2-1 人工智能在药物递送领域的年度出版物数量

检索策略：[TOPIC：（"Artificial intelligence" OR "AI" OR "Machine learning" OR "Deep learning"）AND TOPIC：（"Drug delivery" OR "Drug formulation" OR "Pharmaceutical formulation" OR "Pharmaceutics"）]，并从Web of Science数据库中获取了截至2021年的已发表文献

与人工智能的结合促进了众多剂型的研发，包括亲水凝胶骨架缓释片、口腔速崩膜和片剂、环糊精复合物、固体分散体、纳米晶体等[20-29]。例如，2018年深度神经网

络（deep neural network，DNN）被用于药物制剂处方的开发[30]。2019年和2020年科学家们通过使用机器学习和各种计算方法，对一些剂型（如环糊精包合物、固体分散体和纳米晶体）进行了体内外特性的预测[31-34]。2021年人工智能被用于辅助开发预防病毒感染的mRNA疫苗[35]。此外，一个基于注意力机制的深度神经网络被用于处理药剂学表格数据，并在环糊精包合物上进行验证，模型体现了良好的性能，并对某些问题提供了合理的解释[36]。

药剂学领域可以从各种AI技术中受益，包括专家系统和机器学习算法。数据驱动的方法可以应用于药剂学的各个方面，包括处方前研究、处方筛选和临床精准医学。一个精心设计的专家系统可以优化药物制剂处方，缩短时间和样品消耗，确保产品质量一致，并积累药物制剂专家的知识。机器学习可以通过算法从大量数据中获取模型，然后使用训练好的模型对新样本进行定量预测。

人工智能正进入制药产业，正在改变药品研发领域和药物递送系统开发的研究范式和观念，因此有必要回顾目前在药剂学中应用人工智能和机器学习算法的情况，以了解我们的当前位置以及如何进一步发展。

2.2 机器学习算法

在1959年，Arthur Samuel提出了"机器学习"这一术语。机器学习被定义为"一门研究赋予计算机学习能力而无需显式编程的领域"[37]。如今，机器学习已被视为人工智能的一个分支，旨在研究与算法和统计模型相关的科学问题。机器学习使用现有数据通过学习算法生成数学模型，这些经过充分训练的模型能够为新样本提供预测，以指导实际决策的制定。因此，机器学习已被认为是实现人工智能的一种重要方法。

根据用于训练机器学习模型的数据集是否具有标签，学习任务可以分为两个主要类别：监督学习和无监督学习。在监督学习中，使用带有标签的数据集，让机器学习正确答案。机器学习之前通常需要大量资源来手动标记这些样本。然而，在无监督学习中，使用没有标签的数据集，机器学习的目标是建模这些数据的概率分布。监督学习在药物制剂处方开发中经常被采用，包括预测药物制剂处方的体内外性能。此外，根据标签数据是连续的还是离散的，监督学习任务可以分为分类任务和回归任务两个主要类别。

此外，机器学习包含多种学习算法。表2-1简要总结了在药物制剂处方开发领域常用的经典机器学习算法，包括线性模型、ANN、决策树、集成学习、随机森林（random forest，RF）和XGBoost[38,39]。

图2-2展示了在药剂学领域中机器学习建模的一般流程。在机器学习任务中，典型的建模过程通常包括以下六个步骤：（a）确定机器学习问题和任务，并定义评估标准；（b）通过文献检索或实验进行高质量数据的收集；（c）数据的提取和预处理；（d）选择适用的机器学习算法并将整个数据集划分为子集；（e）进行模型训练和调整模型的超参数配置；（f）在未见数据上进行最终模型泛化性能的测试。

表2-1　药物制剂处方优化和预测中常用的机器学习和优化算法简要概述

机器学习/优化算法		学习任务	优点	缺点
线性模型		回归/分类	透明的模型结构，易进行优化	仅构建线性关系
人工神经网络（ANN）		回归/分类	对于数据的微小变化敏感，具备强大的表征能力	需要更多数据和计算资源来调整内部权重；其预测难以解释
深度学习		回归/分类	具有基于大数据的自动特征提取能力、端到端的学习能力，以及强大的模型表征能力 卷积神经网络（CNN）和循环神经网络（RNN）适用于非结构化数据，如图像数据和序列数据	需要大规模数据来训练网络，容易出现过拟合，并需要大量计算资源来训练模型。此外，还需要精心设计的网络架构，并手动调整多个超参数
遗传算法		—	不受制于问题的数学性质，不会陷入局部最小值	只能搜索近似解。当受到变异影响的元素数量较多时，搜索空间的大小会呈指数级增长
模糊神经网络		分类	能够从数据中学习参数，同时保留模糊系统的基于规则的可解释性	不能保证所学的模式具有真实的物理含义。随着规则的增加，模糊神经网络的可解释性会降低
支持向量机		回归/分类	能够解决高维问题，适用于小数据的机器学习任务 能够通过核函数处理非线性关系	当样本数量较多时，其训练效率较低 没有通用方案来选择适合特定问题的核函数
决策树		回归/分类	透明的模型结构使得树中的数据分割可以被解释为易于理解的规则	单独使用一个决策树的模型表征能力不足
集成学习	随机森林	回归/分类	通常情况下，对于结构化和混合类型数据，该模型在许多实际任务中表现出优越的性能，超越了其他算法，如常用的表格数据	不适用于非结构化数据的任务，如图像数据和序列数据
	XGBoost	回归/分类		

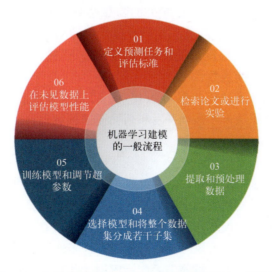

图2-2　在药剂学领域中进行机器学习建模的一般流程

2.2.1 线性模型

线性模型是一类基本的机器学习模型，包括线性回归和逻辑回归。线性回归建立了输入变量与输出变量之间的线性关系。逻辑回归主要用于解决二元分类问题，其预测结果可以视为概率值。因此，在药剂学领域，线性回归通常用于回归任务，而逻辑回归则广泛应用于分类任务。尽管由于历史原因，逻辑回归被称为"回归"，但实际上它是一种用于分类任务的方法。

对于线性回归，如果样本特性可以用一个特征来描述，相应的线性回归模型将包含一个独立变量。这种类型的线性回归模型称为简单线性回归。如果样本特性需要用多个特征来表示，那么相应的线性回归模型将包含多个独立变量，被称为多元线性回归（mixed logistic regression，MLR）模型。通常情况下，线性模型的优化使用最小二乘法。应用线性回归有两个主要优点：首先，线性模型的形式相对简单，计算不复杂；其次，线性模型具有透明性，易于解释。线性模型的权重可以被视为在预测输出变量时相应输入特征的重要性。然而，线性模型的缺点在于其难以很好地拟合非线性关系。对于逻辑回归，在映射数据从实数范围到[0,1]的过程中采用了逻辑函数，因此其输出可以被解释为某事件发生的概率。这在药物开发和递送领域中具有重要的应用。

2.2.2 人工神经网络

神经网络（ANN）是一种模仿生物神经网络的结构和功能的数学模型[40]。ANN由人工神经元构成，这些神经元接收输入数据，通过加权求和并应用激活函数来产生输出（激活值），从而模拟神经元的行为。根据神经元之间的连接方式，可以构建不同的ANN模型。近年来，ANN在预测性能方面表现出色，已被广泛应用于解决许多实际问题。

1958年，感知机（perceptron）被提出，它是一种ANN模型，仅由输入层和输出层两层神经元构成[41]。然而，基本感知机被证明无法解决逻辑异或（XOR）问题[42]。后来，研究人员为基本感知机添加了一个额外的隐藏层神经元，这构成了所谓的多层感知机（multilayer perceptron，MLP），它包含三层神经元。这种MLP能够成功解决逻辑XOR问题。位于输入层和输出层之间的神经网络层被称为隐藏层。研究表明，只有一个隐藏层的ANN可以无限逼近任意复杂的连续函数。

神经网络的训练过程涉及迭代调整ANN权重，以适应训练数据。常用的ANN优化算法是反向传播梯度下降优化算法，在药物开发和药物递送领域也有广泛应用[11, 43, 44]。

2.2.3 深度学习

近来，深度学习引起了广泛关注，特指具有多个隐藏层的深度人工神经网络模型。鉴于其深度网络结构，深度神经网络具备强大的表征能力。随着计算能力的迅速发展和高效算法的应用，深度神经网络的模型训练变得可行。与此同时，随着大数据的涌现和正则化技术的不断发展，深度神经网络的过拟合风险逐渐降低。在许多实际应用中，深度学习展示出与人类专家相当甚至超越的性能[14, 45]。深度学习广泛应用于计算机视觉、自然语言处理、生物信息学、药物设计与开发以及医学诊断等领域[15, 46]。

深度学习的主要优势在于其自动特征提取能力[15]。传统机器学习技术的性能依赖于领域专家设计和选择的输入特征的质量,这一过程被称为特征工程。特征工程在传统机器学习建模中扮演重要角色,但其耗时且昂贵。此外,特征的选择可能受到专家主观看法的影响,最终可能误导模型。在深度学习中,特征提取不再依赖于人类,而是由深度神经网络自动完成。深度学习的多层结构可视为通用的自动特征提取器[11, 47]。深度神经网络通过多层结构自动将原始输入转化为高层级的抽象特征,这使得深度学习能够完成复杂的学习任务,并展现出比传统机器学习技术更出色的泛化性能。此外,深度学习具备强大的学习和表征能力,以及良好的可迁移性。然而,深度学习的不足之处在于其对大规模数据、大量计算资源和强大硬件的需求。另外,深度神经网络的设计和超参数调优也需要较多时间。

深度神经网络(DNN)的类型包括全连接神经网络、卷积神经网络(CNN)和循环神经网络(RNN)。全连接神经网络适用于处理结构化表格数据,而CNN和RNN则专为处理图像数据和序列数据而设计。例如,2018年Yang Yilong及其合作者首次将深度学习应用于药物制剂处方预测[30],该研究涉及两种剂型,分别是基于羟丙甲纤维素(HPMC)的口服缓释骨架片和口腔速崩膜的快速释放剂型。与深度学习模型相比,多元线性回归(MLR)、偏最小二乘回归(partial least squares regression,PLSR)、支持向量机(SVM)、ANN、RF和K最近邻等模型也被开发用于比较。此外,为解决数据分布不均衡问题,自动数据集选择算法被提出,该算法可均衡划分整个数据集以选择代表性数据。深度学习模型的预测准确度能够满足药物制剂处方设计的要求。2018年,Christopher P. Calderon及其合作者采用CNN算法对蛋白质药物制剂处方中基于流动成像显微镜图像数据的亚可见颗粒进行分类[48]。亚可见颗粒指尺寸小于25 μm的颗粒,训练样本包括20万张图像。CNN模型经过训练,将流动成像显微镜图像中的颗粒分为4个类别,包括通过将单克隆抗体暴露于冻融应激、搅拌应激、泵A中静脉免疫球蛋白和泵B中静脉免疫球蛋白等产生的颗粒。在相同颗粒生成条件下,CNN模型可以实现95%的分类准确度。2020年,Ma Xiangyu及其合作者应用CNN算法基于X射线微型计算机断层扫描图像数据检测片剂内部的裂纹[49]。原始训练数据集包含573张图像,通过增强策略将原始训练数据集中的数据数量扩大至43548张图像。基于该数据集开发了两个CNN模型,用于构建自动片剂内部缺陷检测分析程序。其中一个CNN模型用于区分瓶中的片剂,另一个CNN模型用于识别片剂内部的裂纹。该程序实现了94%的平均准确度。

深度模型具有较大的模型容量。正则化技术被用于解决模型过拟合问题,包括早停、L1和L2正则化技术、批归一化和Dropout。通常使用的优化算法包括Adam和RMSprop[50]。ReLU、Tanh和Sigmoid常被用作激活函数[51]。

2.2.4 遗传算法

遗传算法(GA)并非机器学习算法,而是一种优化方法。由于其广泛应用于神经网络和药物制剂处方的优化,我们也需要了解其基本概念。1960年,John Holland提出了一种基于达尔文进化理论的遗传算法[52]。1989年,David E. Goldberg对遗传算法进行了扩展[53]。遗传算法通过模拟自然选择和生物进化过程来寻找近似最优解。

遗传算法的工作原理是从一个可能的解决方案集合开始,形成一个基因编码的个体种群。在初始种群生成后,根据"适者生存"的原则,遗传算法迭代地进化,生成越来越好的近似最优解。在每一代中,根据个体的适应度评分选择适应度更高的个体,这些评分是通过目标函数计算的。此外,个体的基因组会通过交叉和突变进行修改,以生成新一代。新种群就像自然物种的演化一样，更适应环境。最后一次迭代中，选择具有最高适应度的个体作为问题的最终近似最优解。

遗传算法的优点是对搜索问题的数学性质要求较低。然而，遗传算法的局限性在于它只能寻找近似解而非最优解。当遗传算法处理复杂问题时，需要突变的元素数量较多，搜索空间的大小会呈指数级增加。

2.2.5　模糊神经网络

模糊神经网络，也被广泛称为神经模糊逻辑、神经模糊系统和神经模糊混合，是一种算法，结合了模糊逻辑和ANN的要素[54]。模糊神经网络依赖领域专家的知识来定义规则，模拟人类的推理过程。其学习能力则利用了人工神经网络的特性。

在实际操作中，模糊神经网络首先通过模糊层将数据转化为模糊集合[55]。随后，模糊神经网络通过训练数据学习模糊系统的规则。学习算法被用于调整模糊系统的权重。最终，模糊神经网络结合不同规则以生成结果。

模糊神经网络的优点在于其参数不受人类专家的限制，而是从数据中学习这些参数。此外，它保持了基于规则的模糊系统的可解释性。然而，模糊神经网络的局限性是模型无法保证从数据中学到的模式在实际应用中具有实际意义。此外，随着规则的增加，模糊神经网络的可解释性逐渐降低。

2.2.6　支持向量机

1995年，Corinna Cortes和Vapnik基于万普尼克-泽范兰杰斯理论（Vapnik-Chervonenkis theory，简称VC理论）发布了当前标准的支持向量机（SVM）[56]。作为一种监督学习算法，最初的SVM在给定的数据集上进行训练，以进行非概率性线性分类。随后引入了核技巧（Kernel trick）[57]。核函数隐式地将数据映射到高维空间，以实现非线性预测。此外，Platt缩放方法可以将SVM用作概率分类器。随着算法的扩展，支持向量回归被用于回归任务设定[58]。

支持向量机选择了最佳的超平面来分离不同类型的输入样本。距离超平面最近的样本被称为支持向量，超平面和支持向量之间的距离称为间隔。一般认为，间隔越宽，泛化误差越低[59]。因此，SVM学习算法搜索能够在两个类别之间获得最宽间隔的超平面。SVM的目标是最大化这一间隔，支持向量支持或定义了超平面。

SVM在处理小数据学习任务和高维模式识别方面具有独特的优势。此外，通过使用核函数，SVM可以处理非线性关系。然而，SVM的局限性体现在样本数量较多时，其训练效率不高。此外，虽然有许多核函数可供选择，但没有通用的选择方案。在2020年，Theresa K. Cloutier及其合作者将SVM算法应用于基于分子模拟数据的单克隆抗体与辅料的优先相互作用的预测[60]。数据集包括山梨醇、脯氨酸、蔗糖、海藻糖、精氨酸盐酸盐和氯化钠六种辅料。他们开发了包含182个特征的特征集，以定量描述单克隆抗体的表面局部区域。使用了来自41种抗体的43816个残基的数据集来训练SVM模型。SVM模型可以提供准确性高达86%的预测。

2.2.7　决策树

决策树是一种基于二叉树或多叉树数据结构的机器学习模型[61, 62]。在决策树模型中，包含根节点、内部节点和叶子节点。根节点和内部节点包含数据分割规则。此外，决策树模型的输入可以是离散值或连续值。当输入特征为连续值时，会采用离散化技术来处理这些输入数据。

在优化算法方面，主要关注如何选择最佳的分割特征。随着树的生长，节点中包含的样本应趋向于同一类别。信息增益、信息增益比和基尼系数被用作评估指标，以度量样本的纯度[61, 63, 64]。举例来说，如果以信息增益作为纯度评估指标，决策树会选择具有相同或相似特征值的样本。因此，随着树的生长，信息增益会不断增大。为了解决模型过拟合问题，决策树模型可以采用剪枝策略。剪枝策略会删除一些不必要的节点和分支，以简化树结构，从而减轻过拟合问题。决策树的剪枝策略包括预剪枝策略和后剪枝策略。

决策树还可以用作规则挖掘的方法。这些用于划分样本的规则可能容易被专家理解。此外，集成学习方法在许多数据竞赛中展现了出色的性能。决策树经常被用作集成学习中的基础学习器，以构建更为精密的集成模型，从而获得更好的性能。

2.2.8 集成学习

集成学习的目标是通过将多个基础学习器结合在一起，获得更强大、更全面的集成学习器[65]。它利用训练数据集来构建多个个体基础学习器，然后采用一种组合策略来生成最终输出。在实践中，关键在于同时构建高准确性和多样性的个体基础学习器，以实现高性能的整合。因此，具有良好准确性和多样性的训练策略是集成学习领域的研究焦点。

在集成学习中，存在两种主要策略：串行策略和并行策略。串行策略的代表算法是Boosting，而并行策略的代表算法是Bagging。

XGBoost是Boosting算法的一种重要变体[39]。XGBoost在许多实际应用中展现出卓越的预测性能，赢得了许多大数据竞赛。XGBoost的优势包括在枚举最佳分割特征和特征值时能够并行计算，从而提高计算效率。此外，XGBoost还支持行和列抽样、后修剪以及缩减技术，有助于减轻过拟合问题。Bagging则基于自助采样方法（Boostrap）生成基础学习器[66]。随机森林（RF）是Bagging的扩展版本，其模型训练过程中引入了随机因素到特征选择过程中[38]。首先，RF会随机选择一定数量的特征，然后从这些特征中选择最优的特征，而不是使用所有特征。在实际机器学习应用中，RF通常表现出比其他机器学习模型更好的预测性能。

2.3 机器学习在药剂学中的应用

目前，药剂学领域越来越多地采用机器学习技术，涵盖了处方前研究、各种剂型的体内外特性研究以及体内-体外相关性（in vitro-in vivo correlation，IVIVC）研究。随着药物数据积累的增加、机器学习算法的不断改进以及计算能力的快速增长，机器学习模型的性能得到了显著提升。在这些机器学习算法中，ANN广泛用于预测压片性质、药物溶解和溶出特性以及构建体内-体外相关性。ANN已经在药物制剂领域有一段时间的应用历史。表2-2总结了机器学习模型在药物制剂处方开发中的最新进展。图2-3提供了一个将计算技术应用于药物制剂处方设计、优化和预测的高级概述框架。

表2-2 药物制剂处方开发领域已发表的机器学习研究的总结

年份	药物剂型	机器学习算法和统计方法	目标特性	参考文献
\multicolumn{5}{c}{速释片}				
1995	盐酸氢氯噻嗪速释片	ANN，多项式回归	药物溶出速率、硬度	[67]
1996	咖啡因速释片	ANN	几何平均粒径、流动性、堆密度、振实密度、崩解时间、厚度、硬度、脆碎度	[68]
1998	未披露化合物速释片	ANN，RSM	推片力	[69]
1998	未披露化合物速释片	ANN，RSM	流动性、Kawakita方程的斜率、Kawakita方程的截距、堆密度、振实密度	[70]
1998	205种不同处方的速释片	ANN，RSM	抗张强度、崩解时间、脆碎度、顶裂以及15 min、30 min、45 min和60 min的药物溶出度	[71]
2003	地尔硫䓬速释片	ANN，MLR	Weibull方程的参数	[72]
2006	205种不同处方的速释片	ANN，模糊神经网络	抗张强度、崩解时间、脆碎度、顶裂以及15 min、30 min、45 min和60 min的药物溶出度	[73]
2007	205种不同处方的速释片	模糊神经网络，决策树	抗张强度、崩解时间、脆碎度、顶裂以及15 min、30 min、45 min和60 min的药物溶出度	[74]
2007	205种处方的速释片	ANN，决策树	抗张强度、崩解时间、脆碎度、顶裂以及15 min、30 min、45 min和60 min的药物溶出度	[75]
2009	泼尼松速释片	模糊神经网络，MLR	权重变异系数、抗压强度、脆碎百分比、崩解时间以及30 min的药物溶出度	[76]
2010	对乙酰氨基酚、茶碱、抗坏血酸、美芬酸和盐酸氯丙嗪速释片	集成ANN	抗张强度和崩解时间	[77]
2012	依普利尔速释片	ANN，遗传编程	抗张强度、30 min的药物溶出度	[78]
2013	依普利尔速释片	ANN，RSM	抗张强度、30 min的药物溶出度	[79]
\multicolumn{5}{c}{硬明胶胶囊}				
2005	卡马西平、氯磺丙脲、地西泮、布洛芬、洛索洛芬、萘普生和吡罗昔康硬明胶胶囊	ANN	10 min、30 min、45 min的药物溶出度	[80]
\multicolumn{5}{c}{口服缓释制剂}				
1991	盐酸氯苯那敏缓释骨架胶囊	ANN，RSM	药物溶出度：Peppas方程 ($\frac{M_t}{M_\infty}=kt^N$) 的释放指数 N 和药物溶出半衰期 $t_{0.5}$	[17]
1994	双氯芬酸钠、萘普生钠、水杨酸钠、硫酸奎尼丁、咖啡因、茶碱、对乙酰氨基酚、盐酸苯海拉明、盐酸普萘洛尔、盐酸四氢氨基吖啶和盐酸苯丙醇胺缓释骨架片	ANN	1 h、3 h、6 h、12 h的药物溶出度	[81]

续表

年份	药物剂型	机器学习算法和统计方法	目标特性	参考文献
1997	马来酸氯苯那敏和对乙酰氨基酚/伪麻黄碱缓释骨架胶囊	ANN	药物溶出度：Peppas 方程（$\frac{M_t}{M_\infty}=kt^N$）的释放指数 N 和药物溶出半衰期 $t_{0.5}$	[82]
1997	三嘧啶缓释骨架片	ANN，RSM	药物溶出度：Peppas 方程（$\frac{M_t}{M_\infty}=kt^N$）的释放指数 N 和释放常数 k	[83]
1999	某药物的缓释骨架片	ANN	IVIVC 的构建	[84]
1999	某交感神经药物的缓释骨架片	ANN	1 h、2 h、4 h、6 h、8 h、10 h、12 h、16 h、20 h 和 24 h 的药物溶出度	[85]
2000	茶碱缓释骨架片	ANN	药物溶出度：药物溶出方程（$C=100-\left[W_{f_0}e^{-k_f t}+(100-W_{f_0})e^{-k_s t}\right]$）中零时刻的快速释放分数 W_{f_0}、快速释放速率常数 k_f、缓慢释放速率常数 k_s	[86]
2000	茶碱缓释骨架颗粒	ANN	0.25 h、0.5 h、1 h、1.5 h、2 h、3 h、4 h、6 h、8 h、10 h 的药物溶出度	[87]
2002	茶碱缓释骨架颗粒	RNN	0.25 h、0.5 h、1 h、1.5 h、2 h、3 h、4 h、6 h、8 h、10 h 的药物溶出度	[88]
2002	阿司匹林缓释骨架片	ANN	1 h、2 h、4 h、8 h 的药物溶出度；药物溶出度：Peppas 方程（$\frac{M_t}{M_\infty}=kt^N$）的释放指数 N 和释放常数 k	[89]
2003	阿司匹林缓释骨架片	ANN	1 h、2 h、4 h、8 h 的药物溶出度	[90]
2007	对乙酰氨基酚缓释骨架片	ANN	IVIVC 的构建	[91]
2007	阿司匹林缓释骨架片	ANN	药物稳定性：在 60℃、50℃、40℃、30℃下药物含量降低的表观零级动力学常数	[92]
2008	盐酸普萘洛尔缓释骨架片	遗传编程	1 h、6 h、12 h 的药物溶出度	[93]
2009	双氯芬酸钠缓释骨架片	RNN，MLP	0.5 h、1 h、1.5 h、2 h、3 h、4 h、6 h、7 h、8 h 的药物溶出度	[94]
2010	尼莫地平缓释骨架片	ANN，MLR	90% 的药物溶出所需时间，2 h 和 8 h 的药物溶出度	[95]
2010	硫酸沙丁胺醇缓释骨架片	ANN	1 h、2 h、4 h、6 h、8 h、12 h 的药物溶出度	[96]
2012	双氯芬酸钠和咖啡因缓释骨架片	ANN，决策树	0.5 h、1 h、1.5 h、2 h、3 h、4 h、6 h、7 h、8 h 的药物溶出度	[97]
2012	卡维地洛缓释骨架片	ANN	0.5 h、1 h、1.5 h、2 h、2.5 h、3 h、4 h、6 h、8 h、10 h、12 h、24 h 的药物溶出度	[98]
2000	硫酸沙丁胺醇渗透泵片	ANN	前 8 小时的平均药物释放速率 v 和累积药物释放量与时间的相关系数 r	[99]
2014	硝苯地平渗透泵片	ANN	IVIVC 的构建	[100]

续表

年份	药物剂型	机器学习算法和统计方法	目标特性	参考文献
乳液、微乳和纳米乳液给药系统				
2001	五元微乳系统，包含 n-醇和 1,2-癸二醇 2 种共表面活性剂	ANN	相行为：微乳、层状液晶、O/W 粗乳液、W/O 粗乳液类别	[101]
2005	利福平和异烟肼微乳	ANN	药物稳定性：利福平、异烟肼、吡嗪酰胺在 9 种药物组合中的占比	[102]
2008	普布可油溶液、自乳化药物递送系统和自纳米乳化药物递送系统	模糊神经网络	IVIVC 的构建	[103]
2008	布地奈德纳米乳液	ANN	粒径	[104]
2008	四元微乳系统，其中聚氧乙烯 40 或聚甘油-6 异硬脂酸酯作为共表面活性剂	ANN	水溶性极限 W_{max}	[105]
2008	四元微乳系统，其中癸酸甘油酯作为共表面活性剂	ANN	相行为：O/W 微乳、双连续微乳、W/O 微乳、O/W 乳液或 W/O 乳液类别	[106]
2008	水包油包水乳液	ANN	乳液稳定性：离心后保留的乳液体积百分比	[107]
2010	布地奈德纳米乳液	ANN	纳米乳液稳定性：第 30 分钟和第 30 天纳米乳液粒子的尺寸差异	[108]
2016	四元纳米乳液，其中乙醇作为共表面活性剂	ANN	纳米乳液稳定性（冻融循环实验），对 MCF-7 细胞的细胞毒性	[109]
水凝胶透皮递药系统				
1999	褪黑素水凝胶	ANN, RSM	药物通量、滞后时间	[110]
1999	洛索洛芬水凝胶	ANN	药物通量、滞后时间、皮肤刺激分数	[111]
2001	洛索洛芬水凝胶	ANN，多项式回归	药物通量、皮肤刺激分数	[112]
纳米颗粒				
2011	载纳曲酮的基于 PLA-PEG-PLA 三嵌段的聚合物纳米粒	ANN	粒径	[113]
2012	基于壳聚糖的聚合物纳米粒	ANN	粒径	[114]
2014	载紫杉醇的基于 PLGA-PMBH 的聚合物纳米粒	ANN	粒径	[115]
2014	金纳米粒和银纳米粒	PLSR	细胞连接	[116]
2015	载盐酸维拉帕米的固体脂质纳米粒	ANN, RSM	包封率、粒径	[117]
2016	载姜黄素的基于三磷脂的固体脂质纳米粒	高斯过程	结合自由能	[118]
2017	载芬戈莫德的基于 PHBV 的聚合物纳米粒	ANN	粒径、PDI、包封率、载药量	[119]

续表

年份	药物剂型	机器学习算法和统计方法	目标特性	参考文献
2017	载白蛋白的基于壳聚糖的聚合物纳米粒	ANN	粒径、包封率、对MRC-8细胞的细胞毒性	[120]
2017	基于不同聚合物的聚合物纳米粒，包括EC、PCL、PLA、PLGA、Eudragit RS、PVAc	ANN	粒径、PDI	[121]
2019	金纳米粒	SVM	纳米粒阳性细胞数目	[122]
2019	球形核酸	MLR，逻辑回归，XGBoost	分泌性胚胎碱性磷酸酶浓度	[123]
2019	金纳米粒	ANN	半衰期、脾脏和肝脏中的积累情况	[124]
2020	652种不同处方的纳米粒	RF	巨噬细胞的细胞内摄取和细胞因子释放	[125]
2020	910种不同处方的纳米晶体	LightGBM，RF，深度学习，SVM，K最近邻，决策树，PLSR，MLR	粒径、PDI	[33]
固体分散体				
2005	布洛芬固体分散体	ANN，模糊神经网络	2 min、5 min、10 min和20 min的药物溶出度	[126]
2012	非洛地平固体分散体	ANN	15 min的药物溶出度	[127]
2013	替布隆固体分散体	ANN	30 min的药物溶出度	[128]
2013	布洛芬钠、吲哚美辛、卡马西平、对乙酰氨基酚固体分散体	集成ANN，RSM	工艺产量、出口温度、粒径	[129]
2014	布洛芬钠、吲哚美辛、伊曲康唑、布洛芬、卡马西平、对乙酰氨基酚固体分散体	集成ANN，RSM	工艺产量、出口温度、粒径	[130]
2019	涉及50种药物的646种不同处方的固体分散体	深度学习，RF，LightGBM，SVM，ANN，K最近邻，决策树，朴素贝叶斯分类器	3个月和6个月的物理稳定性	[32]
环糊精复合物				
2001	347种不同处方的α-环糊精复合物和β-环糊精复合物	组贡献模型	结合自由能	[131]
2015	218种不同处方的β-环糊精复合物	ANN，MLR	结合自由能	[132]
2017	76种手性化合物的β-环糊精复合物，40种手性化合物的am-β-环糊精复合物	集成MLR	结合自由能	[133]

续表

年份	药物剂型	机器学习算法和统计方法	目标特性	参考文献
2019	3000 种不同处方的环糊精复合物，其中涉及 8 种环糊精和 1320 种化合物	LightGBM，ANN，RF	结合自由能	[31]

注：ANN，人工神经网络；RSM，响应面法；MLR，多元线性回归；IVIVC，体内-体外相关性；MLP，多层感知机；O/W，水包油；W/O，油包水；W/O/W，水包油包水；PLA-PEG-PLA，聚乳酸-聚乙二醇-聚乳酸；PLGA-PMBH，聚乳酸-聚乙二醇-聚乳酸-对甲酰基苯甲酰肼；PHBV，聚（3-羟基丁酸-co-3-羟基戊酸酯）；PDI，多分散指数；EC，乙基纤维素；PCL，聚ε-己内酯；PLA，聚乳酸；PLGA，聚乳酸-羟基乙酸共聚物；PVAc，聚乙酸乙烯酯；SVM，支持向量机；RF，随机森林；PLSR，偏最小二乘回归。

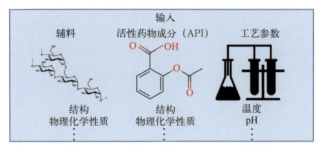

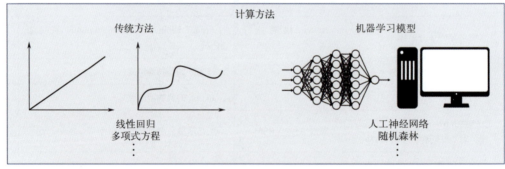

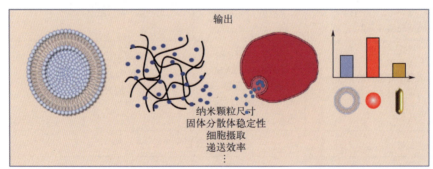

图2-3 一个应用计算技术分析药物制剂处方中体内和体外相互作用数据关系的框架

2.3.1 速释片剂

速释片剂是一种能够迅速崩解并释放其活性药物成分（API）的药片，无须特定的药物释放速率控制特征，如羟丙甲纤维素（HPMC）凝胶或薄膜涂层技术。一些研究中采用了机器学习技术，以优化和预测速释片的性能[67, 69-71, 77, 79]。例如，1996年Jothi G. Kesavan和Garnet E. Peck分别开发了两个ANN模型，用于预测制粒过程和压片过程，共使用了32种处方[68]。对于制粒过程的ANN模型，回归分析了四个输出变量，包括几何平均粒径、流动性、堆积密度和振实密度；对于压片过程的ANN模型，预测了四个输出变量，包括硬度、脆碎度、厚度和崩解时间。最后，针对小数据和输入特征不足问题进行讨论，这都可能导致模型性能不佳。2003年，Pradeep M. Sathe和Jurgen Venitz对一组包括28种地尔硫䓬片剂处方的数据集进行了ANN和多元线性回归（MLR）模型的训练[72]，拟合"Weibull"函数的参数用于评估模型性能，最终结果表明ANN模型优于MLR。2006年，Shao Qun及其合作者在一个包含205个实验处方数据的速释片数据集上比较了模糊神经网络和ANN[73]。模型用于预测药片的抗拉强度、崩解时间、脆碎度、顶裂以及15 min、30 min、45 min和60 min内的药物溶出情况。研究结果表明，ANN模型在数据集上的预测精度高于模糊神经网络。2007年，Shao Qun及其合作者利用模糊神经网络和决策树算法生成了速释片的开发规则，与之前的研究相同的是，使用了相同的处方数据集和目标变量[74]。两种方法都成功地建立了有用的规则，而且这两种方法生成的规则相似。2007年，Shao Qun及其合作者在速释片数据集上进行了决策树与人工神经网络的比较研究。与之前的研究相同，数据集和目标变量保持一致[75]。研究结果表明，决策树的性能略低于人工神经网络。不仅如此，由于决策树具有透明的模型结构，它能够将其工作过程解释为人类可理解的规则，这些规则可能会给药物制剂处方开发提供更多洞见。2009年，Mariana Landín及其合作者应用模糊神经网络算法研究了直压片[76]。与多元线性回归相比，模糊神经网络表现出更高的准确性。更重要的是，模糊神经网络生成的规则被发现具有重要的可重复利用经验和药剂专家共识。2012年，Buket Aksu及其合作者采用了人工神经网络、模糊神经网络和遗传规划方法，基于QbD理念开发了雷米普利片[78]。雷米普利是用于治疗充血性心力衰竭和高血压的药物。该研究调查了处方变量对片剂质量的影响，包括羟丙甲基纤维素比例、润滑剂类型和润滑剂浓度。将15%的数据作为验证集进行模型评估，并选择破碎强度、30 min内的药物溶出百分比、API含量、杂质六水合雷米普利以及杂质雷米普利二酮哌嗪作为输出变量。

2.3.2 硬明胶胶囊

在2005年，Wendy I. Wilson及其团队将ANN和专家系统技术应用于硬明胶胶囊的研发。该ANN是基于历史数据进行训练的[80]。研究中选择了7种生物制药分类系统（BCS）Ⅱ类药物作为模型药物，包括卡马西平、氯磺丙脲、地西泮、布洛芬、酮洛芬、萘普生和吡罗昔康。BCS Ⅱ类药物具有高渗透性和低溶解度，因此这些药物的吸收可能受到药物溶解度差的限制。人工神经网络用于预测在10、30和45分钟内溶解的药物百分比。三个输出的测试集R^2分别为69、70和88。此外，基于ANN模型的预测，构建了一个基于规则的专家系统，可推荐优化的硬胶囊处方。在该研究中，进行了一些简化假设，例如，假定所使用的辅料与药物相容，并且仅使用微晶纤维素和乳糖混合物作为稀释剂。由于处方数据有限，网络训练过程中应用了30000次迭代，这个数量可能过大，可能导致过拟合问题。

2.3.3 口服缓释制剂

口服缓释制剂的设计旨在使药物在一段时间内以低释放速率持续释放。口服缓释制剂包括口服缓释骨架片和颗粒，以及口服渗透泵片，可减缓药物的释放速率，以降低药物治疗的副作用和用药频率。机器学习已经用于协助开发缓释药物递送系统的研究[81-83, 86-88, 90, 92, 93, 95-98]。在这些研究中，主要关注点包括预测药物的释放行为和构建IVIVC模型。例如，1999年James A. Dowell及其合作者采用多种ANN结构，建立了用于缓释片的IVIVC模型[84]。药物的溶出曲线直接映射到药物在体内的浓度随时间变化的曲线。对于药物溶出测试，选取了两种含有7个时间点的缓释片处方作为输入。对于药物在体内的研究，采用了来自9名患者的1512个PK时间点数据作为输出，这些PK数据在15个时间点进行采样。研究引入了常规ANN、RNN和跳跃连接ANN来构建IVIVC模型。1999年，Chen Yixin及其合作者引入了ANN和PK模拟方法，以预测控释制剂的体外药物释放和体内行为[85]。他们以一种交感药物为模型药物，制备了22种药物处方。在机器学习建模方面，使用了7个处方变量和3个片剂特性变量作为输入。此外，模型输出了10个时间点的药物溶解百分比。最后，在模型验证中，4种处方中有3种显示出了模型预测与实际观察之间的良好一致性。2002年，Svetlana Ibrić及其合作者构建了一个广义回归神经网络，用于优化缓释骨架片的制备[89]。他们根据中心复合设计并制备了10种阿司匹林骨架片处方。Eudragit RS PO的用量和片剂硬度被测量并用作输入。ANN模型预测了Peppas方程中4个时间点的药物溶解，包括释放指数N和释放常数k。为了评估模型的性能，引入了差异因子f_1和相似性因子f_2作为标准。2007年，Jelena Parojčić及其团队针对两种托烷司琼缓释片建立了体内-体外相关性（IVIVC）模型[91]。这两种托烷司琼处方基于Carbopol 971P和71G两种聚合物制备而成。通过IVIVC的建立，成功降低了体内研究的需求，从而有效降低了药物开发的成本。IVIVC模型的构建采用了FDA推荐的反卷积方法和ANN方法，两种计算工具都被应用并进行了比较。为了表示体内药物释放情况，研究人员使用了来自9名人体志愿者的累积尿液排泄-时间曲线，这些曲线作为体内药物动力学参数，并用作ANN模型的响应函数。两种方法均成功建立了可靠的IVIVC模型。2009年，Jelena Petrović及其同事们采用了具有长短期记忆（LSTM）单元的RNN模型，用于预测体外药物溶出曲线[94]。研究中采用了二甲基双氯酚酸钠作为模型药物，并制备了12种该药物的聚乙二醇控释片剂处方。随后进行了体外溶出试验和片剂特性实验，构建了一个小型制药数据集。研究中的体外药物释放数据以10个时间点的时间序列形式用作ANN模型的输出，而f_1和f_2则作为评估指标。结果表明，与多层感知机（MLP）相比，RNN模型在数据集上表现更为出色。

ANN算法还被广泛应用于口服渗透泵片的研究中[100]。以2000年为例，Wu Tao及其合作者开发了ANN模型，以优化沙丁胺醇硫酸盐渗透泵片的设计[99]。他们制备了30种不同的沙丁胺醇硫酸盐渗透泵片处方，并测试了它们的药物溶出性能。模型的输入参数包括羟丙甲纤维素用量、包衣溶液中的PEG 1500含量以及包衣重量。通过ANN模型，预测了前8小时的体外药物释放速率的平均值以及累积药物释放量与时间的相关系数。这些研究对于药物开发和药物递送领域具有重要的意义。

2.3.4 乳液、微乳液和纳米乳液药物递送系统

乳液、微乳液和纳米乳液药物递送系统是由两种或更多不相溶的液体（通常为水和油）组成的。乳液是一种异质且在热力学上稳定的系统。通常乳液用于局部或经皮的药物递送系统，有助于促使药物递送或渗透到皮肤中。微乳液或纳米乳液则是微观或纳米级别的乳液。

在制剂开发中，一个关键步骤是寻找适用于该系统的合适乳化剂和稳定剂。机器学习方法已应用于计算辅助制剂设计[101-105, 108, 109]。例如，2008年F. Podlogar及其合作者通过ANN努力预测微乳液的相行为[106]。通过制备不同的微乳液，确定这些微乳液的类型，建立了ANN模型来对这些微乳液进行分类。首先，将制剂成分用作ANN模型的输入。其次，因为微乳液的热力学特性显示出不同的内部亚稳态形态，所以差示扫描量热法（DSC）的曲线也被用作训练另一个ANN模型的输入。这些ANN模型是通过遗传算法进行训练的。具有5个输出的ANN模型用于多类别分类，可表示5种微乳液的概率，包括O/W型微乳液、双连续微乳液、W/O型微乳液、O/W型乳液和W/O型乳液。结果发现两个ANN模型均表现出高准确性。在2008年，Wei Huixian将ANN应用于预测带有不同乳化剂的W/O/W型乳液的物理稳定性[107]。其通过测量离心后新制备产品的乳液体积来表示乳液的物理稳定性。期间共使用了39个实验数据来训练ANN。结果表明，ANN模型对乳液即时稳定性的预测具有良好的准确性。因此，ANN可以作为一个筛选乳化剂的有用工具。

2.3.5 水凝胶经皮给药系统

水凝胶经皮给药系统是由交联的三维聚合物网络构成，其中含有大量水分。水凝胶制剂呈固体状，由于其水含量高，具有出色的生物相容性，因此能够在药物应用于组织时维持一段时间内的高局部药物浓度。机器学习也被广泛应用于水凝胶处方的优化[110]。例如，1999年Kozo Takayama及其合作者使用ANN[111]研究了酮洛芬经皮制剂的优化。在酮洛芬乙醇水凝胶中，O-乙基薄荷脑被用作经皮吸收增效剂，而O-乙基薄荷脑和乙醇的用量则是关键的处方变量，它们被用作ANN模型的输入。研究发现，少量的O-乙基薄荷脑能够促进酮洛芬从水凝胶向皮肤的分配，而较高剂量的O-乙基薄荷脑则能提高药物的扩散性。将穿透速率、滞后时间和刺激评分被作为输出参数，结果显示ANN模型在预测穿透速率和刺激评分方面与实际观察结果高度一致，从而实现了快速的处方优化。2001年Wu Pao-Chu及其合作者开发了机器学习模型，用于优化酮洛芬水凝胶给药系统[112]。在制剂实验中，采用了三因素球形二阶复合实验设计，共进行了16个实验，包括1个重复中心实验和15种不同的处方。这些处方由不同比例的1-O-乙基-3-正丁基环己醇、二异丙基己二酸二酯和异丙醇组成，它们的用量被用作预测穿透速率和刺激评分的输入参数。此外，还采用了ANN模型和多项式回归（二阶）。研究结果表明，ANN模型在数据集上的表现优于二阶多项式函数。

2.3.6 纳米药物递送系统

在药剂学领域，对脂质体和聚合物纳米粒的研究已经有超过40年的时间。目前，在纳米颗粒技术的发展方面取得了进展，包括固体脂质纳米粒、胶束和纳米晶等。药物通常被嵌入到纳米尺度的载体材料中，以实现独特的性能，如高表面积体积比、防止降解和主动靶向。纳米药物存在的主要问题是脱靶[134]。纳米颗粒药物的递送受到多种因素的影响，包括但不限于尺寸、形状、分布、化学成分和表面化学性质。为了将药物传递到特定靶标，设计最佳的纳米药物递送系统仍然具有挑战性。

当纳米颗粒被注射到人体内时，它们便在体内开启独特的命运轨迹。在这个过程中，纳米颗粒需穿越多个屏障，不同的分子将与它发生相互作用。首先，蛋白质会立即吸附到纳米颗粒表面形成蛋白质包被。蛋白质包被的性质取决于生物分子和纳米颗粒的物理化学性质，并影响着纳米颗粒的体内行程。例如，纳米颗粒表面的配体的靶向效应可能被掩盖。研究发现，与未包被蛋白质的纳米颗粒相比，包被血清蛋白的纳米颗粒具有较低的细胞特异性靶向效应[135]。

在靶向组织中的细胞之前，纳米颗粒必须通过血管系统传输，然后穿出血管。这一过程取决于纳米颗粒的物理化学特性以及血管生理学。不同组织的血管生理学各异。例如，肝脏和肾脏的血管具有窗孔，纳米颗粒的有效截止尺寸分别约为100 nm和6 nm[136, 137]；在大脑中，血脑屏障结构中的血管非常紧密，可防止纳米颗粒将药物输送到大脑[138]；在实体肿瘤中，纳米颗粒使用被动或主动的传输机制来通过血管外渗[139]。此外，纳米颗粒的物理化学特性也应进行设计和优化。

在目标组织的血管外渗后，纳米颗粒必须穿过细胞外基质。在进入其靶细胞之前，纳米颗粒可能会受到细胞外基质的阻碍。细胞外基质的结构在不同组织和疾病条件下存在差异。此外，结缔组织细胞和其他非靶细胞可能会阻止纳米颗粒将药物输送到其预定的靶细胞。例如，肿瘤组织中的巨噬细胞会捕获纳米颗粒，以防止其达到癌细胞[140]。因此，纳米颗粒的设计还应考虑如何避免被细胞外基质和细胞截留。

当达到靶细胞时，纳米颗粒需要通过各种细胞摄取机制进入细胞，并到达细胞内的最终靶亚细胞位置。细胞表型、表面受体类型和表达水平决定了细胞摄取途径和速率。例如，A549细胞依赖小窝蛋白途径，而132N1细胞依赖于网格蛋白介导的内吞作用[141]。纳米颗粒的物理化学特性也会影响摄取。此外，应使用允许逃逸内体的策略，如pH敏感性聚合物[142]。

体循环中的纳米颗粒主要通过肝脏和网状内皮系统（RES）进行清除。这些器官的作用是防止纳米颗粒达到其目标部位并保持长时间循环。当纳米颗粒经过时，肝窦内的库普弗细胞（Kupffer cell，亦称为肝巨噬细胞）可以夺取大部分纳米颗粒[143]，从而降低了静脉注射纳米颗粒的递送效率。因此，关键是设计纳米颗粒的理化特性，以避免肝脏和网状内皮系统的清除，同时提高纳米颗粒到达目标部位的递送效率。此外，其他器官也可以清除纳米颗粒，例如肾脏可以排泄尺寸小于6 nm的纳米颗粒[137]。这些屏障可以降解和清除纳米颗粒，从而防止纳米颗粒将药物递送到其作用部位。在小鼠模型中发现，仅有0.7%的受配体包被的纳米颗粒到达实体肿瘤，而0.0014%到达癌细胞[140]。了解纳米颗粒的物理化学特性与生物屏障之间的相互作用可以帮助预测、优化和设计高效的纳米颗粒药物递送系统。

最近的实验进展越来越聚焦于体内、体外以及疾病部位的纳米颗粒表征，这为纳米医学领域的机器学习应用提供了丰富的数据资源。纳米颗粒的数据集正在迅速积累，这使得人工智能算法能够建立纳米颗粒与生物系统之间复杂的关联[134]。机器学习技术已广泛应用于纳米颗粒的预测，对加速设计过程具有显著意义[114, 115, 117, 118, 120]。在物理化学特性方面，许多研究专注于预测颗粒大小和多分散指数（PDI），因为它们对纳米颗粒的药代动力学特性有重要影响。此外，机器学习还用于识别纳米颗粒的其他特性，如载药能力、包封效率以及细胞摄取和毒性[144, 145]。例如，2011年H. Asadi及其团队研究了可生物相容且可降解的聚合物材料作为纳米颗粒载体，并确定了控制颗粒大小的关键因素[113]。他们采用纳米沉淀法制备了聚乳酸-聚乙二醇-聚乳酸（PLA-PEG-PLA）三嵌段聚合物。多个因素被认为会影响颗粒大小和分布，如聚合物浓度、药物剂量、溶剂比例和混合速率，从而影响纳米颗粒在体内的行为。最终，通过ANN进行训练，将这些因素与颗粒大小建立了关联。此外，还确定了聚合物浓度是控制纳米颗粒大小的最关键输入因素。2014年，Carl D. Walkey及其团队发现，基于蛋白冠特性，可以使用基于偏最小二乘回归（PLSR）模型预测金和银纳米颗粒与细胞的相互作用[116]。他们构建了包含105个纳米颗粒的数据集，采用液相色谱串联质谱法确定血清蛋白冠。2017年，Shadab Shahsavari及其团队研究并优化了一种载芬戈莫德的聚合物纳米颗粒药物递送系统[119]。他们使用可生物降解的聚（3-羟基丁酸-co-3-羟基戊酸酯）（PHBV）作为药物载体，采用ANN作为预测模型，将纳米颗粒的颗粒大小、PDI、载药能力和包封率四个关键特性设定为输出。此外，还在模型训练过程中使用了三种优化算法，分别是梯度下降、Levenberg-Marquardt方法和贝叶斯正则化。2017年，John Youshia及其合作者引入了ANN模型，用于预测聚合物纳米颗粒的粒径和PDI[121]。之前的研究侧重于聚合物浓度的优化。在本次研究中，作者们汇集了包括乙基纤维素（EC）、聚乳酸（PLA）、聚乙酸乙烯（PVAc）、Eudragit RS、聚乳酸-羟基乙酸共聚物（PLGA）和聚ε-己内酯（PCL）等不同聚合物的数据集，并应用人工神经网络实现了聚合物筛选和处方预测。通过计算网络内部连接权重，对输入因素的贡献进行了排名。2019年，Benjamin R. Kingston及其合作者使用SVM模型，基于三维显微镜图像数据，预测金纳米颗粒在微转移中的传递[122]。他们构建了包含1301个微转移数据的数据集，利用光片显微镜测量了转移瘤的形态。经过良好训练的SVM模型能够准确预测纳米颗粒阳性细胞的数量，其RMSE为27，相关系数为0.94。高通量筛选方法被用于探索纳米颗粒开发的扩展化学空间。2019年，Gokay Yamankurt及其合作者建立了高通量筛选方法，用于合成和分析球状核酸[123]。此项研究确定了包括核直径、脂质组成、抗原类型、位置和密度、寡核苷酸序列、共轭化学、共轭末端、骨架和密度以及互补密度在内的11个球状核酸性质；鉴定了约1000个球状核酸纳米颗粒，并使用XGBoost模型训练了数据集，以预测免疫活性和分泌的胚胎碱性磷酸酶浓度；通过识别纳米晶体的蛋白质包被组成，预测了纳米颗粒的积聚和细胞摄取。2019年，James Lazarovits及其合作者利用机器学习方法，基于金纳米颗粒的蛋白质包被形成，预测了纳米颗粒的半衰期及其在脾脏和肝脏的积累[124]。从大鼠血液中提取金纳米颗粒，分别在1小时、2小时、4小时、8小时和24小时内进行隔离；构建了包含63630个蛋白质无标记定量强度的数据集，并利用神经网络进行训练，其预测准确度达到94%。在2020年，Zhan Ban及其合作者使用RF算法，从纳米颗粒蛋白质包被中预测细胞识别属性[146]。他们预测了巨噬细胞的细胞摄取和细胞因子释放这两个细胞识别属性。从56篇文献中提取了包含652种不同纳米颗粒蛋白质包被的数据，并分析了其中的21个定量和定性特征，包括颗粒形状、类型、修饰类型、动态光散射等。最终模型能够以R^2值超过0.75的性能预测细胞识别。同年，He Yuan及其合作者使用机器学习技术来开发纳米晶体[33]。纳米晶体可以将药物尺寸缩小到纳米尺度，从而增加颗粒的表面积，提高不溶性药物的溶解度和生物利用度。他们从文献中提取了共910个制剂颗粒尺寸数据和310个处方PDI数据。研究包括了湿球磨法、高压均质法和反溶剂沉淀法三种纳米晶体制备方法。在多个机器学习算法中，LightGBM表现出对湿球磨法和高压均质法制备的纳米晶体预测准确性最高，这是因为反溶剂沉淀制备方法的实验重复性较差。使用LightGBM对输入特征的贡献进行排名，并作为计算方法为纳米晶体的开发提供更多见解。

此外，纳米医学也是实现精准医学进化的有用工具[147]。精准医学旨在根据患者的遗传和表观特征，为个体患者量身定制适合的治疗方案。机器学习促进了个性化和靶向纳米医学的合理设计，还能够预测纳米颗粒与药物、生物组分和癌细胞的相互作用效率。

2.3.7 固体分散体

固体分散体是包括两种或更多API和聚合物的非晶态分散体。在药物开发和药物递送领域，固体分散体是一种常见的制剂类型，通过增加表面自由能来提高不溶性药物的溶解度和溶出度。聚合物用于维持固体分散体的物理稳定性。制备固体分散体可以采用熔融法、溶剂法和溶剂熔融法。机器学习技术已广泛应用于预测固体分散体的药物释放和稳定性[126, 128-130]。例如，2012年Sofia A. Papadimitriou及其合作者研究了PVP/PEG混合物作为固体分散体的载体，非洛地平作为模型药物，通过熔融技术制备了固体分散体[127]。在处方优化过程中采用了通用的因子设计，研究了载体对固体分散体药物溶解度的影响。结果表明，通过人工神经网络模型预测了非洛地平固体分散体在15分钟时的累积药物释放百分比（percent of release，PR）。2019年，Han Run及其合作者利用机器学习技术预测了固体分散体的物理稳定性，收集了来自同行评审论文的相对庞大的物理稳定性数据集[32]。他们建立了包括深度学习、RF、LightGBM、SVM、人工神经网络、K最近邻、DT和朴素贝叶斯分类器在内的八种算法的机器学习模型。这些机器学习模型成功地预测了3个月和6个月的物理稳定性，并通过制剂实验验证了模型性能的可靠性。此外，他们还使用分子模拟来模拟二元和三元固体分散体的原子水平的分子机制。

2.3.8 环糊精

环糊精（CD）是由淀粉制成的，已经被发现并研究了大约100年。CD分子是具有氢供体和受体的环状寡糖。CD分子的外表面具有亲水性，而内腔则是亲脂性的。在制药工业中，CD分子通常被用作复合剂。CD复合物可以通过CD分子与化合物分子之间可逆结合来形成。这些复合物有助于提高不溶性药物的溶解度和稳定性。机器学习方法也已应用于环糊精制剂设计中。在CD处方开发方面，CD复合物的结合自由能通常被用作评估结合强度和稳定性的重要指标。在CD领域的机器学习应用中，常常将主体分子与客体分子之间的结合自由能作为模型预测的目标[132, 133]。例如，2001年，Takahiro Suzuki采用了定量结构-性质关系（QSPR）方法来开发α-环糊精或β-环糊精的复合物[131]。该研究使用了包括102个α-环糊精数据和218个β-环糊精数据的数据集，最后还使用了额外的27个数据进行模型测试。他们训练了一种基于组贡献的模型，这种模型属于多元线性回归（MLR）模型。该模型假设每个化学基团的贡献可以累加以计算化合物的性质，且各基团之间线性独立且无相互作用。2019年，Zhao Qianqian及其合作者收集了一个包含CD复合物结合自由能的大型制剂数据集，总共涵盖了超过3000个不同的处方[31]。该数据集包括八种不同类型的环糊精，例如2-羟基丙基-β-环糊精、随机甲基化的β-环糊精、2,3,6-三-*O*-甲基-β-环糊精、2,6-二-*O*-甲基-β-环糊精以及磺基丁醚-β-环糊精等。为了更好地解释模型，他们采用了LightGBM模型获得了特征的重要性排序。这个排序为我们提供了关于哪些制剂因素主要影响复合物结合的见解。此外，他们还测试了模型性能与数据规模之间的关系。

2.4 大模型在药物发现和药物开发领域的应用

药物发现与开发领域目前面临着多种挑战。深度学习已经崭露头角，成为解决这些挑战的有力工具。最近，大规模模型，如大型语言模型（LLM），生成式预训练Transformer（GPT）模型（如ChatGPT），以及其他基于Transformer和基于Transformer的双向编码器（BERT）的模型，包括计算机视觉（CV）领域的视觉Transformer（ViT）模型，已经在药物发现与开发领域的各种任务中展现出巨大潜力[148]。大规模模型通常指具有大量可训练参数的深度学习模型。这些模型通常拥有数十亿个权重，使它们能够有效地捕捉数据中微妙的模式和复杂的关联关系。大规模模型需要在海量数据上进行迭代训练，优化众多权重，并用于解决复杂问题。一些著名的大规模模型，包括GPT、路径语言模型（PaLM）、分割模型（SAM）和ViT，已经得到了发展，并在各种应用领域产生了广泛影响。

药物发现与开发领域的传统机器学习方法依赖于人工设计的分子描述符和指纹，需要药学专家的知识积累。深度学习通过从大规模数据集中学习已经显示出独特的优势。例如，大规模模型可以通过预训练有效地捕获化合物的结构信息，并将其应用于特定的下游任务。根据文献综述，目前大规模模型在药物发现与开发中的应用主要集中在以下几个方面：①用于下游药物发现与开发任务的语言模型预训练；②用于下游药物发现与开发任务的多任务学习与多性质预测预训练；③药物-靶标相互作用（DTI）预测；④抗菌肽（AMP）预测；⑤药代动力学性质预测；⑥新分子设计的生成模型；⑦临床医学图像处理；⑧医学文档检索与推荐；⑨临床合理用药和药物相互作用（DDI）预测。这些研究主题对于解决药物发现与开发中的关键挑战至关重要。在这些主题中，DTI预测和分子生成与设计是最引人关注的，可能是因为它们与当前成功发现药物的挑战密切相关。在本节中，我们将通过概述开发大规模模型所采用的方法（预训练策略、输入与输出），总结已取得的成就和关键发现。

大规模模型使得自动化、快速、成本效益的模型预训练和微调策略成为可能。在这个领域的研究中，使用了各种预训练策略的组合，其中包括：

（1）语言模型预训练策略：这一策略涉及使用语言建模任务对大规模模型进行预训练。这些预训练模型从大量文本数据中捕获了句法和语义信息，使其可以在药物发现和开发领域的下游任务中得以应用。

（2）多任务学习和多性质预测预训练策略：这一策略专注于预训练模型以同时预测多个性质。通过在多样化的数据集上进行训练，这些模型可以学习提取相关特征，并在药物发现和开发领域的不同任务中进行泛化。这些预训练策略充分利用了大规模模型的计算能力，以学习数据中的复杂模式和关系，从而有助于它们在后续的药物相关任务中应用。通过综合利用这些策略，研究人员已经在推进药物发现和开发过程方面取得了重大进展。

2.4.1 下游药物发现与开发任务的语言模型预训练

语言模型预训练策略已广泛应用于药物发现与开发领域，充分利用了在大量未标记数据上训练的无监督语言模型。例如，MoLFormer模型采用SMILES序列，经过了对11亿个未标记分子的训练，能够捕获足够的信息以预测各种下游任务的不同性质[149]。另一个例子是

MG-BERT模型[150]，它在大量未标记数据上采用自监督学习策略，即"遮蔽原子预测"，旨在从分子中提取上下文信息。MG-BERT模型生成上下文敏感的原子表示，并将所学知识应用于各种下游分子性质预测任务。在11个ADMET数据集上的实验结果表明其具有出色的性能。通过采用大规模分子语言模型和自监督学习，语言模型预训练策略使模型能够充分利用未标记数据中的丰富信息，用于预测下游分子性质，从而为药物发现与开发提供了有力支持。这些方法在药物发现与开发任务中具有重要意义。

2.4.2 多任务学习和多性质预测的预训练在药物发现与开发领域的应用

研究人员还提出了一种创新的预训练方法，即多任务学习和多性质预测的预训练策略。MTL-BERT模型采用了大规模预训练、多任务学习以及SMILES枚举[151]。该方法首先利用自监督预训练从大量未标记数据的SMILES中提取化学信息，然后通过在多个下游任务之间共享信息来微调预训练模型。SMILES枚举被用作数据增强方法。MTL-BERT在60个数据集上展现出卓越的性能。基于原子特征预测、分子特征预测和对比学习任务的K-BERT从SMILES字符串中提取上下文信息[152]。在15个数据集上的结果表明，K-BERT优于基于描述符和基于图的模型。生成的指纹K-BERT-FP在这些数据集上表现出与MACCS相当的性能，同时还能够发现分子大小和手性信息。这些方法通过利用大规模预训练、多任务学习和数据增强，从分子中提取信息，在实验中表现出卓越的性能，为人工智能药物发现与开发领域提供了新的研究途径和深入见解。

2.4.2.1 药物-靶标相互作用预测

药物-靶标相互作用（DTI）预测是一个重要的研究领域。深度学习模型能够准确预测药物与靶标之间的相互作用。近年来，研究人员提出了各种基于Transformer和BERT的预训练模型与架构，以提高对DTI的预测与理解。这些基于Transformer和BERT的模型利用自注意机制捕获药物与靶标的信息，并采用交叉注意机制促进信息交流，从而提升了预测性能。其中，有一项研究引入了ChemBERTa模型，该模型利用基于BERT的预训练模型进行DTI预测[153]。通过特定案例研究验证了模型性能，涉及13对化合物与细胞色素P450（CYP）酶，结果表明其具有出色的DTI预测能力。另一项研究提出了基于Transformer的端到端架构[154]。利用注意模块，该架构能够自动提取不同级别的DTI信息并进行预测与解释。此外，一项研究利用了83000000种分子的分子文本表示[155]，通过迁移学习对有限标记数据的靶标的亲和性进行预测。基于Transformer和BERT的预训练模型在DTI预测方面展现出巨大的潜力。这些方法通过充分利用大规模数据和注意机制，能够提取分子之间复杂的关系，提供准确的预测与解释。这些研究有望加速药物发现过程。

2.4.2.2 抗菌肽预测

还有许多其他引人关注的研究方向和应用领域。其中一个重要的研究方向是预测抗菌肽（AMP）的功能[156]。AMP是一类具有生物活性的肽段，拥有抗微生物特性，对细菌耐药问题具有关键作用。深度学习模型可以用来提取肽段序列中结构和功能方面的信息，以预测一个肽段是否具有抗微生物活性。这种模型有助于鉴定潜在的AMP候选分子，促进新型抗微生物药物的研发。

2.4.2.3 药代动力学性质预测

一个重要的研究领域聚焦在药代动力学性质上，包括吸收、分布、代谢、排泄以及毒性（ADMET）。ADMET性质对于药物研发（R&D）和安全性评估至关重要。在药物的探索和开发过程中，平衡药理学和药代动力学特性一直是一项挑战。ADMET预测有助于在药物研发的早期阶段评估候选化合物的潜在风险。有一项研究提出了一种基于Graph BERT的ADMET模型，这个Transformer模型可以在考虑多种性质约束的情况下执行结构转化。通过这种方法，可以有选择地修改初始分子，同时保留其核心骨架结构。这基于Graph BERT的ADMET模型不仅能考虑药理学效应，还能优化药代动力学性质。

2.4.2.4 生成模型在新药分子设计中的关键作用

生成模型在新药分子设计领域扮演着至关重要的角色。常用的SMILES分子表示法可以与高级自然语言处理（NLP）模型（如Transformer）相结合，用于分子设计。例如，带有Mask自注意机制训练的Transformer（如MolGPT），可以生成和验证全新的分子结构。此外，科学家们还提出了一种有条件的分子生成预训练Transformer模型（cMolGPT），用于设计与特定靶标蛋白相互作用的化合物[159]。这一模型能够设计特异性靶向的分子，为有针对性的药物设计提供了支持。此外，生成模型还可以生成具有所需理化性质的新型分子。多重约束分子生成（MCMG）模型采用有条件Transformer，以探索满足化学空间内多个性质限制的全新化合物[160]。MCMG通过知识蒸馏技术降低模型复杂度，并通过强化学习增强了分子结构的多样性。此外，这些模型还整合了用于分子设计和评估的搜索算法。例如，生成模型和束搜索算法已被应用于设计维甲酸受体相关孤儿受体（ROR）的全新反激动剂[161]。这些设计出的分子能够以少数反应步骤合成，并表现出很高的效能。

在临床医学领域，大规模模型也被用于疾病预测、诊断和个性化治疗。通过分析临床试验数据、医学影像以及药物相互作用数据，这些大规模模型能够帮助医疗专业人员做出诊断决策，并为个性化治疗提供建议。

2.4.2.5 临床医学图像处理

大规模模型也广泛应用于临床医学图像处理领域，包括医学图像分割和COVID-19感染诊断。通过与视觉Transformer（ViT）结合，研究人员能够从图像中提取关键特征，实现高效准确的分割和诊断。在精准医学研究领域，医学图像分割具有重要意义。为了提高分割的准确性和泛化能力，研究人员提出了TSE DeepLab，该模型增强了全局特征的提取能力[162]，表现出更高的分割准确性和泛化能力。另一个挑战是在肺炎诊断中准确识别病理性肺部纹理，尤其是毛玻璃影像。研究人员引入了基于ViT的PneuNet[163]，用于准确诊断肺部X光图像。TSE DeepLab和PneuNet利用了Transformer和ViT，以提高医学图像分割和肺炎诊断的准确性。这有望在未来的临床实践中发挥重要作用。

2.4.2.6 医学文档检索与推荐

在医学文档检索与推荐领域，临床试验搜索是一项至关重要的任务。将患者与相关的经验性证据匹配起来是一项复杂的任务，需要具备临床和生物学知识。为了解决这个问题，研究人员探索了在检索平台中基于BERT的排名模型的应用[164]。这为精准医学提供了一个有效的工具。

2.4.2.7 临床合理用药和药物相互作用预测

药物相互作用（DDI）的目标是在生物医学文献中识别药物之间的潜在相互作用。研究人员提出了一种基于Transformer的模型，用于从生物医学文献中提取信息进行DDI预测[165]。这类模型为药剂师提供了参考，并确保了患者用药的安全性。

2.4.2.8 自动化实验平台和机器学习可解释性

最近的一项研究探索了将聚合物-蛋白质混合物应用于增强蛋白质在非自然环境中的稳定性[166]。通过设计和合成随机共聚物，采用主动机器学习策略，成功地识别出在热变性条件下保持甚至增强了三种不同酶的活性的共聚物。尽管筛选结果有所不同，但主动学习恰如其分地识别了有效的共聚物组合，以稳定每种酶的活性。这项研究提高了设计强大的聚合物-蛋白质混合材料的能力，为蛋白质稳定性和混合材料的应用提供了新的见解。

机器学习的可解释性在机器学习研究中具有重要意义。尽管深度学习模型在预测准确性方面表现出色，但其黑盒特性使解释决策过程变得具有挑战性。因此，研究人员正在努力开发可解释的机器学习方法，以提高模型的可解释性。深度学习和大规模模型已经在药物发现、药物开发和临床医学领域展现出重要的潜力。这些方法通过学习来自大规模化学、生物学和医学信息数据集的知识，提高了药物属性预测、新分子设计和临床医学任务的准确性和效率。因此，它们也为药物发现、药物开发和精准医学带来了新的机遇。

2.5 人工智能在临床与精准医学领域的应用

随着科学技术的进步，我们人类的预期寿命不断延长，老龄化社会正在迅速到来。老龄人口的急剧增长将对社会保障、退休制度、医疗保健、制药产品服务以及健康护理等众多社会问题产生深远影响。尽管近几十年来死亡率持续下降，但我们仍需应对癌症和影响老年人群寿命的退行性疾病。

在2015年，精准医学这个概念被提出，自那时起，这个概念引起了广泛关注。事实上，精准医学可以追溯到对个体化医疗的更深层理解。个体化医疗的概念早在古代就存在，古代医学已反映了医学治疗的个性化理念。从个体化医疗到精准医学，疾病的预防、诊断和治疗经历了许多变革。正如美国国立卫生研究院（NIH）所建议的那样，精准医学越来越强调个体因素，如个人基因、生活方式和周围环境。

机器学习在精准医学中发挥着至关重要的作用，它是实现精准医学的有力工具。我们将关注AI在精准医学和药物递送领域的重要价值和作用。例如，AI在为糖尿病患者提供正确剂量的胰岛素方面发挥着关键作用。糖尿病分为1型和2型，1型糖尿病患者需要胰岛素治疗。自动化胰岛素泵被提出作为自动化药物递送装置[167]。该装置由智能控制算法、连续葡萄糖监测传感器、计量泵和胰岛素四个组成部分。该装置通过密切监测患者的餐饮时间、食物类型和血糖来获取数据，然后计算出正确的剂量并递送胰岛素。这使得患者能够更好地控制血糖水平，甚至过上正常的生活。类似的医疗设备还可以对体内数据进行监测、计算个性化措施、进行医疗干预和动态调整。

此外，机器学习还被应用于其他临床医学领域[168]，如乳腺癌的治疗建议[169]、心血管疾病的治疗[170]和皮肤癌的诊断[171]。此外，AI 还被用于临床试验设计[172]。

精准医学的目标是为个体患者提供个性化的医疗诊断和治疗，能够利用个体患者的数据指导医疗实践，从而实现前所未有的整体医疗成果。医生、患者和医疗机构都可以受益于这些前沿技术，这些技术也将不断演进。

2.6 机遇与挑战

随着人工智能技术的发展，人工智能和机器学习算法正越来越多地应用到药物开发领域。人工智能和机器学习在药物开发的自动化方面不断凸显其重要性，这带来了机遇和挑战。机遇在于，在现代制药历史的 70 多年里，人工实验试错一直是主导的开发范式，人工智能和机器学习为自动化整个药物产品开发过程提供了可能性。这将体现在未来的一系列制药过程中，包括高通量预实验、自动处方筛选、数据标准化和规范化、建模、预测、控制和优化。与此同时，这也带来了一些挑战，以下是一些参考挑战。

一个常见问题是由于实验时间和样品不足导致的数据不足。对于小数据问题，迁移学习可能会有所帮助。迁移学习在大型原始数据集上训练模型，然后将经过训练的模型或层迁移到特定的小数据任务上[173]。在实践中，需要对迁移模型进行微调以适应特定任务。目前，已经在药物 PK 参数的预测中使用了迁移学习[174]。基于对抗的迁移学习也已应用于知识传递[175-178]。此外，生成对抗网络（GAN）中的数据增强方法也是一个选择[179-181]。GAN 中的生成网络可以学习样本的分布并生成新样本。生成的新样本可以进一步用于数据增强，从而有助于减轻模型过拟合的风险。此外，降维和特征选择方法也非常有用。当训练样本不足时，模型容易过拟合。降维和特征选择方法可以去除重要性较低的特征，降低过拟合的风险。此外，集成机器学习和多尺度模拟，如量子化学、分子动力学、蛋白质构象模拟和基于生理的药代动力学（PBPK）建模，不仅可以从微观角度提供额外的洞察力，还可以作为良好的模拟器生成数据。

不平衡的数据分布问题日益显著。不平衡数据或数据长尾的情况往往与小数据问题相伴随。在药物产品开发领域，通常会聚焦于几种化学分子。一些常用的模型药物已经被深入研究，而其他化学分子的数据却稀缺。这最终带来了训练具有良好泛化性能的机器学习模型的挑战。为迎接这一挑战，可以引入高通量筛选技术，例如针对药物溶解度、溶剂与稳定剂的组合、经皮制剂的膜透过性等进行实验[182-186]。此外，对于分类任务，模型的评估应该采用多个指标，包括准确率、精确度和召回率等。也可采用重新采样（如欠采样和过采样）或权重调整边缘数据的方法（如修改神经网络中的损失函数或对决策树中的小数据样本信息增益进行加权）。

机器学习可解释性是一个重要议题。可解释的机器学习方法能够为药物产品开发和药物递送领域提供更多洞察，协助找到自变量与因变量之间的因果关系，发现关键的处方组分和工艺参数，甚至指导合理的实验设计。如今，人们不再仅满足于机器学习模型的准确预测，而是追求理解模型背后的运作机制[187]。在高风险领域，如生物医学，理解模型决策过程变得极其重要。早期的线性模型具有透明度和可解释性，但随着复杂的决策系统的兴起，如深度学习，模型变得越来越难以理解。深度学习模型或基于树的集成模型可能包含数以万计的参数或成千上万棵树。尽管它们在实现人工智能应用方面取得了巨大成功，甚至在许多领域超越了人类，但我们很难理解模型操作行为背后的原因。数据和模型的可解释性变得至关重要。通常有三种常用的可解释方法：首先是建模前的可解释机器学习方法，其次是自解释机器学习模型，最后是建模后的可解释机器学习方法。建模前的可解释机器学习方法通常使用统计方法可视化数据并计算相关系数。自解释机器学习模型包括线性回归和决策树模型，其中线性模型中自变量的权重可解释为输入特征的重要性，决策树的树结构可解释为数据分割规则。然而，随着输入特征数量和决策树深度的增加，这两种模型变得难以理解。建模后的可解释机器学习方法将机器学习模型视为黑盒子，通过不同输入得到模型输出，以探查可能的内部机制。常用的建模后算法包括 LIME 和 SHAP[188-190]。特别对于深度学习，常用的可解释方法包括中间隐藏层的可视化、消融实验和基于注意力机制的方法。对于基于树的集成学习模型，特征重要性排名非常有用。

在制药产品开发中，不同数据类型的表征是多维的。药物具有多种关键质量属性，仅使用单一类型的数据可能无法充分代表药物产品的性质，数据融合解决了这个问题。数据融合的目的是整合不同类型的数据，消除可能的冗余信息，相互补充，最终提高数据的可靠性。例如，结构化或非结构化数据，可以首先使用深度神经网络提取关键特征，然后，提取的特征可以进行进一步的预测。前馈全连接神经网络适用于处理二维表格数据，循环神经网络适用于处理时间序列数据，如药剂学中的药物溶解曲线和血浆药物浓度，而卷积神经网络适用于分析图像和图形数据，如分子图[191, 192]。

目前，在药物制剂领域，人工智能的应用逐渐增多。然而，药剂科学家通常不是计算机或统计学专家，因此难以轻松应用机器学习算法解决问题，其中一个障碍是从众多的超参数配置中进行选择。而对于药剂科学家来说，模型的超参数往往难以理解和调整。对于机器学习工程师来说，调整最佳的超参数也需要大量的工作。近年来，人工神经网络的成功应用高度依赖于精心设计的网络架构，但人工神经网络中的众多网络结构超参数导致了组合爆炸问题。此外，每个任务的最佳超参数配置也各不相同，因此自动优化模型的过程变得必不可少。自动优化模型是在高维空间中寻找最佳参数配置。超参数优化方法和网络架构搜索算法（NAS）可以自动化和加速这一过程。首先，需要定义搜索空间，然后根据优化和搜索策略搜索超参数配置，最后在进行下一轮之前评估模型性能。常用的超参数优化方法包括网格搜索、随机搜索和贝叶斯优化方法。此外，网络架构搜索算法（NAS）受到越来越多的关注[193]。目前，已经提出了许多新的策略来部署 NAS，其中常用的方法包括基于强化学习的算法[194, 195]、基于进化的算法[196, 197]和基于梯度的算法[198, 199]。

2.7　总结

在过去的七十年里,人们见证了药物和制剂产品领域的不断进步。药物和制剂产品开发的显著进展,为人类寿命的延长做出了重要贡献。这进一步促使我们需要开发更多的药物产品,以满足患者需求并治疗各种疾病。通过研发创新和复杂的药物递送系统,药剂科学家们可以在治疗更多疾病方面发挥重要作用。药物递送系统能够将不溶、生物利用度低和不稳定的药物候选物转化为具有治疗效力的药物产品,将半衰期短的药物制成控释制剂,甚至能够制造出基于生物分子的mRNA疫苗。

在最近的十年中,药物和制剂产品开发的范式正在发生变革。这个迅速变化的趋势已经导致了制药行业的范式和文化发生了巨大的转变。人工智能现在为我们提供了独特的机会,有可能超越过去所取得的成就。与此同时,我们也面临着一系列的机遇和挑战。要解决这些问题,我们需要保持好奇心,深入思考,积极采用先进技术,并坚持不懈地进行科学研究。

参考文献

[1] Ku M S, Dulin W. A biopharmaceutical classification-based Right-First-Time formulation approach to reduce human pharmacokinetic variability and project cycle time from First-In-Human to clinical Proof-Of-Concept[J]. Pharm Dev Technol, 2012, 17(3), 285-302.

[2] Beg S, Swain S, Rizwan M, et al. Bioavailability enhancement strategies: Basics, formulation approaches and regulatory considerations[J]. Curr. Drug Deliv. 2011, 8(6): 691-702.

[3] Eichhorn C, Gräni C. Diagnosing and sports counselling of athletes with myocarditis[J]. Swiss Sports and Exercise Medicine 2019, 67(2): 28-36.

[4] Landin M, Rowe R C. Formulation tools for pharmaceutical development[M]. Amsterdam: Elsevier Ltd, 2013: 7-37.

[5] Wang W, Ye Z, Gao H, et al. Computational pharmaceutics : A new paradigm of drug delivery[J]. J Control Release, 2021, 338: 119-136.

[6] Juran J M. Juran on quality by design: the new steps for planning quality into goods and services[M]. New York : Maxwell Macmillan International, 1992.

[7] International Conference on Harmonisation; guidance on Q8(R1) Pharmaceutical Development; addition of annex; availability. Notice Fed Regist, 2009, 74: 27325-27326.

[8] Zomer S, Gupta M, Scott A. Application of multivariate tools in pharmaceutical product development to bridge risk assessment to continuous verification in a quality by design environment[J]. J Pharm Innov, 2010, 5: 109-118.

[9] Armstrong N A. Pharmaceutical experimental design and interpretation, second edition[M]. London: CRC Press, 2006.

[10] Wehrlé P, Stamm A. Statistical tools for process control and quality improvement in the pharmaceutical industry[J]. Drug Dev Ind Pharm, 1994, 20(2): 141-164.

[11] Hinton G E, Osindero S, Teh Y W. A fast learning algorithm for deep belief nets[J]. Neural Comput, 2006, 18(7): 1527-1554.

[12] Hinton G E, Salakhutdinov R R. Reducing the dimensionality of data with neural networks[J]. Science, 2006, 313: 504-507.

[13] Silver D, Huang A, Maddison J C, et al. Mastering the game of go with deep neural networks and tree search[J]. Nature, 2016, 529: 484-489.

[14] Silver D, Schrittwieser J , Simonyan K, et al. Mastering the game of Go without human knowledge[J]. Nature, 2017, 550(7676): 354-359.

[15] Lecun Y, Bengio Y, Hinton G. Deep learning[J]. Nature, 2015, 521(7553): 436-444.

[16] Jumper, J, Evans R, Pritzel A, et al. Highly accurate protein structure prediction with AlphaFold[J]. Nature, 2021, 596: 583-589.

[17] Hussain A S, Yu X, Johnson R D. Application of neural computing in pharmaceutical product development[J]. Pharm Res,

1991, 8: 1248-1252.

[18] Bannigan P, Aldeghi M, Bao Z, et al. Machine learning directed drug formulation development[J]. Adv. Drug Deliv. Rev., 2021, 175: 113806.

[19] He S, Leanse L G, Feng Y. Artificial intelligence and machine learning assisted drug delivery for effective treatment of infectious diseases[J]. Adv Drug Deliv Rev, 2021, 178: 113922.

[20] Erb R J. Introduction to backpropagation neural network computation[J]. Pharm Res, 1993, 10: 165-170.

[21] Rowe R C, Roberts R J. Artificial intelligence in pharmaceutical product formulation: Neural computing and emerging technologies[J]. Pharmaceutical Science and Technology Today, 1998, 1(5): 200-205.

[22] Rowe R C, Roberts R J. Artificial intelligence in pharmaceutical product formulation: knowledge-based and expert systems[J]. Pharmaceutical Science and Technology Today, 1998, 1(4): 153-159.

[23] Takayama K, Fujikawa M, Nagai T. Artificial neural network as a novel method to optimize pharmaceutical formulations[J]. Pharmaceutical Research , 1999, 16(1): 1-6.

[24] Sun Y, Peng Y, Chen Y, et al. Application of artificial neural networks in the design of controlled release drug delivery systems[J]. Adv Drug Deliv Rev, 2003, 55(9): 1201-1215.

[25] Takayama K, Fujikawa M, Obata Y, et al. Neural network based optimization of drug formulations[J]. Adv Drug Deliv Rev, 2003, 55(9): 1217-1231.

[26] Ekins S, Shimada J, Chang C. Application of data mining approaches to drug delivery[J]. Adv Drug Deliv Rev, 2006, 58(12): 1409-1430.

[27] Colbourn E A, Rowe R C. Novel approaches to neural and evolutionary computing in pharmaceutical formulation: Challenges and new possibilities[J]. Future Med Chem, 2009, 1(4): 713-726.

[28] Ibrić S, Djuriš J, Parojčić J, et al. Artificial neural networks in evaluation and optimization of modified release solid dosage forms[J]. Pharm, 2012, 4(4): 531-550.

[29] Dai S, Xu B, Shi G, et al. SeDeM expert system for directly compressed tablet formulation: A review and new perspectives[J]. Powder Technol, 2019, 342: 517-527.

[30] Yang Y, Ye Z, Su Y, et al. Deep learning for in vitro prediction of pharmaceutical formulations[J]. Acta Pharm Sin B, 2019, 9: 177-185.

[31] Zhao Q, Ye Z, Su Y, et al. Predicting complexation performance between cyclodextrins and guest molecules by integrated machine learning and molecular modeling techniques[J]. Acta Pharm Sin B, 2019, 9(6): 1241-1252.

[32] Han R, Xiong H, Ye Z, et al. Predicting physical stability of solid dispersions by machine learning techniques[J]. Journal of Controlled Release, 2019, 311-312: 16-25.

[33] He Y, Ye Z, Liu X, et al. Can machine learning predict drug nanocrystals？[J] Journal of Controlled Release, 2020, 322: 274-285.

[34] Ye Z, Yang Y, Li X, et al. An integrated transfer learning and multitask learning approach for pharmacokinetic parameter prediction[J]. Mol Pharm 2019, 16(2): 533-541.

[35] Wang W, et al. Prediction of lipid nanoparticles for mRNA vaccines by the machine learning algorithm[J]. Acta Pharm Sin B, 2022, 12(6): 2950-2962.

[36] Ye Z, Yang W, Yang Y, et al. Interpretable machine learning methods for in vitro pharmaceutical formulation development[J].Food Frontiers, 2021, 2(2): 195-207.

[37] Samuel A L. Some studies in machine learning using the game of checkers[J]. IBM J Res Dev, 2000, 44, 206-226.

[38] Breiman L. Random forests[J]. Mach Learn, 2001, 45: 5-32.

[39] Chen T, Guestrin C. XGBoost: A Scalable Tree Boosting System[C]. In: Proceedings of the 22 nd ACM SIGKDD International Conference on Knowledge Discovery and Data Mining(2016): 785-794.

[40] McCulloch W S, Pitts W. A logical calculus of the ideas immanent in nervous activity[J]. Bulletin of Mathematical Biophysics, 1943, 5: 115-133.

[41] Rosenblatt F. The perceptron: A probabilistic model for information storage and organization in the brain[J]. Psychol Rev, 1958, 65: 386-408.

[42] Minsky M, Papert S A. Perceptrons: An introduction to computational geometry[M]. Massachusetts: MIT press, 1969.

[43] Kelley H J. Gradient theory of optimal flight paths[J].ARS Journal, 1960, 30: 947-954.

[44] Bryson A E. A gradient method for optimizing multistage allocation processes. Proceedings of the Harvard Univ. Symposium on digital computers and their applications(1961).

[45] Krizhevsky A, Sutskever I, Hinton G E. 1097-1105.

[46] Schmidhuber J. Deep learning in neural networks: An overview[J]. Neural Netw, 2015, 61: 85-117.

[47] Bengio Y, Courville A, Vincen P. Representation learning: A review and new perspectives[J]. IEEE Trans Pattern Anal Mach Intell, 2013, 35: 1798-1828.

[48] Calderon C P, Daniels A L, Randolph T W. Deep convolutional neural network analysis of flow imaging microscopy data to classify subvisible particles in protein formulations[J]. J Pharm Sci, 2018, 107: 999-1008.

[49] Ma X, et al. Application of deep learning convolutional neural networks for internal tablet defect detection: high accuracy, throughput, and adaptability[J]. J Pharm Sci, 2020, 109: 1547-1557.

[50] Kingma D P, Ba J. Adam: a method for stochastic optimization[J]. arXiv e-prints, 2014, arXiv: 1412.6980.

[51] Nair V, Hinton G E. Rectified linear units improve restricted boltzmann machines, in: ICML'10: Proceedings of the 27 th International Conference on International Conference on Machine Learning, 2010, 807-814.

[52] Holland J H. Adaptation in Natural and Artificial Systems: An Introductory Analysis with Applications to Biology, Control and Artificial Intelligence[M]. Massachusetts: MIT Press, 1992.

[53] Goldberg D E. Genetic Algorithms in Search, Optimization and Machine Learning[M].Massachusetts: Addison-Wesley Longman Publishing Co., Inc., 1989.

[54] Jang J S R, Sun C T. Neuro-fuzzy modeling and control[J]. Proc IEEE, 1995, 83: 378-406.

[55] Zadeh L A. Fuzzy sets. Information and Control[J].1965, 8(3): 338-353.

[56] Cortes C, Vapnik V. Support-vector networks[J]. Mach Learn, 1995, 20: 273-297.

[57] Boser B E, Guyon I M, Vapnik V N. A training algorithm for optimal margin classifiers[M]. New York: Association for Computing Machinery, 1992: 144-152.

[58] Drucker H, Surges C J C, Kaufman L, et al. Support vector regression machines[J]. Neural Information Processing Systems., 1996: 155-161.

[59] Hastie T, Tibshirani R, Friedman J H. The elements of statistical learning: data mining, inference, and prediction[M]. Berlin: Springer, 2009.

[60] Cloutier T K, Sudrik C, Mody N, et al. Machine learning models of antibody-excipient preferential interactions for use in computational formulation design[J]. Mol Pharm, 2020, 17: 3589-3599.

[61] Breiman L, Friedman J H, Olshen R A, et al. Classification and regression trees[M]. Boca Raton: CRC Press, 2017.

[62] Wu X, Kumar V, Quinlan J R, et al. Top 10 algorithms in data mining[J]. Knowl. Inf Systems Syst, 2008, 14: 1-37.

[63] Quinlan J R. Induction of decision trees[J]. Mach Learn, 1986, 1: 81-106.

[64] Salzberg S L. C4.5: Programs for Machine Learning by J. Ross Quinlan. Morgan Kaufmann Publishers, Inc., 1993[J]. Mach Learn, 1994, 16: 235-240.

[65] Dietterich T G. Ensemble Methods in Machine Learning. In: International workshop on multiple classifier systems[J]. LNCS, 2000, 1587: 1-15 .

[66] Breiman L. Bagging predictors[J]. Mach Learn, 1996, 24: 123-140.

[67] Turkoglu M, Ozarslan R, Sakr A. Artificial neural network analysis of a direct compression tabletting study[J]. Eur J Pharm Biopharm, 1995, 41: 315-322.

[68] Kesavan J G, Peck G E. Pharmaceutical granulation and tablet formulation using neural networks[J]. Pharm Dev Technol, 1996, 1: 391-404.

[69] Bourquin J, Schmidli H, Van Hoogevest P, et al. Advantages of Artificial Neural Networks (ANNs) as alternative modelling technique for data sets showing non-linear relationships using data from a galenical study on a solid dosage form[J]. European Journal of Pharmaceutical Sciences, 1998, 7: 5-16.

[70] Bourquin J, Schmidli H, Van Hoogevest P, et al. Pitfalls of artificial neural networks (ANN) modelling technique for data sets containing outlier measurements using a study on mixture properties of a direct compressed dosage form[J]. Eur J Pharm Sci, 1998, 7: 17-28.

[71] Bourquin J, Schmidli H, Van Hoogevest P, et al. Comparison of artificial neural networks (ANN) with classical modelling techniques using different experimental designs and data from a galenical study on a solid dosage form[J]. Eur J Pharm Sci, 1998, 6: 287-300.

[72] Sathe P M, Venitz J. Comparison of neural network and multiple linear regression as dissolution predictors[J]. Drug Dev Ind Pharm, 2003, 29: 349-355.

[73] Shao Q, Rowe R C, York P. Comparison of neurofuzzy logic and neural networks in modelling experimental data of an immediate release tablet formulation[J]. European Journal of Pharmaceutical Sciences, 2006, 28: 394-404.

[74] Shao Q, Rowe R C, York P. Comparison of neurofuzzy logic and decision trees in discovering knowledge from experimental data of an immediate release tablet formulation[J]. Eur J Pharm Sci, 2007, 31: 129-136.

[75] Shao Q, Rowe R C, York P. Investigation of an artificial intelligence technology-Model trees. Novel applications for an

immediate release tablet formulation database[J]. Eur J Pharm Sci, 2007, 31: 137-144.

[76] Landín M, Rowe R C, York P. Advantages of neurofuzzy logic against conventional experimental design and statistical analysis in studying and developing direct compression formulations[J]. European Journal of Pharmaceutical Sciences, 2009, 38: 325-331.

[77] Takagaki K, Arai H, Takayama, K. Creation of a tablet database containing several active ingredients and prediction of their pharmaceutical characteristics based on ensemble artificial neural networks[J]. J Pharm Sci 2010, 99: 4201-4214.

[78] Aksu B, Paradkar A, Matas M, et al. Quality by design approach: Application of artificial intelligence techniques of tablets manufactured by direct compression[J]. AAPS PharmSciTech, 2012, 13: 1138-1146.

[79] Aksu B, Paradkar A, Matas M, et al. A quality by design approach using artificial intelligence techniques to control the critical quality attributes of ramipril tablets manufactured by wet granulation[J]. Pharm Dev Technol, 2013, 18: 236-245.

[80] Wilson W I, Peng Y, Augsburger L L. Generalization of a prototype intelligent hybrid system for hard gelatin capsule formulation development[J]. AAPS PharmSciTech, 2005, 6(3): E449-457.

[81] Hussain A S, Shivanand P, Johnson R D. Application of neural computing in pharmaceutical product development: Computer aided formulation design[J]. Drug Dev Ind Pharm, 1994, 20: 1739-1752.

[82] Ebube N K, McCall T, Chen Y, et al. Relating formulation variables to in vitro dissolution using an artificial neural network[J]. Pharm Dev Technol, 1997, 2: 225-232.

[83] Takahara J, Takayama K, Nagai T. Multi-objective simultaneous optimization technique based on an artificial neural network in sustained release formulations[J]. J Control Release, 1997, 49: 11-20.

[84] Dowell J A, Hussain A, Devane J, et al. Artificial neural networks applied to the in vitro-in vivo correlation of an extended-release formulation: Initial trials and experience[J]. J Pharm Sci, 1999, 88: 154-160.

[85] Chen Y, McCall T W, Baichwal A R, et al. The application of an artificial neural network and pharmacokinetic simulations in the design of controlled-release dosage forms[J]. J Control Release, 1999, 59: 33-41.

[86] Takayama K, Morva A, Fujikawa M, et al. Formula optimization of theophylline controlled-release tablet based on artificial neural networks[J]. J Control Release, 2000, 68: 175-186.

[87] Peh K K, Lim C P, Quek S S, et al. Use of artificial neural networks to predict drug dissolution profiles and evaluation of network performance using similarity factor[J]. Pharmaceutical Research, 2000, 17: 1384-1388.

[88] Goh W Y, Lim C P, Peh K K, et al. Application of a recurrent neural network to prediction of drug dissolution profiles[J]. Neural Comput Appl, 20002, 10: 311-317.

[89] Ibri S, Jovanovi M, Djuri Z, et al. The application of generalized regression neural network in the modeling and optimization of aspirin extended release tablets with Eudragit® RS PO as matrix substance[J]. J Control Release, 2002, 82: 213-222.

[90] Ibrić S, Jovanoviċ M, Djuriċ Z, et al. Artificial neural networks in the modeling and optimization of aspirin extended release tablets with Eudragit L 100 as matrix substance[J]. AAPS PharmSciTech, 2008, 4: 62-67.

[91] Parojčić J, Ibrić S, Djuriċ Z, et al. An investigation into the usefulness of generalized regression neural network analysis in the development of level A in vitro-in vivo correlation[J]. Eur J Pharm Sci, 2007, 30: 264-272.

[92] Ibriċ S, Jovanoviċ M, Djuriċ Z, et al. Generalized regression neural networks in prediction of drug stability[J]. J Pharm Pharmacol, 2007, 59: 745-750.

[93] Do D Q, Rowe R C, York P. Modelling drug dissolution from controlled release products using genetic programming[J]. Int J Pharm, 2008, 351: 194-200.

[94] Petrović J, Ibrić S, Betz G, et al. Application of dynamic neural networks in the modeling of drug release from polyethylene oxide matrix tablets[J]. Eur J Pharm Sci, 2009, 38: 172-180.

[95] Barmpalexis P, Kanaze F I, Kachrimanis K, et al. Artificial neural networks in the optimization of a nimodipine controlled release tablet formulation[J]. Eur J Pharm Biopharm, 2010, 74: 316-323.

[96] Chaibva F, Burton M, Walker R B. Optimization of salbutamol sulfate dissolution from sustained release matrix formulations using an artificial neural network[J]. Pharmaceutics, 2010, 2: 182-198.

[97] Petrović J, Ibrić S, Betz G, et al. Optimization of matrix tablets controlled drug release using Elman dynamic neural networks and decision trees[J]. International Journal of Pharmaceutics, 2012, 428: 57-67.

[98] Aktas E, Eroglu H, Kockan U, et al. Systematic development of pH-independent controlled release tablets of carvedilol using central composite design and artificial neural networks[J]. Drug Development and Industrial Pharmacy, 2013, 39: 1207-1216.

[99] Wu T, Pan W, Chen J, et al. Formulation optimization technique based on artificial neural network in salbutamol sulfate osmotic pump tablets[J]. Drug Dev Ind Pharm, 2000, 26: 211-215.

[100] Ilić M, Crossed D Signuriš J, Kovačević I, et al. In vitro-In silico-In vivo drug absorption model development based on mechanistic gastrointestinal simulation and artificial neural networks: Nifedipine osmotic release tablets case study[J]. European Journal of Pharmaceutical Sciences, 2014, 62: 212-218.

[101] Agatonovic-Kustrin S, Alany R G. Role of genetic algorithms and artificial neural networks in predicting the phase behavior of colloidal delivery systems[J]. Pharmaceutical Research, 2001, 18: 1049-1055.

[102] Glass B D, Agatonovic-Kustrin S, Wisch M H. Artificial neural networks to optimize formulation components of a fixed-dose combination of rifampicin, isoniazid and pyrazinamide in a microemulsion[J]. Curr Drug Discov Technol, 2005, 2: 195-201.

[103] Fatouros D G, Nielsen F, Douroumis D, et al. In vitro-in vivo correlations of self-emulsifying drug delivery systems combining the dynamic lipolysis model and neuro-fuzzy networks[J]. Eur J Pharm Biopharm, 2008, 69: 887-898.

[104] Amani A, York P, Chrystyn H, et al. Determination of factors controlling the particle size in nanoemulsions using Artificial Neural Networks[J]. Eur J Pharm Sci, 2008, 35: 42-51.

[105] Djekic L, Ibric S, Primorac M. The application of artificial neural networks in the prediction of microemulsion phase boundaries in PEG-8 caprylic/capric glycerides based systems[J]. International Journal of Pharmaceutics, 2008, 361: 41-46.

[106] Podlogar F, Šibanc R, Gašperlin M. Evolutionary artificial neural networks as tools for predicting the internal structure of microemulsions[J]. J Pharm Pharm Sci, 2008, 11, 67-76.

[107] Wei H, Zhong F, Ma J, et al. Formula optimization of emulsifiers for preparation of multiple emulsions based on artificial neural networks[J]. J Dispersion Sci Technol, 2008, 29: 319-326.

[108] Amani A, York P, Chrystyn H, et al. Factors affecting the stability of nanoemulsions-use of artificial neural networks[J]. Pharmaceutical Research, 2010, 27: 37-45.

[109] Seyedhassantehrani N, Karimi R, Tavoosidana G, et al. Concurrent study of stability and cytotoxicity of a novel nanoemulsion system: an artificial neural networks approach[J]. Pharm Dev Technol, 2017, 22: 383-389.

[110] Kandimalla K K, Kanikkannan N, Singh M. Optimization of a vehicle mixture for the transdermal delivery of melatonin using artificial neural networks and response surface method[J]. J Control Release, 1999, 61: 71-82.

[111] Takayama K, Takahara J, Fujikawa M, et al. Formula optimization based on artificial neural networks in transdermal drug delivery[J]. J Control Release, 1999, 62, 161-170.

[112] Wu P C, Obata Y, Fujikawa M, et al. Simultaneous optimization based on artificial neural networks in ketoprofen hydrogel formula containing *O*-ethyl-3-butylcyclohexanol as percutaneous absorption enhancer[J]. J Pharm Sci, 2001, 90: 1004-1014.

[113] Asadi H, Rostamizadeh K, Salari D, et al. Preparation of biodegradable nanoparticles of tri-block PLA-PEG-PLA copolymer and determination of factors controlling the particle size using artificial neural network[J]. J Microencapsulation, 2011, 28, 406-416.

[114] Esmaeilzadeh-Gharedaghi E, Faramarz M A, Amini M A, et al. Effects of processing parameters on particle size of ultrasound prepared chitosan nanoparticles: An Artificial Neural Networks Study[J]. Pharm Dev Technol, 2012, 17, 638-647.

[115] Mostafavi S H, Aghajani M, Amani A, et al. Optimization of paclitaxel-loaded poly(D, L-lactide-*co*-glycolide-*N-p*-maleimido benzoic hydrazide) nanoparticles size using artificial neural networks[J]. Pharm Dev Technol, 2015, 20, 845-853.

[116] Walkey C D, Olsen J B, Song F, et al. Protein corona fingerprinting predicts the cellular interaction of gold and silver nanoparticles[J]. ACS Nano, 2014, 8: 2439-2455.

[117] Li Y, Abbaspour M R, Grootendorst P V, et al. Optimization of controlled release nanoparticle formulation of verapamil hydrochloride using artificial neural networks with genetic algorithm and response surface methodology[J]. Eur J Pharm Biopharm, 2015, 94: 170-179.

[118] Hathout R M, Metwally A A. Towards better modelling of drug-loading in solid lipid nanoparticles: Molecular dynamics, docking experiments and Gaussian Processes machine learning[J]. Eur J Pharm Biopharm, 2016, 108: 262-268.

[119] Shahsavari S, Rezaie Shirmard L, Amini M, et al. Application of artificial neural networks in the design and optimization of a nanoparticulate fingolimod delivery system based on biodegradable poly(3-Hydroxybutyrate-*co*-3-Hydroxyvalerate)[J]. J Pharm Sci, 2017, 106: 176-182.

[120] Baharifar H, Amani A. Size, Loading efficiency, and cytotoxicity of albumin-loaded chitosan nanoparticles: An artificial neural networks study[J]. J Pharm Sci, 2017, 106: 411-417.

[121] Youshia J, Ali M E, Lamprecht A. Artificial neural network based particle size prediction of polymeric nanoparticles[J]. Eur J Pharm Biopharm, 2017, 119: 333-342.

[122] Kingston B R, Syed A M, Ngai J, et al. Assessing micrometastases as a target for nanoparticles using 3D microscopy and

[123] Yamankurt G, Berns E J, Xue A, et al. Exploration of the nanomedicine-design space with high-throughput screening and machine learning[J]. Nat Biomed Eng, 2019, 3: 318-327.

[124] Lazarovits J, Sindhwani S, Tavares A J, et al. Supervised learning and mass spectrometry predicts the in vivo fate of nanomaterials[J]. ACS Nano, 2019, 13: 8023-8034.

[125] Bansal A K, Munjal B, Koradia V, et al. Role of Innovator Product Characterization in Generic Product Development. In: Excipient Applications in Formulation Design and Drug Delivery[M]. Berlin: Springer International Publishing, 2015: 521-538.

[126] Mendyk A, Jachowicz R. Neural network as a decision support system in the development of pharmaceutical formulation-Focus on solid dispersions[J]. Expert Sys Appl, 2005, 28: 285-294.

[127] Papadimitriou S A, Barmpalexis P, Karavas E, et al. Optimizing the ability of PVP/PEG mixtures to be used as appropriate carriers for the preparation of drug solid dispersions by melt mixing technique using artificial neural networks: I[J]. Eur J Pharm Biopharm, 2012, 82: 175-186.

[128] Barmpalexis P, Koutsidis I, Karavas E, et al. Development of PVP/PEG mixtures as appropriate carriers for the preparation of drug solid dispersions by melt mixing technique and optimization of dissolution using artificial neural networks[J]. Eur J Pharm Biopharm, 2013, 85: 1219-1231.

[129] Patel A D, Agrawal A, Dave R H. Development of polyvinylpyrrolidone-based spray-dried solid dispersions using response surface model and ensemble artificial neural network[J]. J Pharm Sci, 2013, 102: 1847-1858.

[130] Patel A D, Agrawal A, Dave R H. Investigation of the effects of process variables on derived properties of spray dried solid-dispersions using polymer based response surface model and ensemble artificial neural network models[J]. Eur J Pharm Biopharm, 2014, 86: 404-417.

[131] Suzuki T. A nonlinear group contribution method for predicting the free energies of inclusion complexation of organic molecules with α-and β-cyclodextrins[J]. J Chem Inf Comput Sci, 2001, 41, 1266-1273.

[132] Xu Q, Wei C, Liu R, et al. Quantitative structure-property relationship study of β-cyclodextrin complexation free energies of organic compounds[J]. Chemometr Intelligent Lab Syst, 2015, 146: 313-321.

[133] Solovev A, Solov'ev V. 3D molecular fragment descriptors for structure-property modeling: predicting the free energies for the complexation between antipodal guests and β-cyclodextrins[J]. Journal of Inclusion Phenomena and Macrocyclic Chemistry, 2017, 89: 167-175.

[134] Poon W, Kingston B R, Ouyang B, et al. A framework for designing delivery systems[J]. Nat Nanotechnol, 2020, 15: 819-829.

[135] Salvati A, Pitek A S, Monopoli M P, et al. Transferrin-functionalized nanoparticles lose their targeting capabilities when a biomolecule corona adsorbs on the surface[J]. Nat Nanotechnol, 2013, 8: 137-143.

[136] Poon W, Zhang Y, Ouyang B, et al. Elimination pathways of nanoparticles[J]. ACS Nano, 2019, 13, 5785-5798.

[137] Soo Choi H, Liu W, Misra P, et al. Renal clearance of quantum dots[J]. Nat Biotechnol, 2007, 25: 1165-1170.

[138] Saraiva C, Praça C, Ferreira R, et al. Nanoparticle-mediated brain drug delivery: Overcoming blood-brain barrier to treat neurodegenerative diseases[J]. J Control Release, 2016, 235: 34-47.

[139] Sindhwani S, Syed A M, Ngai J, et al. The entry of nanoparticles into solid tumours[J]. Nat Mater, 2020, 19: 566-575.

[140] Dai Q, Wilhelm S, Ding D, et al. Quantifying the ligand-coated nanoparticle delivery to cancer cells in solid tumors[J]. ACS Nano, 2018, 12: 8423-8435.

[141] dos Santos T, Varela J, Lynch I, et al. Effects of transport inhibitors on the cellular uptake of carboxylated polystyrene nanoparticles in different cell lines[J]. PLoS One, 2011, 6(9): e24438.

[142] Hu Y, Litwin T, Nagaraja A R, et al. Cytosolic delivery of membrane-impermeable molecules in dendritic cells using pH-responsive core-shell nanoparticles[J]. Nano Lett, 2007, 7: 3056-3064.

[143] Tsoi K M, MacParland S A, Ma X, et al. Mechanism of hard-nanomaterial clearance by the liver[J]. Nat Mater, 2016, 15: 1212-1221.

[144] Jones D E, Ghandehari H, Facelli J C. A review of the applications of data mining and machine learning for the prediction of biomedical properties of nanoparticles[J]. Comput. Methods Programs Biomed, 2016, 132: 93-103.

[145] Sason H, Shamay Y. Nanoinformatics in drug delivery[J]. Isr J Chem, 2019, 60(12): 1108-1117.

[146] Charoo N A, Shamsher A A A, Zidan A S, et al. Quality by design approach for formulation development: A case study of dispersible tablets[J]. Int J Pharm, 2012, 423: 167-178.

[147] Adir O, Poley M, Chen G, et al. Integrating Artificial Intelligence and Nanotechnology for Precision Cancer Medicine[J]. Adv Mater, 2020, 32(13): 1901989.

[148] Savage N. Drug discovery companies are customizing ChatGPT: here's how[J]. Nat Biotechnol, 2023, 41: 585-586.
[149] Ross J, Belgodere B, Chenthamarakshan V, et al. Large-scale chemical language representations capture molecular structure and properties[J]. Nat Mach Intell, 2022, 4: 1256-1264.
[150] Zhang X C, Wu C K, Yang Z J, et al. MG-BERT: Leveraging unsupervised atomic representation learning for molecular property prediction[J]. Brief Bioinform, 2021, 22(6): bbab152.
[151] Zhang X C, Wu C K, Yi J C, et al. Pushing the boundaries of molecular property prediction for drug discovery with multitask learning bert enhanced by SMILES enumeration[J]. Res, 2022, 2022(5): : 0004.
[152] Wu Z, Jiang D, Wang J, et al. Knowledge-based BERT: a method to extract molecular features like computational chemists[J]. Brief Bioinform, 2022, 23(3): bbac131.
[153] Kang H, Goo S, Lee H, et al. Fine-tuning of BERT model to accurately predict drug-target interactions[J]. Pharmaceutics, 2022, 14(8): 1710.
[154] Monteiro N R C, Oliveira J L, Arrais J P. DTITR: End-to-end drug-target binding affinity prediction with transformers[J]. Comput Biol Med, 2022, 147: 105772.
[155] Morris P, St Clair, R, Hahn W E, et al. Predicting binding from screening assays with transformer network embeddings[J]. J Chem Inf Model, 2020, 60: 4191-4199.
[156] Lee H, Lee S, Lee I, et al. AMP-BERT: Prediction of antimicrobial peptide function based on a BERT model[J]. Protein Sci, 2023, 32(1): e4529.
[157] Yang L, Jin C, Yang G, et al. Transformer-based deep learning method for optimizing ADMET properties of lead compounds[J]. Phys Chem Chem Phys, 2023, 25: 2377-2385.
[158] Bagal V, Aggarwal R, Vinod P K, et al. MolGPT: Molecular generation using a transformer-decoder model[J]. J Chem Inf Model, 2022, 62(9): 2064-2076.
[159] Wang Y, Zhao H, Sciabola S, et al. cMolGPT: a conditional generative pre-trained transformer for target-specific de novo molecular generation[J]. Molecules, 2023, 28(11): 4430.
[160] Wang J, Hsieh, C Y, Wang M, et al. Multi-constraint molecular generation based on conditional transformer, knowledge distillation and reinforcement learning[J]. Nat Mach Intell, 2021, 3: 914-922.
[161] Moret M, Helmstädter M, Grisoni F, et al. Beam search for automated design and scoring of novel ROR ligands with machine intelligence[J]. Angew Chem Int Ed, 2021, 60: 19477-19482.
[162] Yang J, Tu J, Zhang X, et al. TSE DeepLab: An efficient visual transformer for medical image segmentation[J]. Biomed Signal Process Control, 2023, 80: 104376.
[163] Wang T, Nie Z, Wang R, et al. PneuNet: deep learning for COVID-19 pneumonia diagnosis on chest X-ray image analysis using Vision Transformer[J]. Med Biol Eng Comput, 2023, 61: 1395-1408.
[164] Rybinski M, Xu J, Karimi S. Clinical trial search: Using biomedical language understanding models for re-ranking[J]. J Biomed Informatics, 2020, 109: 103530 .
[165] Zaikis D, Vlahavas I. TP-DDI: Transformer-based pipeline for the extraction of drug-drug interactions[J]. Artif Intell Med, 2021, 119: 102153.
[166] Tamasi M J, Patel R A, Borca C H, et al. Machine Learning on a robotic platform for the design of polymer-protein hybrids[J]. Adv Mater, 2022, 34(30): 2201809.
[167] Bergenstal R M, Garg S, Weinzimer S A, et al. Safety of a hybrid closed-loop insulin delivery system in patients with type 1 diabetes[J]. JAMA, 2016, (13): 1407-1408.
[168] Ahmed Z, Mohamed K, Zeeshan S, et al. Artificial intelligence with multi-functional machine learning platform development for better healthcare and precision medicine[J]. Database(Oxford), 2020: baaa010.
[169] Somashekhar S P, Sepúlveda M J , Puglielli S, et al. Watson for oncology and breast cancer treatment recommendations: Agreement with an expert multidisciplinary tumor board[J]. Ann Oncol, 2018, 29: 418-423.
[170] Krittanawong C, Zhang H, Wang Z, et al. Artificial intelligence in precision cardiovascular medicine[J]. J Am Coll Cardiol, 2017, 69: 2657-2664.
[171] Esteva A, Kuprel B, Novoa R, et al. Dermatologist-level classification of skin cancer with deep neural networks[J]. Nature, 2017, 542, 115-118.
[172] Harrer S, Shah P, Antony B, et al. Artificial intelligence for clinical trial design[J]. Trends Pharmacol Sci, 2019, 40: 577-591.
[173] Pan S J, Yang Q. A survey on transfer learning[J]. IEEE Trans Knowl Data Eng, 2010, 22: 1345-1359.
[174] Ye Z, Yang Y, Li X, et al. An integrated transfer learning and multitask learning approach for pharmacokinetic parameter prediction[J]. Mol Pharm, 2019, 16: 533-541.

[175] Ganin Y, Lempitsky V. Unsupervised domain adaptation by backpropagation[C]. In: Proceedings of the 32 nd International Conference on Machine Learning, PMLR , 2015, 37: 1180-1189.

[176] Long M, Cao Y, Wang J, et al. Learning Transferable Features with Deep Adaptation Networks[C].In: Proceedings of the 32 nd International Conference on Machine Learning, PMLR, 2015, 37: 97-105 .

[177] Liu M Y, Tuzel O. Coupled Generative Adversarial Networks[C]. 30 th Conference on Neural Information Processing Systems, 2016: 469-477.

[178] Tzeng E, Hoffman J, Saenko K, et al. Adversarial Discriminative Domain Adaptation[C]. In: 2017 IEEE Conference on Computer Vision and Pattern Recognition(CVPR), Honolulu, HI, USA, 2017: 2962-2971.

[179] Goodfellow I J, et al. Generative adversarial nets[C]. In: NIPS'14: Proceedings of the 27 th International Conference on Neural Information Processing Systems, 2014, 2: 2672-2680.

[180] Radford A, Metz L, Chintala S. Unsupervised Representation Learning with Deep Convolutional Generative Adversarial Networks[C].International Conference on Learning Representations, 2016.

[181] Zhang H, Xu T, Li H, et al. StackGAN: Text to Photo-Realistic Image Synthesis with Stacked Generative Adversarial Networks. In: 2017 IEEE International Conference on Computer Vision, ICCV[C]. Institute of Electrical and Electronics Engineers Inc., 2017: 5908-5916.

[182] Gardner C R, Almarsson O, Chen H, et al. Application of high throughput technologies to drug substance and drug product development[J]. Comput Chem Eng, 2004, 28(6-7): 943-953.

[183] Morissette S L, Almarsson Ö, Peterson M L, et al. High-throughput crystallization: Polymorphs, salts, *co*-crystals and solvates of pharmaceutical solids[J]. Adv Drug Deliv Rev, 2004, 56(3): 275-300.

[184] Bevan C D, Lloyd R S. A high-throughput screening method for the determination of aqueous drug solubility using laser nephelometry in microtiter plates[J]. Anal Chem, 2000, 72: 1781-1787.

[185] Buchanan N L, Buchanan C M. High throughput screening method for determination of equilibrium drug solubility[J]. In: Polysaccharide Materials Performance by Design. ACS Symposium Series, 2009, 1017: 65-80.

[186] Wohnsland F, Faller B. High-throughput permeability pH profile and high-throughput alkane/water logP with artificial membranes[J]. J Med Chem, 2001, 44: 923-930.

[187] Gilpin L H, et al. (eds T. Eliassi-Rad et al.) 80-89(Institute of Electrical and Electronics Engineers Inc.).

[188] Ribeiro M T, Singh S, Guestrin C. "Why Should I Trust You？": Explaining the Predictions of Any Classifier[C]. In: Proceedings of the 2016 Conference of the North American Chapter of the Association for Computational Linguistics: Demonstrations. San Diego, California: Association for Computational Linguistics, 2016: 97-101.

[189] Lundberg S M, et al. Explainable machine-learning predictions for the prevention of hypoxaemia during surgery[J]. Nat Biomed Eng, 2018, 2: 749-760.

[190] Lundberg S M, Erion G, Chen H, et al. Explainable AI for Trees: From Local Explanations to Global Understanding[J]. arXiv e-prints, 2019, arXiv: 1905.04610.

[191] Lusci A, Pollastri G, Baldi P. Deep architectures and deep learning in chemoinformatics: The prediction of aqueous solubility for drug-like molecules[J]. J Chem Inf Model, 2013, 53: 1563-1575.

[192] Li X, Yan X, Gu Q, et al. DeepChemStable: Chemical stability prediction with an attention-based graph convolution network[J]. J Chem Inf Model, 2019, 59: 1044-1049.

[193] Elsken T, Hendrik Metzen J, Hutter F. Neural Architecture Search: A survey[J]. arXiv e-prints, 2018, arXiv: 1808.05377.

[194] Baker B, Gupta O, Naik N, et al. Designing neural network architectures using reinforcement learning[J]. arXiv e-prints, 2016, arXiv: 1611.02167.

[195] Zoph B, Le Q V. Neural architecture search with reinforcement learning[J]. arXiv e-prints, 2016, arXiv: 1611.01578.

[196] Real, E. *et al.* 4429-4446 (International Machine Learning Society(IMLS)).

[197] Real E, Aggarwal A, Huang Y, et al. Regularized evolution for image classifier architecture search[J]. arXiv e-prints, 2018, arXiv: 1802.01548.

[198] Liu H, Simonyan K, Yang Y. DARTS: Differentiable architecture search[J]. arXiv e-prints, 2018, arXiv: 1806.09055.

[199] Luo R, Tian F, Qin T, et al. Neural architecture optimization[J]. arXiv e-prints, 2018, arXiv: 1808.07233.

第3章

药剂学计算资源

董 界 中南大学,中国

3.1 计算药剂学的概念

近年来,随着包衣技术、微囊化技术、固体分散体技术、脂质体技术以及纳米技术等的蓬勃发展,新剂型的开发和质量的提升取得了显著进展。尽管新的药物制剂技术和方法不断涌现,大多数药物处方的设计和筛选在一定程度上仍然依赖于药剂学的基本理论和研究人员的经验。在没有充分预测药物与辅料之间相互作用关系的情况下,处方开发仍然是一个耗时、昂贵且不可预测的实验室试错过程。因此,迫切需要发展新的技术与之结合,提升处方开发的准确度和效率。

计算药剂学(computational pharmaceutics)是将计算机模拟技术与药剂学经典理论相结合,将量子力学(QM)、分子动力学(MD)模拟、过程模拟和药动学模拟等多尺度模拟相结合,通过构建和应用不同尺度的计算模型[1,2],研究药物体系中各组分在生产、储存甚至生理状态下的聚集、运动和扩散行为,并寻求规律,最终应用于药物处方设计、生产以及药物递送的学科。它和药剂学现有的分支相结合,有利于形成一种合理的、演绎的、以实验为基础的策略,具有很大的应用潜力。

到目前为止,计算药剂学在固体分散体、包合物、胶束药物递送系统、脂质体、纳米颗粒等方面已经取得了阶段性成果。例如,纳米颗粒药物递送系统凭借其药效好、副作用小等优势常用于给药,但载体的选择以及最佳药物负荷的确定相对繁琐,对此,Metwally和Hathout[3]提出了计算机辅助药物制剂设计(CADFD),用于组合多种信息学工具以及统计学方法来评估不同药物在其潜在载体上的负载。这种计算方法可用于设计新的药物载体系统,减少实验室试错实验的同时大大提高研发效率。另一个例子是Rio等[4],将三种聚合物按不同比例组合,获得了热敏性和黏膜黏附性水凝胶,并使用人工神经网络进行建模来预测水凝胶的性能。结果显示,人工智能工具对水凝胶的黏附能力和释放能力进行了充分表征,使用这类工具可以确定每种聚合物对处方性能的影响,能够促进具有免疫刺激特性的新型水凝胶的开发。Chaibva等[5]利用人工神经网络优化了硫酸沙丁胺醇处方,以改善其在药物制剂中的溶解度。通过优化隐藏层中的节点数来优化ANN模型,从而指导硫酸沙丁胺醇的处方设计,将ANN的预测溶出曲线与参考曲线进行对比,结果表明,预测制剂与制成制剂之间存在一致性,进一步说明了人工神经网络在优化具有理想性能特征的药物制剂方面的可能效用。

综上所述,将计算机模拟技术与药剂学相结合,预测药物与辅料可能形成的稳定的新结构及其物理化学性质,可以从分子水平上研究聚集体的稳定机制,从而完成药物制剂的处方设计、筛选、工艺优化和某些特定给药系统的理论研究。通过计算机模拟,既能提高工作效率、缩短试验周期,同时又能节省试验成本,是一项具有重要意义的工作。计算药剂学与传统药剂学的结合将促进制剂新技术的发展,为药剂学理论研究开辟新的方向。

3.2 计算药剂学数据库

3.2.1 数据库技术推动药物制剂领域快速发展

当今世界是一个被各类数据包围的互联网世界,数据可以说无处不在。数据的来源有很多,当用社交软件聊天、网上购物、打车出行、手机支付、打电话、发短信时,这些内容都将转化为数据进行存储。所谓数据(data),是指对事物或过程的原始测量值,是对事物的初步认识,除了文本类型的数据,图像、声音、视频、音乐等都是数据。数据借助人的思维或者信息技术处理后,揭示出事实中事物之间的关系,称为信息(information);经过实践不断处理和反复验证,事实中事物之间的关系被正确揭示出来,最终形成知识(knowledge)。从数据到信息到知识的过程,是一个数据不断变得有序,不断得到验证,并最终揭示实际存在的固有逻辑规律的过程。

数据在进入数据库之前需要经过数据挖掘和处理,使其形成可供存储的数据形式。当前大部分生物医药数据库均为结构化数据库。在数据库框架方面,常用的数据库管理软件包括Oracle、Microsoft SQL Server、IBM Db2、MySQL等。其中MySQL应用较为广泛,在大中型数据库中表现稳健。例如:专门针对药物的DrugBank数据库[6]中使用开源Ruby-on-Rails Web应用程序框架构建数据库系统,采用MySQL作为数据库引擎,该数据库及时更新和记载了最新的药物数据。在数据库输入输出方面,不同于普通信息数据库,大部分药物相关数据库的输入除了文本和数字等常规格式之外,还包括各类分子文件格式,例如序列和蛋白质的FASTA格式,小分子的SMILES、MOL和SDF格式。DrugBank和ChEMBL数据库不仅支持常规的关键字模糊查询,还可以直接输入分子各类信息和SMILES格式进行检索。输出方面,大部分数据库一般以图表和数字形式输出。但不同的数据库根据其目的也会输出网络图以及其他格式的文件。在功能层面,大部分数据库具备各种查询功能,也具备一些基本的比较和导出功能。值得注意的是,一些数据库也具备了先进的预测功能,实现根据已有信息推测新的规律和知识。

药物开发过程涉及大量的数据,并且在不同的研发阶段,产生的数据也不一样。在药物开发的前期,基因、蛋白质以及各类组学信息应用广泛。在靶标发现和验证阶段,各种生物分子,例如蛋白质和小分子之间的各类基础信息、相互作用信息,以及各类计算预测信息也需要数据库进行存储和共享。进入药效以及药理学研究阶段,各种药物信息,包括理化性质、生物活性、毒性、药代动力学性质等信息也非常丰富。这些研究阶段产生的各类数据信息汇成了各类重要数据库供研究者查询和挖掘。进而,这些数据库联合化学信息学和生物信息学技术为早期药物筛选和优化提供了重要的数据基础。这些数据库中极具代表性的包括:NCBI基因相关系列数据库,蛋白质信息代表性数据库Uniprot,蛋白质结构晶体数据库RCSB,蛋白质相互作用数据库STRING,信号通路数据库KEGG,小分子综合性数据库ZINK和ChEMBL,专门的在研和批准药物信息数据库DrugBank。单细胞测序(SNS)技术在靶标发现中变得越来越重要,特别是在精准医疗时代。在这方面,一些公共和私人数据库在学术研究和工业发展中被广泛使用,例如SCPortalen和scRNASeqDB。对读者来说,了解这些进展将是有帮助的。

值得注意的是，药物开发进入药物制剂阶段，往往是基础研究走向应用的重要阶段和转折阶段，这部分数据与前述的药物发现和设计阶段的数据存在较大区别。主要区别包括两点：第一，药物制剂阶段的数据的主体不仅仅是对于活性药物成分（active pharmaceutical ingredient，API），还包括各类辅料（填料、黏合剂、崩解剂、稳定剂等）的各种信息，以及制剂工艺中的各类信息。第二，药物制剂数据相对保守。在药物发现和设计阶段，许多高校和研究院所贡献了极其丰富的数据，但除了一些纳米制剂等新型剂型，常规制剂更贴近于实用性，这些制剂在高校和研究院所不再是研究热点。制剂数据更加贴近于工业界，这些数据往往是工业界的核心知识产权或者说是公司命脉。制药公司通常拥有自己的内部数据库，用于管理和分析其处方数据，具体来说，这些数据库包括活性药物成分、辅料、溶剂、稳定剂、沉淀剂等的处方比例和相关性质，涉及化学结构、分子权重、溶解度、密度、毒性、热稳定性等多个属性，这些属性可用来评估处方的药物相容性、稳定性和活性，相关人员可根据需求进行查询和筛选。例如，根据特定药物类别、特定疾病领域、剂型、药物相容性等条件进行搜索。数据库的规模大小不一，规模大的可包含成千上万个处方数据，规模小的可能只包含几百个甚至几十个数据。由于这些数据库不对外公开，因此可供获取的公共数据资源还是相对较少的。也正是由于这些原因，药物制剂数据库的发展显得尤为重要。尤其是在当前人工智能和科学计算快速发展的今天，药物制剂数据库将为智能化的剂型研发和工艺优化提供坚实的数据基础。

3.2.2 药剂学数据库资源

前文已提到药物制剂专门的数据库资源相比于药物发现和药物设计的专门数据库而言相对较少。但当前也有一些研究者已开发了相关的数据库用于药物制剂的信息查询与处方设计。这里本文将药剂学数据库资源整理总结在表3-1中。

表3-1 药剂学数据库资源总结

年份	名称	特色	数据量	参考文献
2006	Drugbank（V2.0）	提供丰富的药物结构、药物靶标以及药物代谢等信息，方便用户进行信息查询。也可用于分子对接，药物筛选以及靶标预测等方面	包含4900种药物的相关信息，每个条目包含100多个数据字段	[6]
2007	RNAJunction	提供有关RNA结构的详细信息，用户可根据序列、关键词等公开进行搜索，用于分析RNA结构以及设计纳米级的新型RNA结构	12000多个RNA连接以及吻环结构，每个结构提供详细注释	[12]
2009	OpenCDLig	创建OpenCDLig作为与环糊精复合物相关的实验数据来源。可下载3D复合物结构用于计算机辅助研究，检索与环糊精相关的文献，发布高质量数据等	含434个复合体和626个实验	[7]

续表

年份	名称	特色	数据量	参考文献
2010	Tablets database	创建一个用于标准处方和预测药物特性的片剂数据库	300个实验结果	[8]
2010	Cyclodextrin knowledgebase	建立一个包含已发表文献（论文、书籍、专利等）的专用环糊精复杂数据库。可以快速检查已发表的数据并对有关环糊精-配体复合物的现有文献进行结构搜索，结合易于使用的预测工具进行环糊精复合物的计算研究	数据库包含四个模块：发布模块（包含47235个条目）；交互模块（包含10847个条目）；手性模块（包含5123个条目）；分析模块（内置95种环糊精主体的结构）	[11]
2016	Cyclo-lib	提供了天然和修饰环糊精在水溶液中的原子级结构动力学信息，并提供工具用于在轨迹的特定时间间隔内对不同环糊精进行比较分析	提供对70多种修饰环糊精分子动力学模拟轨迹的深入分析	[9]
2018	Lhasa Database	提供一个大规模数据库，包含对药品中药用辅料元素测定的高质量数据，以支持根据相应指南对此类杂质的风险评估	包含了201种辅料的26723次元素测定结果	[14]
2019	vGNP database	使用新方法来开发虚拟金纳米颗粒（vGNP）库，通过表面模拟精确预测新纳米材料的纳米疏水性	41个GNP数据集	[10]
2021	SAPdb	以表格方式一目了然地提供关于肽自组装纳米结构的全面信息，集浏览、搜索和分析模块于一体，便于用户进行数据检索、数据比较和属性检查	包含301篇文献中的1049个条目	[13]

总的来说，纳入上表的药剂学数据库资源共有9个，从研发年份来看，主要开发于2006年至2010年以及2016年至2021年之间。2006年之前以及2011年至2015年之间未发现关于药剂学数据库的报道。这些数据库涵盖了纳米颗粒、片剂、环糊精、药用辅料等各个领域。其中，大多数数据库专注于环糊精和纳米颗粒。例如，OpenCDLig、Cyclodextrin knowledgebase、Cyclo-lib与环糊精相关，而RNAJunction、vGNP database、SAPdb则侧重于纳米制剂。这9个数据库均旨在收集和储存现有的实验数据，方便用户搜索和查询，但总数据规模相比药物设计领域数据库而言明显较少。其中，Cyclodextrin knowledgebase数据条目最多，涉及四个不同模块。

这里我们选择一些有代表性的数据库进行详细描述。

（1）与环糊精相关数据库

环糊精是具有环状结构的多糖分子，其特殊的分子构造使其能与一些小分子物质形成水溶性包合物。随着对环糊精研究的不断深入,研究人员积累了大量的实验数据,构建了两个Web应用程序来检索和分析与环糊精相关的数据。OpenCDLig[7]是与环糊精复合物相关的实验资源来源,该数据库包含626个实验和434个复合物。该数据库的数据检索功能相对有限,个体研究人员不太可能将旧的结果提交到该数据库中。为解决OpenCDLig数据库的不足,创建了Cyclodextrin knowledgebase[11]。Cyclodextrin knowledgebase包含四个模块:①发布模块,包含47235个条目,允许通过标题、摘要、作者和出版年份等关键字在数据库中进行文本搜索;②交互模块,包含10847个条目,提供结构搜索;③手性模块,包含5123个条目,提供与对映体分离有关的热力学数据;④分析模块,建立一个涵盖95个环糊精主分子结构概况的数据库,并使用分子对接工具预测小分子-环糊精复合物的几何形状,以探索包合物的结构和相互作用能。该数据库可以用作一个强大的集成系统,快速检查已发表的数据,进行现有文献中环糊精-配体复合物的结构搜索,并使用用户友好的预测工具进行环糊精复合物的计算研究。遗憾的是,这两个数据库目前均已无法访问。

(2) 与纳米颗粒相关数据库

2008年Eckart等[12]开发了RNAJunction数据库用于分析RNA结构并设计纳米级的新型RNA结构。2019年Wang等为促进新型纳米材料,特别是纳米药物的开发,构建了一个虚拟纳米颗粒库(VGNP database)[10],通过表面模拟精确预测新纳米材料的纳米疏水性。该数据库具有41个GNP数据集,这41个GNP具有较高的纳米结构多样性,形状、大小、密度、表面配体以及疏水性多样性,基于此数据库建立纳米疏水性模型用来指导纳米材料设计。2021年Mathur等[13]开发了SAPdb数据库来存储由肽自组装形成纳米颗粒的全面信息。SAPdb拥有1049个实验验证的纳米结构条目,其中,701个条目为二肽,328个条目为三肽,20个条目为单个氨基酸,每个条目都包含有关肽的全面信息,例如化学修饰,形成的纳米结构类型等。SAPdb在Linux系统上运行,使用Apache作为代理软件,后端由MySQL执行数据存储,前端使用HTML5、PHP和JavaScript开发,实现了在移动设备、平板电脑和桌面设备上的跨平台兼容性。SAPdb将促进小型自组装肽作为纳米载体或纳米材料的研究。

(3) 与药用辅料相关数据库

药用辅料在药物开发中发挥着举足轻重的作用,Lhasa Database数据库[14]的建立,旨在提供一个包含高质量数据的广泛资源库,涵盖了药用辅料的元素分析。这一资源有助于根据ICH Q3D指南评估药品中的杂质风险(图3-1)。该数据库包含了201种辅料的26723次元素测定结果,覆盖了处方中大部分常用的赋形剂。在数据库构建过程中,使用客户端-服务器结构,成员用户能够通过本地浏览器界面查询、显示和导出数据,终端用户不能以任何方式修改数据库的内容。KNIME分析平台用于分析该辅料元素数据库中的杂质数据。在缺乏其他信息来源的情况下,用该数据库中的数据来预测辅料成分的元素杂质浓度及其波动。

总之,这些药剂学相关数据库为药物研究人员提供了信息交流和共享的基础平台。随着研究领域的不断发展和深化,一些数据库开始附加各种实用且针对性强的工具和插件,帮助开发人员实现信息检索之外的高级功能,如性能计算和材料筛选。

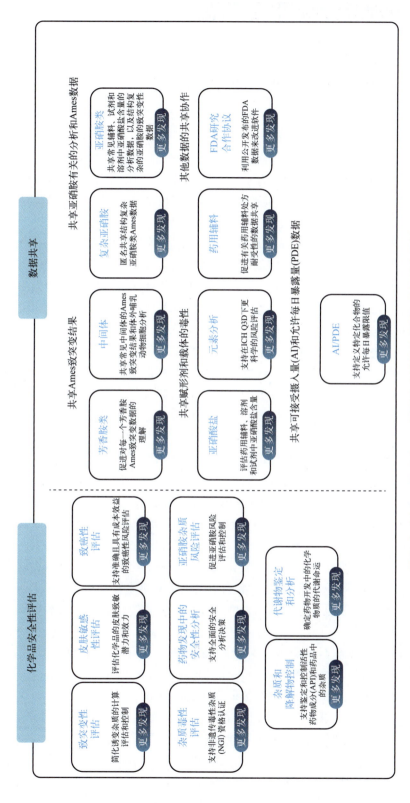

图3-1 Lhasa Database涵盖安全性评估范围和数据共享领域

3.3 药物制剂计算平台资源

3.3.1 人工智能推动药物剂型快速研发和评价

药物研发是一个长周期、高投入、高风险和多环节的过程。为了克服这些挑战和障碍，研究人员开始转向利用计算方法来提升药物开发效率并节省时间和金钱。从较早的定量构效关系（QSAR），到分子对接技术，再到从头计算和分子动力学模拟，这些计算手段极大加速了药物研发的技术迭代。近年来，人工智能技术快速发展，在建模预测和分子生成领域被证实是一种强大的工具。在药物制剂领域，人工智能也逐渐应用于药物理化性质预测、处方评价以及药物筛选等方面。

人工智能，亦称机器智能，指的是让机器来做需要人类智力才能完成的事情，比如学习、推理、思考、决策等，是数据驱动的计算机程序。人工智能包含三个核心要素：数据、算法和算力。仅有算法不足以支持人工智能，还必须依赖大数据和计算能力的支持。机器学习是人工智能的一个重要研究分支，是指赋予机器学习的能力，以让机器完成直接编程无法完成的任务。它可以基于大数据拟合高维非线性相关性，并发现输入的微小方差对目标标签差异的影响。机器学习可分为有监督学习和无监督学习。有监督学习适用于输入数据包含有标签的情况，标签用于训练机器学习模型，最终给出特定模式；无监督学习适用于输入数据的标签未知的情况，从输入数据的特征中学习相应的模式；半监督学习适用于标签不完整的情况，利用标记数据推断未标记数据的标签，或利用未标记数据获得关于训练数据集结构的信息。

机器学习建立在统计分析的基础之上，因此，早期的机器学习算法主要是基于概率论或者统计分析方法，如决策树（decision tree，DT）、线性回归（linear regression）、逻辑回归（logistic regression）、偏最小二乘法（partial least squares，PLS）等；随着计算机技术和应用数学的不断发展，新的算法包括支持向量机（support vector machine，SVM）、随机森林（random forest，RF）、梯度提升算法（XGBoost，LightGBM）等应运而生，这些经典的机器学习算法各有不同的特点和优势。有些算法具备较好的可解释性，有些算法是所谓的"黑盒"；有些算法对参数调整要求较少，而有的需要复杂的参数调整才能实现更高的准确率。但这些算法在处理表格型数据方面具备天然的优势，并且在相对较小的数据集上通常优于一些深度学习方法。

当前发展最快的算法是基于人工神经网络的深度学习（deep learning），已发展出多种深度学习类型，如卷积神经网络（convolutional neural network，CNN）、循环神经网络（recursive neural network，RNN）、自动编码器（autoencoder）等。

人工智能、机器学习以及深度学习三者之间各有侧重，一般根据应用场景进行准确表达。这里为了方便，我们统一归为人工智能算法。这些算法目前已应用于药物设计和开发过程的各个领域中，从简单的理化性质预测，到靶标预测和虚拟筛选，再到分子模拟和分子生成，以及药代动力学性质研究和药物重定向等药物设计和开发过程。这些算法的应用形式主要包括相关/相似性判定、模型预测以及新化学实体生成。

3.3.2 计算药剂学中的人工智能模型

预测模型是人工智能算法应用的一种主要形式。预测模型的构建也可以看成一个广义的先归纳、后演绎的过程，即收集现有的样本，提取这些样本的共同特征作为输入，利用算法训练并得到最优模型，再用该模型去预测新样本的终点。对于药物制剂领域，预测模型的应用可以减少试错实验的进行，在较短时间内寻找最优处方，缩短处方研发周期；可以快速预测药物的溶出度，评估药物的稳定性以及各种相关性能，显著节约时间和成本并提高效率。

3.3.2.1 人工智能预测模型构建的一般原理和步骤

（1）数据集构建

数据的准确性是模型成功构建的关键，因此，在数据来源、数据收集、数据处理各个环节都要确保其准确可靠。数据通常有多个来源，包括已出版的书籍、已发表的期刊、专利、已开发的数据库以及在线工具和在线网站，如 DrugBank、PubMed、Web of Science 等。数据来源确定后，根据研究目标制定关键词，并在公共数据库中进行文献检索，筛选和收集符合要求的数据。随后，进行数据处理。需要对不同来源的数据进行对比，通常会出现数据收集重复的情况，这些冗余数据应被去除，以保证数据的唯一性。同时，对缺失信息的数据进行补充，剔除异常值。经过预处理后的数据按照一定比例划分为三个数据集：训练集（training set）、测试集（test set）和验证集（validation set）。其中，训练集用于训练模型，验证集用于调整超参数以优化模型性能，测试集用于评估模型对未知数据的预测能力。

（2）数据描述/分子描述符计算

当前，在药剂学中，化学信息学主要用于识别和表征药物及辅料分子，并计算分子特征。在数据处理过程中，计算机如何快速有效地识别和存储不同的药物分子呢？这依赖于一些常用的分子文件格式。化学小分子常采用 MOL、SDF 和 SMILES 格式进行储存，大分子通常采用 PDB 格式。MOL 文件包含纯文本信息，存储了构成分子的原子和化学键的相关信息。它可以存储二维（2D）结构和三维（3D）结构，是当前应用最广泛的小分子结构存储文件格式。SDF 文件可以看作是多个 MOL 文件的集合，区别在于 SDF 文件能够同时存储多个分子。SMILES 文件在不涉及 3D 结构的情况下是最方便且节约空间的选择，即利用线性的字符或数字组合来表示化合物的结构，化合物的立体化学信息，如顺反异构和旋光异构也可以被表示。一个 SMILES 只能表示一个分子，但一个分子可以有多个 SMILES，但也可以用标准化 SMILES 进行统一。

分子结构识别并存储到计算机后，需要转换为数学描述来进一步处理信息，以获得分子的特征（feature）。常见的数学描述包括分子描述符（molecular descriptor）和分子指纹（molecular fingerprint）。分子描述符（molecular descriptor）是一组表示化学物质结构特征或化学性质的描述符。它们将编码在分子符号表示中的化学信息转换为数字或标准化的实验结果。分子描述符可分为定量描述符和定性描述符，而分子指纹是一种定性描述符，通过特定的编码方法表示分子的结构、性质、分子片段或子结构信息。分子描述符可以根据计算的复杂度进行分类，包括零维（0D）、一维（1D）、二维（2D）和三维（3D）描述符。0D描述符包括分子量、原子数和原子类型、摩尔折射率等；1D描述符涉及氢键受体和供体数、极性表面积（PSA）、片段数等特征；2D描述符解释了原子的结构特征和连接方式（如邻接和连接）；3D描述符包括分子几何形状和分子体积等。目前已开发出许多商业和开源软件用于分子描述符计算，如Dragon、MODEL、MOE、ChemDes、CDK、RDKit、OpenBabel、PyBioMed等。

在解决药剂学问题时，通常不仅需要考虑活性药物成分（API）的分子特征，还需要考虑辅料的分子特征。不同的研究人员有不同的处理方式。其中一种方法是直接基于辅料单体的化学结构计算小分子描述符。对于聚合物，则增加与聚合度和相关性质有关的特定描述符。最后将药物和辅料的描述符按照不同的需求进行组合[15,16]。

（3）数据预处理和特征选择

数据预处理主要指处理输入特征矩阵的缺失值，并剔除高相关性和低方差描述符的过程。特征选择是从初始的描述符集合中选择最有效特征的过程，以减少特征数量并提高学习算法的性能。特征选择是一个搜索寻优的过程，从原始特征中搜索特征子集提交给评价函数进行评价，当评价函数值达到停止准则的阈值后即可停止搜索，再在验证集上验证选出来的特征子集的有效性。特征选择一方面可以减少特征数量和维度，提高模型的泛化能力，减少过拟合；另一方面可以增强对特征和特征值之间的理解。欠拟合和过拟合是评价模型泛化能力的两个指标，对于模型而言，我们的目标是使其在训练集和测试集上都具有较强的拟合能力。欠拟合意味着模型在训练集和测试集上的预测性能都较差。过拟合则表明模型预测训练集时表现较好，但在测试集上的预测性能较差。

特征选择方法包括三种：过滤法、包装法和嵌入法。

① 过滤法：根据特征的发散性或相关性指数对每个特征进行评分。设定评分阈值或期望特征数量，选择符合标准的特征。主要方法有相关系数法、方差选择法、卡方检验、信息增益等。

② 包装法：生成各种特征子集进行评分，然后比较这些子集。这一过程涉及在每次迭代中基于目标函数（通常是预测性能评分）选择或排除某些特征。常用方法为递归特征消除（RFE）法。

③ 嵌入法：在预定义的模型结构内选择最佳特征以提高模型准确性。在这种方法中，机器学习模型被训练，得到每个特征的权重系数，根据权重系数（通常按降序排列）选择特征。嵌入法类似于过滤法，但它是通过机器学习算法和模型评估特征的相关性，而不是直接依据统计学指标进行判断。

（4）模型构建

模型主要分为两类：定性分类模型和定量回归模型。定性分类模型根据样本数据中的分类标准和特定类别，预测后续给出的对象属于哪一类；定量回归模型则以定量方式描述统计关系。在实际问题中，首先需确定要构建的模型的数量和实际意义，然后选择合适的算法训练模型，最后，比较和分析不同算法的结果以获得最优模型。

（5）模型评价

模型评价方法包括内部验证和外部验证。内部验证使用与训练数据同源的数据评价模型，而外部验证使用在模型开发过程中未使用的数据来评估模型在新数据上的表现。用于外部验证的数据应与用于构建模型的数据在数据空间上相似。

内部验证主要包括两种：留出法和交叉验证法。在留出法中，数据集被划分为两个互斥的集合，即训练集和测试集。大约2/3到4/5的数据被划分到训练集，剩下的1/3到1/5的数据被划分到测试集。在使用算法的预设参数在训练集上训练模型后，使用测试集来评估模型的预测性能，根据测试结果调整算法参数，并重复建模和验证模型，直到获得最优模型。然而，留出法存在易过拟合且不便矫正的问题。交叉验证法与留出法相比更具优势。交叉验证法可分为K折交叉验证法（K-CV）和留一法交叉验证（LOO-CV）。K折交叉验证（K-CV）将包含N个样本的数据集随机划分成K个互斥的子集，每个子集包含N/K个样本。选取其中一个子集作为测试集，剩下K-1个子集作为训练集。在训练集上训练模型后，在测试集上进行评估以计算模型的泛化误差。交叉验证重复K次，K次结果的平均值作为模型的最终泛化误差。K的取值可以为5、10、15等，其中，10折交叉验证最为常用。K折交叉验证适用于样本量较大的情况，当样本量较小时，采用留一法。通常，外部验证在模型验证中起主导作用，预测模型在实际应用前必须经过外部验证，只有对外部验证表现较好时才能说明模型的泛化能力好。

定性分类模型和定量回归模型的评价指标有所不同。灵敏度（SE）、特异性（SP）、准确率（ACC）、马修斯相关系数（MCC）、AUC（ROC曲线下面积）是用于评估定性分类模型性能的几个指标。其中，SE、SP、ACC和MCC是基于模型测试结果的四个统计值得到的，分别为真阳性（TP）、假阴性（FN）、真阴性（TN）和假阳性（FP）。采用二分类方法将样本分为阳性样本和阴性样本，当阳性样本被正确预测为阳性时为真阳性（TP），阳性样本被错误预测为阴性时为假阴性（FN）；当阴性样本被正确预测为阴性时为真阴性（TN），阴性样本被错误预测为阳性时为假阳性（FP），它们的计算公式如下：

$$SE = \frac{TP}{TP+FN}$$

$$SP = \frac{TN}{TN+FP}$$

$$ACC = \frac{TP+TN}{TP+TN+FP+FN}$$

$$MCC = \frac{TP \times TN - FN \times FP}{\sqrt{(TP+FN)(TP+FP)(TN+FN)(TN+FP)}}$$

灵敏度（SE）衡量模型在预测阳性样本集时的准确性，特异性（SP）评估模型在预测阴性样本集时的精度，准确率（ACC）反映模型对所有样本集的预测准确性，马修斯相关系数（MCC）则评估模型的综合预测能力。AUC以FP作为横轴，TP作为纵轴，表示ROC曲线下的面积，取值范围为0.5到1之间。

决定系数（R^2）和均方根误差（RMSE）是用于评估定量回归模型性能的指标。决定系数是用来衡量回归模型拟合度和解释性的统计指标，均方根误差是预测值与真实值之间偏差的平方与样本数量（n）比值的平方根，它们的计算公式如下：

$$R^2 = 1 - \frac{\sum(y_i - \widehat{y_i})^2}{\sum(y_i - \bar{y})^2}$$

$$\text{RMSE} = \sqrt{\frac{\sum_{i=1}^{n}(y_i - \widehat{y_i})^2}{n}}$$

式中，y_i、$\widehat{y_i}$、$\bar{y}$ 分别表示样本的实验值、模型预测值和实验值的平均值；n 表示数据集中的样本数目。

3.3.2.2 计算药剂学中的预测模型

预测模型在药物处方设计和优化、剂型开发、理化性质预测、溶出和释放、药物和辅料相互作用等方面都有重要应用。例如，在处方设计和优化方面，Yang 等[17]基于处方数据建立了六种传统机器学习模型和一种深度学习模型，用于口服快速崩解膜（OFDF）和缓释基质片（SRMT）的处方预测。深度学习相比于传统机器学习算法展现出更优的预测准确性，可用于在小数据集上预测药物处方，从而缩短药物开发时间并节省资源。Gao 等[18]使用 LightGBM 模型预测穿心莲内酯（AG）与环糊精（CD）的结合自由能，开发了一种新型 AG-CD-TPGS 三元处方，显著改善其水溶性、溶出速率以及口服生物利用度。

在制剂开发方面，Ahuva 等[19]基于K-最近邻（KNN）、迭代随机消除（ISE）和支持向量机（SVM）构建了两种类型的QSPR模型。这些模型旨在识别潜在的新型候选分子用于脂质体药物递送。QSPR模型可以作为一种可靠和有用的工具，用于加速新型药物递送系统的开发。纳米晶体由于其尺寸可达纳米级在提高水不溶性药物的溶出速率方面表现出很大的优势，He 等[20]利用八种机器学习算法建立纳米晶体粒径和PDI的预测模型，用于简化和加速纳米晶体开发。

在药物理化性质预测方面，Han 等[21]从数据库中收集了646个固体分散体（SD）稳定性数据，并使用八种机器学习算法构建预测模型。随机森林（RF）对SD物理稳定性的预测准确率达到82%，并揭示了每个处方特征的重要性，这对SD处方设计有显著的帮助。此外，Youshia 等[22]基于人工神经网络（ANN）构建预测模型，以聚合物的分子量、疏水性等作为输入，粒径的多分散指数作为输出，成功预测了由各种聚合物制备的粒径在70~400 nm范围的纳米颗粒。

在药物溶出和释放方面，Takayama 等[23]测量了112种片剂的溶出度，并将其整合到一个包含活性药物成分理化性质和粉末特性以及片剂基本物理属性的数据库中，应用四层人工神经网络（4LNN）根据活性药物成分（API）的物理化学性质和粉末特性预测溶解速率，有助于确定具有良好溶出曲线的可靠处方，并改善其基本特性，如拉伸强度和崩解时间等。同样，2019 年 Galata 等[24]使用从近红外和拉曼光谱中收集的数据以及测量的压缩力作为 ANN 模型的输入，来预测缓释片剂的体外溶出曲线。2021 年，Tosca 等[25]建立了基于人工神经网络（ANN）的QSPR模型来预测类药分子的固有溶解度。

综上所述，基于人工智能算法的一系列预测模型在药剂学中取得了显著进展，这不仅可以优化药物处方设计、加速新型制剂开发，还能改善药物溶出速率、增强物理稳定性以及提高生物利用度。预测模型的建立和应用为药剂学的发展指明了新的方向。

3.3.3　计算平台/网络服务器

前文介绍了一系列药剂学中的计算预测模型。较为遗憾的是，大部分的模型仅仅发表了论文，仅有少量的模型进行了应用转化。计算平台/网络服务器是这种转化的重要体现形式。现有的药剂学计算平台总结见表3-2。

表3-2　药剂学中的计算平台/网络服务器

年份	计算平台	特色	参考文献
2013	ME_expert 2.0	提供了一个工具来协助微乳剂（ME）的处方开发并减少实验室试验的负担。该工具利用人工神经网络和随机森林算法对微乳剂的形成进行建模，从而指导微乳剂的开发	[30]
2014	MemBuilder	为了自动化和简化各种脂质双层膜的构建，并根据联合力场和全原子力场为内含脂质提供分子拓扑结构，推出了基于Web的图形用户界面工具MemBuilder。MemBuilder兼容18种脂质分子，支持4种力场	[35]
2017	Micelle Maker	Micelle Maker为一种在线工具，旨在利用多种脂质（目前支持25种脂质类型）创建胶束，并在经过最小化和平衡处理后，将其直接输入后续的分子动力学模拟中	[27]
2020	M3DISEEN	旨在使用人工智能机器学习技术加快熔融沉积建模（fused deposition modeling，FDM）处方开发过程。共设计了614种载药处方，采用了145种不同的药物辅料。利用人工智能模型能够高精度地预测关键的制造参数，在较小的误差范围内准确预测高熔融挤出和FDM温度	[31]
2021	PharmSD	收集了目前最全面的数据集，并开发了一个新的固体分散体（SD）处方预测平台。该平台可独立预测SD的物理稳定性、溶出类型和溶出速率，并整合预测结果形成一个虚拟筛选管道，用于SD制剂的虚拟设计。此外，提供两种工具使研究人员能评估模型的应用域并计算溶出曲线的相似性	[15]
2021	Polymer Builder	提供了一个通用且自动化的构建程序，以帮助用户使用Web浏览器轻松、交互地构建复杂的聚合物系统。为分子动力学程序提供验证良好的全原子模拟输入，允许用户使用熟悉的包执行分子动力学模拟	[28]
2023	FormulationAI	开发了首个基于人工智能的虚拟处方评价系统，涵盖药物-环糊精、固体分散体、纳米晶体、自乳化、脂质体给药和磷脂复合物六大系统。构建了先进的预测平台，可根据基本信息预测和分析稳定性、结合能等17种处方评估参数	[29]

从表3-2中可以看出，药剂学领域已经开发了一些计算平台，其中大多数是在最近几年发布的。还可以看出，人工智能技术与药剂学的结合受到越来越多的关注，人工智能技术已被用来解决剂型开发、处方优化等一系列问题。在研究内容方面，这些平台涵盖了相对广泛的领域，涉及乳剂、脂质、固体分散体、聚合物等各个领域。这些平台不仅能简化步骤，提高处方设计的效率，还能集中资源，统一标准，拓宽应用场景。例如，PharmSD平台不仅通过比较不同的机器学习算法和描述符成功建立了稳健的SD模型，还提供了一个用户友好的免费服务器，使得对给定分子与多达26种不同聚合物的行为进行快速、简便的预测成为可能。尽管这些服务器的应用刚刚起步，但可以预见的是，计算平台的使用能大大加快药物研发速度。

以下是一些具有代表性的计算平台的详细介绍。

(1) ME_expert 2.0[30]

它是针对微乳剂（ME）开发的一种决策支持系统（DSS）。严格来说，它不是一个计算平台/网络服务器，而是一个工具。微乳剂是一种易于制备、毒性和刺激小且应用范围广的剂型，与固体分散体（SD）处方设计一样，微乳剂的开发也依赖于实验室试错或配方者的经验来进行，因此，迫切需要将药物研究的范式从依赖经验的研究转变为数据驱动的方法。2013年Mendyk等[30]用人工神经网络（ANN）和随机森林（RF）分类器对微乳剂（ME）的形成进行建模，开发了微乳剂处方开发的决策支持系统。该支持系统的构建包含以下几个过程：首先，收集并处理了一个包含300多万条记录的大型数据库；其次，采用ANN模型搜索最小输入向量大小，之后使用RF和ANN模型构建DSS推理引擎。结果表明，ANN和RF都适合作为ME处方开发的DSS推理引擎。其中，ANN被用作预测和数据挖掘工具，而RF仅被用于预测ME的相位边界。最后，再将模型实现到软件中。

(2) PharmSD[15]

PharmSD[15]是一个专门为固体分散体设计的配方预测平台。该平台于2021年7月首次发布，旨在通过应用机器学习模型预测SD关键性质来提高水不溶性药物的溶解度和口服生物利用度。由于许多辅料和药物描述符依赖于从不同资源手动收集的数据，研究人员面临着如何利用已发布模型的挑战，因此急需提供一个用户友好的服务来实施稳健的模型预测服务。该平台的构建流程如下：首先，通过系统的数据收集得到最全面的数据集，包括SD物理稳定性数据、溶解类型和溶解速率；然后，使用MOE和PybioMed等工具计算多种分子描述符；最后，利用RF、SVM和LightGBM算法建立溶解速率回归模型。使用RF、SVM、XGBoost和LightGBM算法建立物理稳定性和溶解类型的分类模型。为了获得最佳模型，采取了几种有效的策略，这些模型和相关数据随后被集成到平台中，创建了一个用户友好的界面。用户只需提交药物结构，平台即可快速预测与26种聚合物的药物行为，从而大大扩展了优选解决方案的范围，并为SD处方设计提供了多种可能性（图3-2）。

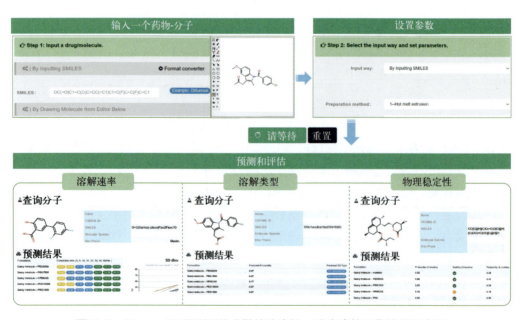

图3-2　PharmSD预测固体分散体稳定性、溶出度的工作流程示意图

（3）FormulationAI[29]

它是目前首个综合性的基于人工智能的药物处方设计平台。该平台由与PharmSD平台[11]相同的研究团队构建。研究人员通过数据挖掘，从公开出版物和数据库中收集了近10年的大量的药物剂型的处方数据。通过规范数据来源、去除重复以及标准化结构和数据等一系列操作，得到全面的数据集。构建了截至本文撰写时间点、最全面的6大药物制剂增溶处方体系数据集。此外，在构建人工智能预测模型之前，研究人员还统一了不同辅料的类型结构和规格标准，构建了全新的针对药物-辅料关系对描述符。然后，通过系统性研究比较不同AI算法和分子表征算法，实现了药物-环糊精、固体分散体、磷脂复合物、纳米晶体、自乳化、脂质体递送6大体系17种重要性质的智能预测与评估。最后，采用先进的平台开发技术，构建了一套功能强大的预测平台，使用者只需要提供药物和辅料的基本信息就可以预测和分析上述重要的处方评价参数（图3-3）。

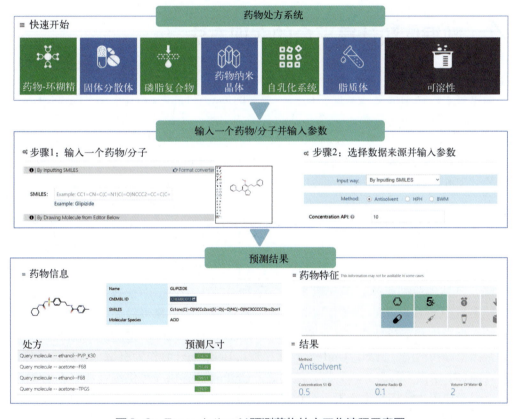

图3-3　FormulationAI预测药物处方工作流程示意图

（4）M3DISEEN[31]

它是利用内部3D打印实验和从已发表文献中提取的数据来增强各种机器学习技术的性能，以预测熔融沉积建模（FDM）、3D打印（3DP）加工温度、可打印性和灯丝机械特性。3D打印又称增材制造，最早是在1980年由Chuck Hull发明了第一种3D打印技术形式——立体光刻[32]。3D打印技术凭借其灵活性、定制性、个性化等特点在药剂学各个领域均有应用，包括剂型优化、处方开发、药物递送等。3D打印技术可以通过调整打印材料、设备工艺等参数，对药物剂量实现精准控制，实现药物的缓释、速释以及靶向释放。此外，3D打印技术可以将多种药物同时载入剂型中，实现多药物的组合制备，为复杂疾病的治疗提供方便性和精确性，加速药物制剂研发进程，减少实验室试错实验的进行。M3DISEEN是在这个基础上开发的，通过挤出和印刷从145种不同的材料中制备载药制剂，并从制备的载药制剂数据集中选取614个符合挤出和打印条件的处方，建立人工智能模型预测关键参数，包括挤出温度、机械特性、印刷温度和印刷适性等，实现了良好的预测性能，可用于指导药物处方开发，简化并推动3D打印技术成为药物开发中的一项重要技术。

计算平台/网络服务器基于现有数据建立预测模型，并在高性能计算中心或云平台部署这些模型。巧妙之处在于，来自世界各地的用户可以通过简单的鼠标点击获取计算结果。这避免了实验室中的盲目试错，通过人工智能将药物开发从基于知识的理论设计转变为基于数据的方法，从而节省资源并提高效率。

3.4 数据库和计算平台的实现方法

数据库对于药物制剂研究来说，提供了重要的信息存储和交流媒介。但总的来说，这类资源还是比较稀缺，尤其是相比于当前蓬勃发展的生物医药数据库和化学数据库。这里面的原因，除了我们提到的工业界数据保守之外，药物制剂在应用场景方面的限制是另一个原因。此外，还有一个不容忽视的原因，那就是数据库的构建和使用对于药物学家来说是有专业门槛的。因此，我们来谈一谈，前述数据库的主要实现方式。

对于一般的数据库，其在搭建过程中，选用的软件层和应用层主要与数据库的数据量、数据库用途以及维护计划密切相关。数据库引擎主要分为关系型数据库和非关系型数据库。前者代表性产品包括MySQL、Oracle、SQLServer以及PostgreSQL等，后者代表性产品包括MongoDB、Redis和CouchDB等。前文我们总结了计算药剂学相关的数据库，大部分数据库无从知晓其具体的驱动引擎。但一般来说，生物医药大型数据库往往比较复杂，涉及多个主体甚至是数组资源之间的交叉存取和查询，所以数据库引擎可以是多种。这类数据库除了常规的数据查询和下载功能，往往提供了多种数据库下载方式，以便研究者使用不同的方式进行数据挖掘和清洗。例如，UniProt数据库使用Berkeley DB作为引擎，并提供了包括多种数据格式的FTP站点下载服务。更为方便的是，UniProt还提供了可供编程和整合的REST API服务。这对于使用本地环境进行数据分析的研究者以及在开发新的软件产品中整合UniProt的服务是非常友好的[33]。类似的数据库还包括DrugBank[6]和PDB数据库[26]。对于一般中小型数据库一般会采用结构化的数据库软件，例如Cyclodextrin knowledgebase[11]、OpenCDLig[7]、RNAJunction[12]，便使用了MySQL作为数据库引擎。

对于计算平台/网络服务器，其实现过程通常包括：服务器的选取、域名解析、服务端计算程序的编写、数据存储、用户界面和可视化等。对于服务器的选取，早期许多计算平台选择研究机构的本地主机，但这种服务往往受到网络环境以及机构变迁等因素影响，因此不太稳定。后期，多数服务器都搭建在专门的服务器管理机构。这种方式大大提升了计算平台的稳定性。在域名方面，当前的服务器，绝大多数的网址并没有进行事先规划，缺乏可读性和实际含义，并往往在网址中附带各类不必要的技术信息以及逻辑符号，这大大影响了服务器访问的方便性。这一现象，不仅限于药剂学领域，其他研究领域的计算平台也是如此。服务端计算程序的编写是核心，决定了计算平台的功能和效率。目前大部分计算平台的这部分内容是无法直接获取的。核心计算程序的编写最主要考虑数据的动态获取以及变量存储，这对计算负载和计算速度很重要。此外，还需要考虑前后端交互的数据类型和功能区分。在数据存储方面，当前大部分计算服务器不会像数据库有那样高的数据存储需求，因此可以采用轻量化的SQLite或者稍微复杂的MySQL。前者在高并发的情况下往往不能胜任。在用户界面和可视化方面，前后端分离是非常重要的，选择MVC构架的形式（例如Django）是较好的选择，这有利于后期的维护以及将来的业务拓展。在前文总结的计算药剂学平台中，计算平台数量相对较少，这些规律体现并不是很明显。

在编程语言方面，早期的数据库有些是基于Perl语言以及Ruby语言，例如OpenCDLig[7]使用了Ruby语言。在PHP语言流行的相当长一段时间，PHP语言也是网站制作的主要选择之一，例如Cyclodextrin knowledgebase[11]和RNAJunction[12]是采用PHP语言实现的。近些年，Python语言也变得流行，PharmDE[34]就是采用Python语言构建的。而对于大型数据库，例如UniProt数据库[33]，基于Java的构架往往在处理复杂业务逻辑和高负载的情况下显得更有优势。对于计算平台/网络服务器来说，编程语言的选择与数据库类似。主要的区别在于计算平台/网络服务器通常需要在服务器端调用计算程序。因此，网站前端与服务器端往往会采用不同的编程语言，例如MemBuilder Ⅱ[35]在后端处理完数据后，在前端通过PHP语言编写用户界面。当然，由于人工智能的预测模型通常是在Python环境下构建的，因此在前端基于Python编写的网络服务器也越来越多。例如，PharmSD[15]和FormulationAI[35]均是采用这种形式。

此外，数据库和计算平台在设计的过程中需要选择适合其业务逻辑的网站构架。为了方便大家理解。图3-4简单描述了传统网站构架和现代化网站构架的区别。图3-4（A）显示的是传统的网站构架示意图，其主要特点是用户端和服务端的通信请求是相对独立和低效的，同时传输数据的形式是多种多样的，并且由于数据任务和可视化业务是串行的，所以容易发生阻塞。图3-4（B）显示的是改进后的构架，这种构架主要是在数据通信方面进行了优化，通常引入异步获取技术和消息中间件（例如AJAX和Redis），使得前端可以在无刷新情况下实时更新数据状态，并且可以利用消息队列提升任务分配的效率，避免阻塞。图3-4（C）显示的是当前比较流行的构架，其主要是在后端进行了优化，将后端划分为模型-控制-视图（MVC），从而剥离了业务逻辑、数据模型以及可视化，使得网站实现不同程度的模块化，更加有利于维护和扩展。此外，在数据存储部分，丰富了数据库的选择和管理模式，这对于大中型计算平台是尤其重要的。

在将来的发展过程中，需要解决数据库和计算平台稳定访问和稳定支持的问题。因为许多服务器在论文出版后不久就无法访问，这可能是网址缺乏规划也可能是没有及时维护，这大大降低了数据库和计算平台的实用价值。当然，我们也需要看到几个趋势：首先，多种新的技术，包括HTML5、VUE等前端技术以及Python语言社区的不断增强，轻量化、美观化的数据库和计算平台会成为趋势，一体化和高效率的数据库或计算资源会不断涌现。其次，未来的数据资源和计算资源无疑都是朝着可移植的方向发展，各类规范化的数据接口（API）将是这类资源标配。

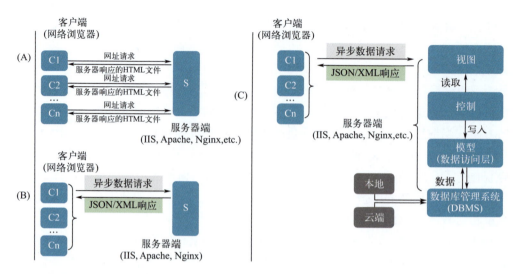

图3-4 不断发展的网站构架简略示意图。从（A）到（C），网站构架在速度、效率、扩展性以及用户友好等方面得到不断提升

3.5 总结

综上所述，人工智能和药剂学的跨学科结合使得计算药剂学取得了快速的发展，药物研发从传统上依赖于实验室试错和药学专家经验逐步转向于通过人工智能和机器学习方法处理药物研发中的复杂问题。计算药剂学目前已渗透到药物研发的各个领域，如通过机器学习和深度学习建模来优化片剂、胶囊剂、乳剂、微囊等各种剂型的药物处方设计；采用基于生理的药代动力学建模来预测药物在体内的吸收、分布、代谢和排泄；根据定量结构-性质关系预测药物复合物的结合常数等。此外，人工智能方法还能在海量的数据中进行数据挖掘，构建知识数据库储存药物研发中的各项数据，方便用户查询和使用；构建各种计算平台和在线工具预测药物的溶出度、质量稳定性，指导难溶性药物开发、评估药物-辅料不相容性等；未来，需要进一步开发更具体、更全面的计算资源。前者可以解决更具体的问题，而后者可以加速行业内的数据共享和知识连接。

计算药剂学在取得巨大发展的同时也面临着许多挑战。第一，在数据层面，开发数据库或构建模型需要大量数据支持。目前，制药行业的数据相对缺乏，数据收集主要依赖于手动从相关文献、专利和数据库中挖掘，费时费力，数据质量也无法得到保证。因此，亟需建立一个既能提供数量又能确保质量的数据社区，或者在数据存储和识别方面达成共识，以应对这一挑战。此外，药物在体内的复杂作用导致数据多样且复杂，如何提取和转换这些数据以构建适合人工智能算法的数据表示也是一个难题。第二，在计算方法层面，大多数药物开发使用单一的机器学习方法进行预测建模，如何将多种机器学习方法和PBPK模型、MD模拟等集成使用仍是需要思考的问题。第三，在人才培养上，药剂学和计算机在此之前是两个独立的学科，利用计算机和药剂学来解决药物问题需要精通计算机科学和药学的专业人才。因此，人工智能方法在药学中的应用需要不断探索，仍然面临许多挑战。第四，计算模型的精度需要进一步提高，预测的准确性仍然存在不足。

在计算药剂学的未来发展过程中，需要坚持理论与创新。首先，应简化数据收集流程，统一复杂的数据标准，强化数据存储的安全性，并加强数据共享建设。其次，应培养创新型人才，在药学学科内开设计算机课程，将药学与计算机科学相结合，这对人工智能在药学中的发展大有裨益。最后是增强计算能力，提高模型预测精度，考虑集成多种机器学习方法并应用多尺度建模。此外，随着ChatGPT等通用大型语言模型（LLM）的快速发展，如何接受并充分利用大型人工智能模型的能力也将带来新的机遇和增长。当然，回归本源，药剂学本身也需要改革创新，开发新型制剂。相信在不久的将来，人工智能将为制剂在内的药物研发各个环节带来革命性的进步。

参考文献

[1] Wang W, Ye Z, Gao H, Ouyang D. Computational pharmaceutics: a new paradigm of drug delivery[J]. Journal of Controlled Release, 2021, 338: 119-136.

[2] Wang N, Zhang Y, Wang W, et al. How can machine learning and multiscale modeling benefit ocular drug development[J]? Advanced Drug Delivery Reviews, 2023, 196: 114772.

[3] Metwally A A, Hathout R M. Computer-assisted drug formulation design: novel approach in drug delivery[J]. Molecular Pharmaceutics, 2015, 12(8): 2800-2810.

[4] Rio L G, Diaz-Rodriguez P, Landin M. Design of novel orotransmucosal vaccine-delivery platforms using artificial intelligence[J]. European Journal of Pharmaceutics and Biopharmaceutics, 2021, 159: 36-43.

[5] Chaibva F, Burton M, Walker R B. Optimization of salbutamol sulfate dissolution from sustained release matrix formulations using an artificial neural network[J]. Pharmaceutics, 2010, 2(2): 182-198.

[6] Wishart D S, Knox C, Guo A C, et al. DrugBank: a knowledgebase for drugs, drug actions and drug targets[J]. Nucleic acids research, 2008, 36: D901-D906.

[7] Esposito R, Ermondi G, Caron G. OpenCDLig: a free web application for sharing resources about cyclodextrin/ligand complexes[J]. Journal of Computer-Aided Molecular Design, 2009, 23(9): 669-675.

[8] Takagaki K, Arai H, Takayama K. Creation of a tablet database containing several active ingredients and prediction of their pharmaceutical characteristics based on ensemble artificial neural networks[J]. Journal of Pharmaceutical Sciences, 2010, 99(10): 4201-4214.

[9] Mixcoha E, Rosende R, Garcia-Fandino R, et al. Cyclo-lib: a database of computational molecular dynamics simulations of cyclodextrins[J]. Bioinformatics, 2016, 32: 3371-3373.

[10] Wang W, Yan X, Zhao L, et al. Universal nanohydrophobicity predictions using virtual nanoparticle library[J]. Journal of Cheminformatics, 2019, 11(1): 6.

[11] Hazai E, Hazai I, Demko L, et al. Cyclodextrin knowledgebase a web-based service managing CD-ligand complexation data[J]. Journal of Computer-Aided Molecular Design, 2010, 24(8): 713-717.

[12] Eckart B, Robert H, Yingling Y G, et al. RNAJunction: a database of RNA junctions and kissing loops for three dimensional structural analysis and nanodesign[J]. Nucleic acids research, 2008, 36, D392-D397.

[13] Mathur D, Kaur H, Dhall A, et al. SAPdb: A database of short peptides and the corresponding nanostructures formed by self-assembly[J]. Computers in Biology and Medicine, 2021, 133(5-6): 104391.

[14] Boetzel R, Ceszlak A, Day C, et al. An Elemental Impurities Excipient Database: A Viable Tool for ICH Q3D Drug Product Risk Assessment[J]. Journal of Pharmaceutical Sciences. 2018, 107(9): 2335-2340.

[15] Dong J, Gao H, Ouyang D. PharmSD: A novel AI-based computational platform for solid dispersion formulation design[J]. International Journal of Pharmaceutics, 2021, 604: 120705.

[16] Dong J, Yao Z J, Zhang L, et al. PyBioMed: a python library for various molecular representations of chemicals, proteins and DNAs and their interactions[J]. Journal of Cheminformatics, 2018, 10(1): 16.

[17] Yang Y, Ye Z, Su Y, et al. Deep learning for in vitro prediction of pharmaceutical formulations[J]. Acta Pharmaceutica Sinica. B, 2018, 9: 177-185.

[18] Gao H, Su Y, Wang W, et al. Integrated computer-aided formulation design: A case study of andrographolide/cyclodextrin

ternary formulation[J]. Asian Journal of Pharmaceutical Sciences 2021, 16(4): 494-507.

[19] Cern A, Barenholz Y, Tropsha A, et al. Computer-aided design of liposomal drugs: In silico prediction and experimental validation of drug candidates for liposomal remote loading[J]. Journal of Controlled Release, 2014, 173: 125-131.

[20] He, Y, Ye Z, Liu X, et al. Can machine learning predict drug nanocrystals[J]? Journal of Controlled Release, 2020, 322: 274-285.

[21] Han R, Xiong H, Ye Z, et al. Predicting physical stability of solid dispersions by machine learning techniques[J]. Journal of Controlled Release, 2019, 311-312: 16-25.

[22] Youshia J, Ali M E, Lamprecht A. Artificial neural network based particle size prediction of polymeric nanoparticles[J]. European Journal of Pharmaceutics and Biopharmaceutics, 2017, 119: 333-342.

[23] Takayama K, Kawai S, Obata Y, et al. Prediction of dissolution data integrated in tablet database using four-layered artificial neural networks[J]. Chemical & Pharmaceutical Bulletin, 2017, 65(10): 967-972.

[24] Galata D L, et al. Fast, spectroscopy-based prediction of in vitro dissolution profile of extended release tablets using artificial neural networks[J]. Pharmaceutics.2019, 11(8): 400.

[25] Tosca E M, Bartolucci R, Magni P. Application of artificial neural networks to predict the intrinsic solubility of drug-like molecules[J]. Pharmaceutics, 2021, 13(7): 1101.

[26] Noguchi T, Akiyama Y. PDB-REPRDB: a database of representative protein chains from the Protein Data Bank(PDB) in 2003[J]. Nucleic acids research, 2003, 31: 492-493.

[27] Kruger D M, Kamerlin S C L. Micelle maker: An online tool for generating equilibrated micelles as direct input for molecular dynamics simulations[J]. Acs Omega, 2017, 2(8): 4524-4530.

[28] Choi Y K, et al. CHARMM-GUI polymer builder for modeling and simulation of synthetic polymers[J]. Journal of Chemical Theory and Computation, 2021, 17: 2431-2443.

[29] Dong J, Wu Z, Xu H, Ouyang D. FormulationAI: a novel web-based platform for drug formulation design driven by artificial intelligence[J]. Brief Bioinform, 2023, 25(1): bbad419.

[30] Mendyk A, Szlęk J, Jachowicz R. 3-ME_expert 2.0: a heuristic decision support system for microemulsions formulation development[M]. In: Formulation Tools for Pharmaceutical Development, ed Aguilar J E. London: Woodhead Publishing, 2013: 39-71.

[31] Elbadawi M, Castro B M, Gavins F K H, et al. M3DISEEN: A novel machine learning approach for predicting the 3D printability of medicines[J]. Int J Pharm, 2020, 590: 119837.

[32] Slotwinski J A, Campbell T A. Metrology for additive manufacturing-opportunities in a rapidly emerging technology, 2013.

[33] Jain E, Bairoch A, Duvaud S, et al. Infrastructure for the life sciences: design and implementation of the UniProt website[J]. BMC bioinformatics, 2009, 10: 136.

[34] Wang N, Sun H, Dong J, et al. PharmDE: A new expert system for drug-excipient compatibility evaluation[J]. International Journal of Pharmaceutics, 2021, 607: 120962.

[35] Ghahremanpour M M, Arab S S, Aghazadeh S B, et al. MemBuilder: a web-based graphical interface to build heterogeneously mixed membrane bilayers for the GROMACS biomolecular simulation program[J]. Bioinformatics, 2014, 30(3): 439-441.

第4章

干粉吸入给药方式的计算机数值模拟技术

胡驾纬　萨里大学，英国
张　凌　萨里大学，英国
邬传宇　萨里大学，英国

4.1 引言

干粉吸入是一种通过干粉吸入器（dry powder inhaler，DPI）等装置进行药物给药的方法[1]，它可以递送包括小分子药物和蛋白质类药物（如胰岛素）等多种药物成分。这些药物成分通常以细粉末的形式制备，可以直接送入肺部，从而在局部发挥作用或被吸收入体循环（即血液循环），实现快速药物输送，产生疗效。此外，与体内给药相比，干粉吸入给药方式可以最小化所需药物量，即以较少的剂量达到与其他方式相似甚至更好的治疗效果。因此，DPI在治疗慢性阻塞性肺疾病、哮喘以及其他呼吸系统疾病方面的应用越来越广泛。

在干粉吸入器中，细粉末通常储存于储库、胶囊或泡罩中，并在患者吸入时从装置中释放出来。与定量吸入器（metered dose inhaler，MDI）通常使用的推进剂不同，DPI不涉及任何推进剂。MDI中使用的推进剂可能对环境有害，同时还可能对某些患者产生刺激作用。因此，与MDI相比，DPI不仅对环境更友好，对患者也更友好。此外，相较于MDI，DPI在患者吸入时即可释放药物，不需要在吸入后进行太多操作协调，使用更加简便。然而，从DPI中释放细粉末是一个复杂的过程，其受到处方特性、装置设计和患者操作的影响。

DPI的性能取决于其药物处方特性，如颗粒大小、形状和含水量等。在这些特性中，干粉颗粒的大小是最为关键的，因为它决定了DPI中干粉的雾化行为，从而影响了在肺部的沉积和药物递送效率。一般来说，用于DPI处方的颗粒粒径必须足够小，以保证干粉可以悬浮在气流中，被患者吸入并沉积在肺部；同时干粉颗粒粒径也不应太小，以免被吸入后再被呼出。研究表明，直径在1~5 μm的颗粒通常具有最高的肺部沉积效率[2]。此外，颗粒形状、表面积和表面电荷也会影响DPI的性能。研究发现，相同体积的细长颗粒比球形颗粒更有利于肺部沉积[3]；同时，拥有更大表面积和更高表面电荷的干粉颗粒有助于增强与肺组织之间的接触或静电作用，从而提高干粉在肺部的沉积效率[4]。另外，颗粒的含水量也是影响DPI性能的重要因素。高含水量可能导致粉末结块和团聚，从而降低DPI的稳定性和有效性[5]。

药物干粉吸入器（DPI）的性能不仅受药物处方特性影响，还受到装置设计的重要影响。DPI的工作机制依赖于患者产生的吸入气流，将药物粉末雾化并沉积在肺部。然而，不同患者的吸入气流能力存在差异。研究表明，气流阻力较低的DPI装置比阻力较高的装置具有更高的药物递送效率[6]和更好的剂量一致性[7]。此外，Baloira等[8]比较了不同DPI装置的性能，发现装置的设计显著影响了药物在肺部的沉积效率，其值可以在7.6%和69.3%之间变化。

DPI的药物递送效率还受患者的操作和吸入技术影响，即患者能否正确吸入所需剂量。这里的操作包括患者正确使用DPI、产生足够的吸入气流以有效地将药物颗粒送入肺部的技术和能力。研究表明，不论使用何种类型的干粉吸入器，患者的吸入技术都会极大地影响药物颗粒在肺部的沉积效率[9]。吸入气流速度较低的患者可能无法产生足够的气流来有效地雾化颗粒，导致输送到肺部的药物减少[7]。Lavorini等[10]、de Boer等[11]以及Clark和Hollingworth[12]的研究表明，吸入气流速度对不同DPI性能的影响显著，特别是对细颗粒剂量和肺部沉积效率的影响。具体而言，较高的吸入气流速度会导致较低的细颗粒分数（fine particle fraction，FPF），即达到肺部的颗粒比例降低。这意味着吸入过快的患者可能从其

DPI中获得较低的药物剂量，而缓慢而深的吸入则会获得更高的肺部沉积效率。

从力学角度上讲，DPI的性能和效率取决于药物颗粒在团聚、分散（或解聚）和沉积过程中的行为[13]。DPI的性能通常需要使用撞击器进行体外测试来评估[14]。然而，这些体外测试方法由于其自身局限性，对于理解处方特性、装置设计和患者操作之间的相互作用的帮助有限。DPI的数值模拟技术，尤其是利用离散元法（discrete element method，DEM）和离散元法与计算流体动力学（CFD）耦合的方法，即DEM-CFD方法，越来越受到研究的关注[15-19]。本章将介绍DEM和DEM-CFD在DPI数值模拟中的应用，包括：(a) 颗粒团聚模拟；(b) 颗粒团聚体解聚模拟；(c) DPI装置中颗粒的沉积模拟。

4.2 离散元法

离散元法（DEM）是一种用于研究颗粒系统（如制药粉末、农作物颗粒和沙粒等）行为的数值方法。其中，每个颗粒都被单独处理，而颗粒系统被建模为由多个相互作用的颗粒与边界组成的组合体。系统中每个颗粒的运动由牛顿第二定律控制，颗粒之间以及颗粒与壁面之间的相互作用则由接触定律来描述，并通过特定的接触检测算法进行识别[20]。

DEM最初由Peter Cundall在1971年提出，用于模拟岩石在岩土工程中的运动。Cundall的工作奠定了DEM发展的基础，现在被广泛认为是DEM的开创性工作，激发了其他学者对DEM的进一步发展和扩展。DEM能够严格考虑颗粒之间的相互作用力，包括范德华力[22]、静电作用力[23]和液桥力[24]，具备模拟复杂的颗粒行为的能力，如凝聚、颗粒团聚和颗粒破碎。因此，如今DEM发展为一种强大的数值工具，并在制药、矿业、化工和土木等工程在内的各个领域广泛应用。

此外，DEM还可以基于单个颗粒的特性预测颗粒系统的整体行为，这在制药过程建模和在制药生产中识别关键物料属性和关键工艺参数方面特别有吸引力[25]。例如，DEM数值模拟技术被用于研究制药压片中的粉末流动[26]、压模填充[27, 28]和粉末压缩[29]等过程中粉体特性和操作参数的影响。此外，DEM模拟还用于分析连续混合[30]、湿法制粒[31]、双螺杆制粒[32]和粉碎[33]过程中的粉末流动行为，以探索颗粒特性（如颗粒大小、形状和密度）和工艺条件[34]对制药生产过程的影响，并评估装置设计[35]对制药生产性能的影响。研究表明，DEM在模拟各种制药生产过程方面功能强大，可以为颗粒行为和相互作用提供有价值的信息，并可用于优化制药处方、工艺和装置设计，提高工艺效率和产品质量。

在过去几十年中，DEM还通过与其他模拟流体的数值模拟技术，如计算流体动力学（CFD）[36, 37]、平滑粒子流体动力学（SPH）[38]和格子Boltzmann方法（LBM）[39]等，进行耦合的方式进一步发展，从而可以考虑流体（如液体和气体）的存在对颗粒行为的影响。在这些耦合方法中，DEM-CFD是一种非常流行的用于模拟颗粒-流体系统的数值方法。如图4-1所示，颗粒的运动使用DEM来模拟，而流体流动使用CFD来描述，并且通过双向耦合方案考察流体流动和颗粒运动的相互影响。关于DEM-CFD方法的详细描述可以参考Guo等的论文[36]。与其他耦合方法（如DEM-SPH和DEM-LBM）相比，DEM-CFD是一种更高效的计算方法，并被广泛应用在模拟干粉吸入过程中，其中颗粒与流体流动之间的相互作用决定了干粉吸入器的性能和药物输送效率。

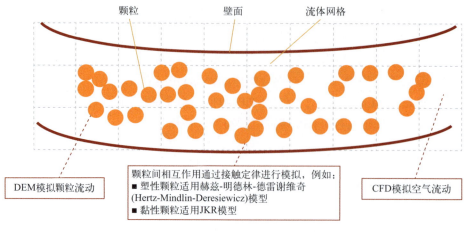

图4-1 DEM-CFD原理图解

4.3 颗粒团聚模拟

干粉吸入器（DPI）中使用的粒径为几微米的细药粉，其具有很强的聚结性和较差的流动性和可加工性。为了克服这些问题，通常需要对药物粉末进行团聚处理：使药物颗粒与大粒径载体颗粒（通常约为70 μm）混合形成基于载体的团聚体，或药物颗粒间彼此聚集形成仅药物颗粒的团聚体[40]。因此，药物颗粒团聚是决定DPI递送效率的关键过程。通常，在药物颗粒团聚过程中使用搅拌器[41, 42]进行再混合，原本细小的药物颗粒由于静电力、范德华力或两者的组合而附着在一起或附着在载体颗粒的表面上[43]。DPI处方的团聚和解聚过程决定了其雾化性能，即细颗粒分数（FPF）[44, 45]。因此，深入了解团聚和解聚过程对于开发DPI处方至关重要。而DEM数值模拟技术可以在微观和宏观水平上阐释团聚机制。

4.3.1 仅药物颗粒团聚体的形成

对于仅存在药物颗粒的处方，使用DEM生成虚拟团聚体，以便探索处方特性在分散（即解聚）过程中对雾化性能的影响。在DEM模拟中，团聚体通常是通过施加特定的向心力场和范德华力来创建的。向心力场促进颗粒向中心聚集，而范德华力在颗粒之间产生强大的内聚力，最终形成稳定的团聚体[45-48]。当所有颗粒的动能趋近于零时，向心力场被重力场取代或完全移除。许多研究人员使用这种组合方法来生成虚拟团聚体。例如，Thornton等[46]使用表面能为3.0 J/m^{2}的1000个初级颗粒模拟了团聚过程，然后分析了由于碰撞而导致的团聚体的破碎。Yang等[48]也在DEM中使用单一尺寸的初级颗粒模拟了类似的团聚过程，并发现随着团聚体直径的增加，配位数和堆积密度以指数形式递减。之后，Tong等[45]使用相同的方法创建了具有多分散颗粒系统的虚拟团聚体。van Wachem等[49]则通过将所有初级颗粒以特定速度移动向域中心来生成仅药物颗粒的团聚体，并发现采用这种方法可以生成与物理实验中相同孔隙率的团聚体。

4.3.2 基于载体的团聚体的形成

许多研究人员也使用DEM对基于载体的处方进行了建模[19, 50-53]。基于载体的团聚体的形成与前面描述的仅药物颗粒团聚体的形成类似。例如，Yang等[19]最初围绕载体颗粒随机生成了一定数量的药物颗粒，如图4-2（A）所示。然后，将所有药物颗粒设置为以特定速度向载体颗粒的中心移动。一旦药物颗粒与载体颗粒接触，就施加内聚力以确保药物颗粒附着在载体颗粒的表面上，从而形成稳定的团聚体 [图4-2（B）]。另外，药物颗粒也可以在向心力作用下移动到载体颗粒的表面[50]，或直接生成在载体颗粒上[51-53]。

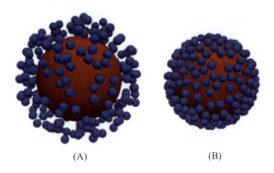

(A)　　　　　(B)

图4-2　采用离散元法（DEM）生成基于载体的团聚体：（A）初始设置；（B）虚拟团聚体[19]（已获Elsevier授权转载）

除了直接生成虚拟团聚体外，DEM还可用于模拟自然团聚过程，以探索处方特性和工艺参数的影响。例如，Yang等[17]通过DEM模拟了垂直振动容器中的药物颗粒与载体颗粒的团聚过程。如图4-3所示，最初药物颗粒和载体颗粒随机生成，并在容器振动时彼此碰撞。由于药物颗粒和载体颗粒之间存在范德华力，一些药物颗粒附着在载体颗粒的表面上 [见图4-3（C）]，形成基于载体的团聚体。研究表明，附着在载体颗粒上的药物颗粒数量取决于振动条件（即振动速度和振幅），在特定频率和振幅下获得了附着在载体颗粒上的最大数量的药物颗粒，该振动条件被确定为最佳频率和振幅。

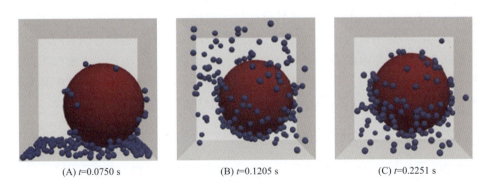

(A) t=0.0750 s　　　　(B) t=0.1205 s　　　　(C) t=0.2251 s

图4-3　离散元法（DEM）模拟在振动容器中载体颗粒（以红色显示）与药物颗粒（以蓝色显示）团聚过程[17]（已获Springer Nature授权转载）

上述团聚体是由具有特定表面能的颗粒间的范德华力相互作用而形成的。此外，Yang 等[15]使用DEM研究了在垂直振动容器中以静电效应主导的载体制剂团聚过程。在这项研究中，药物颗粒和载体颗粒被假设为最初具有相反的电荷。通过研究不同的振动条件（即振动速度幅值和频率）对团聚过程的影响，发现当团聚过程由静电效应主导时，接触数目（即附着在载体颗粒上的药物颗粒数量）随着振动速度幅值和频率的增加而减少（如图4-4所示），这与上文讨论的范德华力主导的情况不同（另见参考文献[17]）。这些研究表明，制剂颗粒的性质，特别是界面和表面性质，在团聚过程中也起着重要作用。

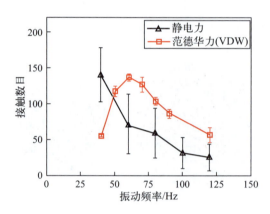

图4-4　垂直振动容器中以静电力和范德华力为主导形成的基于载体的团聚体性能比较[15]
（已获Elsevier授权转载）

4.4　颗粒团聚体解聚模拟

在干粉吸入剂中，团聚体的特性至关重要。这些团聚体既需要具备足够的强度和完整性，以避免在制造过程中发生破裂或磨损，又需要保持一定的松散程度，以便在吸入过程中能够有效地解聚和分散[54]。因此，在干粉吸入的过程中，团聚体的解聚变得至关重要。有研究提出假设，干粉吸入剂中的解聚过程可能受到两种主要因素的影响：一是由空气流引起的空气动力学力；二是团聚体与吸入装置之间的机械冲击[13, 55]。这两种因素的相对大小将决定解聚的效率，而这又与内聚力和分散力的平衡关系密切相关。因此，干粉吸入剂的雾化性能是由多个因素共同决定的，其中包括空气动力学力、机械冲击以及颗粒间的相互作用。在这一背景下，DEM-CFD方法被广泛用于研究颗粒团聚体解聚的过程。

4.4.1　空气动力学力引起的解聚

大多数DPI都是被动装置，即需要通过患者吸入的气流使药物和/或载体颗粒悬浮和解聚。一般情况下，患者吸入气流速度通常相对较低（<100 L/min）[56, 57]。因此，许多研究人员对探索空气动力学力是否会引起药物递送系统的解聚现象十分感兴趣。DEM-CFD模型被广泛使用于研究仅含药物颗粒和基于载体的DPI制剂的解聚过程[19, 58-61]。例如，Tong等[61]

使用了DEM-CFD模型，研究了在旋流流动条件下，由多分散颗粒组成的团聚体是如何在气流速度变化下发生解聚的。此项研究结果表明，空气流速显著影响着解聚行为。特别当团聚体由小的初级颗粒组成时，由于内聚力较强，在较低的流速下更难实现解聚。然而，随着流速的增加，分散效率也随之提高。类似地，Calvert等[58, 60]采用DEM-CFD模型，模拟了仅含药物颗粒的团聚体的解聚过程，并研究了颗粒与气体之间相对速度对解聚行为的影响。研究发现，在某一临界相对速度以上，团聚体会迅速解聚。此外，他们还发现，临界相对速度随着团聚体的尺寸减小而降低。另一方面，Yao等[59]使用了欧拉-拉格朗日（Euler-Lagrange）框架，对由湍流引起的细颗粒松散团聚体的解聚行为进行了建模。该研究关注湍流与颗粒之间的内聚力如何在解聚过程中相互作用。他们的研究发现，解聚现象受团聚体的大小、雷诺数和内聚数的共同影响。

对于基于载体的团聚体，Yang等[19]运用DEM-CFD模型深入研究了空气流对解聚行为的影响。研究结果显示，在特定的空气流动速度下，当基于载体的团聚体受到均匀的空气流冲击时，位于下游空气流方向的药物颗粒相较于其他药物颗粒更容易从载体表面脱落，如图4-5所示。这项研究还揭示，脱落的药物颗粒数量随着表面能的增加和空气流动速度的降低而减少。由此认为，解聚性能由分散力和内聚力共同决定。

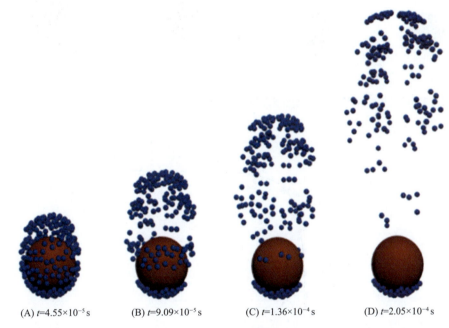

(A) $t=4.55\times10^{-5}$ s (B) $t=9.09\times10^{-5}$ s (C) $t=1.36\times10^{-4}$ s (D) $t=2.05\times10^{-4}$ s

图4-5　DEM-CFD模拟团聚体的解聚过程（通过不同时间点的情况呈现）[19]（已获Elsevier授权转载）

4.4.2　机械冲击引起的解聚

除了空气动力学力可以将颗粒拖入气流中诱发解聚外，团聚体与装置壁面之间的冲击也是DPI中另一个主要的解聚机制[61]，并在过去三十年中激发了越来越多的研究者的兴趣。许多研究人员通过DEM模拟了团聚体与壁面的冲击和团聚体的破裂，并对团聚体的性质和冲击条件（如固体分数[62]、团聚体大小[63]、冲击速度[62, 64-68]和冲击角度[67, 68]）的影响进行了深入研究。研究结果显示，冲击速度是决定破裂性能的最主要参数。Thornton及其合作者[64, 65]确定了一种冲击破裂机制，其中在加载过程中由冲击引起的不可逆塑性变形，以及在卸载过程中某些预先处理过的半子午面的微裂纹形成和融合。Moreno等[68]对等向球形团聚体与目标壁面之间的斜向冲击进行了DEM模拟，并显示冲击速度的切向分量也会影响冲击破裂模式，即使法向分量起主导作用。Tong等[69]通过比较DEM-CFD模拟分析中药物甘露醇团聚体的空气流和壁冲击对解聚行为的影响，显示机械冲击对团聚体的破碎贡献大于空气流引起的剪切效应。

Yang等[16]针对基于载体的团聚体的解聚行为进行了详细的DEM分析，系统地研究了冲击速度、冲击角度和表面能的影响。图4-6展示了载体制剂团聚体在与壁面发生冲击过程中的解聚情况，其中一些药物颗粒（蓝色表示）在冲击过程中脱落，从而实现了分散。他们引入了一个"分散比"的概念，即从载体颗粒上脱落的药物颗粒数与整个载体制剂团聚体的药物颗粒数之比，用以描述解聚行为。研究发现，随着冲击速度和冲击角度的增加，分散比也会增加。解聚行为经过冲击能量和黏附能量的分析，揭示了分散比随着能量比（即有效冲击能量与黏附能量之比）的变化，遵循Weibull分布的趋势（见图4-7）。

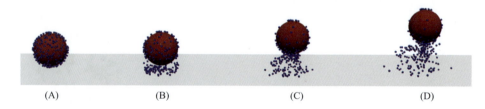

图4-6　通过DEM模拟捕获的载体制剂团聚体与壁面冲击的解聚过程[16]（已获Elsevier授权转载）

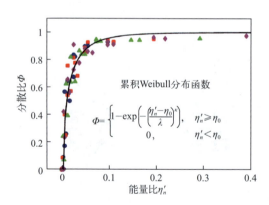

图4-7　分散比随能量比变化的情况（实线代表累积Weibull分布[16]，不同颜色的符号表示使用DEM-CFD模型进行建模的不同情况）（已获Elsevier授权转载）

此外，Ariane等[70]也利用DEM模型研究了基于载体的颗粒团聚体与壁面冲击引起的解聚过程。除了冲击速度和冲击角度外，他们还考察了团聚体的旋转和壁面黏附对解聚的影响。研究结果显示，在这些因素中，团聚体的旋转和壁面黏附对分散比的影响较小。Tamadondar和Rasmuson[71]则研究了载体表面粗糙度对团聚体与壁面冲击过程的影响。研究发现，表面凹凸对解聚性能有显著影响，冲击后剩余的细颗粒主要聚集在载体颗粒表面的空腔中。另一方面，Tong等[50]运用DEM-CFD模型模拟了基于载体的颗粒团聚体与壁面冲击的雾化过程。他们系统地分析了载体-药物颗粒质量比、载体尺寸、气流速度、冲击速度和冲击角度等变量与解聚性能的关联，并研究了这些因素对最终细颗粒分数（FPF）的影响。研究发现，在载体尺寸较大的情况下，载体-药物颗粒质量比对解聚性能的影响比气流速度、冲击速度和冲击角度更为显著。

4.5　DPI中颗粒沉积模拟

除了上述对DPI团聚和解聚机理的分析外，随着计算机硬件的快速发展以及模型的不断优化，DEM和DEM-CFD方法在干粉吸入领域的系统层面研究（即装置尺度上的颗粒行为与气流）得到了越来越广泛的应用[56, 72-75]。这使得装置设计和患者操作对于DPI药物递送效率的影响可以被更加详细地探索和理解。

4.5.1　装置尺度上的DEM-CFD模拟

目前，已有相关文献报道了使用DEM-CFD模拟一些典型商用DPI装置，如Aerolizer®[56, 73]、NextHaler®[74, 75]、Spiriva®[18]和Handihaler® DPI[18]，以及通用的DPI[18]中颗粒的分散行为。

以Aerolizer®为例，Zhou等[56]通过系统性地改变进气口尺寸、嘴管长度和网格空隙率等参数，研究了装置设计如何影响DPI分散性能。研究显示，通过细颗粒分数（FPF）表征的吸入效率在很大程度上依赖于进气口尺寸和网格结构。另一方面，Benque和Khinast[73]也研究了同样的Aerolizer® DPI装置，但着眼于考虑成人、儿童和慢性阻塞性肺疾病（COPD）患者的典型吸入曲线，以及恒定的空气流速对颗粒行为的影响。该研究发现，当考虑患者的吸入模式时，颗粒速度通常会出现较大的波动；而当考虑恒定空气流速时，颗粒倾向于以一致的速度运动。

对于NextHaler®，Ponzini等[74]使用DEM-CFD方法分析了装置内载药颗粒的释放和运动轨迹，并通过已发表的实验数据对模拟结果进行了验证。与此同时，Alfano等[75]则采用两个不同阶段的建模策略对简化的NextHaler®装置中气流的涡流流动进行了研究。在第一阶段，仅考虑了载体颗粒，并利用DEM-CFD模拟得到了载体颗粒在气流中的轨迹和速度。而在第二阶段，模拟了DPI中药物颗粒与载体颗粒的团聚体解聚过程。通过这个策略，可以尽可能多地模拟实际尺寸的DPI中的颗粒行为。

使用CFD-DEM，Zhao等[18]对包括Spiriva®、Handihaler®和通用DPI等不同装置中的大量乳糖载体颗粒（高达7166个）和药物颗粒（高达1713008个）的分散行为进行了建模，并研究了吸入气流速度对这些DPI中释放的空气动力学颗粒尺寸分布的影响。他们还研究了从DPI到气管支气管树的药物递送效率，并探索了颗粒形状，即纵横比，对颗粒空气动力学的影响。研究还表明，载体颗粒形状对DPI的药物递送效率有显著影响。

另外，Liu等[53]开发了粗粒化DEM-CFD方法，以研究L型干粉吸入器的雾化性能。他们提出了两种不同的粗粒化方法，分别是代表性颗粒方法和离散包裹方法。这两种方法的主要区别在于：离散包裹法将载体颗粒和药物颗粒都进行了粗粒化，而代表性颗粒方法仅对药物颗粒采用粗粒化。此外，他们还开展了不进行粗粒化的传统DEM-CFD模拟，以评估这两种粗粒化方法的性能。研究结果显示，当载体颗粒与药物颗粒的尺寸比较小时，两种方法都是有效的。然而，当尺寸比较大时，代表性颗粒方法在模拟DPI性能方面更加准确。他们还发现，使用代表性颗粒方法得到的细颗粒分数（FPF）和分散度分数（dispersion fraction，DF）受药物颗粒特性的影响。

尽管已经在文献中报道了包含数百万颗粒的DPI的DEM-CFD研究，但目前DEM-CFD方法处理的颗粒数量仍然远远低于实际使用的数量，而通常实际使用的颗粒数量可能超过数亿个[51, 52]。另外，目前在装置尺度上的DEM-CFD模拟仅考虑了载体颗粒，而不考虑药物颗粒，或者只考虑了有限数量的药物颗粒。为了克服这些挑战，研究人员引入了多尺度模拟方法来研究DPI的雾化性能[51, 76]。

多尺度模拟方法通常将微观尺度的颗粒间相互作用和流体-颗粒相互作用与装置尺度的宏观建模相结合[13]。例如，Tong等[76]基于DEM-CFD开发了一个多尺度模型，用于研究载体颗粒的分散性能。他们进行了超过200个不同冲击条件下（例如冲击速度和冲击角度）的药物颗粒和载体颗粒脱落过程的模拟。基于这些模拟，使用经验方程式描述了团聚体解聚效果与冲击条件之间的相关性。他们还模拟了Aerolizer®中载体颗粒的运动，以预测与这些经验方程式相结合的雾化性能。通过这种多尺度模拟方法发现，在一定的载体-药物质量比下，DPI的雾化性能随着载体颗粒直径的减小而降低，随着空气流速的增加而增加。

另一个例子是van Wachem等[51]提出的基于DEM-CFD的多尺度模型，涵盖了微观尺度、介观尺度和宏观尺度，用于预测颗粒行为和空气流动动力学。在微观尺度，考虑了载体和药物颗粒在由团聚体-壁碰撞、空气动力学力和团聚体-团聚体碰撞引起的解聚过程中的相互作用；在介观尺度，开发了粗粒化模型，用于描述药物颗粒的相互作用；在宏观尺度，对原型吸入器中载体颗粒的运动和相互作用进行了模拟。通过这个多尺度方法发现，药物颗粒比载体颗粒更容易从吸入器中解聚，整体药物递送效率取决于颗粒之间的黏聚性。

4.5.2　CFD-DPM雾化建模

由于DEM-CFD在模拟DPI中真实颗粒系统时计算能力有限，另一种计算流体动力学与离散颗粒模型（discrete particle model，DPM）耦合的技术，即CFD-DPM，被用来模拟DPI中团聚体分散和雾化过程。CFD-DPM是一种用于模拟多相流的强大数值模拟技术，其中连续的流体相（气体或液体）使用CFD描述，而分散的颗粒或液滴相使用离散颗粒模型（DPM）来模拟。CFD-DPM同时考虑了连续流体相和离散颗粒相之间的相互作用。在这种方法中，将离散颗粒视为具有给定质量的点，其运动由作用在其身上的各种力（如阻力、重力和颗粒间的力）的方程式所调节。离散相方程式包括颗粒质量守恒方程（用于跟踪每个控制体积中的颗粒数目）和颗粒动量方程（用于确定颗粒的运动）。连续流体相与离散颗粒相之间的相互作用通过在流体流动方程中加入适当的源项来建模，这些源项代表颗粒对流体流动的影响，如两个相之间的动量和能量传递。然后，根据颗粒和流体的相对速度和性质计算流体对颗粒施加的力，如曳力（流动阻力的反作用力）和升力。

CFD-DPM被用于分析DPI装置中药物颗粒的分散[77]，以及药物颗粒甚至纳米颗粒在气道中的动力学和沉积[78-81]。它还被用于研究DPI装置中颗粒的运动[82]和指导DPI装置的设计[83]。例如，Kim等[83]使用CFD-DPM研究了六种定制的漩涡型DPI装置和一种商业用漩涡型DPI装置中的气流和颗粒动态行为，并探索了凹槽形状、进气口设计（例如方向和数量）以及吸嘴收缩对颗粒分散行为的影响。研究表明，具有球形凹槽和吸嘴收缩的装置可以达到最佳的分散效率。Sustersic等[84]使用CFD-DPM研究了干粉吸入器Aerolizer®中环流室尺寸对雾化颗粒沉积的影响，并显示最大颗粒速度和沉积颗粒百分比严重依赖于环流室尺寸。Mitani等[81]开发了考虑非球形颗粒的CFD-DPM模型，其中实现了非球形颗粒的阻力模型，以便在CFD-DPM模型中隐式考虑颗粒形状（如纵横比）的影响。然后使用开发的CFD-DPM模型分析了级联撞击器中长条形针靴状颗粒的沉积行为。Islam等[78]对上气道多狭窄部分的纳米颗粒雾输运行为进行了CFD-DPM模拟，采用了喉部模型和Weibel模型的组合。研究表明，在狭窄部分气流通常显现出高速度和低压力，而喉部部分气流通常具有最高压力。此外，气流速度增加时，尤其是在狭窄部分会引起更高的壁面剪切应力。Rahman等[85]采用类似的方法探讨了人体肺部中微米级颗粒的输运和沉积，详细研究了颗粒尺寸和患者年龄老化对颗粒的输运和沉积效率的影响。为了使用CFD-DPM模拟DPI中颗粒的黏附和附着行为，Sustersic等[82, 86]在CFD-DPM模型中引入了黏附和脱落准则，并根据沉积颗粒百分比研究了DPI中颗粒的沉积行为。

相比于DEM-CFD模型，CFD-DPM模型将颗粒视为点，同时忽略或简化了颗粒间的相互作用，因此，无须进行接触检测和建模，具有更高的计算效率。这使得CFD-DPM模型适用于模拟颗粒间接触较少的情况，如稀疏颗粒系统。同时，它还可以处理复杂的几何形状，如复杂的气道系统以及各种流动条件，包括湍流流动。相较之下，DEM-CFD模型更适合用于需要深入了解颗粒行为或模拟稠密颗粒系统的情况。尽管DEM-CFD模型也可以处理复杂几何形状（如人体气道）和不规则形状的颗粒[79]，但目前的计算资源限制了其处理的颗粒数量和模型规模。此外，为了确保DEM-CFD模型和CFD-DPM模型的模拟精度，需要对模型参数进行精确校准，并尽可能结合实验数据对模拟结果进行验证。

4.6 总结

数值模拟技术在分析干粉吸入剂中的聚集、解聚和分散过程分析中表现了强大的实用性和有效性，并取得了显著的进展。通过明确地考虑颗粒行为，数值模拟技术为我们提供了关于DPI性能的详细信息，涵盖了不同尺度上的颗粒运动、颗粒间相互作用、流体颗粒相互作用和气流场。这些数值能够揭示潜在机制，并优化DPI装置的设计，为DPI制剂和装置的开发提供了宝贵的指导。未来，这些模型将进一步考虑更多因素，例如真实的颗粒形状、更加复杂的环境条件（如静电和相对湿度）以及DPI中的湍流流动。此外，我们也将努力在装置尺度上开发更加现实的模型，同时考虑合理数量的颗粒。特别值得关注的是，基于物理的DEM和DEM-CFD模型的进步，将成为DPI数字孪生技术的关键组成部分，为制药工业4.0的实施奠定坚实基础。这些模型与先进的传感器、数字技术和物联网的结合，将推动DPI开发和制造的数字化转型，从而实现更加可持续的DPI制造过程。

参考文献

[1] Wolff R K. Safety of inhaled proteins for therapeutic use[J]. Journal of Aerosol Medicine, 2009, 11: 197-219.

[2] Chaurasiya B, Zhao YY. Dry powder for pulmonary delivery: A comprehensive review[J]. Pharmaceutics, 2021, 13: 31.

[3] Finlay W H. Deposition of aerosols in the lungs: particle characteristics[J]. Journal of Aerosol Medicine and Pulmonary Drug Delivery, 2021, 34: 213-216.

[4] Majid H, Madl P, Hofmann W, Alam K. Implementation of charged particles deposition in stochastic lung model and calculation of enhanced deposition[J]. Aerosol Science and Technology, 2012, 46: 547-554.

[5] Peng T, Lin S, Niu B, et al. Influence of physical properties of carrier on the performance of dry powder inhalers[J]. Acta Pharm Sin B, 2016, 6: 308-318.

[6] Timsina M P, Martin G P, Marriott C, et al. Drug delivery to the respiratory tract using dry powder inhalers[J]. Int J Pharm, 1994, 101: 1-13.

[7] Labiris N R, Dolovich M B. Pulmonary drug delivery. Part Ⅱ: The role of inhalant delivery devices and drug formulations in therapeutic effectiveness of aerosolized medications[J]. Br J Clin Pharmacol, 2003, 56: 600-612.

[8] Baloira A, Abad A, Fuster A, et al. Lung deposition and inspiratory flow rate in patients with chronic obstructive pulmonary disease using different inhalation devices: A systematic literature review and expert opinion[J]. International Journal of COPD, 2021, 16: 1021-1033.

[9] Cochrane M G, Bala M V, Downs K E, et al. Inhaled corticosteroids for asthma therapy: patient compliance, devices, and inhalation technique[J]. Chest, 2000, 117: 542-550.

[10] Lavorini F, Magnan A, Christophe Dubus J, et al. Effect of incorrect use of dry powder inhalers on management of patients with asthma and COPD[J]. Respir Med, 2008, 102: 593-604.

[11] de Boer A H, Hagedoorn P, Hoppentocht M, et al. Dry powder inhalation: past, present and future[J]. Expert Opinion on Drug Delivery, 2016, 14(4): 499-512.

[12] Clark A R, Hollingworth A M. The relationship between powder inhaler resistance and peak inspiratory conditions in healthy volunteers — Implications for in vitro testing[J]. Journal of Aerosol Medicine, 2009, 6: 99-110.

[13] Yang J, Wu C-Y, Adams M. Numerical modelling of agglomeration and deagglomeration in dry powder inhalers: A review[J]. Curr Pharm Des, 2015, 21(40): 5915-5922.

[14] Dorosz A, Żaczek M, Moskal A. Dynamics of aerosol generation and release-Dry powder inhaler performance considerations[J]. J Aerosol Sci, 2021, 151: 105673.

[15] Yang J, Wu C-Y, Adams M. DEM analysis of the effect of electrostatic interaction on particle mixing for carrier-based dry powder inhaler formulations[J]. Particuology, 2015, 23: 25-30.

[16] Yang J, Wu C-Y, Adams M. DEM analysis of the effect of particle-wall impact on the dispersion performance in carrier-based dry powder inhalers[J]. Int J Pharm, 2015, 487(1-2): 32-38.

[17] Yang J, Wu C-Y, Adams M. DEM analysis of particle adhesion during powder mixing for dry powder inhaler formulation development[J]. Granul Matter, 2013, 15: 417-426.

[18] Zhao J, Haghnegahdar A, Feng Y, et al. Prediction of the carrier shape effect on particle transport, interaction and deposition in two dry powder inhalers and a mouth-to-G13 human respiratory system: A CFD-DEM study[J]. J Aerosol Sci, 2022, 160: 105899.

[19] Yang J, Wu C-Y, Adams M. Three-dimensional DEM-CFD analysis of air-flow-induced detachment of API particles from carrier particles in dry powder inhalers[J]. Acta Pharm Sin B, 2014, 4: 52-59.

[20] Seville, Jonathan P K, Wu C-Y. Particle Technology and Engineering, An Engineer's Guide to Particles and Powders: Fundamentals and Computational Approaches[M].Oxford: Butterworth-Heinemann, 2016.

[21] Cundall P A. A computer model for simulating progressive large scale movements in blocky system[J]. Proc Int Symp on Rock, 1971, 2: 2-8.

[22] Thornton C, Ning Z. A theoretical model for the stick/bounce behaviour of adhesive, elasticplastic spheres[J]. Powder Technol, 1998, 99: 154-162.

[23] Pei C, Wu C-Y, England D, et al. DEM-CFD modeling of particle systems with long-range electrostatic interactions[J]. AIChE Journal, 2015, 61(6): 1792-1803.

[24] Zhang L, Wu C-Y. Discrete element analysis of normal elastic impact of wet particles[J]. Powder Technol, 2020, 362: 628-634.

[25] Zheng C, Behjani M A, Hu J, et al. Discrete element modelling of pharmaceutical powder handling processes, In:

Simulations in Bulk Solids Handling[M].Weinheim: Wiley, 2023: 199-230.

[26] Hildebrandt C, Gopireddy S, Technology RS-P. Investigation of powder flow within a pharmaceutical tablet press force feeder: A DEM approach[M]. Amsterdam: Elsevier, 2019.

[27] Wu C-Y. DEM simulations of die filling during pharmaceutical tabletting[J]. Particuology, 2008, 6(6): 412-418 .

[28] Nwose E N, Pei C, Wu C Y. Modelling die filling with charged particles using DEM/CFD[J]. Particuology, 2012, 10: 229-235.

[29] Gao Y, de Simone G, Koorapaty M. Calibration and verification of DEM parameters for the quantitative simulation of pharmaceutical powder compression process[J]. Powder Technol, 2021, 378: 160-171.

[30] Zheng C, Li L, Nitert B J, et al. Investigation of granular dynamics in a continuous blender using the GPU-enhanced discrete element method[J]. Powder Technol, 2022, 412: 117968.

[31] Sarkar S, Chaudhuri B. DEM modeling of high shear wet granulation of a simple system[J]. Asian Journal of Pharmaceutical Sciences, 2018, 13(3): 220-228.

[32] Zheng C, Govender N, Zhang L, et al. GPU-enhanced DEM analysis of flow behaviour of irregularly shaped particles in a full-scale twin screw granulator[J]. Particuology, 2022, 61: 30-40.

[33] Hare C, Ghadiri M, Wu C Y. Discrete element modelling of ribbon milling: A comparison of approaches[J]. Powder Technol, 2021, 388: 63-69.

[34] Hlosta J, Jezerská L, Rozbroj J, et al. DEM investigation of the influence of particulate properties and operating conditions on the mixing process in rotary drums: Part 2—process validation and experimental study[J]. Processes, 2020, 8: 184.

[35] Hildebrandt C, Gopireddy S, et al. A DEM approach to assess the influence of the paddle wheel shape on force feeding during pharmaceutical tableting. Advanced Powder Technology, 2020, 31(2): 755-769.

[36] Guo Y, Wu C Y, Thornton C. Modeling gas-particle two-phase flows with complex and moving boundaries using DEM-CFD with an immersed boundary method[J]. AIChE Journal, 2013, 59: 1075-1087.

[37] Qiu L C, Wu C Y. A hybrid DEM/CFD approach for solid-liquid flows[J]. Journal of Hydrodynamics, 2014, 26: 19-25.

[38] Markauskas D, Kruggel-Emden H, Scherer V. Numerical analysis of wet plastic particle separation using a coupled DEM-SPH method[J]. Powder Technol, 2018, 325: 218-227.

[39] Liu W, Wu C Y. Modelling complex particle-fluid flow with a discrete element method coupled with lattice boltzmann methods(DEM-LBM)[J]. Chem Engineering, 2020, 4: 55.

[40] Chan H. Dry powder aerosol delivery systems: current and future research directions[J]. J Aerosol Med, 2006, 19: 21-27.

[41] Le V, Thi T, Robins E, et al. Dry powder inhalers: Study of the parameters influencing adhesion and dispersion of fluticasone propionate[J]. AAPS PharmSciTech, 2012, 13: 477-484.

[42] Zhou Q T, Morton D A V. Drug-lactose binding aspects in adhesive mixtures: Controlling performance in dry powder inhaler formulations by altering lactose carrier surfaces[J]. Adv Drug Deliv Rev, 2012, 64: 275-2784.

[43] Kaialy W. A review of factors affecting electrostatic charging of pharmaceuticals and adhesive mixtures for inhalation[J]. Int J Pharm, 2016, 503: 262-276.

[44] Smith I J, Parry-Billings M. The inhalers of the future？ A review of dry powder devices on the market today[J]. Pulm Pharmacol Ther, 2003, 16: 79-95.

[45] Tong Z B, Yang R Y, Chu K W, et al. Numerical study of the effects of particle size and polydispersity on the agglomerate dispersion in a cyclonic flow[J].Chemical Engineering Journal, 2010, 164(2-3): 432-441.

[46] Thornton C, Yin K K, Adams M J. Numerical simulation of the impact fracture and fragmentation of agglomerates[J]. J Phys D Appl Phys, 1996, 29: 424-435.

[47] Calvert G, Hassanpour A, Ghadiri M. Mechanistic analysis and computer simulation of the aerodynamic dispersion of loose aggregates[J]. Chemical Engineering Research and Design, 2011, 89: 519-525.

[48] Yang R Y, Yu A B, Choi S K, et al. Agglomeration of fine particles subjected to centripetal compaction[J].Powder Technology, 2008, 184(1): 122-129.

[49] van Wachem B, Thalberg K, Nguyen D, et al. Analysis, modelling and simulation of the fragmentation of agglomerates[J]. Chem Eng Sci, 2020, 227: 115944.

[50] Tong Z B, Yang R Y, Yu A B. CFD-DEM study of the aerosolisation mechanism of carrier-based formulations with high drug loadings[J]. Powder Technol, 2017, 314: 620-626.

[51] van Wachem B, Thalberg K, Remmelgas J, et al. Simulation of dry powder inhalers: Combining micro-scale, meso-scale and macro-scale modeling[J]. AIChE Journal, 2017, 63: 501-516.

[52] Nguyen D, Remmelgas J, Björn I N, et al. Towards quantitative prediction of the performance of dry powder inhalers by multi-scale simulations and experiments[J]. Int J Pharm, 2018, 547: 31-43.

[53] Liu X, Sulaiman M, Kolehmainen J, et al. Particle-based coarse-grained approach for simulating dry powder inhaler[J]. Int J Pharm, 2021, 606: 120821.
[54] Zhou QT, Morton DAV. Drug-lactose binding aspects in adhesive mixtures: controlling performance in dry powder inhaler formulations by altering lactose carrier surfaces[J]. Adv Drug Deliv Rev, 2012, 64: 275-284.
[55] Voss A, Finlay W H. Deagglomeration of dry powder pharmaceutical aerosols[J]. Int J Pharm, 2002: 248: 39-50.
[56] Zhou Q T, Tong Z, Tang P, et al. Effect of device design on the aerosolization of a carrier-based dry powder inhaler—a case study on Aerolizer® Foradile®[J]. AAPS J, 2013, 15: 511.
[57] Islam N, Gladki E. Dry powder inhalers(DPIs)—A review of device reliability and innovation[J]. Int J Pharm, 2008, 360: 1-11.
[58] Calvert G, Hassanpour A, Ghadiri M. Mechanistic analysis and computer simulation of the aerodynamic dispersion of loose aggregates[J]. Chemical Engineering Research and Design, 2011, 89: 519-525.
[59] Yao Y, Capecelatro J. Deagglomeration of cohesive particles by turbulence[J]. J Fluid Mech, 2021, 911: A10
[60] Calvert G, Hassanpour A, Ghadiri M. Analysis of aerodynamic dispersion of cohesive clusters[J]. Chem Eng Sci, 2013, 86: 146-150.
[61] Tong Z B, Yang R Y, Chu K W, et al. Numerical study of the effects of particle size and polydispersity on the agglomerate dispersion in a cyclonic flow[J]. Chemical Engineering Journal, 2010, 164: 432-441.
[62] Mishra B K, Thornton C. Impact breakage of particle agglomerates[J]. Int J Miner Process, 2001, 61: 225-239.
[63] Boerefijn R, Ning Z, Ghadiri M. Disintegration of weak lactose agglomerates for inhalation applications[J]. Int J Pharm, 1998, 172: 199-209.
[64] Kafui K D, Thornton C. Numerical simulations of impact breakage of a spherical crystalline agglomerate[J]. Powder Technol, 2000, 109: 113-132.
[65] Thornton C, Ciomocos M T, Adams M J. Numerical simulations of agglomerate impact breakage[J]. Powder Technol, 1999, 105: 74-82.
[66] Ning Z, Boerefijn R, Ghadiri M, et al. Distinct element simulation of impact breakage of lactose agglomerates[J]. Advanced Powder Technology, 1997, 8: 15-37.
[67] Tong Z B, Yang R Y, Yu A B, et al. Numerical modelling of the breakage of loose agglomerates of fine particles[J]. Powder Technol, 2009, 196: 213-221.
[68] Moreno R, Ghadiri M, Antony S J. Effect of the impact angle on the breakage of agglomerates: a numerical study using DEM[J]. Powder Technol, 2003, 130: 132-137.
[69] Tong Z B, Adi S, Yang R Y, et al. Numerical investigation of the deagglomeration mechanisms of fine powders on mechanical impaction[J]. J Aerosol Sci, 2011, 42: 811-819.
[70] Ariane M, Sommerfeld M, Alexiadis A. Wall collision and drug-carrier detachment in dry powder inhalers: Using DEM to devise a sub-scale model for CFD calculations[J]. Powder Technol, 2018, 334: 65-75.
[71] Tamadondar M R, Rasmuson A. The effect of carrier surface roughness on wall collision-induced detachment of micronized pharmaceutical particles[J]. AIChE Journal, 2020, 66: e16771.
[72] Cui Y, Schmalfuß S, Zellnitz S, et al. Towards the optimisation and adaptation of dry powder inhalers[J]. Int J Pharm, 2014, 470: 120-132.
[73] Benque B, Khinast J G. Estimating inter-patient variability of dispersion in dry powder inhalers using CFD-DEM simulations[J]. European Journal of Pharmaceutical Sciences, 2021, 156: 105574.
[74] Ponzini R, da Già R, Bnà S, et al. Coupled CFD-DEM model for dry powder inhalers simulation: Validation and sensitivity analysis for the main model parameters[J]. Powder Technol, 2021, 385: 199-226.
[75] Alfano FO, Benassi A, Gaspari R, et al. CFD-DEM analysis of the two-phase flow and particle dispersion in carrier-based Dry Powder Inhalers[J]. Chem Eng Trans, 2021, 86: 2021.
[76] Tong Z, Kamiya H, Yu A, et al. Multi-scale modelling of powder dispersion in a carrier-based inhalation system[J]. Pharm Res, 2015, 32: 2086-2096.
[77] Ignjatović J, Šušteršič T, Bodić A, et al. Comparative assessment of in vitro and in silico methods for aerodynamic characterization of powders for inhalation[J]. Pharmaceutics, 2021, 13(11): 1831.
[78] Islam M R, Larpruenrudee P, Rahman M M, et al. How nanoparticle aerosols transport through multi-stenosis sections of upper airways: A CFD-DPM modelling[J]. Atmosphere(Basel), 2022, 13(8): 1192.
[79] Ohsaki S, Mitani R, Fujiwara S, et al. Effect of particle-wall interaction and particle shape on particle deposition behavior in human respiratory system[J]. Chemical & Pharmaceutical Bulletin, 2019, 67(12): 1328-1336.
[80] Rahman M M, Zhao M, Islam M S, et al. Aging effects on airflow distribution and micron-particle transport and deposition

[81] Mitani R, Ohsaki S, Nakamura H, et al. Numerical study on deposition of non-spherical shaped particles in cascade impactor[J]. Advanced Powder Technology 2023；34(6)104045.

[82] Šušteršič T, Bodić A, Ignjatović J, et al[J]. Numerical modeling of particle dynamics inside a dry powder inhaler[J]. Pharmaceutics, 2022, 14(12): 2591.

[83] Kim Y H, Li D D, Yeoh G H, et al. Optimization of swirler type dry powder inhaler device design-Numerical investigation on the effect of dimple shape, inlet configuration and mouthpiece constriction[J]. J Aerosol Sci, 2022, 159: 105893.

[84] Šušteršič T, Vulović A, Filipović N, et al. Effect of circulation chamber dimensions on aerosol delivery efficiency of a commertial dry powder inhaler Aerolizer®. In: 2017 IEEE 17 th International Conference on Bioinformatics and Bioengineering(BIBE)[M], Washington, DC, USA: 2017.

[85] Rahman M M, Zhao M, Islam M S, ET AL. Aging effects on airflow distribution and micron-particle transport and deposition in a human lung using CFD-DPM approach[J]. Advanced Powder Technology, 2021, 32: 3506-3516.

[86] Ignjatovic J, Austersic T, Cvijic S, et al. Comparative assessment of computational vs. in vitro methods for the estimation of dry powders for inhalation emitted fraction.In: BIBE 2021-21 st IEEE International Conference on BioInformatics and BioEngineering, Proceedings[M]. Kragujevac, Serbia: Institute of Electrical and Electronics Engineers Inc., 2021.

第 5 章

药物递送中的分子模拟：
一项聚合物保护修饰的案例研究

亚历克斯·邦克（Alex Bunker）　赫尔辛基大学，芬兰
约瑟夫·克赖因（Josef Kehrein）　赫尔辛基大学，芬兰

5.1 引言

本章将讨论分子动力学模拟理论计算技术在聚合物中的应用,并通过聚合物促进活性药物成分递送作为一种案例来介绍分子模拟在药物递送中的应用:首先,简要概述药物递送和制剂技术发展所涉及的问题,这包括提供保护和携带药物及通过前药的纳米技术用以解决溶解性的问题,然后阐释聚合物在这方面的应用研究。此外,本章也将涵盖药物设计和递送中生物物理角度的机理以及聚合物在其中的特性。然后,介绍分子动力学模拟如何作为一种工具,用以协助实验分析来研究这种机制,以及聚合物应用于药物递送中的情况。本章还讨论了近十年来的相关研究及应用聚乙二醇(PEG)修饰聚合物的金标准,PEG在不同药物递送机制中的应用进展,以及模拟计算应用在除PEG以外的其他修饰聚合物的研究。具体而言,本章主要涉及使用分子动力学模拟研究聚合物与蛋白质的相互作用,因为这是聚合物在蛋白质-聚合物生物偶联物中作为保护修饰的关键应用,从而使其能够抵抗免疫系统的摄取。这也是目前应用于纳米医学的主要形式[1]。通过这项案例研究,希望读者能够洞察药剂学中的机理,并希望读者了解分子动力学模拟是如何与其他实验技术协同作用的。此外,发表于2020年的一篇综述文章[2]概述了分子模拟这种研究工具应用于药物递送研究的进展,主要包括药物递送纳米颗粒和提高药物溶解性的方方面面。如果您对药物递送中的分子模拟细节感兴趣,建议阅读这篇综述文章作为补充材料。

5.1.1 前药和纳米医学:缓解药物递送中的平衡作用

制药研究最早起源于帕拉塞尔苏斯的名言:"Dosis sola facit venenum",即"剂量决定毒性"[3]。简言之,药物是一种能进入人体的分子,然后开始扩散,并以足量的浓度完整地到达目标部位,从而产生预期效果,同时其在人体其他部位的浓度保持在其副作用(即毒性)无法忍受的临界值以下。药物是一种分子,其在保持足够溶解性以通过血液进入目标组织的同时,在平衡药效和毒性的过程中发挥作用。最初,药物设计便是筛选能满足上述要求的分子,但在许多情况下,当一些在目标部位非常有效的药物进入人体后可能无法到达目标部位,再者也可能会在身体其他部位产生毒性。近年来,通过先进的制剂技术,如前药和纳米医学,已经在解决这些问题方面取得了显著成功。

前药(prodrug)是将一个活性药物成分(API)通过共价键连接到另一分子上的药物分子,并在前药到达目标部位时可以断裂共价键释放API发挥药效[4]。而药物纳米技术,也被称为纳米医学[5, 6, 7],主要涉及开发纳米尺度的药物递送载体,通常也被称为纳米颗粒(nanoparticle,NP),以便将药物通过血液输送。药物递送中纳米技术的研发是一个快速发展的领域,多年来已经产生了许多形式(见图5-1)[8-18],若要了解相关细节信息,请阅读2020年出版的综述论文[2]。因为在许多情况下,前药会形成胶束复合物[19],而有些NP是通过与单个大分子偶联而成[20],因此,前药和药物纳米技术之间的界限很模糊:在此我们将这两种方法产生的载体统称为NP。除了改善药物的溶解度以使其能在血液中运输外,将药物封装在NP中还可以实现另外两个目标:①延长药物在血液中的寿命,②靶向递送药物至目标组织。

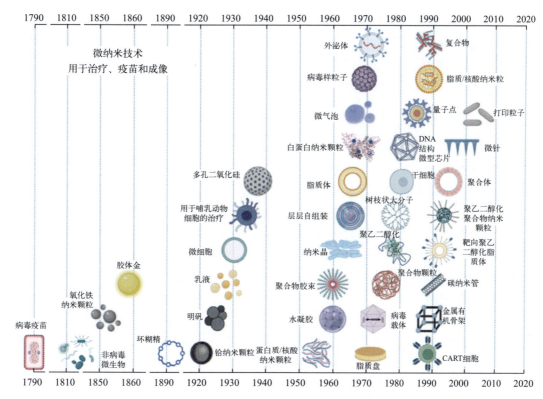

图5-1 微纳米技术在药物递送和成像中应用发展的时间线[15]

（根据CC BY 4.0许可使用）

在众多NP的形式中，值得一提的是基于脂质体的递送系统（liposome-based delivery system，LDS）[21, 22]。脂质体是由磷脂双分子形成的囊泡，同时也是具有多种功能的载体，因为它既可以在膜上携带疏水性药物分子，同时也可以在膜内携带亲水性药物分子。其他类似的由双亲性分子构成的囊泡型药物递送体系也正在研发中，例如泡囊[23, 22, 24]、醇质体[25]、多聚体[26]、不饱和脂肪酸囊泡[27]、外泌体[28]和树状体[29]。然而，LDS是最成熟和应用最广泛的，目前关于囊泡形成[30]及其在药物递送中应用的多篇文章已出版，其内容包括LDS在一般情况下的应用[22]，以及结合分子动力学与实验方法在其研发中的应用[21]。

血液中的外来颗粒，俗称为异物，其大小处于NP范围内，会被单核吞噬细胞系统（MPS）移除[31]，即被血液吸收。吸收的第一步涉及一系列特定蛋白质在NP表面的复杂级联反应，即补体激活[32, 33]。之后，便产生一个特定的蛋白质外壳，被称为蛋白冠[34-45]，覆盖在NP上，然后向吞噬细胞发出信号，吸收并破坏它。特定异物的吸收效率取决于其表面性质，如当NP的表面被设计成干扰补体激活时便可延长其在血液中的寿命。而当NP表面被设计成用于抑制吸收时（也被称为"隐形鞘"）也可延长其在血液中的寿命。由于补体激活是一个极为复杂的过程，隐形鞘的实际作用方式尚不清楚，其可能的机制是它们抑制了蛋白冠的形成，然后加速了错误蛋白冠的聚集，因为目前公认血液中所有异物都会被迅速覆盖上蛋白冠[46]。

通过主动运输或被动运输的方式，可以靶向递送药物至目标组织。主动靶向涉及具有特定结构的分子，并将其设计成与目标组织或细胞中过度表达的受体（也称其为靶标）结合[47]。当这些分子用于修饰NP的表面时，它们可以有效地连接更多的NP到目标细胞，从而增加它们进入目标组织/细胞的比例。在被动靶向中，往往基于靶向组织的整体性质将NP设计更大比例的NP嵌入目标组织。被动靶向的一个例子是所谓的增强渗透和滞留（enhanced permeability and retention，EPR）效应[48, 49]。

5.1.2 药物递送中的聚合物

根据国际纯粹与应用化学联合会（IUPAC）的定义，聚合物由大分子构成，而大分子是由可聚合单体衍生的具有重复构造单元并且分子量较高的分子[50]。这个定义涵盖了广泛的物质，并与许多产业和研究领域相关。目前根据几个不同的标准进行分类，例如化学结构（聚酯，聚烯烃，硅烷，聚酰胺，聚丙烯酸酯，聚氨酯，聚醚），聚合度和聚分散度，单体组成（同聚合物或共聚合物），构架[线性或（超）分支聚合物，树状聚合物]，以及物质的来源[天然或（半）合成][51]。生物体中的聚合物，称为生物聚合物，包括多肽、多糖和寡核苷酸；这些通常是可生物降解的，并在体内有诸多应用[52]。

在生物医学和药学领域，聚合物可用于多种目的，包括医疗器械[53]、表面防污和抗菌[54, 55]、诊断成像[56]、组织工程（也包括新型3D生物打印技术）[57]，以及API（例如泻药或血浆扩容剂）[58]、传统剂型[59]和复杂药物递送系统（drug delivery system，DDS）[60]的辅料。微调聚合物基体，如水凝胶[61]、非晶固体分散体[62, 63]，以及通过温度、pH、光或超声波变化来调控的智能刺激响应系统，可以提供先进的控释机制，应用于多种（肠道）途径释药[64]。另外，涵盖适应范围广泛的极具治疗价值的API已在聚合物基DDS中制剂化，包括化疗药物，特别是紫杉醇（PAC）和多柔比星（DOX），以及抗生素、抗真菌或驱虫药物（如甲硝唑、伊曲康唑、阿苯达唑）[2, 1]。

聚合物的多功能性和实用性主要源于以下三个因素：①聚合物的长度；②单体单元的结构；③易于接枝其他分子到聚合物的末端。聚合物材料的宏观特性由其单体单元的特定相互作用和分子本身的拓扑结构决定，即链长和刚度决定了缠结对整体特性的影响程度[65]。由于聚合物易于修饰到其他分子上，这便形成了一个化学框架，带有许多"隐喻性"的旋钮和开关，用于精细调节性能，由此便形成了可用于构建NP保护修饰的理想材料。在FDA迄今为止批准的大约80种不同的NP中，它们要么是基于聚合物，要么是使用不同聚合度的聚合物进行修饰（表5-1）[8]。接下来，我们将简要描述相关的DDS形式以及那些常用于保护修饰DDS的聚合物。

表5-1 选自多篇综述和多项研究的EMA/FDA批准的聚合物基修饰的DDS[66-71, 8-18]
（目前还有更多的DDS正处在临床试验中[69-74, 12, 1]）

基于脂质体的递送系统				
Doxil®	1995	PEGylated DOX liposome	卡波西肉瘤	[75]
Caelyx®	1996	PEGylated DOX liposome	乳腺癌	[76]
Lipodox®	2013	PEGylated DOX liposome	卵巢癌	[77]
Onivyde®	2015	PEGylated irinotecan liposome	胰腺癌	[78]
Onpattro®	2018	PEGylated siRNA liposome	转甲状腺素蛋白淀粉样变性（ATTR）	[79]
Pfizer-BioNTech vaccine	2020	PEGylated mRNA lipid NP	COVID-19	[80]
Moderna vaccine	2020	PEGylated mRNA lipid NP	COVID-19	[81]

续表

		聚合物基系统		
Verelan® PM	1998	PLGA-verapamil particles	高血压	[82]
Estrasorb®	2003	Polysorbate 80-based estradiol micelle	更年期症状	[83]
Nanoxel®#	2006	PEG-PDLLA docetaxel micelle	骨癌	[72]
Genexol® PM#	2007	PEG-PDLLA PAC micelle	乳腺癌	[72]
Zilretta®	2017	PLGA-TCA hydrogel	膝骨关节炎	[84]
		聚合物–药物偶联物		
Adagen®	1990	PEGylated adenosine deaminase	重症联合免疫缺陷病（SCID）	[85]
Oncaspar®	1994	PEGylated L-asparaginase	白血病	[86]
PegIntron®	2000	PEGylated IFN-α2 b	丙型肝炎	[87]
Pegasys®	2002	PEGylated IFN-α2 a	乙型和丙型肝炎	[88]
Neulasta®	2002	PEGylated G-CSF	中性粒细胞减少症	[89]
Somavert®	2002	PEGylated somatostatin	肢端肥大症	[90]
Macugen®	2004	PEGylated aptamer	黄斑变性	[91]
Mircera®	2007	PEGylated erythropoietin	贫血	[92]
Cimzia®	2008	PEGylated certolizumab	克罗恩病	[92]
Krystexxa®	2010	PEGylated uricase	慢性痛风	[93]
Sylatron™	2011	PEGylated IFN-α2 b	黑色素瘤	[94]
Plegridy®	2014	PEGylated IFN-β1 a	多发性硬化	[95]
Movantik®	2014	PEGylated naloxol	便秘	[96]
Adynovate®	2015	PEGylated factor Ⅷ	血友病 A	[97]
Rebinyn®	2017	GlycoPEGylated factor Ⅸ	血友病 B	[98]
Palynziq®	2018	PEGylated ammonia-lyase	苯丙酮尿症	[99]
Fulphila®	2018	PEGylated G-CSF	中性粒细胞减少症	[100]
Revcovi®	2018	PEGylated adenosine deaminase	重症联合免疫缺陷病（SCID）	[101]
Jivi®	2018	PEGylated factor Ⅷ	血友病 A	[101]
Asparlas™	2018	PEGylated L-aspariginase	白血病	[101]
Ziextenzo®	2018	PEGylated G-CSF	中性粒细胞减少症	[102]
Esperoct®	2019	GlycoPEGylated factor Ⅷ	血友病 A	[103]
Eloctate™	2019	GlycoPEGylated factor Ⅷ	血友病 A	[104]
Empaveli®	2021	PEGylated C3 b inhibitor	阵发性睡眠性血红蛋白尿症	[105]
Skytrofa®	2021	PEGylated hGH	生长激素缺乏症	[106]

续表

无机纳米颗粒				
Infed®	1992	Dextran-coated iron oxide	缺铁	[9]
Dexferrum®	1996	Dextran-coated iron oxide	缺铁	[107]
Ferrlecit®	1999	Gluconate-coated iron oxide	缺铁	[9]
Venofer®	2000	Sucrose-coated iron oxide	缺铁	[9]
Feraheme™	2009	CMD-coated iron oxide	贫血	[9]
Ferinject®	2013	Carboxymaltose-coated iron oxide	贫血	[9]

#= 仅在韩国获得批准，未获得 FDA/EMA 批准；CMD = 羧甲基葡聚糖；G-CSF = 嗜中性粒细胞集落刺激因子；hGH = 人生长激素；IFN = 干扰素；PDLLA = 聚（D, L- 乳酸）；PLGA = 聚乳酸 - 羟基乙酸共聚物；SCID = 重症联合免疫缺陷病；TCA = 三乙酸三醇酯。

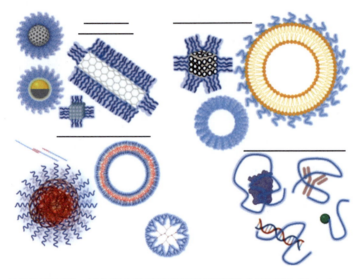

图5-2　DDS示意图，其中聚合物基修饰用作隐形鞘（使用BioRender.com创建）

保护冠以蓝色表示。系统包括基于纳米晶[8]、氧化铁[9]、二氧化硅、金、碳或氮化硼[113]等（无机）固体颗粒，以及脂质体[114]、醇质体[25]、不饱和脂肪酸囊泡[27]、外泌体[28]、非离子脂质体[22-24]、脂质NP[115]和立方体[116, 117]等LDS，以及包括聚合物胶束[109, 72]、聚合物颗粒[17]、树状聚合物[113]、聚合物囊泡[26]、树状聚合物囊泡[29]、多聚物[118]和胶束复合物[119]在内的聚合物基DDS。聚合物直接连接到API可形成聚合物 - 药物偶联物[120- 122]

5.1.2.1　具有聚合物保护修饰的药物递送系统

许多不同的载体可以使用聚合物进行修饰，以增强药物递送（图5-2）。通过将一个或多个聚合物的末端与NP进行共价结合，可为由聚合物材料组成的NP创建隐形鞘。例如，NP可将单个分子修饰为长聚合物。这包括了前药，其中API（包括基于肽或核酸的结构，以及小分子）与单一或多个长（支链）聚合物结合，并将其包裹在里面，这种结构称为聚合物 - 药物偶联物[101]。另一种可能是将几个疏水性分子分别结合到亲水性聚合物上，形成胶束或固体（无机或有机）颗粒，如纳米晶、氧化铁、金、银、硅胶或碳纳米管（CNT），并将聚合物结合到表面上[8, 108]。对于LDS和其他基于囊泡的药物递送系统而言，则是将聚合物修饰到那些形成膜（脂质双分子层）的两性分子的极性头部，从而形成保护性的聚合物隐形鞘。

　　DDS的其中一种形式完全是由聚合物组成，即聚合物胶束。其中NP是由数个AB二聚物或ABA三聚物组成，其中一种类型（即B块）是疏水性的，形成了中心核，而另一种类型（即A块）是亲水性的，从而构成了一个聚合物胶束，形成了隐形鞘。这些两性分子的自组装通常由热力学有利的方式或由减少界面自由能所驱动，从而补偿了聚合物构象熵的损失[109]。一种新兴趋势是应用聚合诱导自组装技术，这在大规模生产聚合物胶束方面具有多种优势[110]。与脂质体类似，这些聚合物胶束也具备多种功能，因为它们可以携带多种API，其中一些主要位于中心的B块内，而另一些可以位于A块内，因此这两种药物可能具有不同的释放路径。然而，根据体系的不同，即使对于相对疏水的荷载物，核心充当药物载体、外壳充当保护性冠层的界限可能也会变得模糊，这也使得简化的核-壳模型面临着挑战[111, 112]。所有组分的复杂相互依赖性主要由疏水相互作用以及其他色散力和静电力（例如氢键、π-π堆叠）所决定，这些力决定了胶束的性质，如形态、尺寸、电荷、稳定性、溶解度、药物分布和负载能力。最终，这些因素决定了制剂的药动学特性以及药物在体内的命运。这种DDS形式的多组分特性有助于药物在单个颗粒体系内的释放，但也可能导致达到靶标的API数量变少。因此，为特定的API选择适当的A和B块对于疾病治疗成功至关重要[72]。

5.1.2.2　用作保护修饰的聚合物

　　目前用于上述方式作为隐形鞘聚合物的金标准是PEG[123, 124]；当将PEG修饰到分子或NP上时，称之为"PEG化"[125, 124, 21, 123, 126]。通过PEG化构建的隐形鞘几乎已经在所有形式的NP中使用[2]；PEG化在药物递送中的应用现在已经非常广泛，例如携带两种已批准的mRNA疫苗的固体脂质纳米颗粒（lipid nanoparticle，LNP）[127]在其处方中都包括PEG化的脂质[128, 129]。然而，在这种情况下，制剂中的PEG聚合物数量不足以提供隐形鞘，而是发挥稳定NP结构的作用。尽管PEG往往是在NP周围形成亲水性壳层，但这是一个过于简化的观点，因为实验测定PEG在极性和非极性溶剂中都是可溶的[130]。通过观察PEG的结构（见图5-3），这一机制将变得更加清晰，即：PEG单体由一个极性氧原子和一个非极性$(CH_2)_2$基团组成。PEG单体的双亲性质还导致了PEG的另一个重要性质，即作为聚合物电解质，能够结合阳离子。早在20世纪80年代，PEG就已经被确定为锂离子电池的电解质[131, 132]，随后于20世纪90年代中期进行了分子动力学模拟测试这种特性背后的机制：它们以螺旋构象缠绕在阳离子周围，极性氧原子与阳离子之间形成盐桥[133, 134]。

　　PEG化脂质体是最早被批准用作药物治疗的NP之一，例如Doxil®[135, 75]是一种由1,2-二硬脂酰-*sn*-甘油-3-磷酸胆碱（DSPC）和胆固醇组成的PEG化脂质体，其PEG化是通过将DSPC的胆碱用乙醇-PEG取代从而产生DSPE-PEG而实现的。也有提出并测试基于LDS药物治疗的其他化学途径来实现PEG化[114]。主动和被动靶向机制也已在PEG化脂质体中进行了考察。例如在化疗领域中，研究者提出通过EPR效应[48, 49, 136]来实现PEG化脂质体的被动靶向，其中PEG化脂质体可以被设计成更容易嵌入肿瘤组织的渗漏血管，然而，实际上最近科学家们已经质疑EPR效应是否能够用作被动靶向策略[137]。主动靶向机制在PEG化脂质体中也进行了研究，即通过将靶向基团修饰到部分PEG链的末端来实现[138]。

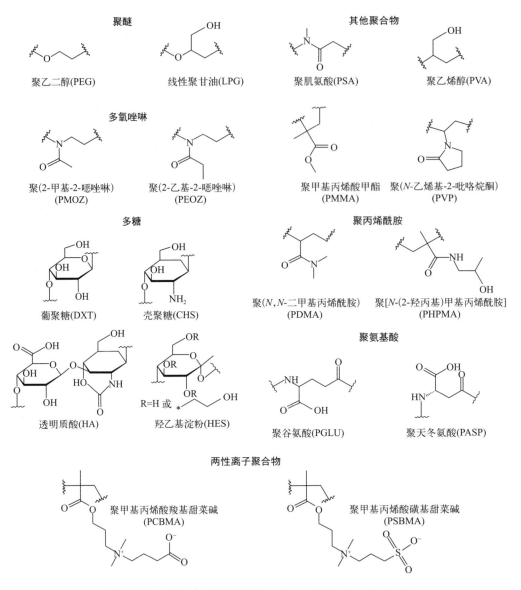

图5-3 目前已被提出和用作药物递送系统的保护性涂层

尽管PEG化是一种成功应用的策略，但它并不是完美的，因此寻找替代PEG的聚合物是一个非常活跃的领域[139]。通过PEG化，血液循环时间得到显著延长，然而，这种延长的程度还可以提高红细胞、血小板和某些抗体的血液循环时间达到1~2个月[135]。此外，最初认为PEG不具有免疫原性，但事实并非如此。早在1983年，Richter等[140]发现PEG能诱导抗体形成，随后的研究还表明这是一个显著的问题[141, 142, 143]，现在被称为加速血液清除（accelerated blood clearance，ABC）现象[144, 145]。近期一个抗PEG抗体与聚合物复合的晶体结构[146]被报道。PEG化还存在其他毒性相关问题[147, 148]。因此，构建隐形鞘的替代聚合物[109, 72, 149, 150]已经被提出并进行了研究。目前，这些替代聚合物包括：聚（2-噁唑啉）（POX）[151-158]；两性离子聚合物[159]；高支化或线性聚甘油（HPG或LPG）[160, 156, 161]；聚寡乙二醇甲基丙烯酸酯（POEGMA）[162]；聚肌氨酸（PSA）[163, 164, 165]；聚（N-乙烯基-2-吡咯烷酮）

(PVP)[166, 167]；聚乙烯醇（PVA）[167]；多种聚丙烯酰胺和聚丙烯酸酯，如聚（N, N-二甲基丙烯酰胺）（PDMA）[168]，聚[N-（2-羟丙基）甲基丙烯酰胺]（PHPMA）[169]，聚甲基丙烯酸甲酯（PMMA）[170]，Eudragit® S100[171]和聚（2-羟乙基甲基丙烯酸酯）（PHEMA）[162]，聚（N-丙烯酰吗啉）（PAcM）[162]；多糖基结构[172]，如葡聚糖（DXT）[173]，壳聚糖（CHS）[60]，透明质酸（HA）[60]，肝素[162]和羟乙基淀粉（HES）[174]；以及多肽[175-179]，包括由脯氨酸、丙氨酸和丝氨酸结构组成的共轭结构（称为PAS化）[180, 181]，以及弹性多肽[182]。关于不同聚合物在DDS中应用的案例研究也列在其他综述中[183, 68, 66]。图5-3中展示了一些聚合物的代表。尽管这些聚合物作为涂层的使用频率没有像金标准PEG那么高，但它们在改善生物相容性、生物活性、药动学、免疫原性和热力学稳定性方面具有益处[162, 149, 161, 156]。进一步研究这些涂层可能为设计新的、更符合个体化治疗需求的制剂开辟新途径[17]。

虽然目前我们已经拥有了各种类型的NP和许多不同的聚合物，并且许多已经获得内部使用批准用作药物递送载体。那么如何在PEG化的基础上进行改进呢？如何确定哪些改进什么会奏效，哪些改进又不会奏效呢？在这样一个复杂的生物体内，显然，经验性测试将使得效率大大降低。因此需要找到一种方法来发展对NP行为及疗效的机制性理解。起点是理解为什么PEG化表现出如此出色效果的机制，然而，对于其作用机制的系统理解目前尚不完全。最初，人们认为PEG化通过抑制蛋白质黏附来抵抗调理作用，即延长血液循环时间[184, 185]，然而后来的研究发现其他证据表明它实际上加速了蛋白冠的形成[186]，仍然有其他研究认为没有影响[187]。目前研究者已经提出的机制之一是，PEG鞘更倾向于结合常见的血液蛋白（白蛋白）[188]，然后形成了一个主要由白蛋白组成的蛋白冠，本身充当新的隐形鞘，从而抑制了补体激活[189]。支持这一观点的证据是蛋白冠的形成在PEG的隐形特性中起着关键作用[190]。其他被提出的机制包括直接抑制巨噬细胞的吸收[187]。最近有关这个主题的三篇综述也已发表[191, 35, 43]。

总而言之，①聚合物是制作隐形鞘的最佳材料，②目前聚合物隐形鞘的金标准是PEG，然而，③它并不是完美的隐形鞘，④仍然存在许多可能的替代物，⑤PEG本身的作用机制，即为什么它作为聚合物隐形鞘的效果如此出色，机制理解尚不全面，⑥虽然通过经验性的试错法尝试开发PEG的替代方案是可行的，但涉及的变量数量使得这种方法很快达到收益亏损点。当前需要了解的是PEG在NP表面时的行为作用方式，PEG替代方案的不同之处以及这种行为如何与其整体NP性质相关。对于这种机制性了解究竟包括哪些内容呢？请继续阅读下文。

5.1.3 机制阐释：制药学中的生物物理学范式

追求机制性理解而不是经验性方法的药物研究意味着什么？在经验性研究中，人们往往通过设计一组实验测量一组数据来确定希望达到的特定值。因此处方会因为多标准优化的过程而变化，以达到最佳值，然而随着系统复杂性的增加，这种方法的进展能力逐渐减弱。实际上，药物递送发生在人体生理极其复杂的环境中。其中API可以被药物递送机制封装，通过与血液中的生物分子相互作用，在体内"旅行"，最终通过细胞膜到达靶细胞，完成API在细胞内的功能。这个过程的各个方面都由分子间相互作用在一个极其复杂的环境中决定，这个环境中存在着各种各样的分子，API在体内的"旅程"中会经历多样的环境，最终到达目的地。因此，机制性理解是为了确定沿着这个旅程发生的事情如何与NP的结构相关联，即在分子水平上发生的相互作用是什么，以及在这个过程中发生的作用与效果有着什么样的关系。这可以将其视为生物物理学应用的范式，即理解生物系统中分子之间的物理相互作用，并应用于药物研究。

药物递送涉及极其复杂的相互作用网络，从生物物理学的角度来看，需要进行细分以便进行理解。当思考其中涉及的内容时，我们会发现一幅简化的图景，即四种不同类型的分子实体之间的相互作用：①小分子药物，尽管尺寸小，但由于其不寻常的人造结构而具有挑战性；②结构强化的生物分子，例如大分子蛋白质和核酸，具有刚性结构，并与其环境具有复杂和特殊的相互作用；③脂质膜，由各种磷脂构成的双层膜；④聚合物，大而不结构化的分子，其性质来自除精确的化学结构外的拓扑结构，例如缠结。在这四种类型结构相互作用时，在物理层面上发生了什么，这些相互作用在药物递送效率中扮演着什么角色，以及如何改善这一过程，这便代表了将生物物理学范式应用于药剂学：追求机制性理解并应用所获得的见解来提高药物递送效率。

许多不同的实验方法可以用来分析这些相互作用。虽然通过联合几种不同的实验分析方法可以获得较高程度的理解，但这种方法毕竟有限。因为每个相互独立的实验针对一个特殊的属性，若将它们结合起来，就会出现类似于"盲人摸象"的情境：一个人碰到象牙，以为是矛；另一个人碰到象鼻，以为是蛇，等等；另外还有一些盲点存在，因此无法得到分子尺度机制的完整理解。故而，目前所需的是一个能够将实验结果统一成一个能提供全面图景的分子模拟视觉模型，即展示分子实际上在做什么，而这便可以由分子动力学模拟提供。

5.1.4　分子动力学模拟：一种机制阐释的工具

分子动力学（MD）模拟是一种理论计算技术，具有直接模拟分子体系相互作用（即形成的结构以及它们的集体运动）的能力，其结果可以被视为在分子尺度上的三维空间影像。这种体系的图像能够照亮盲点并连接实验结果，与实验一起，便可以获得完整的图像。我们希望研究的分子体系实际上是一组核和电子，其相互作用和随时间的运动受一组规则控制：量子力学。精确计算这种行为涉及解一组耦合的偏微分方程，这显然是不可能的。然而，理论量子化学学科的发展，已经提供了数值求解的近似方法。可以通过使用半经验方法进一步简化模型，但是对于我们希望研究的大系统来说，计算过程复杂且计算强度大。因此，可以进行进一步的近似，以得出一种可行的方法，提供模拟我们研究系统行为的全息影像：分子力学范式。

在分子力学范式中，原子和分子被假设为经典粒子，受到其相对位置的经典势能影响。你可以直观地将所产生的原子模型想象成一组黏性的橡胶球（短程吸引的范德华力和更短程的泡利排斥力），带着静电（部分电荷模拟了原子的电负性和氢键行为），原子间通过弹簧（键力）相互连接，并且分子结构的振荡由铰链（键角相互作用）和轴承（二面角势）控制。体系内原子和分子根据牛顿的运动方程响应这些力进而移动，相互碰撞和晃动，最终产生具备原子尺度分辨率的三维空间影像。这就是MD模拟。用于进行这种模拟的势能集被称为"分子力学力场"（图5-4）。正如上面提到的，分子力学模型在观察的现象方面存在限制，许多现象超出了这一模型的范畴。例如，与金属离子的相互作用（如螯合）无法研究。由于键是模型的输入而不是输出，因此只能研究不涉及化学反应的现象。要想观察涉及化学反应（即键的断裂或形成）的现象，则必须考虑使用一定程度的量子力学计算技术，但这会导致计算量显著增加，并显著受限于可以研究的空间长度和时间尺度的增加。在某些情况下，可以在不像研究化学键的断裂和形成那样显著增加计算量的情况下解决的一个问题是pH的影响，即考虑质子化状态的变化。已经开发的所谓"常数-pH MD模拟"就是用来研究分子从一个环境转移到另一个环境时必须考虑的质子化状态的变化。

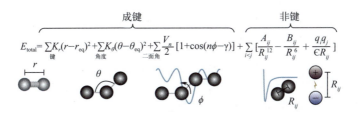

图5-4 力场的典型元素，通过总势能 E_{total} 的导数获得各项。通过测定势能集中指定的平衡值 r_{eq} 和 θ_{eq} 来测定键长 r 和角度 θ 的偏差；二面角可以通过扭曲能垒项 V_n、角度 ϕ、相位 γ 和周期性 n 来进一步描述。非键相互作用通常通过Lennard-Jones和库仑势能来描述，还可以涉及其他项（例如，用于平面外弯曲）[196]（根据CC BY 2.0许可使用）

有关确定此模型[即具备全原子（AA）分辨率的MD模拟]参数方法的讨论可以在其他综述中找到更详细的信息[198-204]。简言之，目前有四大力场用于模拟生物分子（如蛋白质、脂质、糖或核酸）体系，并且这通常也作为研究的基础，例如AMBER[205-210]、CHARMM[211-216]、OPLS-AA[217-219]和联合原子GROMOS力场[220]。这些力场存在差异的地方通常在参数化方式（包括固定原子电荷推导）和推荐的模拟设置方面，例如截断半径和长程相互作用以及1, 4-相互作用的处理[221]。基准测试则会显示各个力场的潜在优缺点[222, 223, 224]。通过使用量子力学（QM）计算或实验结果作为参考数据来开发键参数。例如，AMBER蛋白质力场的最新版本（ff19SB[205]）的二面角参数基于将16个二肽的CMAPs（ϕ/ψ 能量面）与QM数据进行匹配，并通过实验测定的核磁共振（NMR）性质（如螺旋倾向、标量耦合和 S^2 有序参数）来验证该动力学参数。对于研究含其他化学结构的系统，AmberTools的antechamber模块提供了一套程序，用于确定原子类型和初始参数。然而，用户应始终仔细审查其势能集的适用性，以回答特定的研究问题，并最好将结果与实验结果或文献进行比较。根据化学性质，如果在所选的力场集合中找不到合适的类比，可能需要基于进一步的QM计算进行广泛优化（如通过像Gaussian[225]、ORCA[226]或GAMESS[227, 228]这样的流行QM软件），也可以使用更多的支持工具，如ParaMol[229]、paramfit[230]或mdgx[231]。在其他力场方面，与CHARMM兼容的参数通常是基于CGenFF网络服务器的输出端构建[232]，初始的OPLS参数可以通过LigParGen获得[233]，而GROMOS文件可以通过ATB获取[234]。关于聚合物，还出现了构建拓扑结构（和初始结构）的其他辅助工具，包括R.E.D.[235, 236]、PolyParGen[237]、PySoftK[238]、RadonPy[239]、CHARMM-GUI Polymer Builder[240]和PSP[241]。与蛋白质力场类似，文献中可以找到使用不同力场进行聚合物动力学类型比较研究的内容[242]。对于流行的结构元素（例如PEG），已经发布了成功验证实验数据的参数集。CHARMM C35 r醚力场集被证明可以提供与实验值一致的长度和旋转半径[243]。PEG的OPLS-AA参数[244]也已发布。在粗粒化（CG）研究的势能集方面（请参见下文），通常使用参考实验或全原子数据进行验证，并在开发过程中应用不同的技术，包括迭代Boltzmann反演[245]或相对熵最小化[246]（请参阅参考文献[247]以获取更多详细信息）。与之也已经发布了对应的支撑工具，例如PyCGTOOL[248]。

一旦为要模拟的特定分子确定了势能集，则体系也将随之进行构建：设置待模拟分子的初始构型，并且要将待研究的分子进行溶解。对于具有复杂、精确结构的生物分子，迄今为止的起点便是之前确定的结构。对于蛋白质而言，一个包含这些蛋白质结构的数据库是RCSB蛋白质数据库（RCSB PDB），可以从中下载晶体结构[249]。最初，这些结构是通过实验获得的，包括X射线晶体学、核磁共振谱和越来越占主导地位的冷冻电子显微术（cryo-EM）。这个研究领域最近在基于人工智能工具方面取得了突破，可以被视为自双螺旋结构以来生命科学领域最重大的突破：基于整个已通过实验确定结构的蛋白质集合以及来自物理学、化学和进化生物学见解的AlphaFold的发展[250]。在许多情况下，通过AlphaFold获得了足够分辨率的蛋白质结构，可以作为MD模拟的起点，然而各研究工作也存在竞争性，这个领域正在迅速发展，不断改进的是可以通过这种方式成功地确定结构的蛋白质范围以及这些预测的准确性。一旦在模拟中确定了结构化生物分子的构象（包括质子化状态的适当处理），用于构建具有原子级分辨率的生物分子模拟系统的一个直接且日益流行的起点是基于网页的CHARMM-GUI工具[251]。在这个工具中，要研究的分子可以被溶解或纳入所选的脂质膜中。这个网页工具多年来不断扩展，现在还包括构建CG MARTINI系统（见下文）[252]、糖蛋白偶联物[253]、具有不同形状的无机纳米材料[254]或聚合物溶液和熔融体[240]。而用于在广泛构象范围内建立复杂初始配置的另一个流行工具是packmol[255]。它已成功用于构建大系统，例如寨卡病毒[256]。用于生成脂质膜系统的版本，如packmol-memgen[257]，也包含在AmberTools中[231]。在构建聚合物结构模型方面，可以使用程序pysimm，该程序采用线性避免自我交叉的随机行走算法，每一步都将单体连接到增长的链上，及时更新拓扑结构并松弛系统[258]。基于MARTINI势能场开发的程序polyply[259, 260]在随机行走期间使用广度优先搜索算法，并可以包括自定义的几何约束以控制链生长的方向（图5-5）。它包括回映射功能，并且可以轻松定制以包括基于AA或CG力场的构建模块，用于生成所需的模拟参数输入文件。研究者已将其应用于聚合物熔融体系统、环状DNA、聚合物锂离子电池以及包括PEG和葡聚糖的脂质囊泡[261]中。另一个用于准备复杂聚合物（包括树状聚合物）结构的拓扑文件工具是pyPolyBuilder[262]。

对于MD模拟的进一步细节和实际指导，包括处理远程静电相互作用以及使用不同热动力学和压力控制器进行特定温度和压力的采样，读者可以参考其他文献[263-265]。

虽然具有AA级分辨率的MD模拟已成功用于研究广泛的生物物理系统，但仍然受限于大约20 nm的长度尺度和大约1 μs至10 μs的时间尺度（取决于系统大小）；这并不足以获得对某些希望研究的现象的理解。为了研究更大的空间和时间尺度，可以选择粒子来代表比单个原子更大的结构；也就是，原子组、整个分子，甚至一组分子可以由单个粒子代表。这些模型均被称为粗粒化模型。尽管已提出了许多开发粗粒化模型的方案[266]，但其中使用最频繁的两种是MARTINI力场[259, 260]和耗散粒子动力学（DPD）[267, 268]。MARTINI力场使用CG粒子，这些粒子大约是3个原子的组合（对于旧版本的力场，大约4个原子），该模型的势能参数是基于这些组的溶解度参数。而DPD中，粗粒化程度更大：粒子代表软性的"动量载体"，通过恒温器控制温度，以保持在这种更大的空间和时间尺度下流体动力学效应的局部动量。

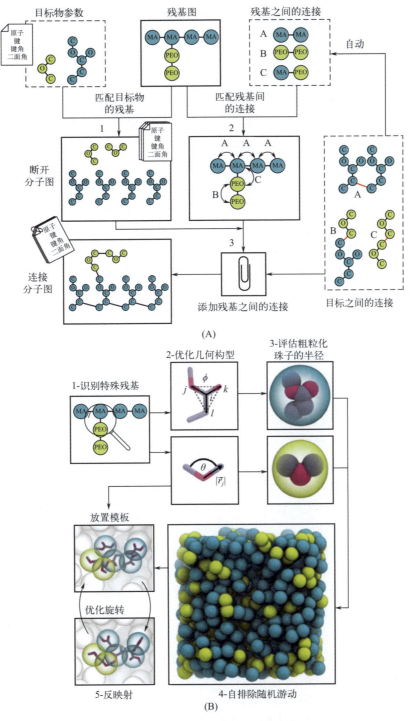

图5-5 polyply程序工作流程的示意图

（A）基于单体构建块输入，构建残基图并生成连接；（B）执行几何优化和自我排斥的随机行走[261]（根据CC BY 4.0许可使用）

使用粗粒化的CG模型进行模拟显然是有代价的。Schulten教授团队描述的"计算显微镜"方法重新聚焦到大空间尺度和长时间尺度，这会降低图像的分辨率。随着粗粒化程度的提高，详细的相互作用会缺失。例如，从AA模型转移到MARTINI势能集时，会失去氢键产生的特定行为，而当AA模型转移到更粗粒化的DPD势能集时，拓扑效应可能会缺失。一个经常被寻求和讨论的想法是"多尺度模拟"——结合不同空间和时间尺度上使用不同方法进行模拟[270]。2013年的诺贝尔化学奖被授予马丁·卡普拉斯、亚里耶·瓦谢尔和迈克尔·莱维特，以表彰他们为"复杂化学系统的多尺度模型开发"所作的贡献[271]。

现在，我们拥有了体系运动的三维轨迹，对于分析不仅仅是可视化，还有几种技术可以分析这段轨迹并从中获得对体系的有用结果。对于许多感兴趣的系统，计算的基本指标是均方根偏差（RMSD）和均方根波动（RMSF）。第一个指标RMSD基于粒子坐标之间的差异，表征了给定时间步长内结构与参考结构（例如起始构象或晶体结构）的相似性。它通常被用作系统收敛的第一个简单评估指标；RMSD值越大则表示蛋白质结构域或配体在结合位点中存在重新排列等情况。第二个指标RMSF是粒子在给定时间间隔内围绕平均结构的波动的度量。例如，蛋白质内的非结构化环通常显示出比更刚性的二级结构元素更高的RMSF值。在下一章中所描述的研究中，径向分布函数（RDF）或成对分布函数（PDF）是提供有关纳米颗粒结构中各个组分分布情况的一个重要工具；对于每个A型粒子，计算在指定的径向距离间隔内位于其中的B型粒子的数量，并随后获得相对于整个系统的归一化密度值，将局部原子密度与整体相密度进行比较。通常，这种技术最常用于溶剂原子。在氢键受体或供体周围，例如蛋白质表面的丝氨酸，通常在一定距离内的特征峰指示第一处和更远的水合层，而在较大距离r时，函数会收敛到一个值$g(r) = 1$，即与整体相溶剂密度相等[231]。也可以从球形胶束的质心开始执行这种计算。因此，可以分析沿不同轴（例如，沿膜法线）的原子分布，以获得质量密度分布。表征特定结构的溶剂暴露情况，可以提供有关药物在DDS中的封装信息。为此，通过探针粒子（半径为1.4Å）在选定原子的自由表面上进行滚动来计算Connolly溶剂可及表面积（SASA）[272]。从这些类型的计算中，可以得出两个选择质点之间的接触面积，以获得有关如哪个区域的聚合物胶束埋藏了大部分药物等的结果。为了提供胶束自组装的整体结构信息，通常计算的一个指标是回转半径，它提供所选原子到其质心的平均距离。这个指标在聚合物化学中非常重要，并且对于某些形状，例如球体，可以转化为物理半径。通常，这些值与散射实验的实验值相关。从这些值和回转半径中，可以计算关于形状表征的进一步描述符：非球度、离心率和相对形状异性，这对于区分例如蠕虫状或球形组装很重要[273]。这些指标的变化可以指示体系中的相变。此外，可以通过计算这些粒子随时间移动的距离来研究溶剂分子、药物或整个DDS的运动，以获得均方位移（MSD）值。通过足够的采样，从这些分析的斜率可以使用爱因斯坦方程导出扩散常数[274]。

近年来，基于机器学习的模式识别算法已经开发出来，可以找到比上述分析技术更精细的结构元素。例如，最近提出的无监督聚类方法[275]，该方法使用从径向-角度三粒子分布函数（g_3）生成的指纹，描述了残基内距离和角度之间的依赖关系[276, 277]（图5-6）。通过t-分布随机邻居嵌入[278]、基于密度的空间聚类应用[279]和主成分分析（PCA）[280]，对脂质的局部结构进行了表征，以有效区分膜中的不同脂质种群。最近另一项研究应用了共同近邻方法来表征局部结构环境[281]，然后通过聚类技术对生成的指纹进行进一步降维，以区分不同形状的纳米颗粒[282]。现已有多种技术用于分析涉及生物大分子模拟的高维MD轨迹数据，例如使用基于神经网络自编码器的降维方法EncoderMap[283]，用于表征蛋白质相互作用[284]。关于大规模轨迹数据分析的更多机器学习方法可以在多个近期发表的综述文章中找到[285-288]。

这些方法涵盖了轨迹分析之外的各种方法，包括粗粒化（CGnet[289, 290]），模拟量子化学相互作用[291]，马尔可夫模型（VAMPnets[292]），增强采样（例如通过学习集体变量[293]）或采样平衡分布的替代方法（Boltzmann生成器[294]）等。随着ChatGPT[295]的出现，语言模型引起了很多关注，并且已经被用于从模拟中学习概率模型[296]。此外，基于这些模型进行了各种生物信息学或化学信息学分析[297]，包括通过学习化学语言进行指标预测（SMILESBERT[298]，ChemBERTa-2[299]，polyBERT[300]和TransPolymer[301]）。机器学习技术在分子模拟领域的应用尚处于初级阶段，但它们的发展和使用程度可能会呈指数级增长。

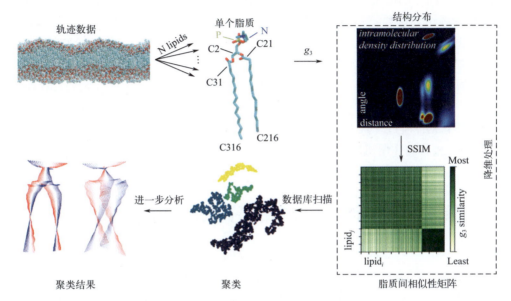

图5-6　基于机器学习的g_3分布分析概述

确定残基内角度和距离，并使用得到的指纹生成脂质相似性矩阵，通过无监督聚类进行降维处理，可以有效地区分膜内不同的脂质种群[275]（已取得Elsevier许可）

为了评估药物与潜在载体的相容性，并调整DPD模拟的参数，许多研究采用了汉森（Hansen）和弗洛里-赫金斯（Flory-Huggins）溶解度参数的概念，这些参数可以通过实验、基团贡献方法或模拟获得。弗洛里-赫金斯参数描述了两种物质的汉森溶解度参数之间的差异。而后者则表征了它们各自的内聚能，可以分为描述氢键、范德华力和偶极-偶极相互作用的各部分。因此，较低的弗洛里-赫金斯参数表明两种物质之间的混溶性或相容性较高[302-304]。基于几何、重量和拓扑的R3m描述符[305, 306]，可作为弗洛里-赫金斯参数的替代。此外，本章中引用的许多工作都应用了分子力学泊松-玻尔兹曼/广义玻恩表面积（MM-PBSA或MM-GBSA）计算，通常在蛋白质-配体复合物上进行，以预测药物在药物传递载体中的结合自由能，从而区分有利和不利的载药过程。该概念基于计算单个分子和复合物的溶剂自由能，以及在气相中的结合自由能，以获得在溶剂中的结合能作为热力学循环的手段[307, 308]。

上述大多数可以计算的指标是静态性质，与动态性质相对，即它们仅依赖于系统不同构象的采样频率，而不依赖于构象空间中的路径。如果只对系统的静态性质感兴趣，而不是动态性质，那么可以使用破坏真实动力学的算法，仅输出构象空间中概率分布的结果。尽管多尺度建模以及上述分析技术能够在一系列空间和时间尺度上提供对系统的理解,但仍存在一个限制:系统仍停留在构象空间中最有利的区域;有时,回答某些问题需要从远离这个区域的信息中获取理解。一旦摆脱了系统真实动力学的约束,就可以使用方法来提供构象空间中特定感兴趣的区域的信息,而不是聚焦于最高概率的区域。借助这些工具,可以确定构象空间中不同区域之间的自由能差异,或者沿着构象空间中的特定路径[通常称为平均力势(PMF)]采样。这种增强采样技术包括扇形采样[309]、元动力学[310]和拉伸分子动力学(SMD)[311]。然而,必须注意的是,从模拟中获取这种先进的准确自由能计算是一项具有挑战性且计算成本高昂的任务。这可以用于高效采样药物分子从胶束中释放的路径,或者观察胶束通过膜的渗透。例如,沿着感兴趣的(多维)反应坐标构建的PMF能量轮廓,可以估计通过结构调控来增强药物从聚合物胶束中释放的情况[312, 2]。关于这些增强采样方法的更多细节可以在最新综述文章中找到[312]。

对于实际应用和提到的表征工具的详细信息,流行模拟软件的手册(例如GROMACS[313]和AMBER[231])可以提供进一步的指导。我们现在已经明确了实现机制性理解的愿景和希望讨论的工具:MD模拟。接下来,将继续专注于使用MD模拟作为工具,以阐释与聚合物基NP的隐形鞘相关的作用机制,并以此作为将MD模拟用作药剂学设计研究工具的案例。

5.2 聚合物在药物递送中的分子动力学模拟

关于PEG化,在本书之前版本的相关章节中讨论了PEG模型的发展历史[124];对于所有聚合物的模型构建,这个主题涉及的内容过于广泛,在此不进行讨论。对此感兴趣的读者可以参考有关纳米颗粒建模的其他相关资源和综述文章[67, 242, 314-322]。现在,DDS中基于聚合物修饰的最近分子模拟研究,大致分为基于脂质、聚合物、蛋白质和无机纳米颗粒(NP)。需要注意的是,在文献中可以找到许多不同的术语来描述相同类型的纳米颗粒。由于界限变得模糊,不可避免地会出现一些重大重叠,例如,多肽可以用作形成聚合物胶束的基础。此外,聚合物结构在DDS中的作用是多方面的,例如,聚合物不仅可以作为载体增强药物溶解性,而且还可以将API从潜在的蛋白质吸附中游离。因此,聚合物辅料的"保护作用"不能总是严格地与系统中的其他目的分开。接下来的几节将总结如何在AA和CG级别上进行特定的PEG化模拟研究。这两种技术相互补充,共同提供了DDS动态作用的更丰富的画面。因此,通过呈现最近研究的结果,读者能清楚地了解到多尺度模拟方法的重要性。实质上,在研究大尺度、以流体动力学为驱动的结构变化时,DPD模型非常有用,例如,用于研究药物装载或聚合物浓度对胶束形态的影响。相比之下,当试图考察分子间相互作用的基础时,例如药物与其递送系统之间的相互作用,建议使用AA模拟。虽然CG级别的模拟在这方面可以提供一些信息,但AA模拟允许对更复杂的相互作用进行详细分析,例如氢键和π-π堆积。因此,模型的选择应该取决于要回答的研究问题。

5.2.1 基于脂质的体系

本部分将从描述研究结果开始,这些研究结果提供了关于PEG化脂质体结构的动态视野，包括功能化的靶向基团以及LNP。

5.2.1.1 聚乙二醇化脂质体

脂质体的模拟[21]和关于PEG化脂质体和小分子药物相互作用的研究工作[125]已发表综述。分子模拟可以阐明PEG化如何影响细胞膜动力学、聚合物与细胞膜的相互作用、表面电荷以及DDS与血液中蛋白质的相互作用。这些现象取决于PEG长度、结构和接枝密度、膜的组成、盐浓度以及可能的血液中蛋白质相互作用的类型[32, 33, 323]。虽然这些可以在实验中进行研究[147]，但AA和CG分辨率下的分子模拟可以补充相关画面[324, 259]。许多文章已经为其中的一些问题提供了答案[124]。此外，PEG的模拟已被用于除药物研究之外的其他领域，例如作为电池电解质[325-341]，在基质中的离子传输[330, 331, 336, 338, 339, 340, 342]，或作为离子液体成分[334, 335]。

早在1998年，Rex等[343]就对PEG化膜进行了模拟，当时的实验工作得到了蒙特卡洛（MC）模拟的补充。然而，那时只能描述一个基本缔合聚合物的图像，与Alexander-de Gennes理论[344-347]一致。该PEG化膜是用这个简化的缔合聚合物表面模型来描述的：根据接枝密度、聚合物长度和刚度，聚合物要么形成"蘑菇"状，在其中与其他聚合物链没有相互作用，该层的厚度与聚合物长度的平方根成比例关系；要么形成"刷子"状，其中由于分子间聚合物相互作用，其厚度与长度成线性比例关系。随后，采用MARTINI力场[348, 349]或DPD方法[350]的CG模拟详细阐述了这一范式，并显示了相行为与聚合物长度和接枝密度的依赖关系。虽然这两种不同状态的图像贯穿整个文献中，但具有亲水性醚基团和疏水性$(CH_2)_2$元素的两性PEG的动力学模拟可能更加复杂。

采用AA级别分辨率进行模拟[244, 351, 138, 125, 352]，研究始于对凝胶状态的简单膜体系进行模拟，使用二硬脂酰磷脂酰胆碱（DSPC）代表凝胶状态，以及使用二亚油酰磷脂酰胆碱（DLPC）代表液晶（LC）状态，然后加入胆固醇以有效模拟Doxil®膜（见表5-1）。对DSPC和DLPC膜进行了PEG化和非PEG化的模拟，然后进行比较。首先在生理水平下采用氯化钠进行模拟，随后在氯化钙和氯化钾存在下进行模拟，其离子强度相似[351]。结果表明在钠离子存在的模拟中，PEG在这些粒子周围缠绕，与大约五个氧原子配位一个带正电的盐离子［图5-7（A）］。这种结合行为因获得诺贝尔奖的冠醚而闻名[354]，并在早些时候观察到[133, 134]。钾在动力学上与钠相似，但复合作用较弱，而对于能促进膜融合的钙离子[355]，取而代之与脂质头部相互作用。这个过程可能会受到保护性PEG冠层的立体阻碍。

在PEG与膜的相互作用方面，聚合物链被发现进入了松散结构的LC膜中，这与PEG在极性和非极性溶剂中的溶解性一致[130]。在10%的接枝密度下，PEG不能进入更有序的凝胶膜，该膜的脂质面积较小。对于这种情况，膜的排斥导致聚合物密度在脂质上方增加，从而将带负电的氯离子排出。相比之下，LC膜的PEG化导致形成PEG层内含氯离子的水团簇。Vucovic等也报告了氯离子的这种现象[356]。这也会在凝胶膜中出现，尤其在更低的PEG接枝密度下（5%）。这些观察结果表明，在引起氯离子排出的较高接枝密度下，表面变为带正电，这曾在未经PEG化的LDS中发现。根据补体激活的决定性因素[323]，更低的5%接枝密度可能代表了更有利于药物递送的膜组成[357]。

Doxil®制剂中也包含胆固醇[135, 75]。尽管在未经PEG化的膜中，胆固醇可以减少脂质分子头基面积，从而导致液态相中的脂质双层浓缩，或者在凝胶状态下进行液化[358, 359]，模拟

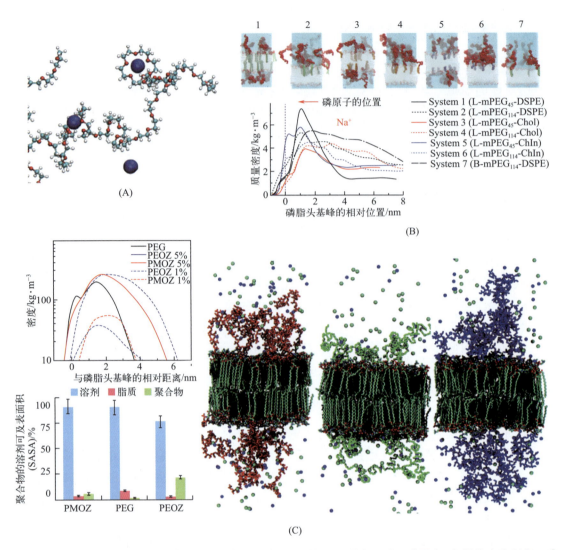

图5-7 （A）PEG围绕钠离子（蓝色球体）建立与其乙醚氧原子的相互作用[图（A）转载自文献[244]，版权2011年，美国化学学会]。（B）具有不同聚合物结构、长度和连接位点的PEG化膜的模拟快照（L-mPEG=线性单甲氧-PEG；B-mPEG=支化单甲氧基-PEG；DSPE=1，2-二硬脂酸-sn-甘油-3-磷酸乙醇胺；Chol=胆固醇；ChIn=氯烷），下方显示磷脂头基周围钠离子的质量密度分布图。对于PEG-氯烷偶联物，头基附近有一个大的次级峰[图（B）转载自文献[114]，版权2020年，美国化学学会]。（C）两种不同制剂密度的质量密度分布图，涉及PMOZ化（红色）、PEG化（绿色）或PMEOZ化（蓝色）脂质膜的模拟快照。PEG质量密度分布图中的次级峰表明PEG穿透了脂质膜，与PMOZ和PMEOZ的发现相反。PEOZ的较大聚合物-聚合物接触区域强调这种聚合物之间的相互作用比穿透膜更强[图（C）转载自文献[155]，版权2017年，得到Elsevier的许可]

工作显示插入在PEG化脂质双层中的胆固醇会导致脂质分子头基面积增加[352]。通过PEG与胆固醇β表面的相互作用，后者的有序效应[358, 359]将被抑制。而在使用CG MARTINI模型[360]进行模拟的研究中，无法观察到这种行为，这也是上述描述的聚合物阳离子相互作用的情况。

最近，研究者还通过计算机模拟补充了关于PEG化脂质体在体内、体外药动学方面的研究[114]。根据保护性涂层的链长、结构和连接位点，重要的鞘层性质发生了变化。与实验结果一致，分支的PEG链在脂质膜周围提供了比线性变体更厚的层，这也通过质量密度轮廓进行了阐释。对于PEG连接到胆烷而不是磷脂或胆固醇的情况，钠离子对磷脂头基的接触反而增加[图5-7（B）]。PEG-胆烷偶联导致了整体上更高的膜紊乱度，从而导致较差的鞘层性质。

此外，基于负载药物的PEG化脂质体的动力学研究[361]，结合相关实验工作发现，模型化合物5, 10, 15, 20-四（4-羟基苯基）卟啉不仅停留在疏水的脂质双层内，还停留在PEG层内。因此，通过与亲脂性载体的相互作用，聚合物的两亲性质影响了载体的药物负载功能；这也适用于对AETP靶向基团的描述[138]（见5.2.1.2）。

正如前面提到的，阐明PEG化DDS在体内的行为也是非常重要的。当进入血液循环时，药物载体会遇到可以改变大小和形状等特性的流体动力学力。这种影响可以使用不同的理论计算方法[362]或称为有限元法的分段连续模型来进行研究[363]。蛋白冠的形成仍然没有完全理解[364]，但应该受到上述基于PEG调节的影响，例如表面电荷的改变。使用当今的计算资源，DDS与生物实体相互作用进行模拟的研究正在迅速增加，并可能有助于在不久的将来更全面地阐释蛋白冠的作用及其机制[365]。

前面已提到CG方法无法捕获AA模拟的一些结果。当使用MARTINI模型时，关键的相互作用细节可能会丧失[366]。然而，CG方法可以在动力学的另一个层面上为研究者提供见解：通过MARTINI模型可以考察PEG长度和密度依赖的混合相、胶束、双胶片或脂质体之间的形态转变[367, 368, 348, 369]，甚至通过DPD模拟也可以观察到更多的LDS形状[370, 371]。利用不同分辨率的多个模型通常可以为所关注的体系提供更大尺度的全貌信息，并将这种方法称为"多尺度模拟"[270]，本章中还会讲述更多应用这种技术的示例研究。

5.2.1.2 具有靶向配体系统

DDS的表面可以连接不同的基团，用于靶向药物递送。这些基团旨在诱导受体介导的内吞作用。可以说，最受欢迎的变体是精氨酰甘氨酰天冬氨酸（RGD），通过与整合素的结合导致细胞黏附[372]。总体而言，这种技术对于靶向药物递送非常有用，可以将药物分子输送到表达某些膜结合受体的癌细胞。另一种提出的靶向基团AETP，虽然在筛选目标受体方面取得了成功，但当修饰PEG化膜时却失败了。与RGD序列相比，AETP更具疏水性，因此认为它会被脂质膜所掩盖。然而，分子动力学模拟结果表明事实并非如此：部分具有疏水性的保护性PEG层才是遮盖更具疏水的AETP基团的原因[138]。

基于此，通过AA分辨率模拟了两种PEG替代物与双层脂质中偶联的情况：一种是更亲水的聚（2-甲基-2-噁唑啉）（PMOZ）[373]，另一种是更疏水的聚（2-乙基-2-噁唑啉）（PEOZ）[155][图5-7（C）]。在PMOZ情况下，靶向基团AETP更易暴露于溶剂中，因此在与PEG情况下的结果相比，可能更有效。此外，与金标准相反，POX变体不会渗透到脂质双层中，也不会与钠离子发生相互作用，这与先前观察到的聚合物电解质PEG[244]的情况相同。然而，对于更亲水的RGD多肽而言，PEG显示出比PMOZ甚至是PEOZ更大的基团暴露。这项研究清楚地证明了保护修饰的选择如何影响靶向基团的活性，以及如何通过分子模拟来研究这种现象。

另一项最近的研究描述了用于靶向非糖基化蛋白受体（ASGPR）治疗肝癌的 N- 乙酰半乳糖胺修饰的 PEG 化脂质体。由此可推测类似的模拟工作未来可以剖析 POX 变体或其他 PEG 替代物是否提高了靶向效率[374]。

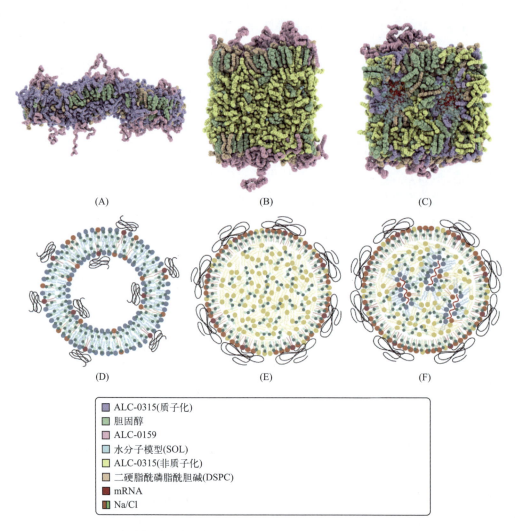

图 5-8　Corminaty 疫苗成分的模拟自组装结果，上部分为模拟快照，下部分为相应纳米载体结构的示意图。（A）和（D）在低 pH 下形成脂质双分子层，其中（ALC-0315）变体被质子化。（B）和（E）形成中性 ALC-0315 变体的单分子层。（C）和（F）在 mRNA 负载后，观察到核酸与 LNP 核心中质子化变体的相互作用。[图（A）~（F）转载自[128]，版权 2022 年，得到 Elsevier 的许可）

5.2.1.3　脂质纳米颗粒

基于 LNP 的基因递送目前引发了科学家的极大关注，尤其是随着两款 mRNA 疫苗的问世，这两款疫苗分别由 Pfizer BioNTech 和 Moderna 两家公司研发。正如之前提到的，PEG 化脂质主要用于 DDS 纳米制剂的稳定性，而不是作为保护性涂层。为了详细分析 mRNA Corminaty 疫苗的组成，Trollmann 等最近在 AA 级别分辨率上进行了模拟，使用微秒级时间尺度模拟包含不同种类NP的多个体系，其中包括用于观察相关脂质的自组装模型，如可质子化的氨基脂质（（4-羟基丁基）氮杂二烷基）双（己烷-6,1-二基）双（2-己基癸酸酯）（ALC-0315）和PEG化脂质2-[（聚乙二醇）-2000-N, N-二十四烷基乙酰胺]（ALC-0159），以及带或不带短mRNA链和不同质子化状态的模型。然后对体系的不同性质如PEG化外层和NP核心的脂质组成、散射强度以及膜弯曲模量进行了分析。模拟脂质双层状体系[图5-8（A）和（D）]的质量密度轮廓表明，在低pH下脂质体系呈现高度无序的组成（与先前[129]的原子水平理解一致）。中性pH的质子化变化，导致相变，将疏水性中性氨基脂质夹在两个高度有序的单分子层之间，因此形成了LNP[图5-8（B）和（E）]。这种内化导致了PEG覆盖的表面积增加。通过脂质/mRNA混合物的自组装研究，并且模拟不同数量质子化状态的氨基脂质发现，对于完全中和的情况，mRNA扩散到水相中，表明需要质子化变体来包裹带负电的核酸以成功实现药物递送。在LNP核心内，只有少量的DSPC分子是这种mRNA封装。此外，还观察到了包含核酸以及水的柱状结构[图5-8（C）和（F）]，类似于倒六角相。对不含mRNA的完整NP的进一步模拟显示了核心和外壳中单个成分的分布情况。无mRNA LNP模拟的散射数据与低q值的实验结果相符。在中性pH条件下，PEG层优先覆盖中性氨基脂质分子，DSPC/胆固醇域在溶剂中的暴露程度增加，因此可能在体内促使其与载脂蛋白E结合。尽管核心和外壳中胆固醇浓度较高（后者接近溶解度极限），但没有观察到晶体形成，核心形成了疏水相。研究者指出，在mRNA存在的情况下不能排除多层结构的存在，基于估计的尺寸（无mRNA，约35 nm；有mRNA，约50 nm），考虑到磷脂含量较低，这似乎不太可能。总之，在低pH条件下，可质子化的氨基脂质充当开关的作用，导致LNP核心在核内体进行解体。随后，由ALC-0315引起的核内体膜不稳定性倒六角相的形成将使mRNA递送到细胞质中。此外，可将上述提到的恒定pH MD方法应用于此体系以进一步阐明其作用机制。

回溯文献中研究的其他模拟的LNP，对负载DOX的DPSC-PEG2000组装进行了NMR研究，并进行了具有PEG2000链（长度为45个单体）的AA模拟。这些模拟补充了NMR实验的结果：球形起始结构转变为椭圆形状，柔性的PEG链形成了冠。NH碳酸酯的回转半径值比磷原子的值小，这表明前者被嵌入脂质头部中，形成了有利的氢键。进一步研究发现NMR实验获得的脂肪酸尾部与磷脂头部的接触是源于脂质链的错开排列[375]。最后，另一项计算机模拟研究考察了树胶和CHS作为天然脂质的替代涂层，用以携带舒尼替尼[376]。基于脂质类型的差异，NP的紧实度、聚合物-脂质相互作用以及聚合物的溶剂暴露情况都有所不同。

5.2.2 基于聚合物的体系

基于聚合物的DDS主要涉及聚合物胶束和树状聚合物，但也包括涉及其他结构（如聚合物颗粒）的模拟研究。

5.2.2.1 聚合物胶束－整体形态和载药行为

正如表5-1所示，目前批准的可作为药物递送系统的聚合物胶束并不多。许多聚合物胶束正在临床试验中，关于这些体系已经发表了大量的实验和模拟研究。通过调整聚合物的组成和结构，可以得到所形成的组装体的化学和形态多样性。模拟技术有助于找到适合特定药物的最佳载体。载药的完整聚合物组装体代表非常庞大的体系，大多数研究采用CG方法。因此，本章提及的大部分分子模拟研究都使用DPD方法，该方法在调整聚合物长度、药物浓度或pH值时可以进行大规模形态转变的研究。随着计算资源的增加，越来越多AA级模拟研究已发表，这也使得科学家们能更详细地研究聚合物与药物之间的特定相互作用。另一种流行的替代方法是模拟较小的体系，其中包含较短的聚合物和较少的药物，然后将所得的结果推广到较大的体系中。

早在2009年，Kuramochi等就对由相对较短的两亲性N-乙酰化PEG-聚（γ-苯乙基-L-谷氨酸）双嵌段共聚物构成的小型胶束模型进行了7 ns的AA级模拟，分别研究了椭圆形胶束中聚合物部分的分布、水含量和扩散性、PDF以及聚合物二面角。结果表明，核心区和外壳区均含有不断与溶剂交换的水分子。在核心区，水分子形成了较小的团簇，并与疏水区域的酯基和酰胺基之间形成氢键；而外层的PEG壳形成了螺旋构象[377]。

Guo等使用DPD方法研究了将药物负载到已自组装成聚合物胶束中的作用机制。药物的负载效率取决于疏水块的长度、与药物的混溶性，还有药物分子的拓扑结构。尺寸较小且分支的化合物比线性且尺寸较大的化合物更容易扩散到内核。如果疏水块的长度过长，保护性的壳不能有效地覆盖内核，从而无法防止胶束的聚集[378]。此外，还使用DPD方法模拟研究了由疏水性二十二碳烯酸（DHA）-组氨酸块和亲水性赖氨酸块组成的DOX负载胶束，以研究聚合物和药物组成对胶束形态的影响[379]。另一项DPD研究考察了不同溶剂中含有PS-PEG嵌段共聚物和NP聚合物胶束的形成。随着亲水性珠子数量的增加，凝聚时间延长[380]。

Loverde等采用了多尺度模拟的方法，分析了紫杉醇在PEG-聚己内酯（PCL）嵌段共聚物胶束中的行为。首先，从低聚物熔体的AA级模拟和正辛醇-水药物分配实验中推导出适用于CG模型的参数。然后，使用CG模型来研究不同的胶束形态。与之前实验得出的相图一致，根据嵌段长度，可以找到蠕虫状、球形、双分子层和聚集体等不同形态[图5-9（A）]。通过研究不同浓度下的药物分布和均方位移（MSD）发现，与实验结果一致，由非平衡动力学将药物从胶束中拉出的结果显示，蠕虫状组装具有最高的药物负载能力。在较高的负载量下，药物与保护冠的相互作用增加，更多的紫杉醇位于两块的界面上，实际上药物在保护冠内的扩散比在内核中更慢。药物-冠层相互作用与观察到的DDS快速释放一致，并且可以通过调节含有乙醇酸重复单元的冠层来进行调整。因此，这项研究成功地演示了分子模拟如何用于检测亲水性外壳的功能，其已不仅仅发挥保护冠的作用[381]。除了通过额外的乙醇酸单元修饰PEG壳外，精氨酸基团最近也被发现具有增强内吞作用[382]。

Kasimova等通过模拟获取弗洛里-赫金斯参数以评估药物负载的能力[303]，并在AA级别上研究了PEG-聚乳酸（PLA）嵌段共聚物在不同亲水性药物分子存在下的紧实度。相较于简单的核-壳模型，在聚合物聚集体中没有明显的亲水性和疏水性聚合物基团之间的分离，同时还含有少量水分子。对于每个模型体系，他们推导出出了弗洛里-赫金斯参数，并成功将其与实验确定的药物负载能力高度相关联。在关于CHS接枝甘油单油酸的计算工作中，亲水性和疏水性块的汉森溶解度参数也成功用于预测药物负载能力[385]。另一项研究也采用了类似的方法：从AA模拟中推导出弗洛里-赫金斯参数，以评估含5-氨基戊二酸甲酯聚合物前药的影响，随后进行了DPD研究以观察胶束的形态。与实验结果一致，前药的更高接枝比与其更高的药物负载能力相关，因为更多的前药基团位于胶束的内核中[386]。

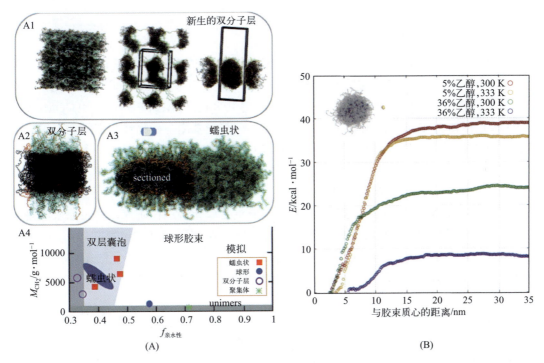

图5-9 （A1）Loverde[381]的粗粒化研究展示PEG1000-PCL3000自组装成新双分子层的过程（PEG为橙色，PCL为黑色，水合层为青色）。（A2）PEG2000-PCL7700的双分子层结构。（A3）PEG2000-PCL5000的蠕虫状组装。（A4）不同形状的粗粒化模拟位置在之前实验确定的相图中的位置[383]，取决于聚合物分子量及其亲水性分数$f_{亲水性}$[图（A1）~（A4）转载自文献[381]，版权2011年，约翰威利父子出版公司]。（B）从PLA-PEG胶束（PLA＝蓝色；PEG＝灰色）中拉出紫杉醇（黄色球体）的温度和共溶剂依赖的PMF曲线[图（B）转载自文献[384]，版权2022年，美国化学学会]

最近研究人员对负载葫芦素的PEG-PLA基胶束进行了AA级模拟，详细分析了不同胶束成分（包括溶剂）之间的氢键数量和寿命。根据MSD分析，扩散可以得到表征。研究结果显示，聚合物-药物氢键的寿命要比与溶剂相关的氢键长得多。与先前仅包含一个聚合物链的药物分子的伪胶束模拟结果相比较，药物和溶剂分子表现出亚扩散运动。因此，该研究显示了如何对较小模型体系进行模拟，它通常用于模拟大型全长聚合物组装以减少计算成本，但并不能总是检测到大型体系中存在的所有运动[387]。通过CG MARTINI方法研究了胶束形状、药物封装和从两性PAC负载的PEG-PLA嵌段共聚物组装中的释放过程发现，从AA模拟中获得的参数与实验玻璃化转变温度的结果相一致，这也用作粗粒化模拟的基础。然后，模拟具有不同摩尔比的聚合物和药物分子的体系，并分析了相关指标，如回转半径、药物封装效率（基于所谓的锥算法[388]）、相对形状各向异性和偏心率，以描述胶束形状、药物分布、随时间变化的聚合物簇数以及SASA。从所提到的形状描述符中发现，未负载药物的胶束呈现球形形态，而负载药物的胶束则可以形成蠕虫状或棒状结构，从某一聚集数开始，各向异性的显著增加可以确定临界相变点。此外，还可使用SMD（从胶束中心拉出单个药物分子）研究胶束的稳定性，从中可以计算出PMF[图5-9（B）]。这些结果表明，较高的温度和增加的乙醇浓度可能会使得递送系统失稳[384]。

5.2.2.2 聚合物胶束 –pH 影响

近期许多模拟研究都涉及 pH 变化对胶束稳定性和相变的影响。这是 DDS 重要研究领域之一，因为抗癌药物针对的通常是形成酸性微环境的肿瘤细胞。Luo 等采用多尺度模拟方法研究了负载喜树碱的两性聚（β-氨基酯）-聚乙二醇共聚物（PAE-PEG）。使用 COMPASS 力场的 AA 级模拟，由 RDF 的结果表明，聚合物中心羧基酯基团与药物羟基之间的氢键有利微环境会在前者质子化后消失。然后，从这些模拟中计算出弗洛里-赫金斯参数，并将其用作 DPD 方法的基础。不同的药物浓度导致了从球形到盘状的不同的胶束组装。从这些观察中得出了一个吸附生长机制，药物负载发生在核心和 PEG 涂层的界面处。除了胶束化，pH 响应性药物释放也可以通过以质子化形式模拟中心酯重复单元来进行研究，这在原子级别上曾开展过[390]。Guo 等使用 DPD 方法作为工具来评估基于胆固醇偶联的组氨酸-精氨酸多肽负载 DOX 后的胶束形态。与实验结果一致，在 pH 低于 6 时，疏水中性组氨酸基团在核心内允许更高的药物负载，然而带电变体的存在导致胶束肿胀，尤其是在较高 pH 下，从而促进药物释放[391]。

使用介观动力学和 DPD（MesoDyn）分析了负载布洛芬的聚合物胶束，该胶束由聚甲基丙烯酸甲酯-co-甲基丙烯酸-b-聚（聚乙二醇甲基醚甲基丙烯酸酯[P（MMA-co-MAA）-b-PPEGMA]组成。模拟结果表明实验形成了核-壳聚合物胶束，随后药物扩散到疏水性核心。不同药物浓度会导致包括层状结构在内的不同的形态。在 pH 高于 5 的条件下对系统进行模拟会导致中心甲基丙烯酸重复单元的去质子化，产生非常疏松的聚集体，从而证实了实验所确定的增强药物释放特性的结构[392]。通过 DPD 研究了 pH 依赖的基于两性 PEG-PAE-PLA 三嵌段共聚物的负载 DOX 胶束的不同形态，以寻找最优的聚合物和药物含量。低 pH 下 PAE 的质子化形成了增强药物释放的特殊结构[393]。类似的研究还在通过 DPD 模拟负载 DOX 的星形共聚物胶束中获得[394, 395]。在类似的方式下，也有研究考察了在疏水/亲水界面处具有化学交联的聚合物胶束，结果表明在酸性 pH 下，pH 响应性三嵌段共聚物组装体中负载的疏水性二环戊二烯持续释放[396]。对于二硒化物星形聚合物，观察到具有持续释放特性的交联胶束具有更高的稳定性[397]。

另一项研究提出了针对 pH 敏感聚合物胶束的合理设计指南：基于药物与聚合物的相容性，不同块的长度可以在不同程度上影响 pH 依赖性的药物释放。较长的疏水块可以导致较大的溶剂接触面积[图 5-10（A）]，从而增强药物释放，然而，这也可能导致核心网络紧凑，进而降低药物扩散。增加亲水块的长度可能会阻碍较大胶束的形成。因此，更多较小的胶束实际上可能会导致更高的药物扩散和释放。最后，如果药物分布在 pH 敏感的块附近显示高浓度，那么聚合物的长度将极大地影响药物释放特性[398]。

另一项通过 DPD 研究关于 pH 敏感的星形聚合物胶束也提出了指南：如上所述，增加 pH 敏感块的长度将增强 pH 依赖性的药物释放。增加疏水块的长度可以增加药物装载量，但对胶束稳定性不利。对于亲水性 PEG 外壳而言，研究报道的情况则相反[400]。基于 DPD 模拟的研究还对 PCL-b-聚二乙基氨乙基甲基丙烯酸酯-b-聚（甲基丙烯酸磺基甜菜碱）（PCL-PDEA-PSBMA）或聚乙二醇甲基丙烯酸酯（PEGMA）三嵌段共聚物胶束的 pH 响应性药物释放进行了研究。不同聚合物浓度和密度分析表明，更亲水和带电荷的新型涂层剂 PSBMA 形成了更均匀的外壳，以及均一球形的负载 DOX 药物的聚集体，这与 PEGMA 涂层的结构相反[401]。在另一项研究中也观察到了类似的情况：通过DPD模拟分析了基于DHA-*b*-聚（γ-苯基-L-谷氨酸）-*b*-聚（甲基丙烯酸羧基甜菜碱）（DHA-PBLG-PCBMA）胶束的pH响应性药物释放过程。与使用PEG作为涂层的变种相比，带电荷的PCB表现出更紧凑的外壳[402]。

基于聚（甲基丙烯酸甲酯-*co*-甲基丙烯酸）-*b*-聚（氨基乙基甲基丙烯酸酯）[poly（MMA-*co*-MAA）-*b*-PAEMA]的聚合物胶束，根据不同的药物负载量和块长度，通过DPD模拟研究了pH响应性药物释放过程，以寻找药物、亲水块和疏水块之间的最佳比例。为完成这一目标，使用了布洛芬（IBU）药物[见图5-10（B）]。与上述多个研究相比，在碱性pH条件下，外部聚集体中的药物浓度较高，这将有助于药物在肠道中的释放[399]。使用混合胶束是实现pH响应性行为的另一途径，例如，基于亲水性PEG块与PCL或甲醚-*b*-聚（*N*，*N*-二乙基氨基乙基甲基丙烯酸酯）结合。虽然后者的质子化可以在酸性pH下导致药物释放，但非质子化的PCL变体提供了持续的释放特性。最近通过DPD方法研究了不同浓度依赖的形态和药物分布的DOX负载变体[403]。另一个混合胶束的例子是聚（*N*，*N*-二乙基氨基乙基甲基丙烯酸酯）-*b*-聚（聚乙二醇甲基醚甲基丙烯酸酯）（PDEAEMA-PPEGMA）和PCL-PPEGMA。这种混合胶束在实验和DPD模拟中的MSD研究结果显示出DOX的初始爆发释放[404]。

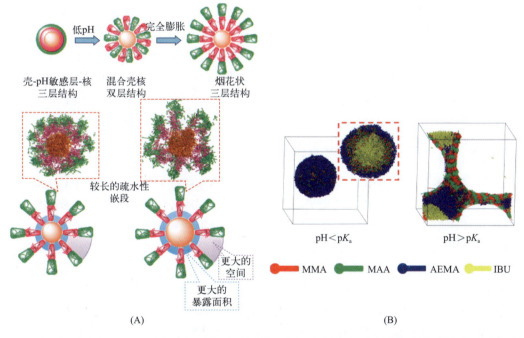

图5-10 （A）酸性条件下，通过DPD模拟观察到的pH敏感的ABC三嵌段共聚物胶束膨胀过程的示意图。pH敏感的B块（粉色）水合增加导致了混合的壳-核结构。随后，亲水性的A块（绿色）进一步膨胀形成三层结构。使用更长的疏水性C块（橙色）在这个膨胀过程后将导致更大的暴露面积[图（A）根据文献[398]的许可转载]。（B）DPD模拟显示负载布洛芬（IBU）的聚甲基丙烯酸甲酯-甲基丙烯酸甲酯嵌段共聚物-*b*-聚[2-（2-氨基乙氧基）乙基甲基丙烯酰胺]系统在碱性pH条件下的形态变化，表明药物在这些条件下释放[图（B）从文献[399]转载，根据CC BY 4.0许可使用]

De Luca等通过全原子模拟研究了pH响应性聚（4-乙烯基咪唑）-b-聚（丙烯酸）（PVI-b-PAA）对肽类的控释，以Gly-Lys（Arg）$_2$作为模型化合物。在pH由7变为4时，由于静电斥力，模拟显示了肽和聚合物载体之间的距离增加[405]。

另有研究者使用DPD模型模拟展示了DOX药物负载的两亲性聚合物胶束的组装和pH依赖性药物释放过程，并对实验结果进行了补充[406]。这些胶束由线性或星形的戊二酸酯-[PLGA-b-聚（N, N-二乙基氨基乙基甲基丙烯酸酯）聚（乙二醇）单甲醚]构成。与实验药物释放曲线一致，在pH低于5时，仍有少量的DOX分子留在聚合物胶束中。

除了pH响应外，某些结构还可以提供温度或氧化还原敏感的相变。例如，由聚{g-2-[2-（2-甲氧基乙氧基）乙氧基]乙氧基-3-己内酯}（PMEEECL）和PAE组成的双响应性聚合物胶束，前者具有温度响应性，在特定温度以上不溶，而后者对pH变化敏感。通过AA级模拟进行了线圈到球体转变温度的评估，并通过计算回转半径进行表示。增加PAE块长度导致这一温度的降低。随后，使用MARTINI力场进行粗粒化模拟，这有助于解析胶束的自组装和pH依赖性的形态转变；通过RDF、药物扩散以及颗粒大小和聚集数的测定等分析研究结果表明，DOX首先被纳入胶束的核-壳界面，然后在保护冠层逐渐积累[407]。

磁响性也在研究范围内，例如，将磁性氧化铁颗粒装载到聚合物胶束中进行实验研究，并通过CG方法进行计算模拟。此外，基于二硫键结合的两性PEG-PCL结构已成功地装载油酸和无机颗粒的聚集体，形成了可对氧化还原敏感的刺激响应释放系统，这可成功用于药物递送[408]。类似的其他研究还包括：通过DPD模拟研究基于氧化还原和pH敏感的由多西他赛（DOC）负载的PEG-聚乳酸-羟基乙酸共聚物（PLGA）-SS-DOX组成的聚合物前药在不同药物浓度下球形胶束的形成过程；通过模拟断裂的二硫键来研究PEG-SS-PPEGMA胶束中的药物释放过程[409]。

5.2.2.3 聚合物胶束-与膜的相互作用

目前，已有多项研究考察了聚合物胶束与膜的相互作用。例如：一项基于CG MARTINI模拟的研究调查了载药聚（乙基乙烯）-聚乙二醇（PEG）聚合物胶束与脂质囊泡的相互作用。虽然只使用单个颗粒来模拟亲水性药物分子，但模拟能够揭示聚合物辅助药物释放到脂质囊泡中的作用机制。聚合物与脂质囊泡融合，显示了亲水块与脂质头基的相互作用，以及核心块与脂质尾部的疏水相互作用。因此，亲水模型药物被释放到囊泡的内部溶剂区域[410]。而另一项基于MARTINI力场的研究也调查了聚合物胶束与脂质双分子层的相互作用。此外，使用无偏和伞形采样法研究PCL和PEG的共聚物，其PMF结果显示出对亲水性和疏水性重复单元之间比率的高度依赖性。此外，对于聚合物胶束在内吸入脂质双分子层中的形态变化也能够观察到，从球形变化为"贾努斯"状，其中亲水性的PEG链伸出到溶剂中，而疏水性的PCL块则埋入脂质双分子层中（图5-11）[411]。

此外，对负载DOX载体的PEG超支化聚合物的药物相互作用[412]研究也已开展。药物与膜的相互作用主要由疏水力（中性DOX）或氢键（带正电的DOX）驱动。带正电的DOX与带负电的脂质间的静电相互作用影响了药物扩散过程。随着聚合物-膜界面区域的过剩电荷不断积累，最终可能导致DDS的凝聚。

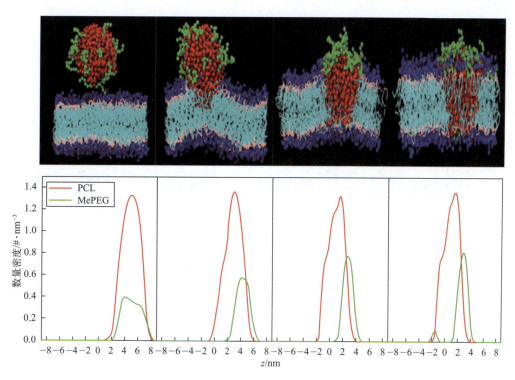

图5-11 模拟快照描绘聚合物胶束在穿过膜时形成"贾努斯"状结构的过程,比较胶束中疏水性PCL和亲水性PEG单元的密度与膜位置的关系(引自文献[411],版权2018,根据Elsevier的许可)

5.2.2.4 聚合物胶束－三嵌段共聚物

两亲性PEG-聚丙烯醚(PEG-PPO)二嵌段或PEG-PPO-PEG三嵌段共聚物(也被称为Pluronic)通常用于形成胶束,并在最近的一些研究中通过分子动力学模拟研究了未载药时的形态。此外,也有研究工作在原子层面考察了不同溶剂和聚合物聚集数对胶束形状的影响,并研究了各个组分的体积分数与胶束中心距离的关系。与三嵌段PEG-PPO-PEG变体相比,二嵌段共聚物和反向嵌段共聚物(PPO-PEO-PPO)显示出PPO的直链构象,而且还观察到EG重复单元的渗透和大量水在核中聚集。虽然添加乙醇会导致后者在核-壳界面处富集,但更疏水的醇类显示出更强的核心渗透(图5-12)。对于核心中的水团簇(发现于Pluronic L64),共溶剂的羟基基团则朝向界面处。甘氨酸和异丁酸体系则显示出更多的聚合物-溶剂间氢键。总的来说,这项研究考察了共溶剂如何以不同程度影响胶束形状和水含量,相关的研究结果在制剂过程中应予以考虑[413]。

之前有研究采用混合粒子场的分子动力学方法来评估混合溶剂对Pluronic P123胶束形状的影响[414]。而另一项研究则通过对不同温度和浓度下Pluronic L64不同相态的CG模拟研究对AA模拟结果进行补充,从聚合物的AA模拟中并通过Boltzmann迭代方法获取了MARTINI参数。从较低到较高的Pluronic浓度,研究者观察到较小的胶束组装体融合成更大的层状相。另外模拟也揭示了聚合物从S形态向U形态的构象转变,末端之间的距离缩短。随着这种转变,水从亲水壳中被排斥出来,其有序性增加。有趣的是,与上述AA模拟研究相比,这些CG模型中低聚合物浓度的球形组装体内没有显著的水团簇现象[415]。

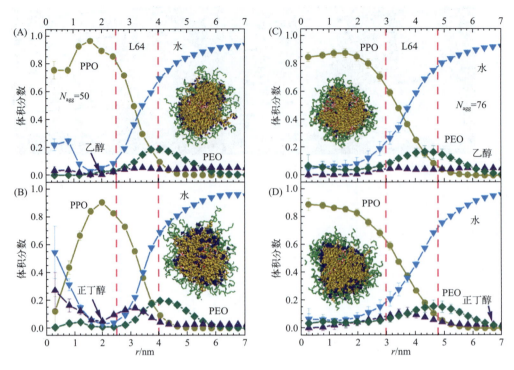

图 5-12 Pluronic L64 模拟中单体、水和醇类共溶剂[（A）和（C）为乙醇；（B）和（D）为正丁醇]的分布，处于两个不同的聚集数[（A）和（B）为 N_{50}；（C）和（D）为 N_{76}]。检测到正丁醇的渗透性较高，核心区域有大量的水[图（A）~（D）转载自文献[413]，根据 American Chemical Society 的许可使用，版权2022]

通过 CG 模拟研究 PEG-PPO-PEG 三嵌段聚合物（Pluronic F127）的 U 形和 S 形[416]组装。质量密度分布结果显示这两种形状具有类似的组成。即使在与 CG 模拟接近的空间和时间尺度上，两种形状之间的大尺度结构转变也无法检测到。由于聚合物链的大小，发生这种转变比较罕见，可能需要使用其他模型来正确评估相应的自由能壁垒。另一项关于负载布洛芬的 Pluronic 胶束研究涉及 DPD 模拟的应用，研究发现随着药物浓度的增加，RDF 结果显示了与体系自由能减少相关的药物分子附近水含量减少。因此，通过减少药物分子和聚合物在溶剂中的数量，以实现热力学稳定化[417]。

基于聚（2-噁唑啉）和聚（2-噁嗪）的两亲性 ABA 三嵌段聚合物可用于治疗相关药物的高含量负载，例如 PAC[151]。近期，这些 DDS 首次在 AA 水平上进行了模拟[418]。早些时候的 DPD 研究是将 β-环糊精接枝的星状嵌段聚合物用于封装金颗粒，其中模拟了聚[寡（2-乙基-2-噁唑啉）甲基丙烯酸酯]基团作为亲水壳的一部分[419]。最近，有研究使用寡（2-乙基-2-噁唑啉）作为新型聚氨酯树状聚合物的涂层剂，但只用寡（乙烯亚胺）壳进行了模拟[420]。与这些模拟方法相辅相成的是，基于机器学习的方法可用于预测从 DrugBank 数据库中筛选出的其他药物负载容量[421]。通过适当的简单描述符表示聚合物-药物混合物，构建基于随机森林的分类模型，显示出高于 0.7 的正确分类率。有趣的是，除了基于计算的描述符外，纳米制药过程中的实验条件信息（薄膜水合过程中的溶剂选择）对生成的模型也很重要[422]。这强调了模型计算在研究共溶剂对胶束形状影响方面的重要性，正如上文对 Pluronic

的研究所述。

5.2.2.5 聚合物胶束－其他研究

最近研究人员通过AA模拟对PEG修饰CHS链的组成进行了优化。观察到构成比例为60∶40（CHS∶PEG）时将会显示复合物最低回转半径值和负载姜黄素分子的RMSD值。通过氢键分析和MM-PBSA计算，聚合物-药物的静电相互作用是优化制剂的驱动力。较小的PEG链会使姜黄素与CHS氨基之间的相互作用增加[423]。

聚合物胶束也可以形成多核心系统，其中多个胶束会聚集成较大的集合体。最近通过DPD模拟[424]显示，高疏水性均聚物、低疏水性均聚物和两性共聚物的混合物会出现这种行为。随着两性共聚物浓度的增加，会形成单个胶束到多核心聚合体的转变。越来越多的两性共聚物出现在胶束表面，更有利于多核心聚合体的形成。因此，所描述的体系代表了一个易于调节的三组分混合物，具有潜在的药物递送应用。

模拟也是阐明纳米制剂动力学过程的有利工具。Styliari等[425]在原子层面模拟了水/丙酮混合物，其中包含吲哚美辛NP和PEG-PCL双嵌段共聚物。在双相起始结构的模拟中，两种溶剂混合，吲哚美辛粒子逐渐溶解到松散形式的聚合物胶束中。然后，丙酮被水分子替代，以模拟制剂过程的某些方面。这会使松散的聚合物-药物组装体更加紧密。然而，短的PEG链并没有在纳米粒子上形成保护冠，取而代之则与药物分子建立了相互作用[425]。

Xu等[426]通过DPD模拟研究调查了接枝不同大小环状刚性或柔性环上的两亲性嵌段共聚物的胶束形态。研究发现接枝具有中心刚性环的PCL-*b*-PAEMA-*b*-PPEGMA链具有高亲水性，而且会组装形成新的通道-层组合聚集体，处于胶束-水界面面积能量最低点。刚性环使得更多疏水空腔用于负载DOC，而相应的柔性环变体则相反。这为中心聚合物环的替代聚合物载体开辟了新的途径。

Wessels等[427]提出了选择合适的聚合物结构以获得所需胶束形态的方案，通过在CG级别上模拟各种线性、刷状或星状聚合物结构发现，与线性和星状变体相比，刷状聚合物在防止分子间疏水接触方面有显著效果，这使得胶束核心尺寸较小。

Rezaeisadat等[428]使用AA模型模拟研究负载姜黄素的聚（*N*-异丙基丙烯酰胺）-*b*-聚乙二醇（PNIPAAm-*b*-PEG）胶束。RDF分析表明PEG链主要位于胶束的冠层，但也会延伸到胶束核心，而姜黄素主要位于胶束的核心区域。相互作用能分析表明药物负载是有利的。SASA计算表明加入聚合物后，疏水药物分子的溶解度增加。

聚（*N*-异丙基丙烯酰胺）-*b*-聚（3，4-二羟基-L-苯丙氨酸）[P（NIPAM）-*b*-P（DOPA）]嵌段共聚物已被研究用于负载DOX。随后通过DPD模拟对其实验结果进行了补充，并显示药物扩散进入DOPA核心层[429]。夫西地酸和PEG的结合物在模拟中发现会自组装成胶束颗粒[430]。外层的PEG壳可防止在体内与HSA产生不利的相互作用。此外，还通过药物与低聚体结合的分子对接进行了考察，不利的接触以及得分不佳的对接评分也会显示出来。

通过DPD模拟，可以研究动态透析过程中的聚合物胶束形成[431]。随后通过用水替换有机溶剂颗粒，模拟了该过程（携带或不携带药物），研究发现，在从分散相中开始胶束化，随后会出现超胶束阶段，并形成柱状形态，最后形成球形胶束。

5.2.2.6 树状聚合物

树状聚合物是一类独特的对称高分支聚合物，已通过理论计算进行表征，并用于药物递送[432]和基因疗法制剂[433]。它们具有分形结构，由分支组成，分支分叉的次数被称为树状聚合物的代数。其尺寸（由代数 G 的数量确定）和表面性质可以容易地进行修改[434, 435]。关于树状聚合物和PEG化变体也在近期的模拟综述中进行了讨论[436, 437]。

使用MARTINI力场对PEG修饰的聚酰胺-胺（PAMAM）树状聚合物的动力学进行了研究，其中回转半径值与中子散射的实验结果相符。稳定的PEG涂层抑制了多个树状聚合物的聚集[438]。在一项后续研究中，考察了更长的PEG链，研究发现涂层聚合物渗透到核心区域，这在一定程度上解释了疏水分子负载的减少。在质子化后，RDF显示核心的扩展和PEG壳密度的增加[439]。核心在PEG化时的扩展和亲水性涂层的折合也在负载5-氟尿嘧啶（5-FU）的PAMAM树状聚合物的AA模拟研究中观察到。超过25% PEG化时，核心中负载的药物显著减少，这对药物递送是不利的。相反，5-FU对于空间受阻的高密度PEG冠层显示出高亲和力[440]。采用DPD模拟方法，解析PEG修饰的聚酯树状聚合物中负载和释放DOC的动力学。研究发现，多个聚合物会合并成更大的组装体，药物位于核心中。降低pH会在外壳中形成孔道，这将有助于药物释放[441]。由PAMAM组成的树状聚合物还可以用其他物质涂层，例如用精氨酸封顶的多个组氨酸。基于MARTINI的模拟显示，因为组氨酸的质子化，在pH等于5时，回转半径值增加，但即使在pH等于7时，核心密度也更大，这表明药物负载能力降低[442]。

Karatasos等[443]开展全原子分辨率的模拟研究PEG化树状聚合物对中性和带电的DOX分子的负载，揭示涂层剂对药物在载体内聚集的影响。Pavan等[444]进行高效率元动力学模拟，增加对PEG化和非PEG化树状聚合物结构的采样，实验结果与光散射数据一致。Tanis等[445]通过研究存在PEG链时PAMAM树状聚合物的相互作用发现，PEG链对树状聚合物的形状会产生影响。在pH依赖的方式下，树状聚合物与水分子间形成的氢键会受到影响，尤其在低pH下，更多的PEG-树状聚合物氢键会使复合物更稳定。

线性-树枝状嵌段共聚物分子通常由亲水性PEG链通过树状赖氨酸（Lys）连接子连接到疏水性胆酸基团上，研究人员对其进行多尺度模拟：首先，基于MARTINI力场构建一个CG模型。在这个层次上，发现未负载和负载PAC变体的胶束形成。然后，进行反映射，将模型缩放到AA级别，并分析药物的分布和封装（通过锥形算法确定）。结果表明超过25%（质量分数）的药物负载量时，观察到水分子流入组装体的核心，使得形成药物-水氢键。胆酸的两性性质，使其在甾烷核心结构周围具有更亲水和更疏水的一侧，这在药物递送系统行使的功能中非常重要，调节这一特性会形成截然不同的胶束形态，尤其是对于更疏水的变体，其中赖氨酸连接子会向外部转移到表面[446]。作为外部PEG修饰的替代方法，Albertazzi等[447]对插入到PAMAM树状聚合物结构中的PEG空间子进行研究，以评估其对荧光染料的负载能力。

Vaisiliu等[448]对新型用于DNA递送的树状聚合物载体进行原子级别的研究。这些树状聚合物由分支的聚乙烯亚胺（PEI）链、可变长度的PEG链和角鲨烯组成。在插入双链DNA（dsDNA）分子之前，对这些载体的聚集进行模拟。与实验观察一致，连接到树状聚合物的较长PEG链导致与核酸的相互作用减少。研究揭示这是由于PEG氧原子与PEI氨基之间的氢键对 PEI-DNA 相互作用形成了有效的立体阻碍。

PAMAM 树状聚合物的性质不仅可以通过连接到末端的 PEG 涂层进行调节，还可以通过改变末端的功能基团来调节。例如，通过在不同 pH 下对乙酰化和非乙酰化的 PAMAM 树状聚合物与不同数量的模型化合物 nateglinide 形成的复合物进行 AA 模拟研究。药物分子最初是通过分子对接方法放置在树状聚合物内部。在模拟过程中发现，在低 pH 条件下封装效率增加。使用 RDF、SASA 和氢键分析来表征树状聚合物形状和聚合物-药物相互作用。尽管在低 pH 条件下，两种树状聚合物变体的药物主要位于疏水核心中，但在中性 pH 下，只有非乙酰化变体才是这种情况（图5-13）。令人惊讶的是，MM-PBSA 计算表明，药物在树状聚合物核心内的位置并不是影响有利结合亲和力的决定因素[449]。

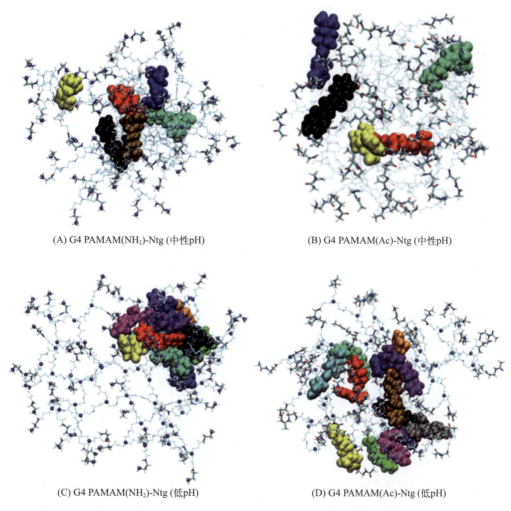

(A) G4 PAMAM(NH$_2$)-Ntg (中性pH)
(B) G4 PAMAM(Ac)-Ntg (中性pH)
(C) G4 PAMAM(NH$_2$)-Ntg (低pH)
(D) G4 PAMAM(Ac)-Ntg (低pH)

图5-13　PAMAM 树状聚合物的模拟快照，分别在中性[（A）和（B）]和低 pH[（C）和（D）]条件下。在低 pH 条件下，观察到树状聚合物核心内药物浓度较高，分别对应于（C）非乙酰化和（D）乙酰化变体，而在中性 pH 条件下，仅观察到与（A）非乙酰化变体相似的分布[图（A）~（D）转载自文献[449]，获得 AIP Publishing 的许可使用]

PAMAM树状聚合物的其他末端也可以影响药物的负载，例如，一项AA研究[450]比较了5-FU与聚合物的相互作用，其中树状分子的末端可以是氨基或羟基。随后分析并计算RDF、SASA、氢键、药物与胶束中心的距离以及MM-PBSA等指标发现，以氨基为末端的树状聚合物包裹的药物分子数量更多，形成的空腔更大。MM-PBSA的结果与等温滴定量热法的实验结果一致，表明疏水作用和静电作用对药物的结合都很重要，因为药物既与羟基又与氨基形成氢键。随后对氨基、乙酰基和羧基末端的变体进行了模拟工作，以评估在不同pH下对小分子chalcon的负载[451]。在中性pH条件下，聚合物会通过疏水相互作用在致密的聚集体中结合chalcon。然而，在酸性环境中，氨基和羧基末端的变体显示出较大的空腔，因此只观察到药物分子的松散协作。伞形采样揭示在中性pH条件下，乙酰化结构与chalcon的最强结合，而在酸性条件下，药物释放得到了增强。这表明乙酰化变体是适用于pH响应性药物递送的载体。

树状聚合物常常用于络合核酸，对此的模拟早在2006年就已经发表过[452]，但运行时间非常有限。Vasumathi等[453]使用AA级模拟研究了不同代数的PAMAM树状聚合物与siRNA的络合，随后通过氨基围绕核酸磷酸盐基团的RDF分析和基于MM-PBSA方法的结合自由能计算进行了研究。结果表明，络合受到周围带电基团的熵排斥影响。更高代的树状聚合物对应于增加的电荷比和结合亲和力。这些观察结果在后来关于dsDNA的研究中得到证实，该研究还显示在络合过程中双链会弯曲，与常见的刚性杆状不同[454]。另一项研究通过调查核酸与CNT和PAMAM树状聚合物的络合发现，抗衡离子的排斥也是决定因素[455]。Su等[456]通过DPD模拟研究展示PAMAM树状聚合物与单链DNA（ssDNA）在中性和低pH下的致密络合。增加的盐浓度对聚合物-DNA的组装不利。另一方面，树状聚合物的代数影响DNA结构的渗透程度，更高的电荷比影响络合物的大小。

聚丙烯亚胺（PPI）基结构是PAMAM树状聚合物的另一种选择。Jain等[457]通过药物-树状聚合物AA级模拟研究，分析了以PPI、PAMAM和二氨基丁烷为核心的不同代数聚合物；还在不同的pH条件下研究法莫替丁、吲哚美辛的载药和保泰松的释放；并对树状聚合物形状、药物分布和氢键行为进行广泛分析，结果发现在低pH下PPI树状聚合物与药物的络合非常低，这解释了观察到的低溶解度。通过PMF分析协作显示药物在这些条件下更有利于释放。更进一步的MM-PBSA计算成功地解析对药物络合有贡献的作用力，对于保泰松而言，相比于G4 PPI树状聚合物，G3 PAMAM树状聚合物因疏水相互作用和更高水平的氢键相互作用而表现出更有利的结合[457]。

尿素-金刚烷基团修饰的PPI树状聚合物的CG模拟是通过从AA模拟中推导出适当的参数，再采用迭代的Boltzmann反演方法进行的。这使得研究人员可以分析多个形状描述符，如回转半径值、单体分布和非球性。更高代数的树状聚合物显示较低的非球性值，而在前三代甚至观察到了类似棒状的形态[458]。此外，研究人员还研究了从稀释到熔融条件下随着浓度增加的树状聚合物形状。通过对结构进行详细分析，包括根据散射实验结果解释原子形状因子，揭示出在非常高浓度下树状聚合物的紧缩以及水含量的降低，溶剂团簇位于堆叠的树状聚合物之间，因此每个聚合物保持单独的实体[459]。Gupta等[460]也通过计算机模拟对PPI树状聚合物的形状和大小进行了研究。在低pH下，氨基的质子化导致尺寸增加，末端向核心的内部折叠减少，但是更高代数的树状聚合物仍显示出高密度的构象。

Kayvani等[461]使用MARTINI力场研究了由PPI-PAMAM组成的混合树状聚合物。虽然

PPI在核心内作为药物载体,但PAMAM杂化导致两个关键差异:树状聚合物体积增加,为药物负载提供更大的空腔,而与PPI树状聚合物相比,外壳层中的聚合物密度由于具有更长的链分支而降低。在树状聚合物的外部区域具有较低的密度可能有利于药物负载[461]。

树状聚合物与细胞膜的相互作用已在多项研究中进行探究。例如,Lee等[463]在CG模拟中发现,与较短的PEG链和乙酰化相比,较长的PEG链能够减少核孔形成,从而有利于减少细胞毒性[462]。通过PMF研究显示,由于正电氨基酸与负电磷酸基头部之间存在静电作用,树状聚合物在低pH下与脂质双层之间存在有利的相互作用。另一项研究则在没有多肽涂层的树状聚合物中得到类似的结论。Lee等[464]通过CG模拟研究树状聚合物与脂质双层的相互作用发现,与细胞渗漏实验一致,膜的变形依赖于聚合物的乙酰化。未乙酰化树状聚合物的正电荷与磷酸基头部之间的相互作用更强。He等[465]通过CG模拟考察了膜结构对树状聚合物相互作用的依赖,并分析了脂质分子头基的面积、膜厚度、曲率以及有序参数等关键性质。在凝胶相中,树状聚合物仅位于膜表面,而在流动相中,它们将渗透到脂质双层的核心区域(图5-14)。将胆固醇添加到膜的凝胶相使其性质更类似于流动相,从而促进与树状聚合物的相互作用。

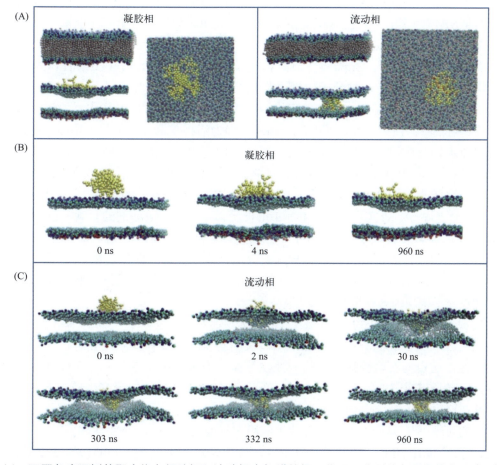

图5-14　不同角度下树状聚合物在凝胶相和流动相中与膜的相互作用,分别从在平衡状态下(A)以及在模拟过程中展示凝胶相(B)和流动相(C)的膜(图(A)~(C)转载自文献[465],已获Elsevier许可)

此外，还存在其他类型的树状聚合物。Ghadari等[466]通过AA模拟研究了不同亚酰胺连接的氨基酸树状聚合物；与外层代数G2和G3的分布受到质子化状态和温度变化的影响不同，G0和G1代相对刚性。带有氢键供体或受体的氨基酸能够与较长的侧链建立更多的相互作用，而较大的非功能性氨基酸则通过增加单体之间的距离来抑制减少的聚合物相互作用。这些观察结果表明，通过选择正确的氨基酸，可以对这些树状聚合物进行微调，以实现特定的药物递送目的。类似地，对由中央功能化富勒烯结构组成的多糖类伪树状聚合物也进行了研究[467]，发现基于MM-GBSA计算的有利结合亲和能取决于所选的模型化合物和糖苷。因此，就像氨基酸树状聚合物一样，选择糖苷的类型可以优化所涉药物的负载。

5.2.2.7 其他聚合物－基于纳米颗粒

本节将讨论其他载体，而这些载体不能简单归类为上述所描述的类别，例如固体聚合物颗粒和凝胶。因为涉及小分子的PEG化，因此计算模拟研究主要围绕着考察药物与一种聚合物的相互作用。其他未在此处描述的聚合物基系统还包括β-环糊精[468]、无定形固体分散体[469]和双面聚合物体[470]。

许多研究探讨了以PLA和PLGA为基础的NP在药物负载方面的适用性。例如，通过对以PLGA NP作为聚酚类表没食子儿茶素没食子酸酯的载体系统进行了实验和计算研究发现[471]，较高的药物负载会导致药物分子与PLGA核心的平均距离更大，因此在表面检测到了更多溶剂暴露的小分子。Stipa等[472]通过分子动力学研究了PLA、PGA和PLGA作为潜在药物载体系统、奎宁用作药物分子的聚合物系统发现，在PLA作为载体的情况下，药物主要在核心内聚集，由药物-药物π-π堆积作用控制；PGA不适合作为载体系统，因为发现药物会扩散到溶剂中；而PLGA表现出最佳性能，因为药物在聚合物组装中均匀分布，并建立了氢键和疏水相互作用。随后，还表征了其他几种药物分子的负载能力，显示了高亲脂性药物封装趋势[473]。(PEG修饰的)PLA也被测试为6-巯基嘌呤的载体。只有在PEG化的NP中观察到药物释放，其中水渗透到聚合物基体中，导致药物分子的溶解[474]。Megy等[475]基于PLA的NP更进一步研究了维生素E和Toll样受体(TLR)激动剂的负载。DPD模拟揭示了TLR激动剂在形成的聚合物NP的外部区域具有更高的浓度，而维生素E位于核心内部。Zatorska等[476]将姜黄素负载到PLA微球和带有两性离子性聚(D/L-乳酸)-b-聚(2-甲基丙烯酸甲酯氧乙基磷酰胆碱)共聚物中，研究发现纯PLA体系更有效地封装了中性疏水药物分子，这些分子不均匀地积聚在核心内部。

在负载不同模型化合物的PLGA(-植物)油NP上进行实验和计算工作，并使用MesoDyn方法研究药物的分布和扩散。结果表明与聚合物载体体系高兼容性的药物分子扩散速率较慢，这也与实验测得结果相一致。然而，应用中尺度模拟方法在捕获强亲水性分子分布方面显示出有限的能力[477]。之前一项应用DPD方法的模拟研究也曾观察到类似的结果，而且在这项工作中，通过将DPD模型与CG模拟相结合，克服了对带电荷基团静电相互作用模拟的限制[478]。这个案例研究强调了应用多尺度模拟方法的必要性。

Guo等[478]使用DPD方法研究了由PAC和PEG-聚(D-乳酸)(PDLA)和/或PEG-聚(L-乳酸)(PLLA)组成的聚合物纤维。药物的结晶棒状结构在没有任何聚合物辅料的情况下通过与作为内部疏水性核心的PLA进行相互作用而破坏，而PEG则在纤维周围形成了一层涂层。有趣的是，PLA块的长度以及它们的立体化学构型影响了药物的分布，这表明在

PLA 立体复合物的情况下，PAC 的释放较慢，因为核心中的药物浓度较高[479]。对于 PEG-PLLA 共聚物的情况，该团队还进行另一项 DPD 研究，以研究在不同聚合物-药物比例下这些复合物的相变[480]。Soto-Figueroa 等[481]利用 DPD 方法研究考察了阿苯达唑作为模型化合物从基于聚（苯乙烯二乙烯基苯）的微球中的释放，观察到膨胀、孔隙形成，最终药物从基质中扩散到酸性溶剂中[481]。此外，使用基于晶格的 MC 模拟核-壳聚合物 NP 释放进入周围血液环境的研究发现，对 pH 敏感的体系具有不稳定的氢键，适用于在肿瘤的酸性环境中改善药物释放[482]。

聚合物 NP 也可以使用 CHS 作为药物载体。例如，对 CHS 与 DOX 在小型模型系统中的相互作用进行研究发现[483]，聚合物氨基与 DOX 的相互作用和药物-药物 π-π 堆积是复合物内的驱动力。在低 pH 下，CHS 会质子化，导致药物释放。另一项研究调查了 CHS 修饰的 NP 中多奈哌齐和卡巴拉汀的载药情况[484]。Eslami 等[485]则通过模拟表征了聚山梨醇酯 80 对 CHS 和聚正丁基氰基丙烯酸酯（PBCA）作为他克林药物载体的影响。在 PBCA 系统中，聚山梨醇酯 80 显示出更有利的溶剂化自由能，药物包封效果得到了增强。在表面活性剂存在下，聚合物 PBCA 的回转半径保持不变，而壳聚糖在表面活性剂存在下显著延伸。使用平衡元动力学方法分别构建水和二甲基亚砜中由单个 CHS 三磷酸分子负载药物 toussantine-A 的自由能轮廓，其中使用两个集体变量：疏水性聚合物-药物接触量和两者之间的质心距离。能量轮廓分析表明，由于与 CHS 的相互作用减少，药物释放相比于水中的条件在二甲基亚砜存在下更有利[486]。而将聚合物一致性力场应用于比较聚正丁基氰基丙烯酸酯和 CHS 基 DDS 中的他克林包封情况发现，与他克林的弗洛里-赫金斯参数相比，聚合物-药物相互作用在前者中更加显著[487]。另一项研究则使用从上述聚合物一致性力场导出的 COMPASS 力场，分析了含有吉西他滨的 CHS 颗粒。RDF 分析结果表明，在没有水的情况下，吉西他滨更接近聚合物载体，而在添加溶剂后，在 40% 的水含量下观察到最高的载药量[488]。

Tokarský 等[489]使用聚合物一致性力场，建立了六种不同环孢素 A 载药的双亲凝胶 NP 的原子模型，这些颗粒基于常用的乳化剂 Cremophor。通过分析聚合物-药物相互作用能量、体积分数以及水含量，以便在计算机模拟中阐明哪种凝胶组合最接近自微乳化递送系统的特性[489]。另一项研究则调查了由 PCL 和不同数量的 HA 链组成的负载异环磷酰胺的纳米复合材料，通过进行包括不同聚合物-药物基团之间的 RDF 计算、汉森溶解度参数、MSD 和药物扩散等在内的广泛分析发现，高比例自由体积会提供更高聚合物运动性以及更容易渗透进入聚合物基体[490]。随后基于 COMPASS 力场也开展了粗粒化模拟，主要研究对象为具有不同长度疏水块的硫酸软骨素-PCL 共聚物。随着疏水块长度的增加，CL 重复单元之间的相互作用增强，而亲水性硫酸软骨素的扩散受到疏水块的影响，此外，在高分子量 PCL 的存在下，棒状聚集物也被观察到[491]。

Hathout 等[492]使用多种不同的数学和计算方法来评估明胶基体的药物负载，即将层次聚类分析、主成分分析以及随后的偏最小二乘回归分析应用于开发模型，预测药物的装载容量；还进行明胶基体的模拟并用于对接研究，以便将结合能量与装载药物质量相关联。

最近通过研究 PEG 作为携带 PAC 和吡罗昔康药物，以及作为血卟啉的隐形鞘功能发现，PEG 在溶剂中正离子周围呈卷曲构象，随后与血卟啉的疏水性成分进行相互作用，然而没有发现与其他药物分子的强相互作用[493]。对于四苯基卟啉和鹰嘴豆素的 PEG 化作用研究，除了熵屏障外，还观察到 PEG 与脂质之间的静电斥力，因此，药物进入细胞膜的过程受到阻碍[494]。作为潜在药物载体，PEG聚合物在抗癌药物dithymoquinone存在下进行模拟，同时进行弗洛里-赫金斯参数的计算[495]。研究结果发现PEG60链是最适合的载体，而较大的链导致聚合物-药物相互作用减弱。

聚合物微针是一种相对较新的基于聚合物的递送体系。Feng等[496]最近对这类结构进行多尺度模拟。从QM计算开始，比较聚合物修饰HA和PVA的电负性，弗洛里-赫金斯参数表明HA与模型化合物磺酰罗丹明B的相容性更好。与这些计算一致，模拟得出的药物与HA的结合能比与PVA更有利。对于基于HA的体系，检测到磺酰罗丹明B的扩散增加，表明药物释放增强。类似的研究也针对胰岛素作为药物负载进行PVA和HA微针的研究[497]。在这种情况下，HA与负载物的相互作用更强，提供更快的药物扩散。

基于超支化多臂共聚物的洋葱状多层囊泡也通过DPD方法进行了模拟，用以研究不同层的自组装[498]。研究表明多层形成的机制和形成的层数取决于体系中的聚合物浓度。这种体系也可能成为未来的DDS形式。

5.2.3 基于蛋白质的体系

将PEG与小分子或多肽偶联是增强药物递送的一种成熟方法[499-501]。表5-1显示，许多聚合物修饰的NP是与蛋白质共价结合的PEG。因此，本章主要关注聚合物-蛋白质生物偶联体系。分子动力学模拟是研究这类体系中潜在的蛋白质-聚合物相互作用的有力工具。与前面章节描述的其他体系一样，AA和CG模型都为二者的动力学机制提供了不同见解。关于蛋白质-聚合物相互作用，最近的一项研究还显示AA和CG（MARTINI 2）模拟PEG时，其力场可能存在差异[502]，尽管使用最新版本（MARTINI 3[260]）的模拟步骤已经发表[503]。

5.2.3.1 蛋白质-聚合物的生物偶联物

最近许多已发表的综述涵盖DDS的实验和计算内容[122, 101, 121, 504]，其中一些聚焦于模拟组分[436, 505, 506, 507]。需要注意的是，PEG化的多肽和蛋白质不仅代表具有治疗价值的药物制剂，还可以在体外使用，例如，用于调节酶的性质（改善溶解度、催化速率），从而实现或改善生物催化工业过程，相关作用机制也在计算机模拟研究中进行了考察[508-513]。PEG的遮蔽效应会通过蛋白质溶解减少免疫反应，而且增加的构象稳定性还可以进一步提高药物的货架期[514, 515, 516]。这与蛋白酶抗性相关，因此也是改善药动学的重要因素[517]。PEG可以进一步提高偶联物的溶解度并减少聚集倾向，因此该技术还可以规避制剂过程中可能出现的问题[515]。所有提到的优势必须超过可能的劣势，首要是显著的生物活性降低，这主要归因于空间位阻[515]，PEG还会降低配体扩散到活性位点的速度[518]。PEG化的IFN-α2a，即Pegasys®，其清除率约为60 mL/h，大约是非PEG化变体的100倍。这种增强的药动学特性弥补了生物活性降低的缺陷（与野生型相比降低了7%），从而使患者可以使用更少的药物[514]。其他缺点可能包括构象稳定性降低，以及（非特异性的）偶联策略导致的不同批次之间出现可变的生物利用度[515]。因此，随着现代位点特异性聚合物连接策略的出现[519]，期望通过合理设计方法来进行构建生物偶联体系，而模拟可以提供必要的机制性理解。

自从第一个PEG化蛋白质的模拟研究发表以来[520]，涉及分子动力学模拟的研究为偶联到生物大分子的聚合物行为提供了有价值的阐释。Yang等[521]使用GROMOS96 43a1联合原子力场研究了PEG化胰岛素，在平衡期间采用模拟退火技术，让聚合物链在蛋白质表面迅速重新定向（图5-15）。通过这项发现蛋白质的二级结构稳定，蛋白质溶剂可及表面积减少。PEG主要通过疏水相互作用与偶联的生物大分子发生相互作用，而与溶剂能形成许多氢键[522]。在PEG化的葡萄球菌溶血酶的研究中应用模拟退火方法，结合分子对接研究，突显了PEG的遮蔽效应——形成偶联蛋白质周围的水合层[523]。另一项研究则在AA水平上考察螺旋结构的PEG化，通过沿螺旋轴施加不同的力，由此观察到聚合物偶联机械性地增强二级结构，这可能是由于蛋白质-蛋白质骨架氢键周围的脱水作用[524]，这也与之前另一项模拟研究结果相符[525]。结合实验研究多肽的纤维化，通过MD模拟研究未结合的PEG-cholane对帕尔米托酰化血管活性肠肽（VIP-palm）二级结构的影响[526]发现，PEG-cholane和VIP-palm以2:1形成的复合物会导致多肽片段的α螺旋结构增加，显示PEG的保护效应。Han等[527]通过计算研究多肽PEG化对膜相互作用的影响发现，通过PEG修饰形成了更多随机卷曲的magainin 2，将会导致多肽和膜产生弱的静电吸引相互作用。

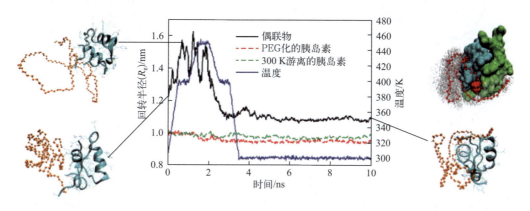

图5-15　采用模拟退火方法对50 kDa聚合物链PEG化的胰岛素进行模拟。具有伸展特性的偶联物作为起始构型（橙色），然后模拟体系在高温下进行，以便让PEG链迅速重新定向到蛋白表面周围。检测到蛋白成分的回转半径。右上方通过插图显示聚合物构象的分布（灰色点），链A为青色，链B为绿色，聚合物和连接位点为红色（引自文献[522]已获许可，版权2011，美国化学学会）

Price等研究基于PEG的脱溶作用。多年来，通过分析不同突变体的小型蛋白质模型，提出了不同的作用机制，阐释PEG如何导致构象稳定：侧链羟基基团[517]和疏水斑块[528]去溶剂化可能导致蛋白表面弱配位结合水的排出，这种特性是熵有益的。此外，通过增强带电氨基酸之间的分子内盐桥[529]和NH-π键[530]，脱溶作用从焓角度更有利。尽管主要是通过实验开展研究工作，但这些研究也包括AA级模拟。围绕羟基的脱溶作用是通过RDF进行的，甚至可以在外部水合层中检测到[517]。此外，对这些偶联物的早期模拟研究还建议，PEG在特定的焓相互作用下稳定蛋白质[531]。基于PEG的构象稳定不仅取决于连接子结构[532]，还取决于连接位点附近的氨基酸序列。而这一点在糖基化中没有观察到[533]，这凸显不同的修饰会改变蛋白质-聚合物偶联物的性质。

最近，Munasinghe等通过AA模拟研究N端连接的PEG化牛血清白蛋白，基于回转半径值，考察了增加PEG链长如何改变哑铃状和收缩状构象之间的平衡[534]。分析聚合物与蛋白质之间的接触模式发现，PEG优先缠绕在带正电的赖氨酸基团周围（图5-16）。因此，溶剂可及表面积（SASA）减少[535]。在后续的研究中，模拟连接到不同位点的PEG。聚合物链末端附近的PEG重复单元与蛋白质保持距离，悬浮在溶剂中，这在熵角度上可能比重新定向到生物表面更有利[536]。随后关于不同PEG链结构和多个偶联位点的分子模拟研究结果显示，使用分支的PEG变体具有更高的接枝密度，与蛋白质产生更大接触面积，部分原因是多个链之间的排斥作用。这可能会增加聚合物涂层的屏蔽效应。此外，梳状PEG替代物POEGMA显示出略微不同的相互作用模式，因为它更容易定位于蛋白质的疏水区域[537]。

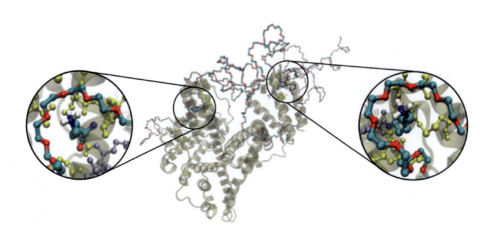

图5-16　模拟快照显示PEG包裹在白蛋白偶联物中带正电的赖氨酸周围
（引自文献[535]已获许可，版权2019，美国化学学会）

通过分子动力学模拟还可以对与胰凝乳蛋白酶结合的两性离子聚合物进行研究。Baker等[508]通过蛋白质RMSD和聚合物灵活性的模拟分析解释了不同pH下偶联物稳定性的差异。从这些研究中推测，聚合物可以充当分子伴侣，有助于蛋白质的重新折叠或稳定部分未折叠的结构。这种功能取决于附加聚合物的电荷和亲水性。对这一相同的聚合物，Munasinghe等[538]进行了一项纯计算研究，并使用接触图分析相互作用，结果表明，与蛋白质相互作用的表面积以及较远重复单元与蛋白质接近的程度，依赖于聚合物的结构，不仅聚合物的选择会影响蛋白质的RMSD，还会影响底物结合口袋内核心残基的构象。Kaupbayeva等[539]随后进行了一项针对这些两性离子变体（PCBMA）不同体系的隐式溶剂原子级模拟，推导出一个接近蛋白质活性位点的胰凝乳蛋白酶抑制剂的扩散常数，从而检测出梳状聚合物具有最佳的屏蔽效应[539]。小型配体朝向结合位点扩散，同时蛋白质与抑制剂或抗体被屏蔽起来，这种效应被称为附加聚合物的"分子筛"效应。最近，有研究人员建立了一种带有多个附加POEGMA链的胰凝乳蛋白酶的CG模型，以评估这种效应。在此过程中，蛋白质被模拟为一个包含额外的圆盘状粒子（表示活性位点）的大球体，而聚合物链则是多个较小的球体。使用MC模拟研究小型底物与结合位点的碰撞，越过POEGMA涂层的间隙将显示出配体在蛋白质表面的聚集，影响"分子筛"效应[540]。

最近通过高斯加速的AA分子动力学模拟与PEG、LPG和PEOZ偶联的IFN-α2a，以进一步研究PEG的替代物[541][图5-17（A）]。虽然PEG的行为与Munasinghe等的报道类似（与带正电氨基酸的相互作用），但LPG和PEOZ的连接形成了不同的相互作用模式。LPG与PEG类似，但更容易与带负电荷的氢键受体（Asp和Glu）发生相互作用。PEOZ有利于与芳香氨基酸（类似于从含芳香元素的聚氧杂环丙烷氧胶凝胶模拟中获得的观察结果[542]）相互作用，同时通过其羧基氧与可用供体基团形成氢键。通过 RMSF 计算[图 5-17（B）]，实验得出的 PEOZ 偶联物热稳定性的降低被进一步解释为蛋白质柔性的增强。通过约束网络分析获得了熔融温度数据[543][图 5-17（C）]。对所有情况都观察到结合位点的空间位阻，这与实验测得的生物活性下降结果相符[156]。

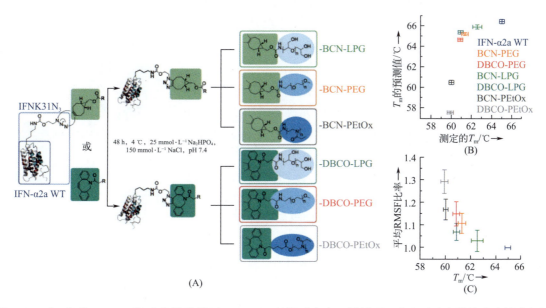

图 5-17 （A）将 10 kDa 聚合物链附着到 IFN-α2a 的偶联方案。模拟显示出实验确定的热稳定性降低与（B）通过约束网络分析得出的熔化温度之间的相关性，以及（C）非结构化环区域的 RMSF 比率（偶联物与野生型）。[图（A）~（C）引自文献[156]，已获许可，版权 2021，美国化学学会]

其他模拟研究侧重于 IFN 偶联物，这些偶联物代表有价值的抗病毒和免疫调节治疗药物。一项关于将不同长度的 PEG 链与 IFN-β1b 偶联的 AA 研究显示，与 apo 蛋白相比，偶联物的亲水性 SASA 增加，这是有效屏蔽蛋白质的一个原因。在关键结合残基的覆盖度方面，可能存在一种理想的链长，以平衡增加的循环时间和降低的生物活性。总体而言，PEG 紧密包裹在蛋白质周围[544]。另一项研究模拟 IFN-α2a 的另一种涂层 PASylation，即连接由脯氨酸、丙氨酸和丝氨酸组成的多肽链。偶联的聚合物没有紧密包裹在蛋白质周围，但也导致亲水性 SASA 增加[181]。

基于带电氨基酸的聚合物材料，例如由谷氨酸和赖氨酸构成的链，通过对其进行模拟，结果显示偶联泛素在较高温度下的稳定性增加，并对附着位点附近的氨基酸产生变构效应[176]。另外一项后续研究考察了此类偶联对另外两种抗糖尿病蛋白质药物胰高血糖素样肽-1（GLP-1）和胰岛素的影响。经过 RMSD、RMSF、二级结构含量分析，报道了由于偶联而导致蛋白质结构重新排列的情况。对于 GLP-1，C 末端偶联导致形成 α 螺旋结构[545]。

现在，蛋白质-聚合物生物偶联的 CG 模型能够以较低的计算成本在更长时间尺度上捕获大尺度构象的变化，故而通过 CG 模拟捕捉到构象变化的动力学行为已远远超越目前 AA 级模拟研究。Wilding 等[546]构建了一个 T4 溶菌酶的 Go 模型[547, 548]，该模型在不同的位点和不同的链长上进行PEG化，并将每个残基表示为单一的珠子。蛋白质的原生接触在不同温度下通过复制交换模拟进行分析，所有模拟在一天内完成。尽管存在关于连接子和聚合物模拟的局限性，但是数据仍然与实验结果呈现相关性[546]。随后的一项研究使用相同的方法对TEM-1 β-内酰胺酶的大量偶联物进行研究，结果显示热稳定性与PEG链附着的二级结构类型无关，而与三级结构（蛋白质结构域）有关。基于这些结果，提出了一个可能的计算筛选工作流程，通过从apo蛋白质的模拟中获得结果，可以过滤掉许多偶联位点[549]。这项计算研究还得到了一些对实验结果的补充。虽然实验结果与计算结果的一致性仅为中度，但提出的工作流程仍然可以用来选择可能的附着位点子集，以进行进一步的实验表征[550]。

随着强化的高通量实验筛选工作流程能快速评估靠近聚合物的蛋白质的性质，从而收集大量数据，基于机器学习的方法正成为生成预测模型的有价值的工具，以选择最佳的聚合物作为蛋白质制剂的载体，最近的一项研究已经说明了这一点[551]。另外，有研究小组还发布另一个预测模型，用于评估赖氨酸位点的多个PEG连接的活性[552]。这些方法可以补充从分子动力学中获得的机制性理解。

总之，蛋白质-聚合物相互作用的分子动力学模拟已成功应用于以原子分辨率获取许多不同体系的关键视野。这些视野包括：检测不同类型聚合物的有利相互作用，研究在改变聚合物长度和结构时的构象变化，并解释构象稳定性和生物活性的变化。值得注意的是，许多提到的研究不仅涉及计算工作，还将该工作与补充性实验相结合，例如使用不同的光散射方法。另外，不同的核磁共振光谱方法可以用来在实验中捕获蛋白质-聚合物接触模式，从而在这一领域补充和验证未来的模拟研究[553-556]。

5.2.3.2　其他蛋白质-聚合物体系

Settanni等使用计算和实验方法研究了两种保护性聚合物PEG和PSA与不同血浆蛋白之间的相互作用[557, 558, 559, 560]。这些相互作用不是氨基酸特异性的，而更多地取决于氨基酸的电荷和极性，以及聚合物与水相互作用的类型。这种方法可以用于其他聚合物涂层的合理设计。

通过分子动力学模拟存在于GLP-1中的其他带电的两性五肽，对相互作用能、氢键、二级结构和SASA的分析揭示，五肽围绕GLP-1形成一个外壳，并增加其螺旋结构含量。VPKEG以静电相互作用方式显示出抗污染性和隐形性质之间的有利平衡，而带有更分散正电荷的VPREG肽在精氨酸侧链上显示出与GLP-1更强的相互作用，这表明可能与氨基酸产生非特异性相互作用[561]。

在许多研究中，基于蛋白质的RMSD和RMSF指标、二级结构含量和相互作用能的分析，并通过AA模拟技术考察了其他聚合物辅料对蛋白质稳定性的影响。例如，IFN-α2在CHS和PLGA存在下稳定，而添加PEG后会不稳定[562]。环糊精或CHS的添加会稳定IL-2[563]，果胶会稳定促红细胞生成素[564]。在抗菌肽GF-17中，CHS聚合物也优于PEG[565]，对于蜂毒肽则PLGA优于PLA[566]。通过PEG、PLGA和PEG-PLGA聚合物对蛙皮素-2进行封装模拟，显示出与芳香和碱性残基有利的蛋白质-聚合物相互作用[567]。同样地，CHS和胆固醇接枝变体对胰岛素的封装模拟显示出与芳香和负电荷残基的有利相互作用[568]。

新型聚丙烯酸/去氧胆酸修饰的CHS聚合物类似于两性共聚物，通过模拟研究评估其与hGH的相互作用，分析接触模式、二级结构含量和RMSF，总体上评估出共聚物通过优先与非结构化环区域相互作用来稳定蛋白质。二者涉及不同类型的相互作用，并通过 MM-PBSA 方法评估出有利的结合自由能[569]。在另一项研究中，对 L-天冬氨酸酶与 PEG 和 PLGA 的相互作用进行了相似分析。尽管蛋白质在这两种情况下都通过封装得到稳定，但 PLGA 显示出更强的静电相互作用，而 PEG-蛋白质相互作用主要由疏水相互作用驱动[570]。为考察蛋白质与聚合物辅料的相互作用，有研究小组研究了 iduronate-2-sulphatase 在三种不同聚合物（PEG、PLGA 和 PLGA-PEG）存在下的相互作用；此外，还评估了聚合物伸展对蛋白质的影响，并对蛋白质-聚合物和聚合物-聚合物接触模式进行了分析。总体上，PLGA 和 PEG-PLGA 与蛋白质的相互作用比 PEG 更有利。不同聚合物链的弛豫时间起着关键作用，而且只有当聚合物-蛋白质相互作用比 LGA-LGA 相互作用更有利时，API 的适当屏蔽才能实现[571]。

使用 MARTINI 力场研究考察蛋白质-聚合物相互作用，可用于筛选优化的水凝胶制剂。在细胞色素 P450 和 PET 酶存在的情况下进行 PS 的模拟。在共聚物中增加亲水性或带电吡啶变体的比例可将聚合物-聚合物和蛋白质-聚合物相互作用的平衡转移到后者。然而，增加吡啶含量超过一定阈值后，观察到聚合物的自聚集和中性单体的延长结构，以及由于带电变体的静电排斥作用而降低蛋白质聚合物共组装。聚合物与蛋白质之间的接触主要由疏水相互作用驱动[572]。其他关于聚合物水凝胶的模拟研究参阅其他文献[573, 574, 575]。

总之，这些研究表明，除了 PEG 外的聚合物选择应该取决于单个蛋白质的表面性质，这可以类比为特定的"指纹"，以用来找到最佳的涂层。

5.2.4　无机纳米颗粒

尽管在市场上，聚合物修饰的 NP 主要是以碳水化合物为基础的氧化铁颗粒（见表 5-1），但其也应用在许多其他材料中，如金、碳纳米管（CNT）或石墨烯。

5.2.4.1　碳基纳米颗粒

Lee 等[436]综述了碳基纳米颗粒在 CNT 上进行的模拟研究进展。例如，通过 AA 模拟研究多肽与（PEG 修饰的）CNT 的相互作用[576]发现，PEG 修饰并未阻止 CNT-多肽的相互作用，因为配体穿透了聚合物层。多肽通过 PEG 层的穿透与增加的 PEG-CNT 接触以及熵有利的水排出相一致。于是得出结论，体系中存在多个现象的相互依赖关系：在低接枝密度下，CNT 上多肽的相互作用位点数量增加，而在高接枝密度下，PEG 外壳中的潜在相互作用位点更常见。然而，在较低的 PEG 密度下，涂层更受到水分的水合作用[576]。

作为对 PEG 的替代，三甲基壳聚糖（TMC）被视作 CNT 和石墨烯的潜在修饰材料[577]。通过分析回转半径值、MSD、RDF 和氢键等指标，评估 TMC 作为 PAC 和 DOX 的递送体系的适用性。与 TMC 的偶联导致药物载体氢键数量增加。PAC-石墨烯-TMC 复合物显示出最有利的性质，表现为快速的药物负载和缓慢释放。在酸性 pH 下，CHS 和 DOX 的氨基之间的静电斥力与 CNT 和石墨烯均有良好的相互作用能，可促进肿瘤环境中的药物释放。类似的智能释放机制在 DOX 负载的 PEI-石墨烯[578]、PAC 负载的 PEI-硅烯纳米片[579]、DOX 负载的 PEI 黑磷片[580]以及 PAC 或 DOX 负载的羧基化二甲基丙烯酰胺-TMC-富勒烯[581]的模拟研究中也进行了描述。另有研究揭示了膜对负载药物的胞吞过程。此外，通过使用直接与药物分子偶联的聚（β-苹果酸）来进行模拟，研究了石墨烯氧化物上 DOX 的 pH 敏感性负载能力[582]；

通过模拟比较CHS修饰的石墨烯与异构素的相互作用发现，相比于纯石墨烯或掺杂P的石墨烯而言，掺杂N的石墨烯具有更好的药物递送性能[583]。而针对PEG化富勒烯的更多模拟研究也已在不同级别上进行了详细分析[584, 585, 586]。

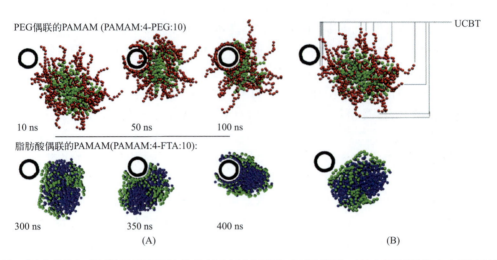

图5-18 （A）PEG或脂肪酸偶联修饰的PAMAM包裹在CNT周围，（B）展开链分支末端（UCBT）[（A）和（B）来源于文献[587]，已获皇家化学学会的许可]

树状聚合物也可用于和CNT进行复合。例如，在一个CG MARTINI模拟研究中，比较连接到PPI、PEG或脂肪酸的PAMAM结构，其中PAMAM仅在这三种变体中的第一种中形成内核。因此在含有脂肪酸的结构中，模拟外部疏水成分。研究结果显示，对于复合材料来说，最稳定的树状聚合物是由PEG组成外壳的树状分子。PEG与CNT和溶剂之间的强烈相互作用成功地将PAMAM的G0结构与CNT分离开来[图5-18（A）]。PEG涂层的亲水性，使它显示出更多展开链分支末端，在接近CNT之前伸展到溶剂中，而不是向核心背折[图5-18（B）]。这实际上有助于与CNT的相互作用，因为通过这些未分支的末端，树状聚合物能够更容易地缠绕在纳米管周围[587]。此研究小组的另一项研究评估了CNT-PAMAM复合物作为蛋白质和小分子的DDS功能。虽然CNT-PAMAM复合物阻止泛素与CNT的相互作用，但在这个复合物中，蛋白质是暴露在溶剂中的。只有添加另一个PAMAM结构后，蛋白质才形成一个稳定的复合物，夹在靠近CNT的两个树状聚合物之间，与溶剂隔离开来。对于小分子芘的情况，模拟结果表明首先通过将芘加载到PAMAM中，然后再形成与CNT的复合物，这可以防止芘在没有PAMAM的情况下更快地吸附到CNT上[588]。

5.2.4.2 硅基纳米颗粒

除了碳基颗粒外，由二氧化硅组成的NP对于各种生物医学应用，包括药物递送和诊断，也具有重要意义。它们复杂的介孔（潜在的多室）结构因大小和形状而异，可以提供大的表面积，并且可以轻松地通过更多的材料进行修改，例如金或铁[589, 590]。各种合成和天然聚合物类型已用于表面修饰，详细概述在文献[591]中提供。例如，使用聚赖氨酸与PEG进行修饰以实现pH依赖的特性[592]，并且通过姜黄素基聚合物等方法引入二氧化硅纳米颗粒的荧光性质，用于成像目的[593]。先前许多原子尺度模拟研究还涉及不同结构的二氧化硅

NP[594]，例如：与含不同末端基团的NP的蛋白质相互作用[595]；在pH响应性递送体系内的二氧化硅-药物相互作用（图5-19）[596]；以及将荧光染料封装在二氧化硅纳米颗粒内用于成像目的的研究[597]。然而，在药物递送领域，涉及模拟接枝到二氧化硅表面的聚合物研究相对较少。

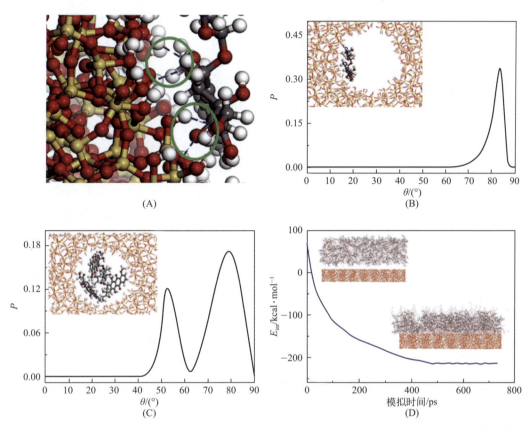

图5-19 （A）DOX分子与介孔二氧化硅的相互作用。（B）单个或（C）多个DOX分子封装在二氧化硅内的接触角分布。（D）DOX-二氧化硅相互作用能在DOX分子最初位于二氧化硅表面上的模拟过程变化。[图（A）~（D）来源于文献[596]，版权2019，已获Elsevier许可]

Ezquerro等[598]研究具有和没有PEG接枝在表面的二氧化硅NP，将其浸入PCL基质中，以调节这种常用于生物医学用途的聚合物机械性能[598]。使用OPLS-AA力场进行AA模拟，以详细研究NP周围的PCL密度以及复合材料的弹性性能。模拟揭示NP周围密集的PCL层，PEG化导致界面区域厚度的增加。因此，尽管与未接枝变体相比，PEG化并未导致复合材料的整体机械性能发生变化，但它增加了PCL对NP的亲和力，从而导致在聚合物基质内的更大分散。Shariatinia和Jalali[599]通过研究二氧化硅填充复合材料，以表征基于COMPASS力场的chorambucil负载的CHS、PLA和PEG水凝胶的性质。此外，RDF、MSD和表面积分析揭示了CHS基系统中最低的药物扩散，表明CHS基系统具有持续释放的特性。

二氧化硅NP可以通过附着蛋白质来进一步实现功能化[600]。Wu等[601]使用分子模拟方法研究了丝蛋白P1及其C端通过PEG连接到二氧化硅表面的相互作用。与溶液中的动力学相比，与硅表面相连的蛋白质二级结构含量没有出现显著变化，因为表面形成足够多的水合层。

其他用于除生物医学以外的聚合物涂层二氧化硅NP的模拟研究也有报道，例如，一项研究显示与硅氧烷基和磺酸基末端基团相比，PEG化NP在油/水界面的油相中渗透性最高[602]。在CG模拟方面，先前进行了DPD研究，以考察存在于聚偏氟乙烯膜-水界面上的二氧化硅NP的动态行为[603]，结果表明NP均匀分散在界面上，但在高接枝比和长度下多个NP的两性聚合物之间因存在相互作用而产生粘聚效应。

5.2.4.3 金基纳米颗粒

PEG化的金NP早期就已经使用AA模拟进行了研究[604, 605]。Oroskar等[606]通过模拟巯基连接的PEG化金颗粒，以研究该药物递送系统与脂质双分子层的相互作用。基于水的渗透，研究者观察到脂质翻转以及离子传输，并对膜的稳定性进行了表征。与烷基硫醇连接链相比，亲水性的PEG外壳将膜的不稳定降至最低。当NP从膜中分离时，脂质不会被移除。随着PEG接枝密度不断增高，大部分卷曲构象会转变为更加延展的结构。总体而言，通过CG方法可以证明PEG修饰对膜不稳定性的最小影响。Zhang等[607]也通过使用疏水性珠子模型颗粒，对PEG-NP-膜相互作用进行了类似的研究，观察到PEG化的NP在模拟不对称的脂质双分子层[由1-棕榈酰-2-油酰-sn-甘油-3-磷酰胆碱（POPC）和1-棕榈酰-2-油酰-sn-甘油-3-磷酸乙醇胺（POPE）组成]时发生转位。通过计算模拟在三个不同温度下的体系，然后分析了膜的不同性质（序参量、横向扩散）以及PEG链的不同性质（回转半径、首尾端距离、体积）。较高的温度导致更快的扩散和增加的颗粒转位。虽然较高的PEG接枝密度使脂质的提取减少，但观察到更多的翻转会将不对称的POPC/POPE单层转变为更对称的膜。因此，可推断接枝密度应该用于平衡这两种观察效应。

Bai等[608]进行了一项DPD研究来调查NP与膜的相互作用。对不同密度的表面活性脂质涂层的颗粒进行模拟，其中膜由脂质和表面活性分子的受体组成，以模拟受体介导的内吞作用。通过考察LNP的负载比，模拟揭示涂层促进了内吞作用。对于这个过程，涂层的变形是必要的。涂覆在NP上的最佳表面活性脂质密度取决于配体-受体结合强度。虽然在较低的强度下，更高的涂层密度是有利的，但在较高的强度下，这会减缓内吞作用。此外，研究结果还表明疏水性表面活性蛋白质的插入会使颗粒的摄取增加。Xia等[609]进行了类似的DPD研究，考察在NP上进行非共价聚合物修饰对正常细胞和癌细胞摄取的影响，并与共价修饰进行比较（图5-20）。通过计算相互作用能和PMF发现，非共价修饰可以代表一种更有利的靶向递送技术，因为只有对正常细胞的吸引力降低，而共价修饰导致正常细胞和癌细胞的摄取都减少。计算模拟结果提出了一种机制：在摄取之前，NP上的配体与聚合物的特定部分发生相互作用，而后者的非特异性块则起到修饰作用。这种修饰在立体上阻碍与正常细胞的相互作用。尽管对于共价修饰，这种立体上的阻碍也会减少对癌细胞的吸引力，但对于非共价结构，这种阻碍增加了配体与膜受体的相互作用，从而导致后者的脱离，增强NP的吞噬。之前有研究也曾对使用PAMAM修饰的金颗粒进行模拟，研究发现在低pH条件下，颗粒的扩散减少，这是因为树状聚合物的伸展和水含量的增加。此外，聚合物-金相互作用和聚合物构象变化都可影响扩散[610]。

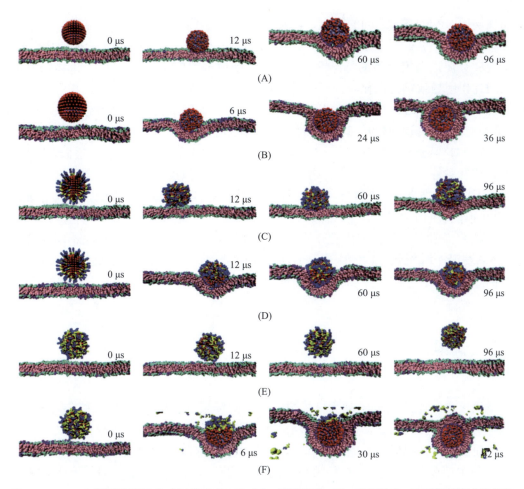

图5-20 DPD模拟快照显示未被修饰的NP（A=正常细胞；B=癌细胞），使用共价聚合物修饰（C=正常细胞；D=癌细胞）和使用有非共价共聚物修饰（E=正常细胞；F=癌细胞）的相互作用

[图（A）~（F）来源于文献[609]，已获英国皇家化学会许可]

5.2.4.4 其他纳米颗粒

银NP是另一种无机纳米颗粒的类型，最近被聚（2-（N,N-二甲基氨基）乙基甲基丙烯酸酯）（PDMAEMA）接枝作为一种可替代的pH敏感修饰剂[611]。在不同pH下进行的AA模拟显示聚合物动力学的明显差异。在高pH下，聚合物氨基是中性的，因此，观察到与银相互作用增强的密集涂层。而在较低pH下，随着质子化基团数目的增加，聚合物伸展到溶剂中，从而增加水-聚合物间氢键的数量，导致颗粒的溶剂暴露增强。

Siani等[612]使用AA模拟对含有环状RGD作为靶向配体的PEG化二氧化钛NP进行了研究。当不考虑接枝密度时，靶向配体位于PEG/水界面上。然而，在高接枝密度下，配体之间的相互作用增加，配体的溶解度减少。因此，基于空间取向，低接枝密度为潜在结合整合素的配体提供最佳暴露环境。同时，这项模拟研究强调了靶向选择配体的最佳接枝密度以优化药物递送。

同样，利用DPD模拟也研究考察了由HSA构成的蛋白冠对细胞摄取的影响[613]。根据不同表面性质的NP与HSA之间的距离，以及由此得出的不同pH下的PMF发现，疏水和带正电的颗粒有利于结合。对于疏水颗粒，HSA修饰可以在免疫反应期间改变细胞摄取的方式，因为蛋白质会促进与膜受体的特异性相互作用（未模拟，仅观察到黏附）。未修饰变体的非特异性相互作用导致颗粒内化，并引发局部脂质破坏。对于带正电的变体，未修饰颗粒无法摄取，而HSA修饰导致膜黏附。对于癌细胞的情况，采用带负电的膜进行模拟，结果表明两种NP类型的细胞摄取减少，这是因为静电排斥效应所致。

Ozmaian等[614]通过CG模拟进一步调整聚合物修饰NP的表面性质，通过插入黏性NP进行研究。这些黏性NP视作异质聚合物基质涂层，但只与涂层中的一种聚合物进行有利的相互作用。因此，这导致了涂层材料中其他聚合物种类更多地暴露在表面上，因此这被认为是调整NP在不同表面上扩散的一种方法。

DPD研究提供了关于包埋模板介导的脂质体指南[615]。通过观察并总结不同封装度的中心无机NP发现，增加聚合物的刚度会减缓胶束组装的速度，并调节封装NP所需的接枝密度和自由脂质数量。

5.3 结论

本章为读者详细介绍分子动力学模拟工具在阐释聚合物应用于药物递送系统方面的研究，重点关注它们作为保护修饰剂的作用。随着聚合物的化学和结构多样性以及新型纳米制剂技术的研发，目前已经在实验和计算方面研究了大量涉及聚合物的载体，无论是其作为涂层材料还是主要成分。尽管PEG仍被视作是实现这种目的的金标准，但是近年来越来越多的替代结构正在研发以克服PEG存在的可能的缺点，并对载体的特性进行精细调整，以适应特定目的。由于将不同重复单元的聚合物块连接到不同类型的化学实体（包括脂质、其他聚合物块、无机物质或生物大分子）具有组合性质，因此可能性几乎是无限的。建立指南以帮助科学家在未来研发优化的纳米制剂变得非常重要。而分子模拟在这一发展愿景中起着核心作用，因为它扮演着必不可少的角色，尤其是用于阐明原子到介观尺度上的相关软物质动力学，这在实验方法中仍然相对难以捉摸，即使到今天也是如此。

本章已经介绍了聚合物修饰在基于脂质的系统中如何影响与药物的相互作用并改变脂质双分子层的动力学。关于PEG化脂质体的AA模拟研究揭示了通过CG模型或实验测量不容易推导出的机制，即：PEG影响表面电荷，调节胆固醇在膜中的作用，同时作为相对亲疏水性药物的替代储库。本章还特别展示了计算模拟如何评估不同成分的靶向效力，以及其如何受到其他聚合物的影响。CG模型还可以让研究者观察到在相变时发生的大尺度构象变化。此外，由于mRNA疫苗的出现用以对抗COVID-19，LNP近年来受到特别关注。在这种情况下，制剂中的PEG链作为稳定剂用于增加药物货架寿命，而分子动力学模拟可以更详细地阐明这种载体的单分子层的结构。这些研究将为未来的LNP基因递送系统的研发提供了更有价值的信息。

由于聚合物胶束具有较大的尺寸，聚合物胶束主要是通过CG方法，特别是DPD方法进行研究。得益于这些模拟研究，胶束的（解）组装过程、药物摄取、分布和释放的基本驱动力被揭露。许多已经提到的出版物展示了如何成功地进行模拟来表征刺激响应性转变。这在新兴的具有质子化聚合物基团的智能pH敏感系统中尤为重要，因为这种体系可用于在酸性肿瘤环境中触发抗癌药物的释放。前面提到的常数pH-MD可以用于这种研究。与脂质体的情况类似，为了表征聚合物胶束内驱动聚合物-药物相互作用的细节过程，需要通过AA模拟进行补充。对于常用作核酸载体的树状聚合物，其中包含可质子化的氨基基团，模拟也很好地表征了改变pH的影响。对聚合物链的微小结构变化，例如将末端氨基换成乙酰化变体或羟基，可能会对药物负载产生巨大影响，使用分子动力学已阐明这些现象背后的原因。计算模拟也已应用于研究基于聚合物的其他体系上，包括水凝胶或固体聚合物颗粒等。

聚合物-蛋白质偶联物代表了当前获得批准的药物纳米技术中聚合物基药物形式的大部分。计算模拟可用于研究聚合物对蛋白质结构产生的可能影响。改变连接位置、结构、链长或偶联聚合物链的数量会调节与药物相关的性质，例如热稳定性、生物利用度和生物活性。分子模拟是解析这些变化背后潜在机制的有利工具，并确定有利的蛋白质-聚合物相互作用位点，而在实验中，这些工作才刚刚开始使用各种NMR技术进行。将来，关于PEG替代物和各种蛋白质的蛋白质-聚合物接触图谱的更多数据可能为开发特定蛋白质（生物）药物的定制聚合物提供普遍适用的合理指南。

纳米技术日益发展，最近几年在这一研究领域的出版物数量呈爆炸式增长。希望本章内容能够向读者提供一个概述，介绍分子动力学模拟工具在这一过程中所扮演的重要角色。通过使用覆盖整个画面的多尺度方法，计算模拟实际上可以有助于合理设计纳米医学疗法的许多关键步骤，包括从体外制剂和药物负载过程到体内现象，如在人体肠道中的溶解、与细胞膜和血清蛋白的黏附和吸收，以及胞吞后的解离。模拟方法可以与其他计算工具结合使用，例如基于QM的计算[616-619]、分子对接[620]，或者随着数据量不断增加，可以利用机器学习生成预测模型[551, 552, 621, 422, 622, 623, 624, 625]。目前所呈现的多项研究展示了如何通过模拟揭露PEG作为金标准的动力学，同时也展示了PEG潜在替代物的不同性质。未来，计算模拟研究将继续揭示有关聚合物、药物和生物实体之间复杂相互作用的有用信息，从而有助于将基于聚合物的药物递送技术范围扩展到PEG之外。

参考文献

[1] Halwani A A. Development of pharmaceutical nanomedicines: From the Bench to the Market[J]. Pharmaceutics, 2022, 14(1), 106.

[2] Bunker A, Róg T. Mechanistic understanding from molecular dynamics simulation in pharmaceutical research 1[J]: Drug delivery. Frontiers in Molecular Biosciences, 2020, 7: 604770.

[3] Rozman K K, Doull J. Paracelsus, Haber and Arndt. Toxicology[J], 2001, 160: 191-196.

[4] Rautio J, Meanwell N A, Di L, et al. The expanding role of prodrugs in contemporary drug design and development[J]. Nature reviews drug discovery, 2018, 17(8): 559-587.

[5] Riehemann K, Schneider S W, Luger T A, et al. Nanomedicine—challenge and perspectives[J]. Angewandte Chemie International Edition, 2009, 48(5): 872-897.

[6] Lammers T, Ferrari M. The success of nanomedicine[J]. Nano Today, 2020, 31: 100853.

[7] Moghimi S M, Simberg D, Anchordoquy T J. Tuning the engines of nanomedicine[J]. Molecular Therapy, 2020, 28(3): 693-694.

[8] Abdellatif A A H, Alsowinea A F. Approved and marketed nanoparticles for disease targeting and applications in COVID-19[J]. Nanotechnology Reviews, 2021, 10(1): 1941-1977.

[9] Nikravesh N, Borchard G, Hofmann H, et al. Factors influencing safety and efficacy of intravenous iron-carbohydrate nanomedicines: From production to clinical practice[J]. Nanomedicine: Nanotechnology, Biology and Medicine, 2020, 26: 102178.

[10] Al Bostami R D, Abuwatfa W H, Husseini G A. Recent advances in nanoparticle-based co-delivery systems for cancer therapy[J]. Nanomaterials, 2022, 12(15): 2672.

[11] Naha P C, Liu Y, Hwang G, et al. Dextran-coated iron oxide nanoparticles as biomimetic catalysts for localized and pH-activated biofilm disruption[J]. ACS nano, 2019, 13(5): 4960-4971.

[12] Shan X, Gong X, Li J, et al. Current approaches of nanomedicines in the market and various stage of clinical translation[J]. Acta Pharmaceutica Sinica B, 2022, 12(7): 3028-3048.

[13] Freire Haddad H, Burke J A, Scott E A, et al. Clinical relevance of pre-existing and treatment-induced anti-poly(ethylene glycol)antibodies[J]. Regenerative Engineering and Translational Medicine, 2021: 1-11.

[14] Shi D, Beasock D, Fessler A, et al. To PEGylate or not to PEGylate: Immunological properties of nanomedicine's most popular component, polyethylene glycol and its alternatives[J]. Advanced drug delivery reviews, 2022, 180: 114079.

[15] Stiepel R T, Duggan E, Batty C J, et al. Micro and nanotechnologies: The little formulations that could[J]. Bioengineering & Translational Medicine, 2023, 8(2): e10421.

[16] Anselmo A C, Mitragotri S. Nanoparticles in the clinic: An update[J]. Bioengineering & translational medicine, 2019, 4(3): e10143.

[17] Mitchell M J, Billingsley M M, Haley R M, et al. Engineering precision nanoparticles for drug delivery[J]. Nature reviews drug discovery, 2021, 20(2): 101-124.

[18] Patra J K, Das G, Fraceto L F, et al. Nano based drug delivery systems: recent developments and future prospects[J]. Journal of nanobiotechnology, 2018, 16: 1-33.

[19] Hao J, Wang J, Pan H, et al. pH-redox responsive polymer-doxorubicin prodrug micelles studied by molecular dynamics, dissipative particle dynamics simulations and experiments[J]. Journal of Drug Delivery Science and Technology, 2022, 69: 103136.

[20] Lu S, Bennett W F D, Ding Y, et al. Design and characterization of a multifunctional pH-triggered peptide C8 for selective anticancer activity[J]. Advanced healthcare materials, 2015, 4(17): 2709-2718.

[21] Bunker A, Magarkar A, Viitala T. Rational design of liposomal drug delivery systems, a review: Combined experimental and computational studies of lipid membranes, liposomes and their PEGylation[J]. Biochimica et Biophysica Acta(BBA)-Biomembranes, 2016, 1858(10): 2334-2352.

[22] Kapoor B, Gupta R, Gulati M, et al. The why, where, who, how, and what of the vesicular delivery systems[J]. Advances in colloid and interface science, 2019, 271: 101985.

[23] Inglut C T, Sorrin A J, Kuruppu T, et al. Immunological and toxicological considerations for the design of liposomes[J]. Nanomaterials, 2020, 10(2): 190.

[24] Khalkhali M, Mohammadinejad S, Khoeini F, et al. Vesicle-like structure of lipid-based nanoparticles as drug delivery system revealed by molecular dynamics simulations[J]. International Journal of Pharmaceutics, 2019, 559: 173-181.

[25] Touitou E, Dayan N, Bergelson L, et al. Ethosomes—novel vesicular carriers for enhanced delivery: characterization and skin penetration properties[J]. Journal of controlled release, 2000, 65(3): 403-418.

[26] Khan S, McCabe J, Hill K, et al. Biodegradable hybrid block copolymer–lipid vesicles as potential drug delivery systems[J]. Journal of colloid and interface science, 2020, 562: 418-428.

[27] Han S. Molecular dynamics simulation of oleic acid/oleate bilayers: an atomistic model for a ufasome membrane[J]. Chemistry and physics of lipids, 2013, 175: 79-83.

[28] Antimisiaris S G, Mourtas S, Marazioti A. Exosomes and exosome-inspired vesicles for targeted drug delivery[J]. Pharmaceutics, 2018, 10(4): 218.

[29] Nummelin S, Selin M, Legrand S, et al. Modular synthesis of self-assembling Janus-dendrimers and facile preparation of drug-loaded dendrimersomes[J]. Nanoscale, 2017, 9(21): 7189-7198.

[30] Šegota S. Spontaneous formation of vesicles[J]. Advances in colloid and interface science, 2006, 121(1-3): 51-75.

[31] Chow A, Brown B D, Merad M. Studying the mononuclear phagocyte system in the molecular age[J]. Nature Reviews Immunology, 2011, 11(11): 788-798.

[32] Ricklin D, Hajishengallis G, Yang K, et al. Complement: a key system for immune surveillance and homeostasis[J]. Nature immunology, 2010, 11(9): 785-797.

[33] Sarma J V, Ward P A. The complement system[J]. Cell and tissue research, 2011, 343(1): 227-235.

[34] Hadjidemetriou M, Kostarelos K. Evolution of the nanoparticle corona[J]. Nature nanotechnology, 2017, 12(4): 288-290.

[35] Zhdanov V P. Formation of a protein corona around nanoparticles[J]. Current opinion in colloid & interface science, 2019, 41: 95-103.

[36] Gupta M N, Roy I. How corona formation impacts nanomaterials as drug carriers[J]. Molecular Pharmaceutics, 2020, 17(3): 725-737.

[37] Casalini T, Limongelli V, Schmutz M, et al. Molecular modeling for nanomaterial–biology interactions: Opportunities, challenges, and perspectives[J]. Frontiers in bioengineering and biotechnology, 2019, 7: 268.

[38] Brancolini G, Tozzini V. Multiscale modeling of proteins interaction with functionalized nanoparticles[J]. Current Opinion in Colloid & Interface Science, 2019, 41: 66-73.

[39] Pederzoli F, Tosi G, Vandelli M A, et al. Protein corona and nanoparticles: how can we investigate on？[J]. Wiley Interdisciplinary Reviews: Nanomedicine and Nanobiotechnology, 2017, 9(6): e1467.

[40] Del Pino P, Pelaz B, Zhang Q, et al. Protein corona formation around nanoparticles–from the past to the future[J]. Materials Horizons, 2014, 1(3): 301-313.

[41] Mahmoudi M. Protein corona: The golden gate to clinical applications of nanoparticles[J]. The international journal of biochemistry & cell biology, 2016, 75: 141-142.

[42] Xi-Feng X, Jiang X Q, Lei-Ji Z. Surface modification of poly ethylene glycol to resist nonspecific adsorption of proteins[J]. Chinese Journal of Analytical Chemistry, 2013, 41(3): 445-453.

[43] Nienhaus K, Nienhaus G U. Towards a molecular-level understanding of the protein corona around nanoparticles–recent advances and persisting challenges[J]. Current Opinion in Biomedical Engineering, 2019, 10: 11-22.

[44] Kharazian B, Hadipour N L, Ejtehadi M R. Understanding the nanoparticle–protein corona complexes using computational and experimental methods[J]. The international journal of biochemistry & cell biology, 2016, 75: 162-174.

[45] Berrecoso G, Crecente-Campo J, Alonso M J. Unveiling the pitfalls of the protein corona of polymeric drug nanocarriers[J]. Drug delivery and translational research, 2020, 10: 730-750.

[46] García-Álvarez R, Vallet-Regí M. Hard and soft protein corona of nanomaterials: Analysis and relevance[J]. Nanomaterials, 2021, 11(4): 888.

[47] Villaverde G, Baeza A. Targeting strategies for improving the efficacy of nanomedicine in oncology[J]. Beilstein Journal of Nanotechnology, 2019, 10(1): 168-181.

[48] Maeda H. The enhanced permeability and retention(EPR)effect in tumor vasculature: the key role of tumor-selective macromolecular drug targeting[J]. Advances in enzyme regulation, 2001, 41(1): 189-207.

[49] Maeda H, Nakamura H, Fang J. The EPR effect for macromolecular drug delivery to solid tumors: Improvement of tumor uptake, lowering of systemic toxicity, and distinct tumor imaging in vivo[J]. Advanced drug delivery reviews, 2013, 65(1): 71-79.

[50] Jenkins A D, Kratochvíl P, Stepto R F T, et al. Glossary of basic terms in polymer science (IUPAC Recommendations 1996)[J]. Pure and applied chemistry, 1996, 68(12): 2287-2311.

[51] Westenhoff S. Macromolecules Volume 1: Chemical Structures and Syntheses[J]. Macromolecular Chmistry an Physics, 2006, 207(6): 636-636.

[52] Baranwal J, Barse B, Fais A, et al. Biopolymer: A sustainable material for food and medical applications[J]. Polymers, 2022, 14(5): 983.

[53] Yin J, Luan S. Opportunities and challenges for the development of polymer-based biomaterials and medical devices[J]. Regenerative biomaterials, 2016, 3(2): 129-135.

[54] Francolini I, Piozzi A. Polymeric systems as antimicrobial or antifouling agents[J]. International Journal of Molecular Sciences, 2019, 20(19): 4866.

[55] Li S J, Shi X. Tailoring antifouling properties of nanocarriers via entropic collision of polymer grafting[J]. ACS nano, 2021, 15(3): 5725-5734.

[56] Elsabahy M, Heo G S, Lim S M, et al. Polymeric nanostructures for imaging and therapy[J]. Chemical reviews, 2015, 115(19): 10967-11011.

[57] Tamay D G, Dursun Usal T, Alagoz A S, et al. 3D and 4D printing of polymers for tissue engineering applications[J]. Frontiers in bioengineering and biotechnology, 2019, 7: 164.

[58] Connor E F, Lees I, Maclean D. Polymers as drugs—Advances in therapeutic applications of polymer binding agents[J]. Journal of Polymer Science Part A: Polymer Chemistry, 2017, 55(18): 3146-3157.

[59] Debotton N, Dahan A. Applications of polymers as pharmaceutical excipients in solid oral dosage forms[J]. Medicinal research reviews, 2017, 37(1): 52-97.

[60] Sung Y K, Kim S W. Recent advances in polymeric drug delivery systems[J]. Biomaterials Research, 2020, 24(1): 12.

[61] Ahmed E M. Hydrogel: Preparation, characterization, and applications: A review[J]. Journal of advanced research, 2015, 6(2): 105-121.

[62] Baghel S, Cathcart H, O'Reilly N J. Polymeric amorphous solid dispersions: a review of amorphization, crystallization, stabilization, solid-state characterization, and aqueous solubilization of biopharmaceutical classification system class II drugs[J]. Journal of pharmaceutical sciences, 2016, 105(9): 2527-2544.

[63] Walden D M, Bundey Y, Jagarapu A, et al. Molecular simulation and statistical learning methods toward predicting drug–polymer amorphous solid dispersion miscibility, stability, and formulation design[J]. Molecules, 2021, 26(1): 182.

[64] Misra A, Shahiwala A. Applications of polymers in drug delivery[M]. Elsevier, 2020.

[65] Grosberg A Y, Khokhlov A R. Giant molecules: here, there, and everywhere[M]. World Scientific, 2010.

[66] Begines B, Ortiz T, Pérez-Aranda M, et al. Polymeric nanoparticles for drug delivery: Recent developments and future prospects[J]. Nanomaterials, 2020, 10(7): 1403.

[67] Procopio A, Lagreca E, Jamaledin R, et al. Recent fabrication methods to produce polymer-based drug delivery matrices(Experimental and In Silico Approaches)[J]. Pharmaceutics, 2022, 14(4): 872.

[68] Khan M I, Hossain M I, Hossain M K, et al. Recent progress in nanostructured smart drug delivery systems for cancer therapy: a review[J]. ACS Applied Bio Materials, 2022, 5(3): 971-1012.

[69] Javia A, Vanza J, Bardoliwala D, et al. Polymer-drug conjugates: Design principles, emerging synthetic strategies and clinical overview[J]. International Journal of Pharmaceutics, 2022, 623: 121863.

[70] Tewari A K, Upadhyay S C, Kumar M, et al. Insights on development aspects of polymeric nanocarriers: the translation from bench to clinic[J]. Polymers, 2022, 14(17): 3545.

[71] Kotta S, Aldawsari H M, Badr-Eldin S M, et al. Progress in polymeric micelles for drug delivery applications[J]. Pharmaceutics, 2022, 14(8): 1636.

[72] Hwang D, Ramsey J D, Kabanov A V. Polymeric micelles for the delivery of poorly soluble drugs: From nanoformulation to clinical approval[J]. Advanced drug delivery reviews, 2020, 156: 80-118.

[73] Campora S, Ghersi G. Recent developments and applications of smart nanoparticles in biomedicine[J]. Nanotechnology Reviews, 2022, 11(1): 2595-2631.

[74] Kiran P, Khan A, Neekhra S, et al. Nanohybrids as protein-polymer conjugate multimodal therapeutics[J]. Frontiers in Medical Technology, 2021, 3: 676025.

[75] Barenholz Y C. Doxil®—The first FDA-approved nano-drug: Lessons learned[J]. Journal of controlled release, 2012, 160(2): 117-134.

[76] Tejada-Berges T, Granai C O, Gordinier M, et al. Caelyx/Doxil for the treatment of metastatic ovarian and breast cancer[J]. Expert review of anticancer therapy, 2002, 2(2): 143-150.

[77] Smith J A, Mathew L, Burney M, et al. Equivalency challenge: Evaluation of Lipodox® as the generic equivalent for Doxil® in a human ovarian cancer orthotropic mouse model[J]. Gynecologic oncology, 2016, 141(2): 357-363.

[78] Drummond D C, Noble C O, Guo Z, et al. Development of a highly active nanoliposomal irinotecan using a novel intraliposomal stabilization strategy[J]. Cancer research, 2006, 66(6): 3271-3277.

[79] Weng Y, Xiao H, Zhang J, et al. RNAi therapeutic and its innovative biotechnological evolution[J]. Biotechnology advances, 2019, 37(5): 801-825.

[80] Oliver S E, Gargano J W, Marin M, et al. Te advisory committee on immunization practices' interim recommendation for use of pfizer-BioNTech COVID-19 vaccine-United States, december 2020[J]. MMWR Morbidity and Mortality Weekly Report, 2020, 69(50): 1922-1924.

[81] Ndwandwe D, Wiysonge C S. COVID-19 vaccines[J]. Current opinion in immunology, 2021, 71: 111-116.

[82] Jain D, Raturi R, Jain V, et al. Recent technologies in pulsatile drug delivery systems[J]. Biomatter, 2011, 1(1): 57-65.

[83] Buster J E. Transdermal menopausal hormone therapy: delivery through skin changes the rules[J]. Expert opinion on pharmacotherapy, 2010, 11(9): 1489-1499.

[84] Rai M F, Pham C T N. Intra-articular drug delivery systems for joint diseases[J]. Current opinion in pharmacology, 2018, 40: 67-73.

[85] Stephan J L, Vlekova V, Le Deist F, et al. Severe combined immunodeficiency: a retrospective single-center study of clinical presentation and outcome in 117 patients[J]. The Journal of pediatrics, 1993, 123(4): 564-572.

[86] Harris J M, Chess R B. Effect of pegylation on pharmaceuticals[J]. Nature reviews Drug discovery, 2003, 2(3): 214-221.

[87] Jacobson I M, Brown Jr R S, Freilich B, et al. Peginterferon alfa-2 b and weight-based or flat-dose ribavirin in chronic hepatitis C patients: a randomized trial[J]. Hepatology, 2007, 46(4): 971-981.

[88] Fried M W, Shiffman M L, Reddy K R, et al. Peginterferon alfa-2 a plus ribavirin for chronic hepatitis C virus infection[J].

[89] Sheridan W P, Fox R M, Begley C G, et al. Effect of peripheral-blood progenitor cells mobilised by filgrastim(G-CSF)on platelet recovery after high-dose chemotherapy[J]. The Lancet, 1992, 339(8794): 640-644.

[90] Leonart L P, Tonin F S, Ferreira V L, et al. Effectiveness and safety of pegvisomant: a systematic review and meta-analysis of observational longitudinal studies[J]. Endocrine, 2019, 63: 18-26.

[91] Ni Z, Hui P. Emerging pharmacologic therapies for wet age-related macular degeneration[J]. Ophthalmologica, 2009, 223(6): 401-410.

[92] Sanchez-Fructuoso A, Guirado L, Ruiz J C, et al. Anemia control in kidney transplant patients treated with methoxy polyethylene glycol-epoetin beta (mircera): the Anemiatrans Group[C]//Transplantation proceedings. Elsevier, 2010, 42(8): 2931-2934.

[93] Nyborg A C, Ward C, Zacco A, et al. A therapeutic uricase with reduced immunogenicity risk and improved development properties[J]. PLoS One, 2016, 11(12): e0167935.

[94] Patel J N, Walko C M. Sylatron: a pegylated interferon for use in melanoma[J]. Annals of Pharmacotherapy, 2012, 46(6): 830-838.

[95] Chaplin S, Gnanapavan S. Plegridy for the treatment of RRMS in adults[J]. Prescriber, 2015, 26(9): 29-31.

[96] Daniali M, Nikfar S, Abdollahi M. Evaluating naloxegol for the treatment of opioid-induced constipation[J]. Expert Opinion on Pharmacotherapy, 2020, 21(8): 883-891.

[97] Turecek P L, Romeder-Finger S, Apostol C, et al. A world-wide survey and field study in clinical haemostasis laboratories to evaluate FVIII: C activity assay variability of ADYNOVATE and OBIZUR in comparison with ADVATE[J]. Haemophilia, 2016, 22(6): 957-965.

[98] Ezban M, Hermit M B, Persson E. FIXing postinfusion monitoring: Assay experiences with N9-GP(nonacog beta pegol; Refixia®; Rebinyn®)[J]. Haemophilia, 2019, 25(1): 154-161.

[99] Lah M, McPheron M. Palynziq clinic: one year and 43 patients later[J]. Molecular Genetics and Metabolism, 2021, 133(3): 250-256.

[100] Aschenbrenner D S. First Pegfilgrastim Biosimilar Approved[J]. AJN The American Journal of Nursing, 2018, 118(10): 19-20.

[101] Kaupbayeva B, Russell A J. Polymer-enhanced biomacromolecules[J]. Progress in Polymer Science, 2020, 101: 101194.

[102] Hoy S M. LA-EP2006: a Pegfilgrastim biosimilar[J]. BioDrugs, 2019, 33: 229-232.

[103] Ezban M, Hansen M, Kjalke M. An overview of turoctocog alfa pegol(N8-GP; ESPEROCT®)assay performance: implications for postadministration monitoring[J]. Haemophilia, 2020, 26(1): 156-163.

[104] Chowdary P, Fosbury E, Riddell A, et al. Therapeutic and routine prophylactic properties of rFactor VIII Fc (efraloctocog alfa, Eloctate®)in hemophilia A[J]. Journal of blood medicine, 2016: 187-198.

[105] Grossi F V, Bedwell P, Deschatelets P, et al. APL-2, a complement C3 inhibitor for the potential treatment of paroxysmal nocturnal hemoglobinuria(PNH): phase I data from two completed studies in healthy volunteers[J]. Blood, 2016, 128(22): 1251.

[106] Chatelain P, Malievskiy O, Radziuk K, et al. A randomized phase 2 study of long-acting TransCon GH vs daily GH in childhood GH deficiency[J]. The Journal of Clinical Endocrinology & Metabolism, 2017, 102(5): 1673-1682.

[107] Wysowski D K, Swartz L, Vicky Borders-Hemphill B, et al. Use of parenteral iron products and serious anaphylactic-type reactions[J]. American journal of hematology, 2010, 85(9): 650-654.

[108] Karatrantos A V, Mugemana C, Bouhala L, et al. From ionic nanoparticle organic hybrids to ionic nanocomposites: Structure, dynamics, and properties: A review[J]. Nanomaterials, 2022, 13(1): 2.

[109] Cabral H, Miyata K, Osada K, et al. Block copolymer micelles in nanomedicine applications[J]. Chemical reviews, 2018, 118(14): 6844-6892.

[110] Penfold N J W, Yeow J, Boyer C, et al. Emerging trends in polymerization-induced self-assembly[J]. ACS Macro Letters, 2019, 8(8): 1029-1054.

[111] Sochor B, Düdükcü O, Lübtow M M, et al. Probing the complex loading-dependent structural changes in ultrahigh drug-loaded polymer micelles by small-angle neutron scattering[J]. Langmuir, 2020, 36(13): 3494-3503.

[112] Haider M S, Lübtow M M, Endres S, et al. Think beyond the core: impact of the hydrophilic corona on drug solubilization using polymer micelles[J]. ACS applied materials & interfaces, 2020, 12(22): 24531-24543.

[113] Mollazadeh S, Sahebkar A, Shahlaei M, et al. Nano drug delivery systems: Molecular dynamic simulation[J]. Journal of Molecular Liquids, 2021, 332: 115823.

[114] Mastrotto F, Brazzale C, Bellato F, et al. In vitro and in vivo behavior of liposomes decorated with PEGs with different

chemical features[J]. Molecular pharmaceutics, 2019, 17(2): 472-487.

[115] Hou X, Zaks T, Langer R, et al. Lipid nanoparticles for mRNA delivery[J]. Nature Reviews Materials, 2021, 6(12): 1078-1094.

[116] Rajesh S, Leiske M N, Leitch V, et al. Lipidic poly(2-oxazoline) s as PEG replacement steric stabilisers for cubosomes[J]. Journal of Colloid and Interface Science, 2022, 623: 1142-1150.

[117] Umar H, Wahab H A, Gazzali A M, et al. Cubosomes: design, development, and tumor-targeted drug delivery applications[J]. Polymers, 2022, 14(15): 3118.

[118] Ita K. Polyplexes for gene and nucleic acid delivery: Progress and bottlenecks[J]. European Journal of Pharmaceutical Sciences, 2020, 150: 105358.

[119] Pereira-Silva M, Jarak I, Alvarez-Lorenzo C, et al. Micelleplexes as nucleic acid delivery systems for cancer-targeted therapies[J]. Journal of Controlled Release, 2020, 323: 442-462.

[120] Thakor P, Bhavana V, Sharma R, et al. Polymer–drug conjugates: Recent advances and future perspectives[J]. Drug Discovery Today, 2020, 25(9): 1718-1726.

[121] Russell A J, Baker S L, Colina C M, et al. Next generation protein‐polymer conjugates[J]. AIChE Journal, 2018, 64(9).

[122] Burridge K M, Page R C, Konkolewicz D. Bioconjugates–From a specialized past to a diverse future[J]. Polymer, 2020, 211: 123062.

[123] Pasut G, Veronese F M. State of the art in PEGylation: the great versatility achieved after forty years of research[J]. Journal of controlled release, 2012, 161(2): 461-472.

[124] Douroumis D, Fahr A, Siepmann J, et al. Computational pharmaceutics: application of molecular modeling in drug delivery[M]. John Wiley & Sons, 2015.

[125] Bunker A. Poly(ethylene glycol)in drug delivery, why does it work, and can we do better？All atom molecular dynamics simulation provides some answers[J]. Physics procedia, 2012, 34: 24-33.

[126] Zhang Z, Zhang Y, Song S, et al. Recent advances in the bioanalytical methods of polyethylene glycols and PEGylated pharmaceuticals[J]. Journal of separation science, 2020, 43(9-10): 1978-1997.

[127] Nanomedicine and the COVID-19 vaccines, Editorial. Nature Nanotechnology, 2020, 15(12), 963.

[128] Trollmann M F W, Böckmann R A. mRNA lipid nanoparticle phase transition[J]. Biophysical Journal, 2022, 121(20): 3927-3939.

[129] Paloncýová M, Čechová P, Šrejber M, et al. Role of ionizable lipids in SARS-CoV-2 vaccines as revealed by molecular dynamics simulations: from membrane structure to interaction with mRNA fragments[J]. The journal of physical chemistry letters, 2021, 12(45): 11199-11205.

[130] Dinç C Ö, Kibarer G, Güner A. Solubility profiles of poly(ethylene glycol)/solvent systems. II. Comparison of thermodynamic parameters from viscosity measurements[J]. Journal of Applied Polymer Science, 2010, 117(2): 1100-1119.

[131] Cha D K, Park S M. Polyethylene glycol as a solid polymer electrolyte[C]//The Twelfth Annual Battery Conference on Applications and Advances. IEEE, 1997: 249-253.

[132] Di Noto V, Lavina S, Giffin G A, et al. Polymer electrolytes: Present, past and future[J]. Electrochimica Acta, 2011, 57: 4-13.

[133] Müller‐Plathe F, van Gunsteren W F. Computer simulation of a polymer electrolyte: Lithium iodide in amorphous poly(ethylene oxide)[J]. The Journal of chemical physics, 1995, 103(11): 4745-4756.

[134] Laasonen K, Klein M L. Molecular dynamics simulations of the structure and ion diffusion in poly(ethylene oxide)[J]. Journal of the Chemical Society, Faraday Transactions, 1995, 91(16): 2633-2638.

[135] Gabizon A, Catane R, Uziely B, et al. Prolonged circulation time and enhanced accumulation in malignant exudates of doxorubicin encapsulated in polyethylene-glycol coated liposomes[J]. Cancer research, 1994, 54(4): 987-992.

[136] Nichols J W, Bae Y H. EPR: Evidence and fallacy[J]. Journal of Controlled Release, 2014, 190: 451-464.

[137] Danhier F. To exploit the tumor microenvironment: Since the EPR effect fails in the clinic, what is the future of nanomedicine？[J]. Journal of Controlled Release, 2016, 244: 108-121.

[138] Lehtinen J, Magarkar A, Stepniewski M, et al. Analysis of cause of failure of new targeting peptide in PEGylated liposome: molecular modeling as rational design tool for nanomedicine[J]. European journal of pharmaceutical sciences, 2012, 46(3): 121-130.

[139] Knop K, Hoogenboom R, Fischer D, et al. Poly(ethylene glycol)in drug delivery: pros and cons as well as potential alternatives[J]. Angewandte chemie international edition, 2010, 49(36): 6288-6308.

[140] Richter A W, Åkerblom E. Antibodies against polyethylene glycol produced in animals by immunization with monomethoxy polyethylene glycol modified proteins[J]. International Archives of Allergy and Immunology, 1983, 70(2): 124-131.

[141] Šroda K, Rydlewski J, Langner M, et al. Repeated injections of PEG-PE liposomes generate anti-PEG antibodies[J]. Cell.

Mol. Biol. Lett, 2005, 10(1): 37-47.

[142] JK A H G, Koling S, Chan L S, et al. Antibody against poly(ethylene glycol)adversely affects PEG-asparaginase therapy in acute lymphoblastic leukemia patients[J]. Cancer, 2007, 110: 103-111.

[143] Yang Q, Lai S K. Anti-PEG immunity: emergence, characteristics, and unaddressed questions[J]. Wiley Interdisciplinary Reviews: Nanomedicine and Nanobiotechnology, 2015, 7(5): 655-677.

[144] Ishida T, Maeda R, Ichihara M, et al. Accelerated clearance of PEGylated liposomes in rats after repeated injections[J]. Journal of controlled release, 2003, 88(1): 35-42.

[145] Ishida T, Kiwada H. Accelerated blood clearance(ABC)phenomenon upon repeated injection of PEGylated liposomes[J]. International journal of pharmaceutics, 2008, 354(1-2): 56-62.

[146] Huckaby J T, Jacobs T M, Li Z, et al. Structure of an anti-PEG antibody reveals an open ring that captures highly flexible PEG polymers[J]. Communications Chemistry, 2020, 3(1): 124.

[147] Nag O K, Awasthi V. Surface engineering of liposomes for stealth behavior[J]. Pharmaceutics, 2013, 5(4): 542-569.

[148] Smyth Jr H F, Carpenter C P, Weil C S. The toxicology of the polyethylene glycols[J]. Journal of the American Pharmaceutical Association(Scientific ed.), 1950, 39(6): 349-354.

[149] Yao X, Qi C, Sun C, et al. Poly(ethylene glycol)alternatives in biomedical applications[J]. Nano Today, 2023, 48: 101738.

[150] Mogoşanu G D, Grumezescu A M, Bejenaru C, et al. Polymeric protective agents for nanoparticles in drug delivery and targeting[J]. International journal of pharmaceutics, 2016, 510(2): 419-429.

[151] Lorson T, Luebtow M M, Wegener E, et al. Poly(2-oxazoline)s based biomaterials: A comprehensive and critical update[J]. Biomaterials, 2018, 178: 204-280.

[152] Sedlacek O, Monnery B D, Filippov S K, et al. Poly(2-oxazoline)s–Are they more advantageous for biomedical applications than other polymers？[J]. Macromolecular rapid communications, 2012, 33(19): 1648-1662.

[153] Viegas T X, Bentley M D, Harris J M, et al. Polyoxazoline: chemistry, properties, and applications in drug delivery[J]. Bioconjugate chemistry, 2011, 22(5): 976-986.

[154] Luxenhofer R, Schulz A, Roques C, et al. Doubly amphiphilic poly(2-oxazoline)s as high-capacity delivery systems for hydrophobic drugs[J]. Biomaterials, 2010, 31(18): 4972-4979.

[155] Magarkar A, Rog T, Bunker A. A computational study suggests that replacing PEG with PMOZ may increase exposure of hydrophobic targeting moiety[J]. European Journal of Pharmaceutical Sciences, 2017, 103: 128-135.

[156] Hauptstein N, Pouyan P, Kehrein J, et al. Molecular insights into site-specific interferon-α2a bioconjugates originated from PEG, LPG, and PEtOx[J]. Biomacromolecules, 2021, 22(11): 4521-4534.

[157] Hauptstein N, Dirauf M, Wittwer K, et al. PEtOxylated Interferon-α2a bioconjugates addressing H1N1 influenza a virus infection[J]. Biomacromolecules, 2022, 23(9): 3593-3601.

[158] Lühmann T, Schmidt M, Leiske M N, et al. Site-specific POxylation of interleukin-4[J]. ACS Biomaterials Science & Engineering, 2017, 3(3): 304-312.

[159] García K P, Zarschler K, Barbaro L, et al. Zwitterionic-coated "stealth" nanoparticles for biomedical applications: recent advances in countering biomolecular corona formation and uptake by the mononuclear phagocyte system[J]. Small, 2014, 10(13): 2516-2529.

[160] Thomas A, Müller S S, Frey H. Beyond poly(ethylene glycol): linear polyglycerol as a multifunctional polyether for biomedical and pharmaceutical applications[J]. Biomacromolecules, 2014, 15(6): 1935-1954.

[161] Hauptstein N, Pouyan P, Wittwer K, et al. Polymer selection impacts the pharmaceutical profile of site-specifically conjugated Interferon-α2a[J]. Journal of Controlled Release, 2022, 348: 881-892.

[162] Hoang Thi T T, Pilkington E H, Nguyen D H, et al. The importance of poly(ethylene glycol)alternatives for overcoming PEG immunogenicity in drug delivery and bioconjugation[J]. Polymers, 2020, 12(2): 298.

[163] Cui S, Pan X, Gebru H, et al. Amphiphilic star-shaped poly(sarcosine)-block-poly(ε-caprolactone)diblock copolymers: one-pot synthesis, characterization, and solution properties[J]. Journal of Materials Chemistry B, 2017, 5(4): 679-690.

[164] Deng Y, Zou T, Tao X, et al. Poly(ε-caprolactone)-block-polysarcosine by ring-opening polymerization of sarcosine N-thiocarboxyanhydride: Synthesis and thermoresponsive self-assembly[J]. Biomacromolecules. 2015；16(10): 3265-74.

[165] Birke A, Ling J, Barz M. Polysarcosine-containing copolymers: Synthesis, characterization, self-assembly, and applications[J]. Progress in Polymer Science, 2018, 81: 163-208.

[166] Torchilin V P, Trubetskoy V S. Which polymers can make nanoparticulate drug carriers long-circulating？[J]. Advanced drug delivery reviews, 1995, 16(2-3): 141-155.

[167] Takeuchi H, Kojima H, Yamamoto H, et al. Evaluation of circulation profiles of liposomes coated with hydrophilic polymers having different molecular weights in rats[J]. Journal of Controlled Release, 2001, 75(1-2): 83-91.

[168] Li Y, Lei X, Dong H, et al. Sheddable, degradable, cationic micelles enabling drug and gene delivery[J]. RSC advances, 2014, 4(16): 8165-8176.

[169] Kopeček J, Kopečková P. HPMA copolymers: origins, early developments, present, and future[J]. Advanced drug delivery reviews, 2010, 62(2): 122-149.

[170] Lili Y, Ruihua M, Li L, et al. Intracellular doxorubicin delivery of a core cross-linked, redox-responsive polymeric micelles[J]. International journal of pharmaceutics, 2016, 498(1-2): 195-204.

[171] De Leo V, Maurelli A M, Giotta L, et al. Polymer encapsulated liposomes for oral co-delivery of curcumin and hydroxytyrosol[J]. International Journal of Molecular Sciences, 2023, 24(1): 790.

[172] Barclay T G, Day C M, Petrovsky N, et al. Review of polysaccharide particle-based functional drug delivery[J]. Carbohydrate polymers, 2019, 221: 94-112.

[173] Kim D H, Kim M D, Choi C W, et al. Antitumor activity of sorafenib-incorporated nanoparticles of dextran/poly(dl-lactide-co-glycolide)block copolymer[J]. Nanoscale research letters, 2012, 7: 1-6.

[174] Liebner R, Mathaes R, Meyer M, et al. Protein HESylation for half-life extension: synthesis, characterization and pharmacokinetics of HESylated anakinra[J]. European Journal of Pharmaceutics and Biopharmaceutics, 2014, 87(2): 378-385.

[175] Hou Y, Lu H. Protein PEPylation: a new paradigm of protein–polymer conjugation[J]. Bioconjugate Chemistry, 2019, 30(6): 1604-1616.

[176] Shao Q. Effect of conjugated(EK)10 peptide on structural and dynamic properties of ubiquitin protein: a molecular dynamics simulation study[J]. Journal of Materials Chemistry B, 2020, 8(31): 6934-6943.

[177] Xing R, Zhang F, Xie J, et al. Polyaspartic acid coated manganese oxide nanoparticles for efficient liver MRI[J]. Nanoscale, 2011, 3(12): 4943-4945.

[178] Romberg B, Oussoren C, Snel C J, et al. Pharmacokinetics of poly(hydroxyethyl-l-asparagine)-coated liposomes is superior over that of PEG-coated liposomes at low lipid dose and upon repeated administration[J]. Biochimica et Biophysica Acta(BBA)-Biomembranes, 2007, 1768(3): 737-743.

[179] Metselaar J M, Bruin P, de Boer L W T, et al. A novel family of L-amino acid-based biodegradable polymer-lipid conjugates for the development of long-circulating liposomes with effective drug-targeting capacity[J]. Bioconjugate chemistry, 2003, 14(6): 1156-1164.

[180] Binder U, Skerra A. PASylation®: a versatile technology to extend drug delivery[J]. Current opinion in colloid & interface science, 2017, 31: 10-17.

[181] Shamloo A, Rostami P, Mahmoudi A. PASylation enhances the stability, potency, and plasma half-life of interferon α-2 a: A molecular dynamics simulation[J]. Biotechnology Journal, 2020, 15(8): 1900385.

[182] van Strien J, Escalona-Rayo O, Jiskoot W, et al. Elastin-like polypeptide-based micelles as a promising platform in nanomedicine[J]. Journal of Controlled Release, 2023, 353: 713-726.

[183] Niculescu A G, Grumezescu A M. Polymer-based nanosystems—A versatile delivery approach[J]. Materials, 2021, 14(22): 6812.

[184] Bradley A J, Devine D V, Ansell S M, et al. Inhibition of liposome-induced complement activation by incorporated poly(ethylene glycol)-lipids[J]. Archives of biochemistry and biophysics, 1998, 357(2): 185-194.

[185] Du H, Chandaroy P, Hui S W. Grafted poly(ethylene glycol)on lipid surfaces inhibits protein adsorption and cell adhesion[J]. Biochimica et Biophysica Acta(BBA)-Biomembranes, 1997, 1326(2): 236-248.

[186] Szebeni J, Baranyi L, Savay S, et al. Role of complement activation in hypersensitivity reactions to doxil and hynic PEG liposomes: experimental and clinical studies[J]. Journal of liposome research, 2002, 12(1-2): 165-172.

[187] Price M E, Cornelius R M, Brash J L. Protein adsorption to polyethylene glycol modified liposomes from fibrinogen solution and from plasma[J]. Biochimica et Biophysica Acta(BBA)-Biomembranes, 2001, 1512(2): 191-205.

[188] Vert M, Domurado D. Poly(ethylene glycol): protein-repulsive or albumin-compatible？[J]. Journal of Biomaterials Science, Polymer Edition, 2000, 11(12): 1307-1317.

[189] Caracciolo G. Liposome–protein corona in a physiological environment: challenges and opportunities for targeted delivery of nanomedicines[J]. Nanomedicine: Nanotechnology, Biology and Medicine, 2015, 11(3): 543-557.

[190] Schöttler S, Becker G, Winzen S, et al. Protein adsorption is required for stealth effect of poly(ethylene glycol)-and poly(phosphoester)-coated nanocarriers[J]. Nature nanotechnology, 2016, 11(4): 372-377.

[191] Li Z, Wang Y, Zhu J, et al. Emerging well-tailored nanoparticulate delivery system based on in situ regulation of the protein corona[J]. Journal of Controlled Release, 2020, 320: 1-18.

[192] Cramar C J. Essentials of Computational Chemistry[M]. John Wiley&Sons, Ltd, 2004: 315.

[193] Thiel W. Semiempirical quantum–chemical methods[J]. Wiley Interdisciplinary Reviews: Computational Molecular Science, 2014, 4(2): 145-157.

[194] Allen M P, Wilson M R. Computer simulation of liquid crystals[J]. Journal of computer-aided molecular design, 1989, 3: 335-353.

[195] Frenkel D, Smit B. Understanding molecular simulation: from algorithms to applications[M]. Elsevier, 2023.

[196] Durrant J D, McCammon J A. Molecular dynamics simulations and drug discovery[J]. BMC biology, 2011, 9: 1-9.

[197] Radak B K, Chipot C, Suh D, et al. Constant-pH molecular dynamics simulations for large biomolecular systems[J]. Journal of chemical theory and computation, 2017, 13(12): 5933-5944.

[198] Brooks B R, Brooks III C L, Mackerell Jr A D, et al. CHARMM: the biomolecular simulation program[J]. Journal of computational chemistry, 2009, 30(10): 1545-1614.

[199] Case D A, Cheatham III T E, Darden T, et al. The Amber biomolecular simulation programs[J]. Journal of computational chemistry, 2005, 26(16): 1668-1688.

[200] Hess B, Kutzner C, Van Der Spoel D, et al. GROMACS 4: algorithms for highly efficient, load-balanced, and scalable molecular simulation[J]. Journal of chemical theory and computation, 2008, 4(3): 435-447.

[201] Karplus M, McCammon J A. Molecular dynamics simulations of biomolecules[J]. Nature structural biology, 2002, 9(9): 646-652.

[202] Phillips J C, Braun R, Wang W, et al. Scalable molecular dynamics with NAMD[J]. Journal of computational chemistry, 2005, 26(16): 1781-1802.

[203] Plimpton S. Fast parallel algorithms for short-range molecular dynamics[J]. Journal of computational physics, 1995, 117(1): 1-19.

[204] van Gunsteren W F, Dolenc J, Mark A E. Molecular simulation as an aid to experimentalists[J]. Current opinion in structural biology, 2008, 18(2): 149-153.

[205] Tian C, Kasavajhala K, Belfon K A A, et al. ff19SB: amino-acid-specific protein backbone parameters trained against quantum mechanics energy surfaces in solution[J]. Journal of chemical theory and computation, 2019, 16(1): 528-552.

[206] Galindo-Murillo R, Robertson J C, Zgarbova M, et al. Assessing the current state of amber force field modifications for DNA[J]. Journal of chemical theory and computation, 2016, 12(8): 4114-4127.

[207] Zgarbová M, Otyepka M, Sponer J, et al. Refinement of the Cornell et al. nucleic acids force field based on reference quantum chemical calculations of glycosidic torsion profiles[J]. Journal of chemical theory and computation, 2011, 7(9): 2886-2902.

[208] Dickson C J, Walker R C, Gould I R. Lipid21: complex lipid membrane simulations with AMBER[J]. Journal of chemical theory and computation, 2022, 18(3): 1726-1736.

[209] Kirschner K N, Yongye A B, Tschampel S M, et al. GLYCAM06: a generalizable biomolecular force field. Carbohydrates[J]. Journal of computational chemistry, 2008, 29(4): 622-655.

[210] He X, Man V H, Yang W, et al. A fast and high-quality charge model for the next generation general AMBER force field[J]. The Journal of Chemical Physics, 2020, 153(11).

[211] Huang J, Rauscher S, Nawrocki G, et al. CHARMM36 m: an improved force field for folded and intrinsically disordered proteins[J]. Nature methods, 2017, 14(1): 71-73.

[212] Hart K, Foloppe N, Baker C M, et al. Optimization of the CHARMM additive force field for DNA: Improved treatment of the BI/BII conformational equilibrium[J]. Journal of chemical theory and computation, 2012, 8(1): 348-362.

[213] Denning E J, Priyakumar U D, Nilsson L, et al. Impact of 2′-hydroxyl sampling on the conformational properties of RNA: update of the CHARMM all-atom additive force field for RNA[J]. Journal of computational chemistry, 2011, 32(9): 1929-1943.

[214] Klauda J B, Venable R M, Freites J A, et al. Update of the CHARMM all-atom additive force field for lipids: validation on six lipid types[J]. The journal of physical chemistry B, 2010, 114(23): 7830-7843.

[215] Guvench O, Mallajosyula S S, Raman E P, et al. CHARMM additive all-atom force field for carbohydrate derivatives and its utility in polysaccharide and carbohydrate–protein modeling[J]. Journal of chemical theory and computation, 2011, 7(10): 3162-3180.

[216] Vanommeslaeghe K, Hatcher E, Acharya C, et al. CHARMM general force field: A force field for drug-like molecules compatible with the CHARMM all-atom additive biological force fields[J]. Journal of computational chemistry, 2010, 31(4): 671-690.

[217] Jorgensen W L, Maxwell D S, Tirado-Rives J. Development and testing of the OPLS all-atom force field on conformational energetics and properties of organic liquids[J]. Journal of the american chemical society, 1996, 118(45): 11225-11236.

[218] Robertson M J, Tirado-Rives J, Jorgensen W L. Improved peptide and protein torsional energetics with the OPLS-AA force field[J]. Journal of chemical theory and computation, 2015, 11(7): 3499-3509.

[219] Robertson M J, Qian Y, Robinson M C, et al. Development and Testing of the OPLS-AA/M Force Field for RNA[J]. Journal of chemical theory and computation, 2019, 15(4): 2734-2742.

[220] Oostenbrink C, Villa A, Mark A E, et al. A biomolecular force field based on the free enthalpy of hydration and solvation: the GROMOS force-field parameter sets 53A5 and 53A6[J]. Journal of computational chemistry, 2004, 25(13): 1656-1676.

[221] Riniker S. Fixed-charge atomistic force fields for molecular dynamics simulations in the condensed phase: An overview[J]. Journal of chemical information and modeling, 2018, 58(3): 565-578.

[222] Abriata L A, Dal Peraro M. Assessment of transferable forcefields for protein simulations attests improved description of disordered states and secondary structure propensities, and hints at multi-protein systems as the next challenge for optimization[J]. Computational and Structural Biotechnology Journal, 2021, 19: 2626-2636.

[223] Petrović D, Wang X, Strodel B. How accurately do force fields represent protein side chain ensembles? [J]. Proteins: Structure, Function, and Bioinformatics, 2018, 86(9): 935-944.

[224] Beauchamp K A, Lin Y S, Das R, et al. Are protein force fields getting better? A systematic benchmark on 524 diverse NMR measurements[J]. Journal of chemical theory and computation, 2012, 8(4): 1409-1414.

[225] Frisch A. gaussian 09W Reference[J]. Wallingford, USA, 25 p, 2009, 470.

[226] Neese F, Wennmohs F, Becker U, et al. The ORCA quantum chemistry program package[J]. The Journal of chemical physics, 2020, 152(22).

[227] Gordon M S, Schmidt M W. Advances in electronic structure theory: GAMESS a decade later[M]//Theory and applications of computational chemistry. Elsevier, 2005: 1167-1189.

[228] Schmidt M W, Baldridge K K, Boatz J A, et al. General atomic and molecular electronic structure system[J]. Journal of computational chemistry, 1993, 14(11): 1347-1363.

[229] Morado J, Mortenson P N, Verdonk M L, et al. Paramol: A package for automatic parameterization of molecular mechanics force fields[J]. Journal of Chemical Information and Modeling, 2021, 61(4): 2026-2047.

[230] Betz R M, Walker R C. Paramfit: Automated optimization of force field parameters for molecular dynamics simulations[J]. Journal of computational chemistry, 2015, 36(2): 79-87.

[231] Case D A, Aktulga H M, Belfon K, et al. Amber 2022. University of California, San Francisco.

[232] Vanommeslaeghe K, Raman E P, MacKerell Jr A D. Automation of the CHARMM general force field(CGenFF) II: assignment of bonded parameters and partial atomic charges[J]. Journal of chemical information and modeling, 2012, 52(12): 3155-3168.

[233] Dodda L S, Cabeza de Vaca I, Tirado-Rives J, et al. LigParGen web server: an automatic OPLS-AA parameter generator for organic ligands[J]. Nucleic acids research, 2017, 45(W1): W331-W336.

[234] Stroet M, Caron B, Visscher K M, et al. Automated topology builder version 3.0: Prediction of solvation free enthalpies in water and hexane[J]. Journal of chemical theory and computation, 2018, 14(11): 5834-5845.

[235] Vanquelef E, Simon S, Marquant G, et al. RED Server: a web service for deriving RESP and ESP charges and building force field libraries for new molecules and molecular fragments[J]. Nucleic acids research, 2011, 39(suppl_2): W511-W517.

[236] Dupradeau F Y, Pigache A, Zaffran T, et al. The REd. Tools: Advances in RESP and ESP charge derivation and force field library building[J]. Physical Chemistry Chemical Physics, 2010, 12(28): 7821-7839.

[237] Yabe M, Mori K, Ueda K, et al. Development of PolyParGen software to facilitate the determination of molecular dynamics simulation parameters for polymers[J]. Journal of Computer Chemistry, Japan-International Edition, 2019, 5: 2018-0034.

[238] Santana-Bonilla A, López-Ríos de Castro R, Sun P, et al. Modular software for generating and modeling diverse polymer databases[J]. Journal of Chemical Information and Modeling, 2023, 63(12): 3761-3771.

[239] Hayashi Y, Shiomi J, Morikawa J, et al. RadonPy: automated physical property calculation using all-atom classical molecular dynamics simulations for polymer informatics[J]. npj Computational Materials, 2022, 8(1): 222.

[240] Choi Y K, Park S J, Park S, et al. CHARMM-GUI polymer builder for modeling and simulation of synthetic polymers[J]. Journal of chemical theory and computation, 2021, 17(4): 2431-2443.

[241] Sahu H, Shen K H, Montoya J H, et al. Polymer structure predictor(PSP): a python toolkit for predicting atomic-level structural models for a range of polymer geometries[J]. Journal of Chemical Theory and Computation, 2022, 18(4): 2737-2748.

[242] Rukmani S J, Kupgan G, Anstine D M, et al. A molecular dynamics study of water-soluble polymers: analysis of force fields from atomistic simulations[J]. Molecular Simulation, 2019, 45(4-5): 310-321.

[243] Lee H, Venable R M, MacKerell A D, et al. Molecular dynamics studies of polyethylene oxide and polyethylene glycol:

hydrodynamic radius and shape anisotropy[J]. Biophysical journal, 2008, 95(4): 1590-1599.

[244] Stepniewski M, Pasenkiewicz-Gierula M, Rog T, et al. Study of PEGylated lipid layers as a model for PEGylated liposome surfaces: molecular dynamics simulation and Langmuir monolayer studies[J]. Langmuir, 2011, 27(12): 7788-7798.

[245] Schommers W. Pair potentials in disordered many-particle systems: A study for liquid gallium[J]. Physical Review A, 1983, 28(6): 3599.

[246] Shell M S. The relative entropy is fundamental to multiscale and inverse thermodynamic problems[J]. The Journal of chemical physics, 2008, 129(14).

[247] Kmiecik S, Gront D, Kolinski M, et al. Coarse-grained protein models and their applications[J]. Chemical reviews, 2016, 116(14): 7898-7936.

[248] Graham J A, Essex J W, Khalid S. PyCGTOOL: automated generation of coarse-grained molecular dynamics models from atomistic trajectories[J]. Journal of chemical information and modeling, 2017, 57(4): 650-656.

[249] Berman H M, Westbrook J, Feng Z, et al. The protein data bank[J]. Nucleic acids research, 2000, 28(1): 235-242.

[250] Jumper J, Evans R, Pritzel A, et al. Highly accurate protein structure prediction with AlphaFold[J]. nature, 2021, 596(7873): 583-589.

[251] Feng S, Park S, Choi Y K, et al. CHARMM-GUI membrane builder: past, current, and future developments and applications[J]. Journal of chemical theory and computation, 2023, 19(8): 2161-2185.

[252] Hsu P C, Bruininks B M H, Jefferies D, et al. CHARMM-GUI Martini Maker for modeling and simulation of complex bacterial membranes with lipopolysaccharides[J]. 2017.

[253] Park S J, Lee J, Qi Y, et al. CHARMM-GUI Glycan Modeler for modeling and simulation of carbohydrates and glycoconjugates[J]. Glycobiology, 2019, 29(4): 320-331.

[254] Choi Y K, Kern N R, Kim S, et al. CHARMM-GUI nanomaterial modeler for modeling and simulation of nanomaterial systems[J]. Journal of chemical theory and computation, 2021, 18(1): 479-493.

[255] Martínez L, Andrade R, Birgin E G, et al. PACKMOL: A package for building initial configurations for molecular dynamics simulations[J]. Journal of computational chemistry, 2009, 30(13): 2157-2164.

[256] Soñora M, Martinez L, Pantano S, et al. Wrapping up viruses at multiscale resolution: optimizing PACKMOL and SIRAH execution for simulating the zika virus[J]. Journal of Chemical Information and Modeling, 2021, 61(1): 408-422.

[257] Schott-Verdugo S, Gohlke H. PACKMOL-Memgen: A simple-to-use, generalized workflow for membrane-protein–lipid-bilayer system building[J]. Journal of chemical information and modeling, 2019, 59(6): 2522-2528.

[258] Fortunato M E, Colina C M. pysimm: A python package for simulation of molecular systems[J]. SoftwareX, 2017, 6: 7-12.

[259] Marrink S J, Risselada H J, Yefimov S, et al. The MARTINI force field: coarse grained model for biomolecular simulations[J]. The journal of physical chemistry B, 2007, 111(27): 7812-7824.

[260] Souza P C T, Alessandri R, Barnoud J, et al. Martini 3: a general purpose force field for coarse-grained molecular dynamics[J]. Nature methods, 2021, 18(4): 382-388.

[261] Grünewald F, Alessandri R, Kroon P C, et al. Polyply; a python suite for facilitating simulations of macromolecules and nanomaterials[J]. Nature communications, 2022, 13(1): 68.

[262] Ramos M C, Quoika P K, Horta V A C, et al. pyPolyBuilder: automated preparation of molecular topologies and initial configurations for molecular dynamics simulations of arbitrary supramolecules[J]. Journal of Chemical Information and Modeling, 2021, 61(4): 1539-1544.

[263] Leach A, Kier L B. Molecular modeling: principles and applications[J]. Journal of Medicinal Chemistry, 1997, 40(18): 2969.

[264] Allen M P, Tildesley D J. Computer Simulation of Liquids[M]. Second edition edn. Oxford, United Kingdom: Oxford University Press, 2017.

[265] Prasad S, Mobley D L, Braun E, et al. Best practices for foundations in molecular simulations[J]. Living Journal of Computational Molecular Science, 2018, 1: 1-28.

[266] Miyazaki Y, Okazaki S, Shinoda W. pSpica: a coarse-grained force field for lipid membranes based on a polar water model[J]. Journal of Chemical Theory and Computation, 2019, 16(1): 782-793.

[267] Groot R D, Warren P B. Dissipative particle dynamics: Bridging the gap between atomistic and mesoscopic simulation[J]. The Journal of chemical physics, 1997, 107(11): 4423-4435.

[268] Espanol P, Warren P B. Perspective: Dissipative particle dynamics[J]. The Journal of chemical physics, 2017, 146(15).

[269] Lee E H, Hsin J, Sotomayor M, et al. Discovery through the computational microscope[J]. Structure, 2009, 17(10): 1295-1306.

[270] Murtola T, Bunker A, Vattulainen I, et al. Multiscale modeling of emergent materials: biological and soft matter[J]. Physical

Chemistry Chemical Physics, 2009, 11(12): 1869-1892.

[271] Committee N. Press release of 2013 Nobel Prize in chemistry.
[272] Connolly M L. Solvent-accessible surfaces of proteins and nucleic acids[J]. Science, 1983, 221(4612): 709-713.
[273] Arteca G A. Molecular shape descriptors[J]. Reviews in computational chemistry, 1996: 191-253.
[274] Maginn E J, Messerly R A, Carlson D J, et al. Best practices for computing transport properties 1. Self-diffusivity and viscosity from equilibrium molecular dynamics[J]. Living Journal of Computational Molecular Science, 2019, 1(1): 6324-6324.
[275] Davies M, Reyes-Figueroa A D, Gurtovenko A A, et al. Elucidating lipid conformations in the ripple phase: Machine learning reveals four lipid populations[J]. Biophysical Journal, 2023, 122(2): 442-450.
[276] Sukhomlinov S V, Müser M H. A mixed radial, angular, three-body distribution function as a tool for local structure characterization: Application to single-component structures[J]. The Journal of Chemical Physics, 2020, 152(19).
[277] Sukhomlinov S V, Müser M H. Stress anisotropy severely affects zinc phosphate network formation[J]. Tribology Letters, 2021, 69(3): 89.
[278] Van der Maaten L, Hinton G. Visualizing data using t-SNE[J]. Journal of machine learning research, 2008, 9(11).
[279] Schubert E, Sander J, Ester M, et al. DBSCAN revisited, revisited: why and how you should(still)use DBSCAN[J]. ACM Transactions on Database Systems(TODS), 2017, 42(3): 1-21.
[280] Buslaev P, Gordeliy V, Grudinin S, et al. Principal component analysis of lipid molecule conformational changes in molecular dynamics simulations[J]. Journal of chemical theory and computation, 2016, 12(3): 1019-1028.
[281] Honeycutt J D, Andersen H C. Molecular dynamics study of melting and freezing of small Lennard-Jones clusters[J]. Journal of Physical Chemistry, 1987, 91(19): 4950-4963.
[282] Roncaglia C, Ferrando R. Machine Learning Assisted Clustering of Nanoparticle Structures[J]. Journal of Chemical Information and Modeling, 2023, 63(2): 459-473.
[283] Lemke T, Peter C. Encodermap: Dimensionality reduction and generation of molecule conformations[J]. Journal of chemical theory and computation, 2019, 15(2): 1209-1215.
[284] Berg A, Franke L, Scheffner M, et al. Machine learning driven analysis of large scale simulations reveals conformational characteristics of ubiquitin chains[J]. Journal of Chemical Theory and Computation, 2020, 16(5): 3205-3220.
[285] Wang Y, Ribeiro J M L, Tiwary P. Machine learning approaches for analyzing and enhancing molecular dynamics simulations[J]. Current opinion in structural biology, 2020, 61: 139-145.
[286] Bernetti M, Bertazzo M, Masetti M. Data-driven molecular dynamics: a multifaceted challenge[J]. Pharmaceuticals, 2020, 13(9): 253.
[287] Glielmo A, Husic B E, Rodriguez A, et al. Unsupervised learning methods for molecular simulation data[J]. Chemical Reviews, 2021, 121(16): 9722-9758.
[288] Noé F, Tkatchenko A, Müller K R, et al. Machine learning for molecular simulation[J]. Annual review of physical chemistry, 2020, 71(1): 361-390.
[289] Husic B E, Charron N E, Lemm D, et al. Coarse graining molecular dynamics with graph neural networks[J]. The Journal of chemical physics, 2020, 153(19).
[290] Wang J, Olsson S, Wehmeyer C, et al. Machine learning of coarse-grained molecular dynamics force fields[J]. ACS central science, 2019, 5(5): 755-767.
[291] Schütt K T, Arbabzadah F, Chmiela S, et al. Quantum-chemical insights from deep tensor neural networks[J]. Nature communications, 2017, 8(1): 13890.
[292] Mardt A, Pasquali L, Wu H, et al. VAMPnets for deep learning of molecular kinetics[J]. Nature communications, 2018, 9(1): 5.
[293] Bhakat S. Collective variable discovery in the age of machine learning: reality, hype and everything in between[J]. RSC advances, 2022, 12(38): 25010-25024.
[294] Noé F, Olsson S, Köhler J, et al. Boltzmann generators: Sampling equilibrium states of many-body systems with deep learning[J]. Science, 2019, 365(6457): eaaw1147.
[295] Liu Y, Han T, Ma S, et al. Summary of ChatGPT/GPT-4 Research and Perspective Towards the Future of Large Language Models.
[296] Tsai S T, Kuo E J, Tiwary P. Learning molecular dynamics with simple language model built upon long short-term memory neural network[J]. Nature communications, 2020, 11(1): 5115.
[297] Zhang S, Fan R, Liu Y, et al. Applications of transformer-based language models in bioinformatics: a survey[J]. Bioinformatics Advances, 2023, 3(1): vbad001.

[298] Wang S, Guo Y, Wang Y, et al. Smiles-bert: large scale unsupervised pre-training for molecular property prediction[C]// Proceedings of the 10 th ACM international conference on bioinformatics, computational biology and health informatics. 2019: 429-436.

[299] Ahmad W, Simon E, Chithrananda S, et al. Chemberta-2: Towards chemical foundation models[J]. arXiv preprint arXiv: 2209.01712, 2022.

[300] Kuenneth C, Ramprasad R. polyBERT: a chemical language model to enable fully machine-driven ultrafast polymer informatics[J]. Nature Communications, 2023, 14(1): 4099.

[301] Xu C, Wang Y, Barati Farimani A. TransPolymer: a Transformer-based language model for polymer property predictions[J]. npj Computational Materials, 2023, 9(1): 64.

[302] Thakral S, Thakral N K. Prediction of drug–polymer miscibility through the use of solubility parameter based Flory–Huggins interaction parameter and the experimental validation: PEG as model polymer[J]. Journal of pharmaceutical sciences, 2013, 102(7): 2254-2263.

[303] Kasimova A O, Pavan G M, Danani A, et al. Validation of a novel molecular dynamics simulation approach for lipophilic drug incorporation into polymer micelles[J]. The Journal of Physical Chemistry B, 2012, 116(14): 4338-4345.

[304] Lübtow M M, Haider M S, Kirsch M, et al. Like dissolves like? A comprehensive evaluation of partial solubility parameters to predict polymer–drug compatibility in ultrahigh drug-loaded polymer micelles[J]. Biomacromolecules, 2019, 20(8): 3041-3056.

[305] Moore M D, Wildfong P L D. Informatics calibration of a molecular descriptors database to predict solid dispersion potential of small molecule organic solids[J]. International journal of pharmaceutics, 2011, 418(2): 217-226.

[306] Gumireddy A, Bookwala M, Zhou D, et al. Investigating and comparing the applicability of the R3 m molecular descriptor and solubility parameter estimation approaches in predicting dispersion formation potential of APIs in a random co-polymer polyvinylpyrrolidone vinyl acetate and its homopolymer[J]. Journal of Pharmaceutical Sciences, 2023, 112(1): 318-327.

[307] Genheden S, Ryde U. The MM/PBSA and MM/GBSA methods to estimate ligand-binding affinities[J]. Expert opinion on drug discovery, 2015, 10(5): 449-461.

[308] Decherchi S, Cavalli A. Thermodynamics and kinetics of drug-target binding by molecular simulation[J]. Chemical Reviews, 2020, 120(23): 12788-12833.

[309] Roux B. The calculation of the potential of mean force using computer simulations[J]. Computer physics communications, 1995, 91(1-3): 275-282.

[310] Laio A, Gervasio F L. Metadynamics: a method to simulate rare events and reconstruct the free energy in biophysics, chemistry and material science[J]. Reports on Progress in Physics, 2008, 71(12): 126601.

[311] Park S, Schulten K. Calculating potentials of mean force from steered molecular dynamics simulations[J]. The Journal of chemical physics, 2004, 120(13): 5946-5961.

[312] Róg T, Girych M, Bunker A. Mechanistic understanding from molecular dynamics in pharmaceutical research 2: lipid membrane in drug design[J]. Pharmaceuticals, 2021, 14(10): 1062.

[313] Abraham M J, Murtola T, Schulz R, et al. GROMACS: High performance molecular simulations through multi-level parallelism from laptops to supercomputers[J]. SoftwareX, 2015, 1: 19-25.

[314] Casalini T. Not only in silico drug discovery: Molecular modeling towards in silico drug delivery formulations[J]. Journal of Controlled Release, 2021, 332: 390-417.

[315] Chen Z, Huo J, Hao L, et al. Multiscale modeling and simulations of responsive polymers[J]. Current Opinion in Chemical Engineering, 2019, 23: 21-33.

[316] Abd-Algaleel S A, Abdel-Bar H M, Metwally A A, et al. Evolution of the computational pharmaceutics approaches in the modeling and prediction of drug payload in lipid and polymeric nanocarriers[J]. Pharmaceuticals, 2021, 14(7): 645.

[317] Angioletti-Uberti S. Theory, simulations and the design of functionalized nanoparticles for biomedical applications: a soft matter perspective[J]. npj Computational Materials, 2017, 3(1): 48.

[318] Stillman N R, Kovacevic M, Balaz I, et al. In silico modelling of cancer nanomedicine, across scales and transport barriers[J]. NPJ Computational Materials, 2020, 6(1): 92.

[319] Ramos M C, Horta V A C, Horta B A C. Molecular dynamics simulations of PAMAM and PPI dendrimers using the GROMOS-Compatible 2016H66 Force Field[J]. Journal of chemical information and modeling, 2019, 59(4): 1444-1457.

[320] Gartner III T E, Jayaraman A. Modeling and simulations of polymers: a roadmap[J]. Macromolecules, 2019, 52(3): 755-786.

[321] Khan P, Kaushik R, Jayaraj A. Approaches and Perspective of Coarse-Grained Modeling and Simulation for Polymer–Nanoparticle Hybrid Systems[J]. ACS omega, 2022, 7(51): 47567-47586.

[322] Dhamankar S, Webb M A. Chemically specific coarse-graining of polymers: Methods and prospects[J]. Journal of Polymer Science, 2021, 59(22): 2613-2643.

[323] Yan X, Scherphof G L, Kamps J A A M. Liposome opsonization[J]. Journal of liposome research, 2005, 15(1-2): 109-139.

[324] Marrink S J, De Vries A H, Mark A E. Coarse grained model for semiquantitative lipid simulations[J]. The Journal of Physical Chemistry B, 2004, 108(2): 750-760.

[325] Annis B K, Kim M H, Wignall G D, et al. A study of the influence of LiI on the chain conformations of poly(ethylene oxide)in the melt by small-angle neutron scattering and molecular dynamics simulations[J]. Macromolecules, 2000, 33(20): 7544-7548.

[326] Borodin O, Smith G D. Molecular dynamics simulations of poly(ethylene oxide)/LiI melts. 2. Dynamic properties[J]. Macromolecules, 2000, 33(6): 2273-2283.

[327] Borodin O, Smith G D. Molecular dynamics simulation study of LiI-doped diglyme and poly(ethylene oxide)solutions[J]. The Journal of Physical Chemistry B, 2000, 104(33): 8017-8022.

[328] Borodin O, Smith G D, Jaffe R L. Ab initio quantum chemistry and molecular dynamics simulations studies of LiPF6/poly(ethylene oxide)interactions[J]. Journal of Computational Chemistry, 2001, 22(6): 641-654.

[329] Borodin O, Smith G D, Douglas R. Force field development and MD simulations of poly(ethylene oxide)/LiBF4 polymer electrolytes[J]. The Journal of Physical Chemistry B, 2003, 107(28): 6824-6837.

[330] Borodin O, Smith G D. Mechanism of ion transport in amorphous poly(ethylene oxide)/LiTFSI from molecular dynamics simulations[J]. Macromolecules, 2006, 39(4): 1620-1629.

[331] Borodin O, Smith G D. Li^+ transport mechanism in oligo(ethylene oxide) s compared to carbonates[J]. Journal of solution chemistry, 2007, 36: 803-813.

[332] Borodin O, Smith G D. Molecular dynamics simulations of poly(ethylene oxide)/LiI melts. 1. Structural and conformational properties[J]. Macromolecules, 1998, 31(23): 8396-8406.

[333] Brandell D, Priimägi P, Kasemägi H, et al. Branched polyethylene/poly(ethylene oxide)as a host matrix for Li-ion battery electrolytes: A molecular dynamics study[J]. Electrochimica acta, 2011, 57: 228-236.

[334] Costa L T, Ribeiro M C C. Molecular dynamics simulation of polymer electrolytes based on poly(ethylene oxide)and ionic liquids. I. Structural properties[J]. The Journal of chemical physics, 2006, 124(18): 184902.

[335] Costa L T, Ribeiro M C C. Molecular dynamics simulation of polymer electrolytes based on poly(ethylene oxide)and ionic liquids. II. Dynamical properties[J]. The Journal of chemical physics, 2007, 127(16): 164901.

[336] Diddens D, Heuer A, Borodin O. Understanding the lithium transport within a rouse-based model for a PEO/LiTFSI polymer electrolyte[J]. Macromolecules, 2010, 43(4): 2028-2036.

[337] Ennari J, Neelov I, Sundholm F. Molecular dynamics simulation of the structure of PEO based solid polymer electrolytes[J]. Polymer, 2000, 41(11): 4057-4063.

[338] Ennari J, Neelov I, Sundholm F. Estimation of the ion conductivity of a PEO-based polyelectrolyte system by molecular modeling[J]. Polymer, 2001, 42(19): 8043-8050.

[339] Ennari J, Pietilä L O, Virkkunen V, et al. Molecular dynamics simulation of the structure of an ion-conducting PEO-based solid polymer electrolyte[J]. Polymer, 2002, 43(20): 5427-5438.

[340] Ferreira B A, Müller-Plathe F, Bernardes A T, et al. A comparison of Li^+ transport in dimethoxyethane, poly(ethylene oxide) and poly(tetramethylene oxide)by molecular dynamics simulations[J]. Solid State Ionics, 2002, 147(3-4): 361-366.

[341] Hektor A, Klintenberg M K, Aabloo A, et al. Molecular dynamics simulation of the effect of a side chain on the dynamics of the amorphous LiPF 6–PEO system[J]. Journal of Materials Chemistry, 2003, 13(2): 214-218.

[342] Karo J, Brandell D. A molecular dynamics study of the influence of side-chain length and spacing on lithium mobility in non-crystalline LiPF6·PEOx; x= 10 and 30[J]. Solid State Ionics, 2009, 180(23-25): 1272-1284.

[343] Rex S, Zuckermann M J, Lafleur M, et al. Experimental and Monte Carlo simulation studies of the thermodynamics of polyethyleneglycol chains grafted to lipid bilayers[J]. Biophysical journal, 1998, 75(6): 2900-2914.

[344] Alexander S. Adsorption of chain molecules with a polar head a scaling description[J]. Journal De Physique, 1977, 38(8): 983-987.

[345] de Gennes P G. Conformations of polymers attached to an interface[J]. Macromolecules, 1980, 13(5): 1069-1075.

[346] de Gennes P G. Polymers at an interface; a simplified view[J]. Advances in colloid and interface science, 1987, 27(3-4): 189-209.

[347] De Gennes P G. Model polymers at interfaces[M]//Physical basis of cell-cell adhesion. CRC Press, 2018: 40-60.

[348] Yang S C, Faller R. Pressure and surface tension control self-assembled structures in mixtures of pegylated and non-pegylated lipids[J]. Langmuir, 2012, 28(4): 2275-2280.

[349] Lee H, Pastor R W. Coarse-grained model for PEGylated lipids: effect of PEGylation on the size and shape of self-assembled structures[J]. The Journal of Physical Chemistry B, 2011, 115(24): 7830-7837.

[350] Thakkar F M, Ayappa K G. Effect of polymer grafting on the bilayer gel to liquid-crystalline transition[J]. The Journal of Physical Chemistry B, 2010, 114(8): 2738-2748.

[351] Magarkar A, Karakas E, Stepniewski M, et al. Molecular dynamics simulation of PEGylated bilayer interacting with salt ions: a model of the liposome surface in the bloodstream[J]. The Journal of Physical Chemistry B, 2012, 116(14): 4212-4219.

[352] Magarkar A, Rog T, Bunker A. Molecular dynamics simulation of PEGylated membranes with cholesterol: building toward the DOXIL formulation[J]. The Journal of Physical Chemistry C, 2014, 118(28): 15541-15549.

[353] Stepniewski M, Bunker A, Pasenkiewicz-Gierula M, et al. Effects of the lipid bilayer phase state on the water membrane interface[J]. The Journal of Physical Chemistry B, 2010, 114(36): 11784-11792.

[354] Pedersen C J. The discovery of crown ethers(Noble Lecture)[J]. Angewandte Chemie International Edition in English, 1988, 27(8): 1021-1027.

[355] Holland J W, Hui C, Cullis P R, et al. Poly(ethylene glycol)- lipid conjugates regulate the calcium-induced fusion of liposomes composed of phosphatidylethanolamine and phosphatidylserine[J]. Biochemistry, 1996, 35(8): 2618-2624.

[356] Vukovic L, Khatib F A, Drake S P, et al. Structure and dynamics of highly PEG-ylated sterically stabilized micelles in aqueous media[J]. Journal of the American Chemical Society, 2011, 133(34): 13481-13488.

[357] Torchilinl V P, Papisov M I. Why do polyethylene glycol-coated liposomes circulate so long？: Molecular mechanism of liposome steric protection with polyethylene glycol: Role of polymer chain flexibility[J]. Journal of liposome research, 1994, 4(1): 725-739.

[358] Martinez-Seara H, Rog T, Karttunen M, et al. Cholesterol induces specific spatial and orientational order in cholesterol/phospholipid membranes[J]. PloS one, 2010, 5(6): e11162.

[359] Pöyry S, Róg T, Karttunen M, et al. Significance of cholesterol methyl groups[J]. The Journal of Physical Chemistry B, 2008, 112(10): 2922-2929.

[360] Lee H, Kim H R, Park J C. Dynamics and stability of lipid bilayers modulated by thermosensitive polypeptides, cholesterols, and PEGylated lipids[J]. Physical Chemistry Chemical Physics, 2014, 16(8): 3763-3770.

[361] Dzieciuch M, Rissanen S, Szydłowska N, et al. PEGylated liposomes as carriers of hydrophobic porphyrins[J]. The Journal of Physical Chemistry B, 2015, 119(22): 6646-6657.

[362] Decuzzi P, Lee S, Bhushan B, et al. A theoretical model for the margination of particles within blood vessels[J]. Annals of biomedical engineering, 2005, 33: 179-190.

[363] Li Y, Stroberg W, Lee T R, et al. Multiscale modeling and uncertainty quantification in nanoparticle-mediated drug/gene delivery[J]. Computational Mechanics, 2014, 53: 511-537.

[364] Ke P C, Lin S, Parak W J, et al. A decade of the protein corona[J]. ACS nano, 2017, 11(12): 11773-11776.

[365] Lee H. Molecular modeling of protein corona formation and its interactions with nanoparticles and cell membranes for nanomedicine applications[J]. Pharmaceutics, 2021, 13(5): 637.

[366] Takada S. Coarse-grained molecular simulations of large biomolecules[J]. Current opinion in structural biology, 2012, 22(2): 130-137.

[367] Lee H, de Vries A H, Marrink S J, et al. A coarse-grained model for polyethylene oxide and polyethylene glycol: conformation and hydrodynamics[J]. The journal of physical chemistry B, 2009, 113(40): 13186-13194.

[368] Rossi G, Fuchs P F J, Barnoud J, et al. A coarse-grained MARTINI model of polyethylene glycol and of polyoxyethylene alkyl ether surfactants[J]. The Journal of Physical Chemistry B, 2012, 116(49): 14353-14362.

[369] Choi E, Mondal J, Yethiraj A. Coarse-grained models for aqueous polyethylene glycol solutions[J]. The Journal of Physical Chemistry B, 2014, 118(1): 323-329.

[370] Aydin F, Uppaladadium G, Dutt M. Harnessing nanoscale confinement to design sterically stable vesicles of specific shapes via self-assembly[J]. The Journal of Physical Chemistry B, 2015, 119(32): 10207-10215.

[371] Aydin F, Uppaladadium G, Dutt M. The design of shape-tunable hairy vesicles[J]. Colloids and Surfaces B: Biointerfaces, 2015, 128: 268-275.

[372] Ruoslahti E. RGD and other recognition sequences for integrins[J]. Annual review of cell and developmental biology, 1996, 12(1): 697-715.

[373] Viegas T X, Bentley M D, Harris J M, et al. Polyoxazoline: chemistry, properties, and applications in drug delivery[J]. Bioconjugate chemistry, 2011, 22(5): 976-986.

[374] Li T, Yu P, Chen Y, et al. N-acetylgalactosamine-decorated nanoliposomes for targeted delivery of paclitaxel to

[375] Hu W, Mao A, Wong P, et al. Characterization of 1, 2-distearoyl-sn-glycero-3-phosphoethanolamine-*N*-[methoxy(polyethylene glycerol)-2000] and its complex with doxorubicin using nuclear magnetic resonance spectroscopy and molecular dynamics[J]. Bioconjugate Chemistry, 2017, 28(6): 1777-1790.

[376] Khaledian S, Kahrizi D, Moradi S, et al. An experimental and computational study to evaluation of chitosan/gum tragacanth coated-natural lipid-based nanocarriers for sunitinib delivery[J]. Journal of Molecular Liquids, 2021, 334: 116075.

[377] Kuramochi H, Andoh Y, Yoshii N, et al. All-Atom molecular dynamics study of a spherical micelle composed of N-acetylated poly(ethylene glycol)−Poly(γ-benzyl l-glutamate)block copolymers: A potential carrier of drug delivery systems for cancer[J]. The Journal of Physical Chemistry B, 2009, 113(46): 15181-15188.

[378] Guo X D, Qian Y, Zhang C Y, et al. Can drug molecules diffuse into the core of micelles？[J]. Soft Matter, 2012, 8(39): 9989-9995.

[379] Wang Y, Zhu D D, Zhou J, et al. Mesoscopic simulation studies on the formation mechanism of drug loaded polymeric micelles[J]. Colloids and Surfaces B: Biointerfaces, 2015, 136: 536-544.

[380] Hpone Myint K, Brown J R, Shim A R, et al. Encapsulation of nanoparticles during polymer micelle formation: a dissipative particle dynamics study[J]. The Journal of Physical Chemistry B, 2016, 120(44): 11582-11594.

[381] Loverde S M, Klein M L, Discher D E. Nanoparticle shape improves delivery: rational coarse grain molecular dynamics(rCG-MD) of taxol in worm-like PEG-PCL micelles[J]. Advanced materials, 2012, 24(28): 3823-3830.

[382] Luo S, Zhang Y, Cao J, et al. Arginine modified polymeric micelles as a novel drug delivery system with enhanced endocytosis efficiency[J]. Colloids and Surfaces B: Biointerfaces, 2016, 148: 181-192.

[383] Rajagopal K, Mahmud A, Christian D A, et al. Curvature-coupled hydration of semicrystalline polymer amphiphiles yields flexible worm micelles but favors rigid vesicles: polycaprolactone-based block copolymers[J]. Macromolecules, 2010, 43(23): 9736-9746.

[384] Duran T, Costa A, Gupta A, et al. Coarse-grained molecular dynamics simulations of paclitaxel-loaded polymeric micelles[J]. Molecular Pharmaceutics, 2022, 19(4): 1117-1134.

[385] Shi C, Sun Y, Wu H, et al. Exploring the effect of hydrophilic and hydrophobic structure of grafted polymeric micelles on drug loading[J]. International Journal of Pharmaceutics, 2016, 512(1): 282-291.

[386] Luo X, Wang S, Xu S, et al. Relevance of the polymeric prodrug and its drug loading efficiency: comparison between computer simulation and experiment[J]. Macromolecular Theory and Simulations, 2019, 28(5): 1900026.

[387] Razavilar N, Hanna G. Molecular-Level Insights into the Diffusion of a Hydrophobic Drug in a Disordered Block Copolymer Micelle by Molecular Dynamics Simulation[J]. Macromolecular Theory and Simulations, 2022, 31(2): 2100060.

[388] Wang Y, Teitel S, Dellago C. Melting of icosahedral gold nanoclusters from molecular dynamics simulations[J]. The Journal of chemical physics, 2005, 122(21).

[389] Sun H. COMPASS: an ab initio force-field optimized for condensed-phase applications overview with details on alkane and benzene compounds[J]. The Journal of Physical Chemistry B, 1998, 102(38): 7338-7364.

[390] Luo Z, Jiang J. pH-sensitive drug loading/releasing in amphiphilic copolymer PAE-PEG: Integrating molecular dynamics and dissipative particle dynamics simulations[J]. Journal of controlled release, 2012, 162(1): 185-193.

[391] Guo X D, Zhang L J, Wu Z M, et al. Dissipative particle dynamics studies on microstructure of pH-sensitive micelles for sustained drug delivery[J]. Macromolecules, 2010, 43(18): 7839-7844.

[392] Zheng L S, Yang Y Q, Guo X D, et al. Mesoscopic simulations on the aggregation behavior of pH-responsive polymeric micelles for drug delivery[J]. Journal of colloid and interface science, 2011, 363(1): 114-121.

[393] Yang C, Sun Y, Zhang L. Dissipative Particle Dynamics Study on Aggregation of MPEG-PAE-PLA Block Polymer Micelles Loading Doxorubicine[J]. Chinese Journal of Chemistry, 2012, 30(9): 1980-1986.

[394] Nie S Y, Sun Y, Lin W J, et al. Dissipative particle dynamics studies of doxorubicin-loaded micelles assembled from four-arm star triblock polymers 4AS-PCL-*b*-PDEAEMA-*b*-PPEGMA and their pH-release mechanism[J]. The Journal of Physical Chemistry B, 2013, 117(43): 13688-13697.

[395] Lin W J, Nie S Y, Chen Q, et al. Structure-property relationship of pH-sensitive(PCL)$_2$(PDEA-*b*-PPEGMA)$_2$ micelles: Experiment and DPD simulation[J]. AIChE Journal, 2014, 60(10): 3634-3646.

[396] Gao J, Wang P, Wang Z, et al. Self-assembly of DCPD-loaded cross-linked micelle from triblock copolymers and its pH-responsive behavior: a dissipative particle dynamics study[J]. Chemical Engineering Science, 2019, 195: 325-334.

[397] Lin W, Xue Z, Wen L, et al. Mesoscopic simulations of drug-loaded diselenide crosslinked micelles: Stability, drug loading and release properties[J]. Colloids and Surfaces B: Biointerfaces, 2019, 182: 110313.

[398] Nie S Y, Lin W J, Yao N, et al. Drug release from pH-sensitive polymeric micelles with different drug distributions: insight

from coarse-grained simulations[J]. ACS Applied Materials & Interfaces, 2014, 6(20): 17668-17678.

[399] Wu Z, Duan M, Xiong D, et al. Mesoscale simulations of pH-responsive amphiphilic polymeric micelles for oral drug delivery[J]. Pharmaceutics, 2019, 11(12): 620.

[400] Wu W, Yi P, Zhang J, et al. 4/6-Herto-arm and 4/6-mikto-arm star-shaped block polymeric drug-loaded micelles and their pH-responsive controlled release properties: a dissipative particle dynamics simulation[J]. Physical Chemistry Chemical Physics, 2019, 21(27): 15222-15232.

[401] Min W, Zhao D, Quan X, et al. Computer simulations on the pH-sensitive tri-block copolymer containing zwitterionic sulfobetaine as a novel anti-cancer drug carrier[J]. Colloids and Surfaces B: Biointerfaces, 2017, 152: 260-268.

[402] Hao L, Lin L, Zhou J. pH-Responsive zwitterionic copolymer DHA-PBLG-PCB for targeted drug delivery: a computer simulation study[J]. Langmuir, 2018, 35(5): 1944-1953.

[403] Yang C, Yuan C, Liu W, et al. DPD studies on mixed micelles self-assembled from MPEG-PDEAEMA and MPEG-PCL for controlled doxorubicin release[J]. Colloids and Surfaces B: Biointerfaces, 2019, 178: 56-65.

[404] Yang C, Liu W, Xiao J, et al. pH-sensitive mixed micelles assembled from PDEAEMA-PPEGMA and PCL-PPEGMA for doxorubicin delivery: experimental and DPD simulations study[J]. Pharmaceutics, 2020, 12(2): 170.

[405] De Luca S, Treny J, Chen F, et al. Enhancing cationic drug delivery with polymeric carriers: The Coulomb‑pH switch approach[J]. Advanced Theory and Simulations, 2021, 4(2): 2000247.

[406] Wen W, Guo C, Guo J. Acid-responsive adamantane-cored amphiphilic block polymers as platforms for drug delivery[J]. Nanomaterials, 2021, 11(1): 188.

[407] Koochaki A, Moghbeli M R, Nikkhah S J, et al. Dual responsive PMEEECL-PAE block copolymers: a computational self-assembly and doxorubicin uptake study[J]. RSC advances, 2020, 10(6): 3233-3245.

[408] Mousavi S D, Maghsoodi F, Panahandeh F, et al. Doxorubicin delivery via magnetic nanomicelles comprising from reduction-responsive poly(ethylene glycol)-*b*-poly(ε-caprolactone)(PEG-SS-PCL)and loaded with superparamagnetic iron oxide(SPIO)nanoparticles: Preparation, characterization and simulation[J]. Materials Science and Engineering: C, 2018, 92: 631-643.

[409] Yang C, Yin L, Yuan C, et al. DPD simulations and experimental study on reduction-sensitive polymeric micelles self-assembled from PCL-SS-PPEGMA for doxorubicin controlled release[J]. Colloids and Surfaces B: Biointerfaces, 2021, 204: 111797.

[410] Srinivas G, Mohan R V, Kelkar A D. Polymer micelle assisted transport and delivery of model hydrophilic components inside a biological lipid vesicle: a coarse-grain simulation study[J]. The Journal of Physical Chemistry B, 2013, 117(40): 12095-12104.

[411] Raman A S, Pajak J, Chiew Y C. Interaction of PCL based self-assembled nano-polymeric micelles with model lipid bilayers using coarse-grained molecular dynamics simulations[J]. Chemical physics letters, 2018, 712: 1-6.

[412] Arsenidis P, Karatasos K. Computational study of the interaction of a PEGylated hyperbranched polymer/doxorubicin complex with a bilipid membrane[J]. Fluids, 2019, 4(1): 17.

[413] Dahanayake R, Dormidontova E E. Molecular structure and co-solvent distribution in PPO-PEO and pluronic micelles[J]. Macromolecules, 2022, 55(23): 10439-10449.

[414] Zhao Y, Ma S M, Li B, et al. Micellization of pluronic P123 in water/ethanol/turpentine oil mixed solvents: hybrid particle–field molecular dynamic simulation[J]. Polymers, 2019, 11(11): 1806.

[415] Bhendale M, Srivastava A, Singh J K. Insights into the phase diagram of Pluronic L64 using coarse-grained molecular dynamics simulations[J]. The Journal of Physical Chemistry B, 2022, 126(25): 4731-4744.

[416] Albano J M R, Grillo D, Facelli J C, et al. Study of the lamellar and micellar phases of pluronic F127: A molecular dynamics approach[J]. Processes, 2019, 7(9): 606.

[417] Kacar G. Thermodynamic stability of ibuprofen loaded poloxamer micelles[J]. Chemical Physics, 2020, 533: 110713.

[418] Lim C, Ramsey J D, Hwang D, et al. Drug‑dependent morphological transitions in spherical and worm‑like polymeric micelles define stability and pharmacological performance of micellar drugs[J]. Small, 2022, 18(4): 2103552.

[419] Zhang X, Lin W, Wen L, et al. Systematic design and application of unimolecular star-like block copolymer micelles: a coarse-grained simulation study[J]. Physical Chemistry Chemical Physics, 2016, 18(38): 26519-26529.

[420] Pinto S N, Mil-Homens D, Pires R F, et al. Core-shell polycationic polyurea pharmadendrimers: New-generation of sustainable broad-spectrum antibiotics and antifungals[J]. Biomaterials Science, 2022, 10(18): 5197-5207.

[421] Wishart D S, Knox C, Guo A C, et al. DrugBank: a comprehensive resource for in silico drug discovery and exploration// nucleic acids research[J]. 2006.

[422] Alves V M, Hwang D, Muratov E, et al. Cheminformatics-driven discovery of polymeric micelle formulations for poorly

soluble drugs[J]. Science Advances, 2019, 5(6): eaav9784.

[423] Sohrabi S, Khedri M, Maleki R, et al. In‑silico tuning of curcumin loading on PEG grafted chitosan: An atomistic simulation[J]. Chemistry Select, 2021, 6(18): 4544-4555.

[424] Nikkhah S J, Sammalkorpi M. Single core and multicore aggregates from a polymer mixture: A dissipative particle dynamics study[J]. Journal of Colloid and Interface Science, 2023, 635: 231-241.

[425] Styliari I D, Taresco V, Theophilus A, et al. Nanoformulation-by-design: an experimental and molecular dynamics study for polymer coated drug nanoparticles[J]. RSC advances, 2020, 10(33): 19521-19533.

[426] Xu J, Wen L, Zhang F, et al. Self-assembly of cyclic grafted copolymers with rigid rings and their potential as drug nanocarriers[J]. Journal of Colloid and Interface Science, 2021, 597: 114-125.

[427] Wessels M G, Jayaraman A. Molecular dynamics simulation study of linear, bottlebrush, and star-like amphiphilic block polymer assembly in solution[J]. Soft Matter, 2019, 15(19): 3987-3998.

[428] Rezaeisadat M, Bordbar A K, Omidyan R. Molecular dynamics simulation study of curcumin interaction with nano-micelle of PNIPAAm-*b*-PEG co-polymer as a smart efficient drug delivery system[J]. Journal of Molecular Liquids, 2021, 332: 115862.

[429] Augustine R, Kim D K, Jeon S H, et al. Chimeric poly(*N*-isopropylacrylamide)-*b*-poly(3, 4-dihydroxy-L-phenylalanine) nanocarriers for temperature/pH dual-stimuli-responsive theranostic application[J]. Reactive and Functional Polymers, 2020, 152: 104595.

[430] Salih M, Walvekar P, Omolo C A, et al. A self-assembled polymer therapeutic for simultaneously enhancing solubility and antimicrobial activity and lowering serum albumin binding of fusidic acid[J]. Journal of Biomolecular Structure and Dynamics, 2021, 39(17): 6567-6584.

[431] Feng Y H, Zhang X P, Li J Y, et al. How is a micelle formed from amphiphilic polymers in a dialysis process: Insight from mesoscopic studies[J]. Chemical Physics Letters, 2020, 754: 137711.

[432] Ma Y. Theoretical and computational studies of dendrimers as delivery vectors[J]. Chemical Society Reviews, 2013, 42(2): 705-727.

[433] Nandy B, Maiti P K, Bunker A. Force biased molecular dynamics simulation study of effect of dendrimer generation on interaction with DNA[J]. Journal of Chemical Theory and Computation, 2013, 9(1): 722-729.

[434] Majoros I J, Williams C R, Baker Jr J R. Current dendrimer applications in cancer diagnosis and therapy[J]. Current topics in medicinal chemistry, 2008, 8(14): 1165-1179.

[435] Sandoval-Yañez C, Castro Rodriguez C. Dendrimers: amazing platforms for bioactive molecule delivery systems[J]. Materials, 2020, 13(3): 570.

[436] Lee H. Molecular modeling of PEGylated peptides, dendrimers, and single-walled carbon nanotubes for biomedical applications[J]. Polymers, 2014, 6(3): 776-798.

[437] Javan Nikkhah S, Thompson D. Molecular modelling guided modulation of molecular shape and charge for design of smart self-assembled polymeric drug transporters[J]. Pharmaceutics, 2021, 13(2): 141.

[438] Lee H, Larson R G. Molecular dynamics study of the structure and interparticle interactions of polyethylene glycol-conjugated PAMAM dendrimers[J]. The Journal of Physical Chemistry B, 2009, 113(40): 13202-13207.

[439] Lee H, Larson R G. Effects of PEGylation on the size and internal structure of dendrimers: self-penetration of long PEG chains into the dendrimer core[J]. Macromolecules, 2011, 44(7): 2291-2298.

[440] Barraza L F, Jiménez V A, Alderete J B. Effect of PEGylation on the structure and drug loading capacity of PAMAM‑G4 dendrimers: A molecular modeling approach on the complexation of 5‑fluorouracil with native and PEGylated PAMAM‑G4[J]. Macromolecular Chemistry and Physics, 2015, 216(16): 1689-1701.

[441] Wen X, Lan J, Cai Z, et al. Dissipative particle dynamics simulation on drug loading/release in polyester-PEG dendrimer[J]. Journal of nanoparticle research, 2014, 16: 1-12.

[442] Lee H, Choi J S, Larson R G. Molecular dynamics studies of the size and internal structure of the PAMAM dendrimer grafted with arginine and histidine[J]. Macromolecules, 2011, 44(21): 8681-8686.

[443] Karatasos K. Self-association and complexation of the anti-cancer drug doxorubicin with PEGylated hyperbranched polyesters in an aqueous environment[J]. The Journal of Physical Chemistry B, 2013, 117(8): 2564-2575.

[444] Pavan G M, Barducci A, Albertazzi L, et al. Combining metadynamics simulation and experiments to characterize dendrimers in solution[J]. Soft Matter, 2013, 9(9): 2593-2597.

[445] Tanis I, Karatasos K. Molecular dynamics simulations of polyamidoamine dendrimers and their complexes with linear poly(ethylene oxide)at different pH conditions: static properties and hydrogen bonding[J]. Physical Chemistry Chemical Physics, 2009, 11(43): 10017-10028.

[446] Jiang W, Luo J, Nangia S. Multiscale approach to investigate self-assembly of telodendrimer based nanocarriers for anticancer drug delivery[J]. Langmuir, 2015, 31(14): 4270-4280.

[447] Albertazzi L, Brondi M, Pavan G M, et al. Dendrimer-based fluorescent indicators: in vitro and in vivo applications[J]. PloS one, 2011, 6(12): e28450.

[448] Vasiliu T, Craciun B F, Neamtu A, et al. In silico study of PEI-PEG-squalene-dsDNA polyplex formation: The delicate role of the PEG length in the binding of PEI to DNA[J]. Biomaterials Science, 2021, 9(19): 6623-6640.

[449] Jain V, Maiti P K, Bharatam P V. Atomic level insights into realistic molecular models of dendrimer-drug complexes through MD simulations[J]. The Journal of Chemical Physics, 2016, 145(12).

[450] Badalkhani-Khamseh F, Ebrahim-Habibi A, Hadipour N L. Atomistic computer simulations on multi-loaded PAMAM dendrimers: A comparison of amine-and hydroxyl-terminated dendrimers[J]. Journal of computer-aided molecular design, 2017, 31: 1097-1111.

[451] Badalkhani-Khamseh F, Ebrahim-Habibi A, Hadipour N L. Influence of dendrimer surface chemistry and pH on the binding and release pattern of chalcone studied by molecular dynamics simulations[J]. Journal of Molecular Recognition, 2019, 32(1): e2757.

[452] Maiti P K, Bagchi B. Structure and dynamics of DNA-dendrimer complexation: role of counterions, water, and base pair sequence[J]. Nano letters, 2006, 6(11): 2478-2485.

[453] Vasumathi V, Maiti P K. Complexation of siRNA with dendrimer: a molecular modeling approach[J]. Macromolecules, 2010, 43(19): 8264-8274.

[454] Nandy B, Maiti P K. DNA compaction by a dendrimer[J]. The Journal of Physical Chemistry B, 2011, 115(2): 217-230.

[455] Nandy B, Santosh M, Maiti P K. Interaction of nucleic acids with carbon nanotubes and dendrimers[J]. Journal of biosciences, 2012, 37: 457-474.

[456] Su Y, Quan X, Li L, et al. Computer simulation of DNA condensation by PAMAM dendrimer[J]. Macromolecular Theory and Simulations, 2018, 27(2): 1700070.

[457] Jain V, Maingi V, Maiti P K, et al. Molecular dynamics simulations of PPI dendrimer-drug complexes[J]. Soft Matter, 2013, 9(28): 6482-6496.

[458] Smeijers A F, Markvoort A J, Pieterse K, et al. Coarse-grained modelling of urea-adamantyl functionalised poly(propylene imine)dendrimers[J]. Molecular Simulation, 2016, 42(11): 882-895.

[459] Smeijers A F, Markvoort A J, Pieterse K, et al. Coarse-grained simulations of poly(propylene imine)dendrimers in solution[J]. The Journal of Chemical Physics, 2016, 144(7).

[460] Gupta S, Biswas P. Effect of pH on size and internal structure of poly(propylene imine)dendrimers: a molecular dynamics simulation study[J]. The Journal of Physical Chemistry B, 2018, 122(39): 9250-9263.

[461] Kavyani S, Amjad-Iranagh S, Dadvar M, et al. Hybrid dendrimers of PPI(core)-PAMAM(shell): A molecular dynamics simulation study[J]. The Journal of Physical Chemistry B, 2016, 120(36): 9564-9575.

[462] Lee H, Larson R G. Membrane pore formation induced by acetylated and polyethylene glycol-conjugated polyamidoamine dendrimers[J]. The Journal of Physical Chemistry C, 2011, 115(13): 5316-5322.

[463] Tu C, Chen K, Tian W, et al. Computational investigations of a peptide-modified dendrimer interacting with lipid membranes[J]. Macromolecular rapid communications, 2013, 34(15): 1237-1242.

[464] Lee H, Larson R G. Coarse-grained molecular dynamics studies of the concentration and size dependence of fifth-and seventh-generation PAMAM dendrimers on pore formation in DMPC bilayer[J]. The Journal of Physical Chemistry B, 2008, 112(26): 7778-7784.

[465] He X, Gu Z, Wang L, et al. Coarse-grained molecular dynamics simulation of dendrimer transmembrane transport with temperature-dependent membrane phase states[J]. International Journal of Heat and Mass Transfer, 2020, 155: 119797.

[466] Ghadari R, Mohammadzadeh Y. MD simulation studies on the effect of the temperature and protonation state on the imide-linked amino acid-based dendrimers[J]. Computational Materials Science, 2018, 151: 124-131.

[467] Ghadari R, Sabri A. In silico study on core-shell pseudodendrimeric glycoside structures in drug delivery related usages[J]. Polyhedron, 2019, 160: 10-19.

[468] Liu Y, Tang P, Pu H, et al. Study on the synthesis and drug-loading optimization of beta-cyclodextrin polymer microspheres containing ornidazole[J]. Journal of Drug Delivery Science and Technology, 2020, 58: 101836.

[469] He Y, Liu H, Bian W, et al. Molecular interactions for the curcumin-polymer complex with enhanced anti-inflammatory effects[J]. Pharmaceutics, 2019, 11(9): 442.

[470] Li S, Yu C, Zhou Y. Computational design of Janus polymersomes with controllable fission from double emulsions[J]. Physical Chemistry Chemical Physics, 2020, 22(43): 24934-24942.

[471] Minnelli C, Stipa P, Sabbatini S, et al. Insights into PLGA-encapsulated epigallocatechin 3-gallate nanoparticles as a new potential biomedical system: A computational and experimental approach[J]. European Polymer Journal, 2023, 182: 111723.

[472] Stipa P, Marano S, Galeazzi R, et al. Molecular dynamics simulations of quinine encapsulation into biodegradable nanoparticles: A possible new strategy against Sars-CoV-2[J]. European polymer journal, 2021, 158: 110685.

[473] Stipa P, Marano S, Galeazzi R, et al. Prediction of drug-carrier interactions of PLA and PLGA drug-loaded nanoparticles by molecular dynamics simulations[J]. European Polymer Journal, 2021, 147: 110292.

[474] Iesavand H, Rahmati M, Afzali D, et al. Investigation on absorption and release of mercaptopurine anticancer drug from modified polylactic acid as polymer carrier by molecular dynamic simulation[J]. Materials Science and Engineering: C, 2019, 105: 110010.

[475] Megy S, Aguero S, Da Costa D, et al. Molecular dynamics studies of poly(Lactic Acid)nanoparticles and their interactions with vitamin E and TLR agonists Pam1CSK4 and Pam3CSK4[J]. Nanomaterials, 2020, 10(11): 2209.

[476] Zatorska M, Łazarski G, Maziarz U, et al. Drug-loading capacity of polylactide-based micro-and nanoparticles– Experimental and molecular modeling study[J]. International Journal of Pharmaceutics, 2020, 591: 120031.

[477] Ghitman J, Stan R, Vlasceanu G, et al. Predicting the drug loading efficiency into hybrid nanocarriers based on PLGA-vegetable oil using molecular dynamic simulation approach and Flory-Huggins theory[J]. Journal of Drug Delivery Science and Technology, 2019, 53: 101203.

[478] Ahmad S, Johnston B F, Mackay S P, et al. In silico modelling of drug–polymer interactions for pharmaceutical formulations[J]. Journal of the Royal Society Interface, 2010, 7(suppl_4): S423-S433.

[479] Guo X D, Tan J P K, Kim S H, et al. Computational studies on self-assembled paclitaxel structures: templates for hierarchical block copolymer assemblies and sustained drug release[J]. Biomaterials, 2009, 30(33): 6556-6563.

[480] Guo X D, Tan J P K, Zhang L J, et al. Phase behavior study of paclitaxel loaded amphiphilic copolymer in two solvents by dissipative particle dynamics simulations[J]. Chemical Physics Letters, 2009, 473(4-6): 336-342.

[481] Soto-Figueroa C, Vicente L. Mesoscopic simulation of the drug release mechanism on the polymeric vehicle P(ST-DVB)in an acid environment[J]. Soft Matter, 2011, 7(18): 8224-8230.

[482] Buxton G A. Simulating the co-encapsulation of drugs in a "smart" core-shell-shell polymer nanoparticle[J]. The European Physical Journal E, 2014, 37: 1-7.

[483] Li J, Ying S, Ren H, et al. Molecular dynamics study on the encapsulation and release of anti-cancer drug doxorubicin by chitosan[J]. International journal of pharmaceutics, 2020, 580: 119241.

[484] Mousavi S V, Hashemianzadeh S M. Molecular dynamics approach for behavior assessment of chitosan nanoparticles in carrying of donepezil and rivastigmine drug molecules[J]. Materials Research Express, 2019, 6(4): 045069.

[485] Eslami M, Nikkhah S J, Eslami E, et al. A new insight into encapsulation process of a drug molecule in the polymer/surfactant system: a molecular simulation study[J]. Structural Chemistry, 2020, 31(5): 2051-2062.

[486] Shadrack D M, Swai H S. Solvent effects on molecular encapsulation of Toussantine-A by chitosan nanoparticle: A metadynamics study[J]. Journal of Molecular Liquids, 2019, 292: 111434.

[487] Eslami M, Nikkhah S J, Hashemianzadeh S M, et al. The compatibility of tacrine molecule with poly(n-butylcyanoacrylate) and chitosan as efficient carriers for drug delivery: a molecular dynamics study[J]. European Journal of Pharmaceutical Sciences, 2016, 82: 79-85.

[488] Razmimanesh F, Amjad-Iranagh S, Modarress H. Molecular dynamics simulation study of chitosan and gemcitabine as a drug delivery system[J]. Journal of molecular modeling, 2015, 21: 1-14.

[489] Tokarský J, Andrýsek T, Čapková P. Molecular modeling of gel nanoparticles with cyclosporine A for oral drug delivery[J]. International journal of pharmaceutics, 2011, 410(1-2): 196-205.

[490] Mazloom-Jalali A, Shariatinia Z. Polycaprolactone nanocomposite systems used to deliver ifosfamide anticancer drug: molecular dynamics simulations[J]. Structural Chemistry, 2019, 30: 863-876.

[491] Chang C Y, Ju S P, Wang L F, et al. Investigation of the self-assembly of CS and PCL copolymers with different molecular weights in water solution by coarse-grained molecular dynamics simulation[J]. Journal of molecular modeling, 2017, 23: 1-12.

[492] Hathout R M, Metwally A K A, Woodman T J, et al. Prediction of drug loading in the gelatin matrix using computational methods[J]. ACS omega, 2020, 5(3): 1549-1556.

[493] Li Y C, Rissanen S, Stepniewski M, et al. Study of interaction between PEG carrier and three relevant drug molecules: piroxicam, paclitaxel, and hematoporphyrin[J]. The Journal of Physical Chemistry B, 2012, 116(24): 7334-7341.

[494] Rissanen S, Kumorek M, Martinez-Seara H, et al. Effect of PEGylation on drug entry into lipid bilayer[J]. The Journal of

Physical Chemistry B, 2014, 118(1): 144-151.

[495] Abdoune Y, Benguerba Y, Benabid S, et al. Numerical investigation of polyethylene glycol polymer(PEG)and dithymoquinone(DTQ)interaction using molecular modeling[J]. Journal of Molecular Liquids, 2019, 276: 134-140.

[496] Feng Y H, Liu J L, Zhu D D, et al. Multiscale simulations of drug distributions in polymer dissolvable microneedles[J]. Colloids and Surfaces B: Biointerfaces, 2020, 189: 110844.

[497] Feng Y H, Zhang X P, Li W X, et al. Stability and diffusion properties of insulin in dissolvable microneedles: A multiscale simulation study[J]. Langmuir, 2021, 37(30): 9244-9252.

[498] Hao T, Tan H, Li S, et al. Multilayer onion-like vesicles self-assembled from amphiphilic hyperbranched multiarm copolymers via simulation[J]. Journal of Polymer Science, 2020, 58(5): 704-715.

[499] Parveen S, Sahoo S K. Nanomedicine: clinical applications of polyethylene glycol conjugated proteins and drugs[J]. Clinical pharmacokinetics, 2006, 45: 965-988.

[500] Veronese F M. Peptide and protein PEGylation: a review of problems and solutions[J]. Biomaterials, 2001, 22(5): 405-417.

[501] Roberts M J, Bentley M D, Harris J M. Chemistry for peptide and protein PEGylation[J]. Advanced drug delivery reviews, 2002, 54(4): 459-476.

[502] Ramezanghorbani F, Lin P, Colina C M. Optimizing protein-polymer interactions in a poly(ethylene glycol)coarse-grained model[J]. The Journal of Physical Chemistry B, 2018, 122(33): 7997-8005.

[503] Grünewald F, Kroon P C, Souza P C T, et al. Protocol for simulations of PEGylated proteins with martini 3[J]. Structural genomics: general applications, 2021: 315-335.

[504] Wang Y, Wu C. Site-specific conjugation of polymers to proteins[J]. Biomacromolecules, 2018, 19(6): 1804-1825.

[505] Lin P, Colina C M. Molecular simulation of protein-polymer conjugates[J]. Current Opinion in Chemical Engineering, 2019, 23: 44-50.

[506] Taylor P A, Jayaraman A. Molecular Modeling and Simulations of Peptide-Polymer Conjugates[J]. Annual Review of Chemical and Biomolecular Engineering, 2020, 11(1): 257-276.

[507] Rouhani M, Khodabakhsh F, Norouzian D, et al. Molecular dynamics simulation for rational protein engineering: Present and future prospectus[J]. Journal of Molecular Graphics and Modelling, 2018, 84: 43-53.

[508] Baker S L, Munasinghe A, Murata H, et al. Intramolecular interactions of conjugated polymers mimic molecular chaperones to stabilize protein-polymer conjugates[J]. Biomacromolecules, 2018, 19(9): 3798-3813.

[509] Heredero M, Beloqui A. Enzyme-Polymer Conjugates for Tuning, Enhancing, and Expanding Biocatalytic Activity[J]. ChemBioChem, 2023, 24(4): e202200611.

[510] Baker S L, Munasinghe A, Kaupbayeva B, et al. Transforming protein-polymer conjugate purification by tuning protein solubility[J]. Nature Communications, 2019, 10(1): 4718.

[511] Noro J, Castro T G, Gonçalves F, et al. Catalytic activation of esterases by PEGylation for polyester synthesis[J]. ChemCatChem, 2019, 11(10): 2490-2499.

[512] Kovaliov M, Wright T A, Cheng B, et al. Toward next-generation biohybrid catalyst design: influence of degree of polymerization on enzyme activity[J]. Bioconjugate Chemistry, 2020, 31(3): 939-947.

[513] Jian Y, Han Y, Fu Z, et al. The role of conformational dynamics in the activity of polymer-conjugated CalB in organic solvents[J]. Physical Chemistry Chemical Physics, 2022, 24(36): 22028-22037.

[514] Veronese F M, Mero A. The impact of PEGylation on biological therapies[J]. BioDrugs, 2008, 22: 315-329.

[515] Lawrence P B, Price J L. How PEGylation influences protein conformational stability[J]. Current opinion in chemical biology, 2016, 34: 88-94.

[516] Turecek P L, Bossard M J, Schoetens F, et al. PEGylation of biopharmaceuticals: a review of chemistry and nonclinical safety information of approved drugs[J]. Journal of pharmaceutical sciences, 2016, 105(2): 460-475.

[517] Lawrence P B, Gavrilov Y, Matthews S S, et al. Criteria for selecting PEGylation sites on proteins for higher thermodynamic and proteolytic stability[J]. Journal of the American Chemical Society, 2014, 136(50): 17547-17560.

[518] Ciepluch K, Radulescu A, Hoffmann I, et al. Influence of PEGylation on domain dynamics of phosphoglycerate kinase: PEG acts like entropic spring for the protein[J]. Bioconjugate chemistry, 2018, 29(6): 1950-1960.

[519] Braun A C, Gutmann M, Lühmann T, et al. Bioorthogonal strategies for site-directed decoration of biomaterials with therapeutic proteins[J]. Journal of Controlled Release, 2018, 273: 68-85.

[520] Manjula B N, Tsai A, Upadhya R, et al. Site-specific PEGylation of hemoglobin at Cys-93(β): correlation between the colligative properties of the PEGylated protein and the length of the conjugated PEG chain[J]. Bioconjugate Chemistry, 2003, 14(2): 464-472.

[521] Daura X, Mark A E, Van Gunsteren W F. Parametrization of aliphatic CHn united atoms of GROMOS96 force field[J].

Journal of computational chemistry, 1998, 19(5): 535-547.
[522] Yang C, Lu D, Liu Z. How PEGylation enhances the stability and potency of insulin: a molecular dynamics simulation[J]. Biochemistry, 2011, 50(13): 2585-2593.
[523] Mu Q, Hu T, Yu J. Molecular insight into the steric shielding effect of PEG on the conjugated staphylokinase: biochemical characterization and molecular dynamics simulation[J]. PLoS One, 2013, 8(7): e68559.
[524] DeBenedictis E P, Hamed E, Keten S. Mechanical reinforcement of proteins with polymer conjugation[J]. ACS nano, 2016, 10(2): 2259-2267.
[525] Jain A, Ashbaugh H S. Helix stabilization of poly(ethylene glycol)-peptide conjugates[J]. Biomacromolecules, 2011, 12(7): 2729-2734.
[526] Ambrosio E, Podmore A, Gomes dos Santos A L, et al. Control of peptide aggregation and fibrillation by physical PEGylation[J]. Biomacromolecules, 2018, 19(10): 3958-3969.
[527] Han E, Lee H. Effects of PEGylation on the binding interaction of magainin 2 and tachyplesin I with lipid bilayer surface[J]. Langmuir, 2013, 29(46): 14214-14221.
[528] Draper S R E, Ashton D S, Conover B M, et al. PEGylation near a patch of nonpolar surface residues increases the conformational stability of the WW domain[J]. The Journal of organic chemistry, 2019, 85(3): 1725-1730.
[529] Xiao Q, Draper S R E, Smith M S, et al. Influence of pegylation on the strength of protein surface salt bridges[J]. ACS chemical biology, 2019, 14(7): 1652-1659.
[530] Draper S R E, Jones Z B, Earl S O, et al. PEGylation increases the strength of a nearby NH-π Hydrogen Bond in the WW Domain[J]. Biochemistry, 2021, 60(26): 2064-2070.
[531] Chao S H, Matthews S S, Paxman R, et al. Two structural scenarios for protein stabilization by PEG[J]. The Journal of Physical Chemistry B, 2014, 118(28): 8388-8395.
[532] Lawrence P B, Billings W M, Miller M K B, et al. Conjugation strategy strongly impacts the conformational stability of a PEG-protein conjugate[J]. ACS chemical biology, 2016, 11(7): 1805-1809.
[533] Price J L, Powers E T, Kelly J W. N-PEGylation of a reverse turn is stabilizing in multiple sequence contexts, unlike N-GlcNAcylation[J]. ACS chemical biology, 2011, 6(11): 1188-1192.
[534] Pai S S, Hammouda B, Hong K, et al. The conformation of the poly(ethylene glycol)chain in mono-PEGylated lysozyme and mono-PEGylated human growth hormone[J]. Bioconjugate Chemistry, 2011, 22(11): 2317-2323.
[535] Munasinghe A, Mathavan A, Mathavan A, et al. Molecular insight into the protein-polymer interactions in N-terminal PEGylated bovine serum albumin[J]. The Journal of Physical Chemistry B, 2019, 123(25): 5196-5205.
[536] Munasinghe A, Mathavan A, Mathavan A, et al. PEGylation within a confined hydrophobic cavity of a protein[J]. Physical Chemistry Chemical Physics, 2019, 21(46): 25584-25596.
[537] Munasinghe A, Mathavan A, Mathavan A, et al. Atomistic insight towards the impact of polymer architecture and grafting density on structure-dynamics of PEGylated bovine serum albumin and their applications[J]. The Journal of Chemical Physics, 2021, 154(7).
[538] Munasinghe A, Baker S L, Lin P, et al. Structure-function-dynamics of α-chymotrypsin based conjugates as a function of polymer charge[J]. Soft Matter, 2020, 16(2): 456-465.
[539] Kaupbayeva B, Boye S, Munasinghe A, et al. Molecular dynamics-guided design of a functional protein–ATRP conjugate that eliminates protein–protein interactions[J]. Bioconjugate Chemistry, 2021, 32(4): 821-832.
[540] Drossis N, Gauthier M A, de Haan H W. Elucidating the mechanisms of the molecular sieving phenomenon created by comb-shaped polymers grafted to a protein——a simulation study[J]. Materials Today Chemistry, 2022, 24: 100861.
[541] Miao Y, Feher V A, McCammon J A. Gaussian accelerated molecular dynamics: unconstrained enhanced sampling and free energy calculation[J]. Journal of chemical theory and computation, 2015, 11(8): 3584-3595.
[542] Hahn L, Zorn T, Kehrein J, et al. Unraveling an alternative mechanism in polymer self-assemblies: an order–order transition with unusual molecular interactions between hydrophilic and hydrophobic polymer blocks[J]. ACS nano, 2023, 17(7): 6932-6942.
[543] Pfleger C, Rathi P C, Klein D L, et al. Constraint network analysis(CNA): a Python software package for efficiently linking biomacromolecular structure, flexibility, (thermo-)stability, and function[J]. 2013.
[544] Xu D, Smolin N, Shaw R K, et al. Molecular insights into the improved clinical performance of PEGylated interferon therapeutics: a molecular dynamics perspective[J]. RSC advances, 2018, 8(5): 2315-2322.
[545] Qiao Q, Cai L, Shao Q. Molecular simulations of zwitterlation-induced conformation and dynamics variation of glucagon-like peptide-1 and insulin[J]. Journal of Materials Chemistry B, 2022, 10(14): 2490-2496.
[546] Wilding K M, Smith A K, Wilkerson J W, et al. The locational impact of site-specific PEGylation: streamlined screening

with cell-free protein expression and coarse-grain simulation[J]. ACS synthetic biology, 2018, 7(2): 510-521.

[547] Karanicolas J, Brooks III C L. The structural basis for biphasic kinetics in the folding of the WW domain from a formin-binding protein: lessons for protein design?[J]. Proceedings of the National Academy of Sciences, 2003, 100(7): 3954-3959.

[548] Karanicolas J, Brooks III C L. Integrating folding kinetics and protein function: Biphasic kinetics and dual binding specificity in a WW domain[J]. Proceedings of the National Academy of Sciences, 2004, 101(10): 3432-3437.

[549] Smith A K, Soltani M, Wilkerson J W, et al. Coarse-grained simulation of PEGylated and tethered protein devices at all experimentally accessible surface residues on β-lactamase for stability analysis and comparison[J]. The Journal of Chemical Physics, 2021, 154(7).

[550] Zhao E L, Soltani M, Smith A K, et al. Assessing site-specific PEGylation of TEM-1 β-lactamase with cell-free protein synthesis and coarse-grained simulation. Journal of Biotechnology, 2022, 345, 55–63.

[551] Tamasi M J, Patel R A, Borca C H, et al. Machine learning on a robotic platform for the design of polymer–protein hybrids[J]. Advanced Materials, 2022, 34(30): 2201809.

[552] Mao L, Russell A J, Carmali S. Moving protein PEGylation from an art to a data science[J]. Bioconjugate Chemistry, 2022, 33(9): 1643-1653.

[553] Watchorn J, Burns D, Stuart S, et al. Investigating the molecular mechanism of protein-polymer binding with direct saturation compensated nuclear magnetic resonance[J]. Biomacromolecules, 2021, 23(1): 67-76.

[554] Xu Y D, Lai R Y, Prochazkova E, et al. Saturation transfer difference NMR spectroscopy for the elucidation of supramolecular albumin–polymer interactions[J]. ACS Macro Letters, 2021, 10(7): 819-824.

[555] Pritzlaff A, Ferré G, Mulry E, et al. Atomic‐scale view of protein‐PEG interactions that redirect the thermal unfolding pathway of PEGylated human Galectin‐3[J]. Angewandte Chemie International Edition, 2022, 61(40): e202203784.

[556] Burridge K M, Shurina B A, Kozuszek C T, et al. Mapping protein-polymer conformations in bioconjugates with atomic precision[J]. Chemical Science, 2020, 11(24): 6160-6166.

[557] Schäfer T, Zhou J, Schmid F, et al. Blood Proteins and Their Interactions with Nanoparticles Investigated Using Molecular Dynamics Simulations[C]//High Performance Computing in Science and Engineering'17: Transactions of the High Performance Computing Center, Stuttgart(HLRS)2017. Springer International Publishing, 2018: 5-19.

[558] Settanni G, Zhou J, Suo T, et al. Protein corona composition of poly(ethylene glycol)-and poly(phosphoester)-coated nanoparticles correlates strongly with the amino acid composition of the protein surface[J]. Nanoscale, 2017, 9(6): 2138-2144.

[559] Settanni G, Zhou J, Schmid F. Interactions between proteins and poly(ethylene-glycol)investigated using molecular dynamics simulations[C]//Journal of Physics: Conference Series. IOP Publishing, 2017, 921(1): 012002.

[560] Settanni G, Schäfer T, Muhl C, et al. Poly-sarcosine and poly(ethylene-glycol)interactions with proteins investigated using molecular dynamics simulations[J]. Computational and Structural Biotechnology Journal, 2018, 16: 543-550.

[561] Teng J, Liu Y, Shen Z, et al. Molecular simulation of zwitterionic polypeptides on protecting glucagon-like peptide-1(GLP-1)[J]. International Journal of Biological Macromolecules, 2021, 174: 519-526.

[562] Moradi S, Hosseini E, Abdoli M, et al. Comparative molecular dynamic simulation study on the use of chitosan for temperature stabilization of interferon αII[J]. Carbohydrate polymers, 2019, 203: 52-59.

[563] Moradi S, Mirzaei S, Khosravi R, et al. Computational investigation on the effects of pharmaceutical polymers on the structure and dynamics of interleukin2 in heat stress[J]. Journal of Biomolecular Structure and Dynamics, 2021, 39(12): 4536-4546.

[564] Kianipour S, Ansari M, Farhadian N, et al. A molecular dynamics study on using of naturally occurring polymers for structural stabilization of erythropoietin at high temperature[J]. Journal of Biomolecular Structure and Dynamics, 2022, 40(19): 9042-9052.

[565] Asadzadeh H, Moosavi A, Arghavani J H. The effect of chitosan and PEG polymers on stabilization of GF-17 structure: a molecular dynamics study[J]. Carbohydrate polymers, 2020, 237: 116124.

[566] Asadzadeh H, Moosavi A. Investigation of the interactions between Melittin and the PLGA and PLA polymers: molecular dynamic simulation and binding free energy calculation[J]. Materials Research Express, 2019, 6(5): 055318.

[567] Jafari M, Doustdar F, Mehrnejad F. Molecular self-assembly strategy for encapsulation of an amphipathic α-helical antimicrobial peptide into the different polymeric and copolymeric nanoparticles[J]. Journal of chemical information and modeling, 2018, 59(1): 550-563.

[568] Salar S, Jafari M, Kaboli S F, et al. The role of intermolecular interactions on the encapsulation of human insulin into the chitosan and cholesterol-grafted chitosan polymers[J]. Carbohydrate polymers, 2019, 208: 345-355.

[569] Khanmohammadi S, Mehrnejad F, Lotfi-Sousefi Z, et al. Design and synthesis of polyacrylic acid/deoxycholic acid-modified chitosan copolymer and a close inspection of human growth hormone-copolymer interactions: An experimental and computational study[J]. Colloids and Surfaces B: Biointerfaces, 2021, 206: 111956.

[570] AL-zuwaini S J, Mehrnejad F, Lotfi-Sousefi Z, et al. The process of L-asparaginase encapsulation by poly(lactic-co-glycolic acid)and methoxy poly(ethylene glycol): A molecular dynamics simulation study[J]. Materials Today Communications, 2022, 31: 103435.

[571] Nyambura C W, Nance E, Pfaendtner J. Examining the Effect of Polymer Extension on Protein-Polymer Interactions That Occur during Formulation of Protein-Loaded Poly(lactic acid-co-glycolic acid)-polyethylene Glycol Nanoparticles[J]. Polymers, 2022, 14(21): 4730.

[572] Cardellini A, Jiménez-Ángeles F, Asinari P, et al. A modeling-based design to engineering protein hydrogels with random copolymers[J]. ACS nano, 2021, 15(10): 16139-16148.

[573] Rukmani S J, Lin P, Andrew J S, et al. Molecular modeling of complex cross-linked networks of PEGDA nanogels[J]. The Journal of Physical Chemistry B, 2019, 123(18): 4129-4138.

[574] Mercado-Montijo J, Anstine D M, Rukmani S J, et al. PEGDA hydrogel structure from semi-dilute concentrations: insights from experiments and molecular simulations[J]. Soft Matter, 2022, 18(18): 3565-3574.

[575] Casalini T, Perale G. From microscale to macroscale: nine orders of magnitude for a comprehensive modeling of hydrogels for controlled drug delivery[J]. Gels, 2019, 5(2): 28.

[576] Benková Z, Čakánek P, Cordeiro M N D S. Adsorption of Peptides onto Carbon Nanotubes Grafted with Poly(ethylene Oxide)Chains: A Molecular Dynamics Simulation Study[J]. Nanomaterials, 2022, 12(21): 3795.

[577] Khoshoei A, Ghasemy E, Poustchi F, et al. Engineering the pH-sensitivity of the graphene and carbon nanotube based nanomedicines in smart cancer therapy by grafting trimetyl Chitosan[J]. Pharmaceutical Research, 2020, 37: 1-13.

[578] Alinejad A, Raissi H, Hashemzadeh H. Development and evaluation of a pH-responsive and water-soluble drug delivery system based on smart polymer coating of graphene nanosheets: an in silico study[J]. RSC advances, 2020, 10(52): 31106-31114.

[579] Razavi L, Raissi H, Farzad F. Assessment of the effect of external and internal triggers on adsorption and release of paclitaxel from the PEI functionalized silicene nanosheet: A molecular dynamic simulation[J]. Journal of Molecular Graphics and Modelling, 2021, 106: 107930.

[580] Hashemzadeh H, Raissi H. Design of new drug delivery platform based on surface functionalization of black phosphorus nanosheet with a smart polymer for enhancing the efficiency of doxorubicin in the treatment of cancer[J]. Journal of Biomedical Materials Research Part A, 2021, 109(10): 1912-1921.

[581] Alimohammadi E, Maleki R, Akbarialiabad H, et al. Novel pH-responsive nanohybrid for simultaneous delivery of doxorubicin and paclitaxel: an in-silico insight[J]. BMC chemistry, 2021, 15: 1-11.

[582] Bina A, Raissi H, Hashemzadeh H, et al. Conjugation of a smart polymer to doxorubicin through a pH-responsive bond for targeted drug delivery and improving drug loading on graphene oxide[J]. RSC advances, 2021, 11(31): 18809-18817.

[583] Shariatinia Z, Mazloom-Jalali A. Chitosan nanocomposite drug delivery systems designed for the ifosfamide anticancer drug using molecular dynamics simulations[J]. Journal of Molecular Liquids, 2019, 273: 346-367.

[584] Hooper J B, Bedrov D, Smith G D. Supramolecular self-organization in PEO-modified C60 fullerene/water solutions: influence of polymer molecular weight and nanoparticle concentration[J]. Langmuir, 2008, 24(9): 4550-4557.

[585] Hooper J B, Bedrov D, Smith G D. The influence of polymer architecture on the assembly of poly(ethylene oxide)grafted C 60 fullerene clusters in aqueous solution: a molecular dynamics simulation study[J]. Physical Chemistry Chemical Physics, 2009, 11(12): 2034-2045.

[586] Bedrov D, Smith G D, Li L. Molecular dynamics simulation study of the role of evenly spaced poly(ethylene oxide)tethers on the aggregation of C60 fullerenes in water[J]. Langmuir, 2005, 21(12): 5251-5255.

[587] Kavyani S, Dadvar M, Modarress H, et al. A coarse grained molecular dynamics simulation study on the structural properties of carbon nanotube–dendrimer composites[J]. Soft Matter, 2018, 14(16): 3151-3163.

[588] Kavyani S, Dadvar M, Modarress H, et al. Molecular perspective mechanism for drug loading on carbon nanotube–dendrimer: a coarse-grained molecular dynamics study[J]. The Journal of Physical Chemistry B, 2018, 122(33): 7956-7969.

[589] Janjua T I, Cao Y, Yu C, et al. Clinical translation of silica nanoparticles[J]. Nature Reviews Materials, 2021, 6(12): 1072-1074.

[590] Kankala R K, Han Y H, Na J, et al. Nanoarchitectured structure and surface biofunctionality of mesoporous silica nanoparticles[J]. Advanced materials, 2020, 32(23): 1907035.

[591] Bansal K K, Mishra D K, Rosling A, et al. Therapeutic potential of polymer-coated mesoporous silica nanoparticles[J].

Applied Sciences, 2019, 10(1): 289.

[592] Mu S, Liu Y, Wang T, et al. Unsaturated nitrogen-rich polymer poly(l-histidine)gated reversibly switchable mesoporous silica nanoparticles using "graft to" strategy for drug controlled release[J]. Acta biomaterialia, 2017, 63: 150-162.

[593] Xu X, Lü S, Wu C, et al. Curcumin polymer coated, self-fluorescent and stimuli-responsive multifunctional mesoporous silica nanoparticles for drug delivery[J]. Microporous and Mesoporous Materials, 2018, 271: 234-242.

[594] Rama P, Abbas Z. The influence of silica nanoparticle geometry on the interfacial interactions of organic molecules: a molecular dynamics study[J]. Physical Chemistry Chemical Physics, 2022, 24(6): 3713-3721.

[595] Sun X, Feng Z, Zhang L, et al. The selective interaction between silica nanoparticles and enzymes from molecular dynamics simulations[J]. PLoS one, 2014, 9(9): e107696.

[596] Peng S, Yuan X, Lin W, et al. pH-responsive controlled release of mesoporous silica nanoparticles capped with Schiff base copolymer gatekeepers: Experiment and molecular dynamics simulation[J]. Colloids and Surfaces B: Biointerfaces, 2019, 176: 394-403.

[597] Gardinier T C, Kohle F F E, Peerless J S, et al. High-performance chromatographic characterization of surface chemical heterogeneities of fluorescent organic–inorganic hybrid core–shell silica nanoparticles[J]. ACS nano, 2019, 13(2): 1795-1804.

[598] Ezquerro C S, Aznar J M G, Laspalas M. Prediction of the structure and mechanical properties of polycaprolactone–silica nanocomposites and the interphase region by molecular dynamics simulations: the effect of PEGylation[J]. Soft Matter, 2022, 18(14): 2800-2813.

[599] Shariatinia Z, Jalali A M. Chitosan-based hydrogels: Preparation, properties and applications[J]. International journal of biological macromolecules, 2018, 115: 194-220.

[600] Brambilla D, Mussida A, Ferretti A M, et al. Polymeric coating of silica microspheres for biological applications: suppression of non-specific binding and functionalization with biomolecules[J]. Polymers, 2022, 14(4): 730.

[601] Wu X, Chang H, Mello C, et al. Effect of interaction with coesite silica on the conformation of Cecropin P1 using explicit solvent molecular dynamics simulation[J]. The Journal of Chemical Physics, 2013, 138(4).

[602] de Lara L S, Rigo V A, Miranda C R. Functionalized silica nanoparticles within multicomponent oil/brine interfaces: a study in molecular dynamics[J]. The Journal of Physical Chemistry C, 2016, 120(12): 6787-6795.

[603] Chen T, Wu F, Chen Z, et al. Computer simulation of zwitterionic polymer brush grafted silica nanoparticles to modify polyvinylidene fluoride membrane[J]. Journal of Colloid and Interface Science, 2021, 587: 173-182.

[604] Barbier D, Brown D, Grillet A C, et al. Interface between end-functionalized PEO oligomers and a silica nanoparticle studied by molecular dynamics simulations[J]. Macromolecules, 2004, 37(12): 4695-4710.

[605] Hong B, Panagiotopoulos A Z. Molecular dynamics simulations of silica nanoparticles grafted with poly(ethylene oxide) oligomer chains[J]. The Journal of Physical Chemistry B, 2012, 116(8): 2385-2395.

[606] Oroskar P A, Jameson C J, Murad S. Simulated permeation and characterization of PEGylated gold nanoparticles in a lipid bilayer system[J]. Langmuir, 2016, 32(30): 7541-7555.

[607] Zhang Z, Lin X, Gu N. Effects of temperature and PEG grafting density on the translocation of PEGylated nanoparticles across asymmetric lipid membrane[J]. Colloids and Surfaces B: Biointerfaces, 2017, 160: 92-100.

[608] Bai X, Xu M, Liu S, et al. Computational investigations of the interaction between the cell membrane and nanoparticles coated with a pulmonary surfactant[J]. ACS applied materials & interfaces, 2018, 10(24): 20368-20376.

[609] Xia Q, Zhu T, Jiang Z, et al. Enhancing the targeting ability of nanoparticles via protected copolymers[J]. Nanoscale, 2020, 12(14): 7804-7813.

[610] Yang P Y, Ju S P, Chuang Y C, et al. Molecular dynamics simulations of PAMAM dendrimer-encapsulated Au nanoparticles of different sizes under different pH conditions[J]. Computational Materials Science, 2017, 137: 144-152.

[611] Blazhynska M M, Kyrychenko A, Kalugin O N. pH-responsive coating of silver nanoparticles with poly(2-(N,N-dimethylamino)ethyl methacrylate): the role of polymer size and degree of protonation[J]. The Journal of Physical Chemistry C, 2021, 125(22): 12118-12130.

[612] Siani P, Frigerio G, Donadoni E, et al. Molecular dynamics simulations of cRGD-conjugated PEGylated TiO_2 nanoparticles for targeted photodynamic therapy[J]. Journal of Colloid and Interface Science, 2022, 627: 126-141.

[613] Ding H, Ma Y. Computer simulation of the role of protein corona in cellular delivery of nanoparticles[J]. Biomaterials, 2014, 35(30): 8703-8710.

[614] Ozmaian M, Freitas B A, Coalson R D. Controlling the surface properties of binary polymer brush-coated colloids via targeted nanoparticles[J]. The Journal of Physical Chemistry B, 2018, 123(1): 258-265.

[615] Shen Z, Loe D T, Fisher A, et al. Polymer stiffness governs template mediated self-assembly of liposome-like nanoparticles:

simulation, theory and experiment[J]. Nanoscale, 2019, 11(42): 20179-20193.

[616] Liang Q. Penetration of polymer-grafted nanoparticles through a lipid bilayer[J]. Soft Matter, 2013, 9(23): 5594-5601.

[617] Adekoya O C, Adekoya G J, Sadiku E R, et al. Application of DFT calculations in designing polymer-based drug delivery systems: An overview[J]. Pharmaceutics, 2022, 14(9): 1972.

[618] Farmanzadeh D, Ghaderi M. A computational study of PAMAM dendrimer interaction with trans isomer of picoplatin anticancer drug[J]. Journal of Molecular Graphics and Modelling, 2018, 80: 1-6.

[619] Moradnia H, Raissi H, Shahabi M. The performance of the single-walled carbon nanotube covalently modified with polyethylene glycol to delivery of Gemcitabine anticancer drug in the aqueous environment[J]. Journal of Biomolecular Structure and Dynamics, 2021, 39(3): 881-888.

[620] Vyas S, Khambete M, Gudhka R, et al. In silico modeling of functionalized poly(methylvinyl ether/maleic acid)for controlled drug release in the ocular milieu[J]. Drug Delivery and Translational Research, 2020, 10: 1085-1094.

[621] Upadhya R, Kosuri S, Tamasi M, et al. Automation and data-driven design of polymer therapeutics[J]. Advanced drug delivery reviews, 2021, 171: 1-28.

[622] Hassanzadeh P, Atyabi F, Dinarvand R. The significance of artificial intelligence in drug delivery system design[J]. Advanced drug delivery reviews, 2019, 151: 169-190.

[623] Boztepe C, Yüceer M, Künkül A, et al. Prediction of the deswelling behaviors of pH-and temperature-responsive poly(NIPAAm-co-AAc)IPN hydrogel by artificial intelligence techniques[J]. Research on Chemical Intermediates, 2020, 46(1): 409-428.

[624] Wang W, Feng S, Ye Z, et al. Prediction of lipid nanoparticles for mRNA vaccines by the machine learning algorithm[J]. Acta Pharmaceutica Sinica B, 2022, 12(6): 2950-2962.

[625] Deng J, Ye Z, Zheng W, et al. Machine learning in accelerating microsphere formulation development[J]. Drug Delivery and Translational Research, 2023, 13(4): 966-982.

第6章

固体制剂3D结构研究

殷宪振　中国科学院上海药物研究所，中国；临港实验室，中国

黄晨夕　临港实验室，中国

曹泽颖　中国科学院上海药物研究所，中国

伍　丽　中国科学院上海药物研究所，中国

肖体乔　中国科学院上海应用物理所，中国

彼得·约克（Peter York）　布拉德福德大学，英国

张继稳　中国科学院上海药物研究所，中国

6.1 引言

药物需经过处方调节制备成可用的剂型,才能方便患者用药。药剂学是一门提供基础科学知识的学科,该学科涉及将原料药转化为制剂过程的不同制备工艺,从而提供安全、高效、高质量的药物递送。药剂学家越来越关注的一个关键挑战是如何从机制上理解原料药和功能性的处方成分从粉末状态过渡到最终剂型的各个阶段的行为,并为患者提供最佳的疗效。预测性计算方法和先进分析技术为应对这些挑战提供了重要的工具。

不同剂型通常按给药途径、物理形态和剂量单位的大小进行分类。从分子层面到宏观层面[1],各种剂型可在不同的尺寸范围内进行定性(见图6-1)。在临床应用中,药物剂型可分为溶液剂、乳剂、悬浮剂、半固体和固体制剂(如微丸、胶囊和片剂)等。从处方工艺研究到最终制剂成型的过程中,还存在晶体、粉末、颗粒等其他中间体结构。此外,在药物释放和溶解过程中,存在水化、溶胀和扩散等行为,这些剂型的内部结构也会发生动态变化。在已上市的给药系统中,固体制剂是最常见的给药形式,绝大多数药品均为固体制剂。

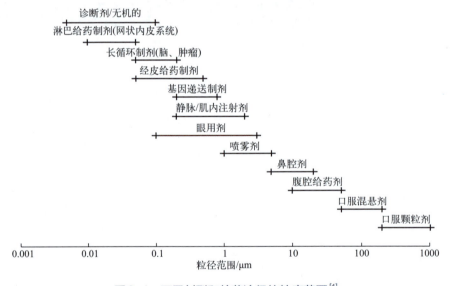

图6-1 不同剂型和给药途径的粒度范围[1]

6.2 固体制剂的结构与研究方法概述

6.2.1 固体制剂的结构

固体制剂的结构对最终药物产品的功能和有效性起着重要作用。原料药和其他非活性成分在大多数固体制剂中以粉末、晶体和固体分散体的形式存在,粒度范围从纳米到毫米级。

粉末和晶体的物理化学和机械特性，如粒度、粒度分布、溶解度、屈服强度等，决定了最终产品的体积特性、药品性能、可生产性、稳定性和外观。特别是药物的粒度和粒度分布对最终产品的关键质量和性能标准如药物含量的均匀性和药物溶出率有重大影响[2]。

颗粒的形态、大小和机械特性会影响其他辅料成分和生产工艺，因此颗粒的表征是处方前研究和处方研究中的一项重要需求。如上所述，药物颗粒的粒径会影响粉末流动性和混合性、剂量单位含量的均匀性、溶出度、生物利用度和稳定性。此外，粒径还对处方、工艺以及最终的临床治疗效果起着重要作用。因此，了解不同批次颗粒之间的差异，有利于进行产品开发和质量控制。在其他方面，常规粒度分析可提供足够的信息来表征样品之间的差异。但如果样品表现出相似的粒度分布，则可能需要识别其他相关特性的细微差别，如颗粒形状或表面积，以确保产品质量和一致性。

固体制剂的结构特征在决定药品质量和性能方面起着主导作用，因此有必要进一步研究这些结构成型过程和评价方法。药物制剂主要由活性药物成分和辅料组成。分子的组装可以是有序状态（即结晶），也可以是无序状态（即无定形），分子结构的类型会对处方设计、工艺选择和最终产品的性能（如药物的稳定性和溶解性）产生影响。固态结晶的复杂性来自药物分子的多态性。如果一种物质的分子在晶格中采用了另一种构象排列，那么这种物质就是多晶型的。多晶型会引起一系列不同的物理化学和机械特性，在处方、工艺选择和药品生产时需注意药物多晶型问题[3-5]。最近，计算药剂学在根据经验化学式预测晶体中不同分子结构的领域中取得了重大进展，描述了药物可能的多晶型范围。计算药剂学结合其他相关领域的预测计算工具，如药物吸收和药动学，在指导和加速固体制剂的开发方面具有重要作用。

6.2.2 固体制剂结构的研究方法

固体制剂制备时，原料药与其他处方成分首先被制备成颗粒形态，再配制成物理混合物（如颗粒填充的硬胶囊）或制剂单元（如微丸、片剂）。在此过程中，通常采用结构表征技术和物理、化学分析方法对制剂单元的结构和物质组成进行分析评价，同时也会对单剂量单元或多剂量单元进行药物的溶出试验。此外，还需要对最终的制剂产品的均匀性、物理特性进行适当的测定，如片剂的重量和硬度。然而，决定制剂产品特性起关键作用的内部结构和微观结构却很少被检测。固体制剂相关的各种细微尺度（从数百纳米到毫米），特别是对于近年来最具吸引力的微球和纳米药物制剂，分析其内部结构无疑是一个巨大的挑战。由于缺乏合适的原位成像技术和方法来量化三维（3D）结构的特征，制剂内部微观结构的研究有待深入。

获取固体制剂的内部结构，可研究制剂功能与结构特征的相关性。研究人员已采取包括原子力显微镜（AFM）、核磁共振（NMR）成像共聚焦显微镜、近红外光谱（NIR）成像和传统显微镜（光学和电子）在内的各种技术进行研究[6]。

扫描电子显微镜（SEM）是观察药物制剂和粉末表面结构（如微囊的形态、粒度分布和热性能）最广泛使用的方法[7]，可以对物体表面进行纳米到亚微米分辨率成像。但SEM不能原位检测制剂内部结构，往往需要破坏样品。

定量超快磁共振成像（MRI）技术，结合 ^{19}F 核磁共振波谱和 1D ^{19}F 图谱，被用于研究基于羟丙甲基纤维素（HPMC）的片剂的溶出过程[8]。水化层的 ^{19}F 1D-MRI 图谱沿轴向长度的像素分辨率为 375 μm，显示了药物在聚合物基质内部的扩散行为。^{19}F 光谱的积分图与紫外含量测定得到的药物释放曲线一致。

然而，上述大多数方法都不是真正的三维方法。拉曼光谱、扫描电镜、核磁共振成像、超声波、振动光谱和近红外光谱等技术通常用于二维观察。小尺寸微球或纳米粒的材料分布可通过激光共聚焦扫描显微镜（CLSM）进行测定，尽管成像尺度有限，但分辨率较高。此外，三维电子衍射也可用于分析纳米晶药物的内部结构，但这种方法通常只适用于晶体样品[9]。这些方法只能揭示表面或表面以下有限深度内部区域的结构信息，要观察内部结构，必须对样品进行切割，从而破坏其原有的三维结构。

这些传统方法除了具有破坏性外，目前该技术还存在其他缺点，如穿透力有限、分辨率低等。虽然二维观测的图像分析在某些情况下可以提供一些定量信息，但真正的原位三维结构研究方法对于真正了解药物剂型的内部微观结构非常重要。

X射线显微断层扫描成像（μCT）是一种强大的非侵入性研究技术，已被用于观察各种物体的三维结构，在提供颗粒状固体制剂的微观结构信息方面具有巨大潜力。与传统技术相比，μCT技术可以微米级分辨率对内部和微观结构细节进行非侵入式可视化[10, 11]。μCT技术是为研究固体制剂和粉末的形态和内部结构而开发的。例如，这种方法可以获得特定粉末的全部空间信息。此外，在对单个颗粒进行图像分析分离后，还可估算出颗粒的大小、形状和空间排列的几何特征分布[12]。这种功能强大的方法可提供详细的形态信息，如多孔颗粒的孔隙形状、空间分布和连通性，这些信息与给药系统的溶解特性相关[13, 14]。

另据报道，μCT与离散元法（DEM）相结合，可用于研究粉末压制法生产药片过程中的颗粒填料[15]。通过硬X射线纳米计算机断层扫描（Nano-CT，简称"纳米CT"）技术重建了聚乳酸-羟基乙酸共聚物（PLGA）微球的微观结构，并揭示了三维结构与药物包封效率之间的定量关系。此外，纳米CT还测定了牛血清白蛋白（BSA）在PLGA微球中的分布和孔隙，实验证明该孔隙与微球中BSA的体外释放相关[16, 17]。

在药物研究中，非侵入式高分辨率对于提取和呈现最精细的结构信息以及最大限度地减少医用计算机断层扫描（CT）典型的局部容积效应至关重要。然而，实验室μCT设备的主要限制是对于药物制剂样本中轻质材料的区分能力不足。同步辐射X射线显微断层扫描成像（SR-μCT）是目前对药物制剂样本成像的"理想"系统。SR-μCT的先进性能得益于其宽广的X射线能量、高强度、高亮度和高偏振。例如，在不同的取样时间，通过SR-μCT对对乙酰氨基酚微球和布洛芬微球的内部精细结构进行了三维可视化分析，通过结构定量分析确定了药物释放的最佳处方[18, 19]。研究表明，结合图像处理和三维重建，基于SR-μCT的三维结构表征从结构角度为药物释放系统的研究提供了新的思路。

6.3 同步辐射X射线显微断层扫描成像技术

计算机断层扫描（CT）是一种非破坏性技术，可提供物体内部结构的三维图像。这种成像技术的基本思想可追溯到J. Radon，他在1917年证明了一个n维物体可以从其$(n-1)$-维投影中重建出来[20]。其物理原理是通常用于CT成像的能量范围内的电离辐射（如X射线）与物质的所谓光效应的相互作用机制。光效应对光子的衰减与元素阶数的三次方成正比，与光子能量的三次方成反比。因此，实际衰减不仅取决于材料，还取决于X射线源的能谱。

同步辐射是一种由径向加速的带电粒子发出的电磁辐射。同步辐射是在同步加速器、贮存环接近光速运动的电子通过磁场发生偏转时产生的。同步辐射的特点是偏振、以窄锥形发射，其频率可覆盖整个电磁波谱[21]。同步辐射X射线显微断层扫描成像（SR-μCT）使用同步辐射X射线作为光源，可实现高速、高强度、高空间分辨率（亚微米或纳米级）和无创透视成像。SR-μCT可以定量评估和观察给药系统（DDS）的三维结构。SR-μCT的先进性能归功于以下几点：①可产生1~200 keV 光子能量的宽X射线能量区；②高强度的总功率（即600 kW），是X射线管的数万倍；③缩短了获取实验数据的时间；④高亮度，其亮度是X射线管的数百倍；⑤完全偏振光，电子轨道面的光为椭圆偏振光。此外，它还是研究生物分子光学活性和磁性材料的良好工具[28]。

6.4 基于SR-μCT的三维结构重建

6.4.1 样品的制备

为了评价固体制剂的结构及其动态变化，需提前进行样品制备，例如药物释放过程中，制剂结构会发生变化。X射线吸收强度、样品含水量、样品稳定性、样品大小和容器等因素都会对SR-μCT的测试结果产生影响。

6.4.1.1 X射线吸收强度

SR-μCT图像的特征强度值由X射线检测系统的透射强度确定，其大小取决于材料的原子质量和X射线能量[11, 23]。药物样品中的不同元素具有不同的X射线吸收强度。为了能够准确检测目标元素，SR-μCT测试的药物样品中的其他元素，都应与目标元素明确区分。样品的物理性质，如堆积密度，也会影响X射线吸收。例如，高于系统分辨率极限或处于亚体素水平的孔隙率将会引起X射线吸收的差异，这些差异被视为不同的灰度值，而这又取决于孔隙率的分布特性、X射线源的点扩散函数和相机像素大小等变量。此外，还需要考虑材料界面，因为其复杂程度决定了是否可以区分边界。

6.4.1.2 密度和密度分布

在进行SR-μCT扫描时，材料密度是一个重要因素。首先，应评估成像材料的基本密度。如果两种相邻材料具有相似的密度，除非存在其他因素（如不同的水化水平）改变基础密度，否则很难有效区分两种材料。

6.4.1.3 样品含水量

水分会干扰SR-μCT样本的成像，因此在图像采集前，样品必须进行干燥以降低含水量。已报道的三种用于SR-μCT样品预处理方法，以去除水分：①烘箱干燥；②冷冻干燥；③用干滤纸吸收尽可能多的水分，并用硅胶室温储存。方法①和③应用于凝胶骨架片时，片剂可能发生收缩，片芯表面形成的凝胶在制备过程中可能塌陷，导致内部凝胶结构发生变化。对于这类样品，冷冻干燥方法可以保持水化层的微观结构，对片芯的结构影响最小。

6.4.1.4 样品稳定性

μCT中X射线具有非常高的能量，因此还需要考虑样品的稳定性。用于SR-μCT扫描的样品需要具有良好的热稳定性，以防样品在测试过程中发生变化。

6.4.1.5 样品固定

为了获取足够多的图像信息，在SR-μCT扫描过程中，样品台通常以一定的速度旋转180°。样品台的旋转可能会引起部分样品（如颗粒样品）的移动或重排，因此应先固定样品。例如，当使用SR-μCT对微晶纤维素和淀粉颗粒样品进行成像时，可以将两个颗粒分别填充到体积为1 mL的圆柱形容器中，填充水平为$F=66\%$[24]，以避免扫描过程中颗粒的移动。

6.4.1.6 样品尺寸

样本大小受限于图像分辨率，根据样本的吸收系数选择图像分辨率。分辨率越高，采集窗口越小。因此，受采集窗口大小的限制，应控制SR-μCT测试样本的大小。

6.4.1.7 容器的选择

用于SR-μCT扫描的样品通常需要固定在某些容器中，如塑料管、胶囊壳等。这些容器应具有一定的刚性和厚度、弱X射线吸收以及成分和结构均匀等。

6.4.1.8 样品数量

根据样本检测的类型和规模，可以选择不同大小的样本。如果目标是宏观尺度，例如对颗粒系统的研究，则应该对相对大量的颗粒进行采样，可能需要几百个。如果是研究微观内部结构，一般只要结果具有统计学意义，可以是几个或几十个单独的颗粒。通过SR-μCT识别两个或多组分系统中的固体单元，可以加入一些吸收较弱的稀释剂将固体单元彼此分离。例如，研究非洛地平缓释片的溶胀、溶蚀时，选取18片，测定9个时间点，每个时间点两片，进行溶出度测试；然后在0.5、1.0、2.0、3.0、4.0、5.0、6.0、7.0和8.0小时，从溶出介质中取出两片，制备样品用于SR-μCT测试[23]。

6.4.1.9 动态过程样本

从经历动态过程（如药物扩散和/或溶解）的材料中，在不同时间提取样品，将其内部结构可视化可以获取样品孔结构和孔隙率的动态特性。SR-μCT可以获取体素大小约为几微米的3D图像，从而展示出具有不同X射线吸收率的材料内部微观结构。体外溶出通常用于评价片剂和其他固体剂型的药物释放行为。可以利用SR-μCT来评价药物释放过程中制剂微观结构随时间的变化。

含有相对高密度金属活性药物成分的片剂，比如硫酸亚铁，可以在溶出过程中使用SR-μCT技术直接成像[14]。溶出介质既不影响片芯的微观结构，也不影响其成像。然而，对于不含金属元素的药物，如非洛地平，其密度与溶解介质相似，溶解介质会干扰成像[25]。

大多数药物都不含有金属元素，因此，从溶出介质中取出的片剂必须在图像采集之前进行干燥。例如，将片剂首先在液氮或超低温制冷剂中冷冻，然后使用冷冻干燥机进行干燥[26]。也可以使用小勺将溶胀的片剂与约 2 mL 的溶出介质一起放置在 24 孔板中，以保持溶胀片剂的初始形状，然后，立即将处于不同水化和溶蚀状态的片剂，置于-80℃的冰箱中冷冻 12 小时，随后在-50℃和 10 mTorr（1 Torr = 133.322 Pa）下干燥 24 小时，再将片剂保存在室温干燥柜（相对湿度20%）中，以便进一步的SR-μCT测试[27]。

在图像采集之前，干燥非洛地平单室渗透泵片应使用相同的方法。然而，由于单片渗透泵片剂的特殊结构，在冷冻时从液体到冰的相变过程中，水的体积膨胀会导致片芯中溶解的药物和悬浮成分在初始冷冻过程中被挤出，因此，冷冻干燥工艺不适用于单室渗透泵片（MOPT）。此外，片芯的残留物主要是基于凝胶的半固体，并且在低温下形成水晶体，这可能会破坏半透膜内的内容物微观结构。因此，内部挤压和晶体形成引起的变形，降低了冷冻干燥法对研究渗透泵片内部结构的适用性。

6.4.2 图像采集和三维重建

6.4.2.1 图像采集

基于在CT扫描期间获取的高质量图像，才能获得准确的实验结果。为了保证图像精度，必须根据实验目的和样品的性质对参数进行优化。这些参数包括：

（1）图像的分辨率：由透镜的放大率和电荷耦合器件（CCD）的像素大小决定。CCD通常是固定的，尝试更高的分辨率意味着采集窗口减小。因此，需在样品尺寸和最小微观结构的预期分辨率之间权衡。

（2）X射线的范围：该范围为1~200 keV。能量越高，不仅穿透样品的能力越高，而且辐射损伤的可能性越大。为了优化X射线能量，应考虑待测样品的元素、分子量、密度和厚度等因素。

（3）曝光时间：它决定了到达探测器的X射线光子的数量。当曝光时间增加时，CCD捕捉投影的通量将增加。CT扫描曝光时间不合适，会降低图像的质量。长时间曝光可能导致过度曝光，会降低材料之间的对比度，并增加每个样本的扫描时间。在曝光不足的情况下，信噪比会降低。此外，应考虑辐射剂量，因为长时间暴露在X射线下，可能会导致样品变形并造成辐射损伤。

（4）样品与检测器之间的距离（DSD）：是SR-μCT扫描的关键因素，对于低密度材料尤其有用。在一定的距离范围内，较长的DSD意味着更好的相位对比度，这有利于区分密度差异较小的材料，而吸收对比度无法区分这些材料。

（5）投影数量：通常由样本的大小和测试的精确度决定。在扫描过程中，样本旋转180°，投影将在多个角度方向上被捕获。投影数量多，有助于提高数据质量并避免伪影，而较多的投影将延长扫描时间并可能导致样品辐射损伤。

准备好的样品可以放在合适的容器中，并固定在样品台上，以防止扫描过程中发生移动。调整样品台的轴心和水平位置非常必要，以确保在旋转过程中水平方向没有偏差。穿透样品后，投影通过衍射限制显微镜光学放大，并通过CCD相机数字化。调整曝光时间和样品到检测器的距离，在样本旋转180°的过程中，采集一定数量的投影图像。在每次采集过程中，还需要光场图像（即在没有样本的光束路径上的X射线照明）和暗场图像（X射线照明关闭），以校正电子噪声和X射线源亮度的变化（图6-2）。

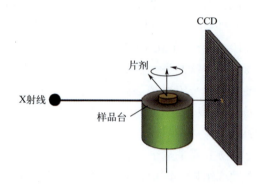

图6-2 同步辐射X射线CT扫描

6.4.2.2 3D重建

3D重建是指渲染物体的真实外观，是由样本的二维图像切片重建起来的。重建过程与从3D图像中获取2D图片相反。图片的本质是从三维物体到2D平面的投影，在此过程中厚度信息会丢失。3D图像中，同一平面相对应的厚度点被约束在同一视线上。从单张图像中，不能确定这个点对应于图像上的哪个厚度位置。如果可以获取两张图像，那么可以找到两条投影射线的交点作为3D点的位置。

使用反投影算法可将投影转换为重建的二维切片。为了提高重建切片的质量，增加了相位检索算法用于相位对比度提取。3D渲染数据可以用已开发的软件进行分析，例如VGStudio Max（Volume Graphics GmbH，德国）、Amira（Visualization Sciences Group，法国）和Image Pro Analyzer 3D（Media Cybernetics，美国），以获取定性和定量信息。图像分割后，去除背景噪声，将切片全部转换为灰度值图像。用分段切片重构三维曲面模型，并调整各参数以优化模型。随后，提取样本中的三维对象，并进行数据分析。

6.4.3 模型构建与分析

模型构建和分析过程需要巨大的计算量，重建的切片被转换为8位灰度值格式，并进行裁剪，以提高准确性和计算效率。然后，对样本切片进行处理以提高图片质量、降低噪声，并分析不同材料和微观结构的灰度值。一般情况下，区分目标对象最重要的定量标准是灰度值，但对于结构或材料含量复杂的样品，形态信息更适合。同一组中所有样本都应使用统一参数进行处理，以确保所有结果都能进行定量分析。

3D模型可以呈现物体的表面形态和内部三维结构。基于材料之间灰度值的差异，可以通过分割从3D模型中提取感兴趣的对象或微结构。利用表面模型，计算三维立体定量参数，如下所示：

（1）体积：以校准单位表示的物体体积。

（2）表面积：以校准单位表示的物体表面积。

（3）宽度：边界框在X方向上的大小。

（4）高度：边界框在Y方向上的大小。

（5）深度：边界框在Z方向上的大小。

（6）中心X：对象中心的X坐标。

（7）中心 Y：对象中心的 Y 坐标。

（8）中心 Z：对象中心的 Z 坐标。

（9）长方体体积：对象边界的体积。

（10）长方体比率：边界的最大大小和最小大小之间的比率。

（11）体积分数：对象体积与长方体体积的比率。

（12）直径：物体的等效直径。

（13）球形度：与物体相同体积的球体的表面积和物体实际表面积的比值。对于球形对象，该参数等于 1，对于其他形状，该参数小于 1。

（14）最大半径：对象中心和曲面之间的最大距离。

（15）最小半径：对象中心和曲面之间的最小距离。

（16）半径比率：最大半径和最小半径之间的比率。

（17）最大费雷特径：对象的两个平行平面之间的最大距离。

（18）最小费雷特径：对象的两个平行平面之间的最小距离。

（19）费雷特径比率：最大费雷特径和最小费雷特径之间的比率。

（20）表面偏差：三角形法线端点的偏差。计算如下：对曲面的所有三角形法线向量进行归一化（长度设置为1），并计算从端点的平均位置到所有其他向量的平均距离。均匀曲面的偏差为0。球体的最大偏差是1.336。

以上参数组合起来，可以推断物体的一些特定物理结构特征，包括孔隙率、比表面积和粗糙度等，它们从不同的角度描述了物体的形态，基于此可以研究所有结构参数与物体性质之间的相关性。样品性质如药物含量、药物释放动力学以及药物加工过程会影响三维结构。此外，可以引入多元分析、数据挖掘和建模方法来构建统计模型。

6.5 三维可视化和定量表征

采集多种固体制剂的 2D 和 3D 图像，可用于研究其功能和结构[64]。以下示例演示了结构信息是如何有利于剂型的设计和测试以及解决相关技术问题的。X射线显微成像提供了定量的结构信息，以及其他技术无法获得的剂型不同区域的形状和大小。该技术适用于测定多层片剂中各层的厚度以及这些层之间各界面的形状和尺寸。它也可用于阐明快速崩解片的微观结构，如使用冷冻干燥技术制造的片剂，其结构特征反映了冷冻干燥前片剂中存在冰晶的大小和形状。该技术可以用于评价药物颗粒的形态和孔径分布，尤其适用于研究湿法制粒颗粒内孔隙的连通性和形状[13, 28]。它还可以用于评价多孔基质结构以及药物从固体剂型释放过程中发生的扩散和溶解过程[14]。

6.5.1 颗粒和颗粒系统的微观结构

6.5.1.1 颗粒的内部结构

药物颗粒的结构信息在产品性能中具有重要意义，包括药物或辅料颗粒的分布、孔隙率、药物或聚合物层的厚度，以及表面的形状和粗糙度。已经有各种实验技术、分析方法来获得这些结构信息。例如，观察颗粒表面结构最常用的方法是SEM[29-32]。拉曼光谱也可以用于揭示制剂表面药物和辅料的分布[33]。然而，这些方法只能揭示被检测颗粒表面或其正下方的结构信息，并且必须切割或破坏样品才能观察内部结构。例如，在SEM的研究中，将样品置于真空下，沉积含有重金属（如铂）的涂层，这会影响样品的表面结构[34]。尽管MRI可以在不破坏样品的情况下揭示药物制剂的内部结构，但由于其低空间分辨率，在固体材料检测中应用受限。由于X射线的高穿透性，CT可以无损伤地表征制剂的3D结构，并对尺寸从厘米到毫米的片剂[35]和颗粒[36]进行结构分析。

在水渗透引起的崩解现象中，片剂内部的空腔结构起着决定性的作用。μCT可以表征微晶纤维素（MCC）片的内部结构，以研究轴向和径向的孔隙和孔隙率。不同MCC片崩解行为的实时可视化表明，崩解模式有两种，可分为层状崩解和分裂型崩解。SR-μCT技术为评价片剂内部结构和阐明崩解机理提供了新的视角[37]。

6.5.1.2 颗粒系统的动力学结构

颗粒的混合和分离是制药、化学和食品工业的基本工艺操作。颗粒在分批搅拌机中混合，如翻滚仓和V型搅拌机。然而，在这种动态过程中，通常很难将颗粒均匀混合。此外，在颗粒处理过程中，成分频繁波动[38,39]。基于这些不均匀现象，如果在片剂压实或胶囊填充之前发生偏析，可能会对含量均匀性产生重大影响，尤其是在药物含量非常低的情况下[2,40]。此外，控制颗粒混合物的均匀性非常重要，因为它会影响药物制剂的重量变化[41]、药物释放[42]和溶解特性[43,44]。因此，颗粒的混合和分离过程，在药品质量控制方面发挥着重要作用。

混合物中各组分的偏析与颗粒特性（如形状、尺寸和表面性质）密切相关。例如，单个成分颗粒之间存在颗粒尺寸和形状变化，则在粉末流入产品容器期间，偏析会成为主要问题[45,46]。因此，量化粉末和颗粒系统物理性质的表征方法，对于解释不同材料在各种工艺条件下的流动行为具有重要的意义。已有几种表征粉末和颗粒系统的方法被报道，包括SEM[47]、NIR[48]和MRI[49,50]等。例如，NIR用于监测粉末混合物的均匀性，并且已经证明NIR可以检测粉末物理化学性质变化的灵敏性[46,48]。然而，很难实现多组分粉末和颗粒系统的内部高分辨率可视化。此外，如探测外表面而非内部结构的SEM，这些技术无法对颗粒进行全面的结构评价[47,51]。且这些方法没有提供定量表征和统计数据信息。μCT在解析颗粒材料的总体（即表面和体积）结构特性方面具有巨大潜力。与传统技术相比，CT技术允许以微米和毫米级分辨率对内部和微观结构细节进行非侵入性可视化[10,11]。

μCT已被开发用于研究固体剂型、粉末和颗粒的外观形态和内部结构。通过这种方法可以获得样品的三维空间信息。此外，对单个颗粒进行图像分析后，可以评价颗粒的大小、形状和空间排列等特征[12]。这种方法还可以提供更详细的结构信息，如孔隙形状、空间分布和多孔颗粒的连接性，而这些信息与药物递送系统中药物的溶解性密切相关[13,14]。例如，CT与DEM相结合可用于研究粉末压片过程中的颗粒填充[15]；SR-μCT可以用于非侵入性地监测二元混合物的均匀性；μCT可分别对微晶纤维素（MCC）和淀粉颗粒样品进行表征；同时，还可以通过计算材料球形度的频率分布，来研究颗粒的尺寸分布。MCC和淀粉颗粒在圆柱形容器中混合，SR-μCT数据可以研究旋转时间（TR）和振动时间（TV）对混合物均匀性的影响，还可以采用混合指数来评估颗粒系统的混合均匀性。结果表明，随着TR的增加，混合物的均匀性得到改善。此外，当颗粒呈现不同的尺寸和形状时，随着TV的延长，偏析增加。非球形的较大淀粉颗粒有上升到顶部的趋势，而较小的球形MCC颗粒有迁移到混合物底部的趋势。因此，SR-μCT技术结合统计方法，可以应用于研究颗粒材料的混合和偏析，而无需从颗粒中去除任何样品（图6-3）。

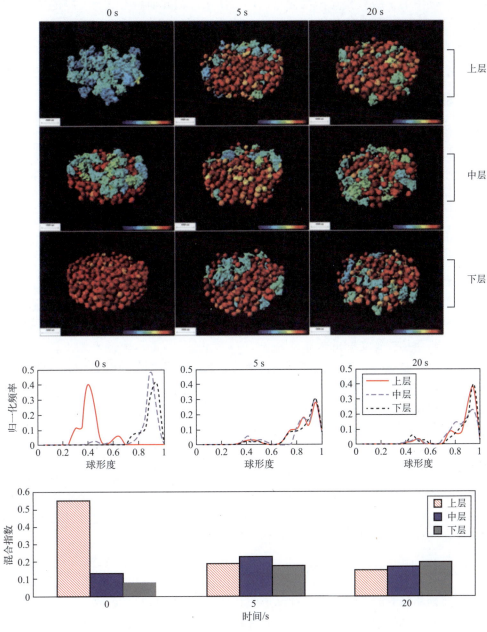

图6-3　颗粒混合和分离的三维重建和量化[24]

6.5.1.3　微晶纤维素颗粒的分类

微晶纤维素（MCC）是一种重要的药用辅料，主要用作口服片剂和胶囊剂的稀释剂和黏合剂。辅料颗粒的结构参数对辅料的质量控制和提高辅料的应用水平具有重要意义。不同制造商、不同规格MCC的结晶度、粒度和形态各不相同，这影响了其流动性、片剂崩解性等性能。通过SR-μCT可以测量MCC颗粒的结构，以区分MCC产品，比较其物理性质差异，并将MCC粉末的结构特性与压缩性、片剂崩解特性和其他制剂行为相关联。MCC压制成片剂后，片剂中的空腔结构对药物分布的均匀性和片剂的崩解方式有一定的控制作用。通过对MCC单颗粒的定量结构研究，首次在单颗粒水平上对辅料粉末的内部结构进行了定量分析，结果表明，辅料结构的差异与制剂的性质有关。因此，SR-μCT高分辨率表征技术结合主成分分析方法可以探索辅料结构、空腔差异、粉末性质和制剂释放行为之间的定量关系[52]。

6.5.2　固体剂型的静态结构和材料分布

高端固体制剂通常具有复杂、特定的结构，这些结构决定了其释放特性并影响体内吸收和生物等效性。现有的制剂创新主要从宏观结构进行，但亚微米到毫米级结构的定量研究严重缺失。由于制剂的内部结构不规则，对制剂的3D结构进行定量表征具有巨大挑战。

6.5.2.1　三维结构对固体制剂溶出度的影响

药物制剂的结构变化决定了其崩解行为和药物释放特性，进而影响药物递送的效率。美托洛尔缓释微丸在溶出过程中，表面出现明显凹陷和变形，但整体结构仍呈球形。颗粒中的药物含量随着溶出时间的延长而逐渐降低。在1小时和4小时，含药层和外涂层之间存在间隙，并且在4小时含药层的中间存在多孔结构。随后，含药层迁移到膜侧，并且在8小时后，在含药层和片芯周围出现大的空隙。最后，在20小时后药物完全释放。这一结果揭示了空间结构和辅料与药物控释之间的关联[53]。

从酸性介质中收集艾司奥美拉唑镁肠溶微丸（ESO）和奥美拉唑镁微丸（OME），并在不同时间间隔通过SR-μCT成像，以探索体外溶出过程中的结构变化。该微丸具有较高的球形度，体外肠溶膜完整。颗粒在体内的三维形状较差，表面明显凹陷。因此，颗粒在体内/体外的结构显著不同。将胃蛋白酶和玻璃微球分别引入溶出介质中，从酶学和力学的角度模拟胃的真实生理环境。同时，对ESO和OME的微丸球形度、孔隙率、微丸体积和片芯体积等结构参数进行定量，使ESO和OME微丸的体内外结构达成一致。基于制剂结构分析方法，通过调节体外溶出条件，揭示了制剂在体内的结构特征。此外，成功桥接了体外培养基和体内条件下颗粒的三维结构特征，并完成了颗粒结构的仿生测定，这可以为新型药物递送系统的设计和体外评价提供新思路（图6-4）[54]。

6.5.2.2　材料的三维空间分布

制剂中药物和辅料的三维分布是制剂形成和药物释放的基础，这决定了药物的特性。新型多单元微丸片剂具有剂量灵活、释药行为选择性和多层次结构等优点。以茶碱微丸为研究对象，SR-μCT可以在没有任何损伤的情况下快速检测片剂的三维结构，并可以与液相色谱-质谱联用（LC-MS）或液相色谱-蒸发光散射检测器（LC-ELSD）相结合用于分析化学成分和确定物质分布。茶碱颗粒主要由灰度值相对较高的基质层（ML）、灰度值相对较低的保护层（PCL）和球形颗粒（PL）三部分组成。与ML相比，PL含有更高比例的茶碱、蔗糖和邻苯二甲酸二乙酯，而乳糖和十二烷基硫酸钠的比例较小。然而，单硬脂酸甘油酯在PCL中的比例要大得多。微观结构表征和三维结构可视化可以指导制剂质量评价,测定化学成分和物质分布有助于开发新型药物递送系统(图6-5)[55]。

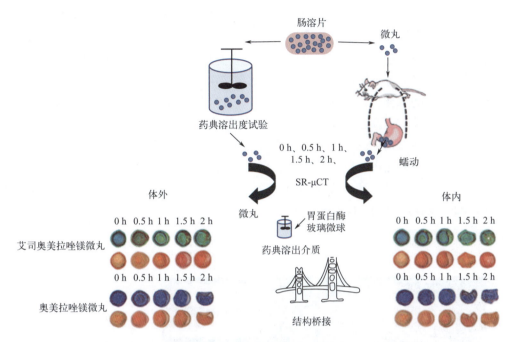

图6-4 肠溶微丸在体外和体内溶解过程中的动态结构差异[54]

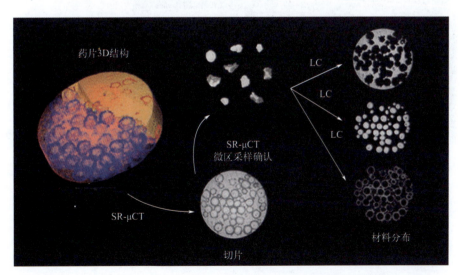

图6-5 通过SR-μCT结合液相色谱法获得多单元球系统的材料空间分布[55]

琥珀酸美托洛尔缓释片是一种复杂的多单元剂型,采用基于同步辐射傅里叶变换红外光谱(SR-FTIR)对涂层中材料的组成和分布进行评价。结果表明,羟丙甲基纤维素分散在乙基纤维素中。此外,颗粒的涂层不含任何药物成分。结构信息和物质分布特征证实,药物的缓释机制是膜控释,这与药物的释放特性一致。该结果为琥珀酸美托洛尔缓释片的质量控制提供了新方法,并为多单元固体剂型的逆向工程设计提供了指导[53]。

6.5.3 亲水性基质片的动态结构

亲水性基质片是口服控释系统最常用的剂型。基于壳聚糖阴离子聚合物的基质片可在胃肠道中发生自组装，然后从原来的基质类型转变为薄膜包衣片。然而，对其在溶出过程中的动力学行为和药物释放过程中内部微观结构的连续变化仍然未知。SR-μCT和相衬成像成功地阐明了壳聚糖-λ-卡拉胶（CHS-λ-CG）基质片在溶出过程中的微观结构。重构的三维图像反映了不同时间点的水化作用和溶胀侵蚀过程。CHS-λ-CG基质片在模拟胃液（SGF）中浸泡2.0小时后，水化层变为凝胶层和固体溶胀层。更重要的是，一旦基质片从SGF（pH 1.2）转移到模拟肠液介质（pH 6.8）中，在片剂表面会形成具有强度和密度增强的新层。3D模型的时空变化进一步为这种交联行为提供了直接证据。新层由CHS-λ-CG聚电解质复合物组成，主导释放机制。总之，通过相衬SR-μCT技术研究CHS-CG基质片的水合动力学，被认为是一种新的药物释放机制（图6-6）[56]。

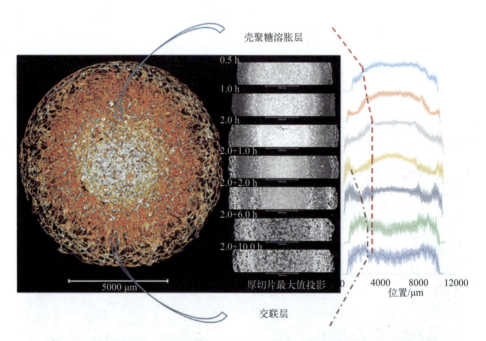

图6-6　通过相衬SR-μCT揭示CHS-λ-CG基质片在溶出过程中的微观结构特征

6.5.3.1　HPMC基质的动态结构

在各种口服控释递药系统中，水溶胀性基质系统，特别是那些含有HPMC的凝胶骨架系统，由于处方组成相对简单、易于制造、成本低，且被监管机构接受，适用于具有不同剂量和溶解度的药物[79]。基于亲水凝胶骨架的药物控释机制已研究较充分，有模型提出在水化层中未溶解的药物和溶解的药物之间界面处的扩散前沿影响药物从基质系统释放的速率。此外，水渗透和/或扩散被认为是高水溶性药物释放的速率限制步骤。对于水溶性较差的药物，基质溶蚀被认为是药物释放的主要机制[80]。例如，已有研究基于SR-μCT定量分析了难溶性药物控制释放中的溶胀和侵蚀机制[27]。

6.5.3.2 非洛地平片表面形态和水化层的可视化

经过SR-μCT评价，水化层、片芯、溶蚀和溶胀前沿随时间的相对运动清晰可见，由此可以观察到片芯的微观结构变化。HPMC基质在吸水后膨胀，导致基质尺寸增大。0.5小时后，水化层清晰可见，并随时间逐渐增大。5.0小时后，水化层变薄。片芯的尺寸在6.0小时时达到最大值，然后随着聚合物水化程度的增加而减小。8.0小时后，基质完全水化，无片芯残留。在1.0小时至6.0小时的时间内，水化层厚度变化不大，表明非洛地平HPMC基质片的释放速率恒定。采用分段切片重构出非洛地平HMPC基质片的3D结构，见图6-7（A）。片剂与溶出介质接触后，片剂的长度、宽度和高度在最初1.0小时内随溶胀而增加。随着HPMC基质的侵蚀，长度和宽度从2.0小时开始减小，然而高度保持不变，片剂的体积和表面积随着时间的推移而减小，如图6-7（B）所示。将重构的切片转换为8位灰度后垂直地重新切片。然后，对不同时间点的片剂垂直切片（包括充分水化的片剂和片芯完全干燥的片剂）并进行分析，确定阈值灰度值，以区分侵蚀前沿、扩散前沿和溶胀前沿[图6-7（C）]。水化层的体积减少比整个片剂的体积减少慢，表明药物释放速率决定了基质侵蚀的影响。

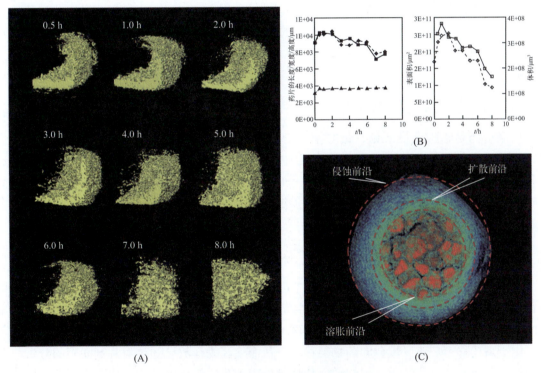

图6-7 非洛地平溶解过程

（A）药物溶解过程中水合层重构的3D图像；（B）药物溶解过程中整片内部结构的变化。[长度（实心菱形）、宽度（实心正方形）和高度（实心三角形）]；（C）非洛地平HPMC片在药物溶解过程中的溶胀前沿、扩散前沿和侵蚀前沿示意图[27]

6.5.3.3 三维水化层参数与药物释放动力学的相关性

基于提取的Iso-Surface模型，通过计算23个3D立体参数，研究了体积和累积释放百分比之间的相关性。所有体积参数,包括整个片剂的体积、玻璃片芯的体积和水化层的体积,都与药物释放的百分比有很好的相关性(R^2=0.90、0.94和0.81)。药物释放速率(dM/dt)值提供了药物递送系统的关键特征。在表面积参数与药物释放速率之间的相关性(R^2)中,片剂表面积为0.45,水化层表面积为0.80,而玻璃片芯表面积与释药速率之间的R^2值为0.87,说明玻璃片芯表面积是决定药物恒定释放的关键因素之一。因此,基质溶胀对药物释放动力学具有重要的控制作用。

此外,采用SPSS PASW统计软件(18.0版)可以构建统计模型用于多变量分析,以不同时间点的药物释放率作为因变量(n=9)。由于无法计算0 h时的比表面积值,故将0 h时的样品排除在外。在考虑R^2、方程显著性、参数系数显著性和变量的物理意义的情况下,进行自变量简化。通过自变量还原法从23个三维结构参数中识别出对非洛地平片释药有主要影响的三个参数,并建立了预测药物释放速率的方程:

$$\frac{dM}{dt} = 420.4 SA_{水化层} + 128.4 SA_{非水化片芯} + 214.9 SSA_{水化层} - 23.4 \quad (6-1)$$

式中,$SA_{水化层}$是水化层的表面积,包括水化层内部的孔隙和通道面积;$SA_{非水化片芯}$是非水化片芯的表面积,这是片芯溶胀成凝胶并发生水合作用的界面;$SSA_{水化层}$是水化层的比表面积,反映了水化层的大小。式(6-1)中的所有相关参数都已归一化,确保所有参数对药物释放率具有相同的决定强度。统计模型显示出相对理想的可预测性,R^2=0.96,具有显著性差异(p<0.001)。

6.5.4 渗透泵片的动态结构

口服给药是临床上最常见、最方便的给药途径之一。渗透泵片可以控制药物的释放速率,保持稳定的疗效,从而弥补传统口服制剂的不足。其中,推拉渗透泵片(PPOP)在递送不溶性药物方面的优势受到了广泛关注。PPOP片剂结构复杂,内部微观结构的变化可能影响药物的释放动力学。然而,目前定义渗透泵片药物释放模型的研究报告没有考虑到这个问题。

6.5.4.1 双层渗透泵片的三维结构

利用高能量、高空间分辨率的SR-μCT可对双层渗透泵片在不同溶出时间点的三维结构进行表征;还能对不同区域NaCl晶体的空间分布和运动路径进行详细的可视化。研究结果表明,溶解的盐会优先向含水量高的外围区域移动,导致外围区域推压层的渗透压较大。随后,由于高迁移率,该区域会向药物层移动,从而使药物释放。通过对片剂间隙的分析,在药物层中发现了通道状结构。根据通道从片剂外围到孔口的动态结构变化确定了药物向孔口运动的路径。在溶解过程中,推动层可分为渗透前沿、渗透区和休眠区。与传统的双层渗透泵片推拉模型不同,这是一种"地下河"模型,结合片剂中晶体从推动层到药物层的三维微观结构变化,阐明双层渗透泵片剂的释放机制,解释药物释放动力学。当推动层在片剂的外围区域触发驱动力时,药物层将通过相同的路径向孔口移动,从而产生可控的药物释放。由实验获得的片剂原位形成的三维结构及其转化行为,揭示了药物的释放机制。因此,片剂三维结构的可视化为表征和解释药物递送系统的潜在机制提供了一种新的工具,为药学领域打开了一扇新的大门(图6-8)[57]。

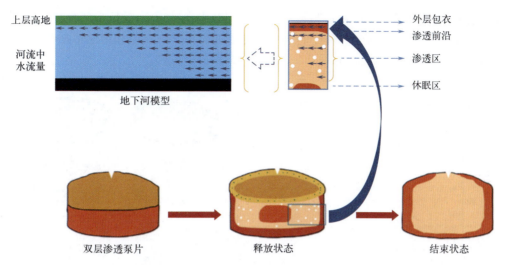

图6-8 基于双层渗透泵片剂三维微观结构的药物释放机制——地下河模型[57]

6.5.4.2 单室型渗透泵片的微观结构

最近，渗透药物递送系统（ODDS）的结构设计取得了进展，已从单室渗透泵发展到多室渗透泵[58]。目前，已有三十多个ODDS产品被开发并投入市场[59]。数百项专利和大量出版物报道了ODDS的处方、临床结果和安全性方面[60]。虽然该单元的整体结构和内部架构是ODDS的关键物理特征，但很少有研究对ODDS片芯在药物释放过程中的内部结构和动态变化进行可视化。

在各种可用的口服控释药物递送系统中，通过恒定内渗透压递送活性剂的ODDS引起了人们的极大兴趣，因为它们与其他口服控释药物递送系统相比具有许多优点。然而，ODDS的药物释放动力学显示出对处方因素的依赖性，包括片芯内药物的溶解度、片芯成分的渗透压、半透膜特性和释药孔大小[61]。因此，对内部3D空间立体数据的微观结构的研究有助于了解整体释放系统的药物释放机制[35]。

6.5.4.3 表面形态和内部3D结构的可视化

在非洛地平单室渗透泵片（MOTS）溶出度测试中，在不同采样时间点（0.5、1.0、3.0、6.0和8.0小时）进行二维单色X射线CT成像，由成像可以看出，半透膜、片芯和释药孔清晰可见，片芯中可见小空隙，还观察到固体内容物在侵蚀和溶胀后从片芯分离。片剂外壳的表面性质在大多数采样时间点都保持原始形态，并且在8.0小时溶出测试后，片剂外壳表面有一些塌陷的迹象。大多数片芯保持固体或半固体形式。在0.5小时和1.0小时出现一些裂纹，而在3.0小时和6.0小时，片芯解聚并形成多个空隙，邻近释药孔的空隙变得越来越大。8.0小时，片芯的内容物几乎是空的。有趣的是，剩余片芯的形状变化不规则，这与药剂学家可能预期的形式和形状明显不同。此外，在8.0小时和10.0小时溶出测试中，一些聚集体黏附在片剂的内壁上，这部分与非洛地平在8.0小时和10.0小时的累积释放曲线和百分比（分别为73.0%和82.4%）相关。

不同药物释放时间点的重建3D断层扫描图像展示了MOTS内部3D结构的动态变化。片芯的形状在0.5小时和1.0小时时为椭圆形。由于片芯水合，3.0小时后形状变得更加不规则，并出现多个空隙。此外，邻近释药孔的形状变化更为显著，这表明非洛地平在释药孔附近的释放比其他位置快得多（图6-9）。

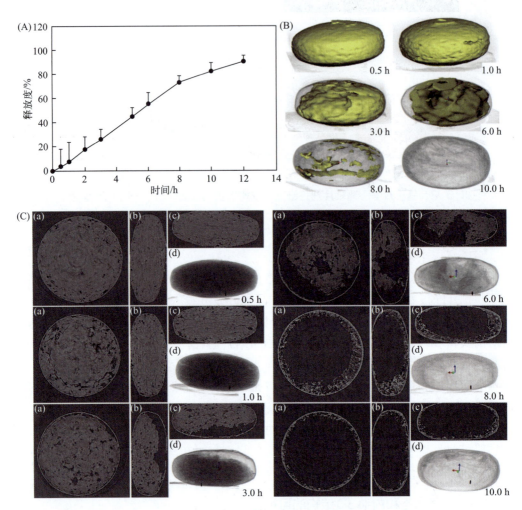

图6-9 （A）非洛地平MOTS的释放量。（B）不同采样时间非洛地平MOTS的三维重建图像（黄色代表片芯的固体部分，空气呈灰色。（C）从不同角度观察非洛地平MOTS的2D单色X射线CT图像[（a）顶部；（b）正面；（c）背面；（d）重建图像；空气显得较暗，灰色代表片芯的固体部分，灰色边缘代表半透膜][35]

6.5.4.4 3D立体参数与片芯中药物剩余百分比之间的相关性

首先，根据重构的3D图像计算剩余药片核心的体积和表面积。然后，根据MOTS的SR-μCT研究，通过100%减去非洛地平体外释放百分比来计算0.5、1.0、3.0、6.0和8.0小时片芯中的剩余药物百分比。结果显示，3D体积与MOTS中非洛地平的剩余百分比有很好的相关性（$R = 0.9988$），这表明3D参数准确地反映了非洛地平MOTS的释放特性。对于MOTS，非洛地平的释放由渗透压和悬浮液中的药物共同控制，而最初由渗透机制控制。吸水后，片芯被液体悬浮液覆盖。片芯的剩余固体成分（含有固体药物）被侵蚀成悬浮液。在3.0小时和6.0小时获得的非洛地平MOTS横截面的二维图像清楚地表明固体成分从片芯到悬浮液的侵蚀。通过渗透压和悬浮液协同机制，悬浮液通过释药孔被泵出。当考虑药物溶解和从MOTS系统释放过程中发生的具体过程时，固体成分与片芯的分离是复杂的，可以表示为：

$$\frac{dM}{dt} = \frac{\pi C}{8} \times \frac{R^4}{\eta} \times \frac{P_1 - P_2}{h} \tag{6-2}$$

对于具有零级药物释放动力学的MOTS，R、η、(P_1-P_2) 和 h 的值几乎恒定。然而，C 的表观值取决于固体含量从片芯分离到悬浮液的程度。这就是侵蚀控制过程，可以表示为：

$$\frac{dM}{dt} = \frac{DAC_s}{l} \tag{6-3}$$

式中，D、A、C_s 和 l 分别是扩散系数、扩散或侵蚀表面积、药物溶解度和边界层厚度。对于给定的药物和片剂，式（6-3）中的 D、l 和 C_s 值为不变参数。因此，式（6-2）中悬浮液中药物的浓度由 A（扩散或侵蚀的表面积，即剩余片芯的表面积）确定。初步评估可能预期片芯的表面积和体积会随着药物释放过程中固体含量的消失而减小。在药物释放过程中，片芯的表面积相当稳定，仅发生少量变化，尽管内部固体内容物的形状确实从椭圆形明显变化为不规则形状，并且如上所述，含有空隙。这导致3D表面积的值几乎恒定。

总之，式（6-2）中的 C、R、η、(P_1-P_2) 和 h 的值在药物释放过程中都是恒定的，这证明了MOTS药物释放动力学的内在机制。因此，3D表面积可以被视为非洛地平MOTS产品质量控制的关键空间参数。

6.5.4.5 单室渗透泵片的分形结构

口服控释药物递送系统的质量通常使用常规参数进行评价，例如药物溶出曲线、含量均一性、相关化合物以及薄膜包衣产品中的包衣增重。在这些参数中，溶出度通常被认为是体内潜在药物释放的指标。体外和体内药动学曲线之间的明确相关性虽然是理想的，但通常不被发现，并且可以在文献中找到具有相似溶出曲线但体内生物活性不同的制剂[62, 63]。这些发现表明，溶出曲线通常缺乏特异性，无法充分理解药物递送系统的内在质量。确定这种所需理解的内在质量的一种方法是开发新的方法来可视化药物递送系统的内部特征，以揭示药物释放过程中片剂内结构发生的动态变化。因此，可以对不考虑内部结构的常规体外释放方法进行校准[64]。断层扫描成像技术，例如X射线计算机显微断层扫描[14, 65]、磁共振成像[66, 67]和太赫兹成像[68]，可以更好地了解固体剂型的结构特征，并提供有关固体剂型的重要信息、药物释放机制与药品质量。通过成像技术还可以进一步了解水合动力学，包括表面形态和内部结构（即前沿位置或层厚度）的可视化、水渗透到聚合物基质中的速率、形成的水凝胶聚合物的浓度以及溶胀过程中药物在水凝胶中的位置[69, 70]。此外，还提出了描述药物释放机制和成功处方设计的关键参数的数学模型[71]。

断层成像技术领域的快速发展也带动了无损3D成像在药剂学中的应用[64]。这些研究大多仅提供药物溶出过程中片剂表面形态和内部结构的定性信息，且这些信息不规则、复杂且不断变化。因此，需要一种定量方法或结构参数来定义药物溶出过程中片剂表面形态和内部结构的复杂性。

分形分析是一种定量分析方法，用于表征自然界物体的形态变异性和复杂性[72, 73]。主体的不规则程度可以高度抽象为非整数分形维数（D_f）。分形分析已应用于医学信号处理和药动学建模。分形维数也已用于根据光学显微镜获取的图像定量评估聚（甲基丙烯酸2-羟乙酯）水凝胶的表面粗糙度[74]。分形维数在溶胀过程中表现出显著的下降，并且与溶胀率高度相关，因此，分形维数提供了与表面粗糙度相关的有趣定量参数。对于固体药物剂型，源自表面成像技术的D_f值已被用来表征颗粒的表面形态，主要集中于二维静态测量，例如扫描电子显微镜和原子力显微镜[75-78]。关于颗粒剂和片剂的表面粗糙度和形状的信息，已经从分形维数的值中获得。然而，很少有出版物关注3D结构的分形分析及其与控释剂型药物溶出的关系。基于SR-μCT获得的逐层2D成像投影研究了非洛地平渗透泵片的表面形态和内部3D结构[1]。因此，基于盒计数方法的3D分形分析被开发，以同时量化非洛地平渗透泵片在药物释放过程中的整体形状、内部多孔通道和表面结构。通过计算3D体积和表面积相关的分形维数值，将其与药物释放动力学相关联，然后，通过3D分形数据阐明非洛地平控释系统的药物释放机制。结果表明，$D_{f,surface}$值与药物释放速率有很好的相关性。$D_{f,surface}$被发现是一种有效的分形参数，可用于表征药物释放过程中片芯发生的复杂变化。分形分析，特别是结构分形分析，最初被用于表征药物释放过程中发生的内部结构变化，这些变化是传统方法所无法测量的。分形维数和药物释放动力学之间的相关程度可能被证明是定量受控药物释放系统的药物溶出中结构变化的作用的一个价值参数（图6-10）。因此，分形维数已被证明是反映药物释放性能的价值的定量指标，并被视为口服控释递药系统质量控制的关键指标[81]。

6.5.4.6 单微丸的释放行为

多微丸固体剂型（例如丸剂和颗粒剂）由众多离散的微丸组成，这些微丸被组合成硬明胶胶囊或压制成片剂，形成单一剂量单位。与用于控释药物递送系统的传统单一单位产品相比，多微丸剂型已获得相当大的普及。建立释放曲线的多微丸系统的传统溶出测试显然不能提供有关单个微丸单独贡献的任何信息，并且是不够的，因为整体的释放动力学是各个单元的复合曲线[82-85]。零级释放单元的集合在某些条件下将表现出一级动力学[86]。单微丸实验的结果也可用于模拟剂量水平上的释放行为[87-90]。例如，最近的一项研究通过SR-μCT技术，将结构细节与盐酸坦索罗辛缓释胶囊（TSH，商品名Harnal）的单丸释放特性相关联。

6.5.4.7 可视化和内部3D参数计算

SR-μCT获得的高分辨率3D图像是再现颗粒形态和微观结构的模型；3D渲染模型显示样品胶囊中每个微丸的完整详细结构信息。随机选择空心微丸和实心微丸来显示形态和微观结构信息，可以清楚地识别出每个微丸的形状、尺寸、形态和内部结构的差异，也可以提取微丸特性，例如直径、表面粗糙度和内部空隙，并用于计算每个微丸的体积和比表面积。在研究药物释放机制时，从CT和3D重构结果中可视化单个微丸的微观结构也特别有价值。

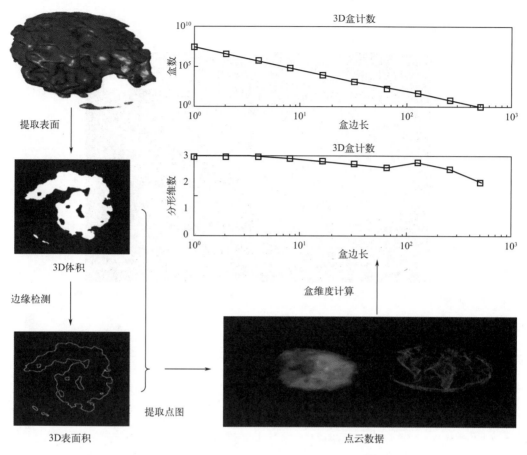

图6-10 非洛地平渗透泵片芯分形维数的计算程序[81]

例如，在尝试描述颗粒时，从重构模型中获得了大约40个空间定量参数。然后选择与释放曲线密切相关的最重要的10个参数。根据得出的数据，每个TSH缓释胶囊中约1000个小丸的大小和形状彼此明显不同。使用频率分布来描述粒子系统。尺寸（体积、表面积和直径）分布范围很宽，并且不呈现高斯分布。此外，大多数微丸的球形度值接近1，而一些微丸仍然不规则。大多数微丸的比表面积在$0.007\sim0.035~\mu m^{-1}$。大约50%的微丸是完全实心的，另一半则具有不同程度的空隙。较小的微丸（相对于表面积和体积）更趋近球形。微丸在成型和包衣过程中受压力效应，造成部分微丸呈椭圆形。当微丸趋近球形时，尺寸偏差减小。然而，在空隙和其他参数之间无较高相关性。空隙率分布与直径呈随机趋势，无显著相关性（图6-11）。

6.5.4.8 单微丸的药物释放动力学

单微丸的载药量分布范围较宽，并且与微丸体积有一定的相关性（$R^2 = 0.7790$）。随着直径的增加，散点图上的点进一步扩散，表明高球形度的微丸中药物含量表现出更好的均匀性。此外，大多数微丸中的药物浓度（单位体积含量）约为$1\sim2~ng\cdot\mu m^{-3}$，单微丸药物含量范围为100~700 ng。这一特征对于理解药物释放机制很重要。然而，几个明显的异常值表明制备过程无法生产完全均匀、一致的微丸。单微丸的溶出度在释放过程中逐渐降低，几乎所有微丸在240分钟后完全释放药物。每个时间点的药物百分比分布相似。

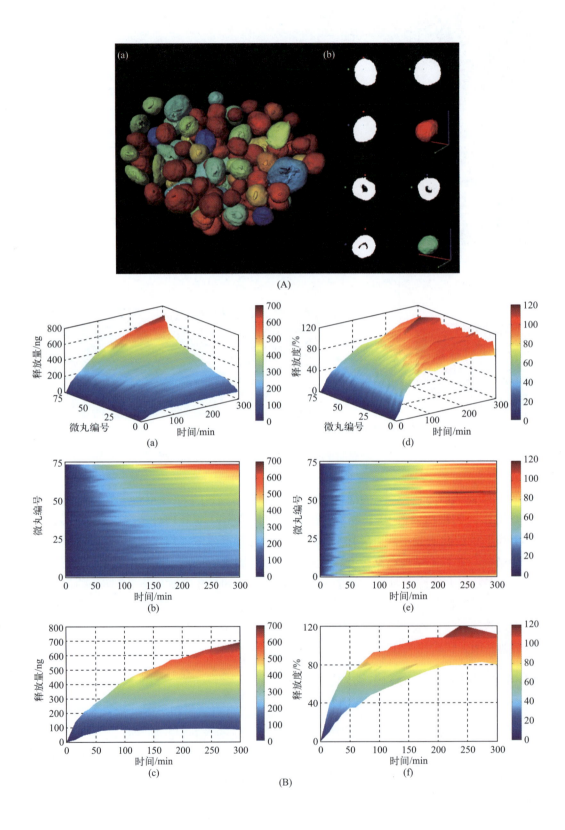

172　计算药剂学——制药4.0中的人工智能和建模

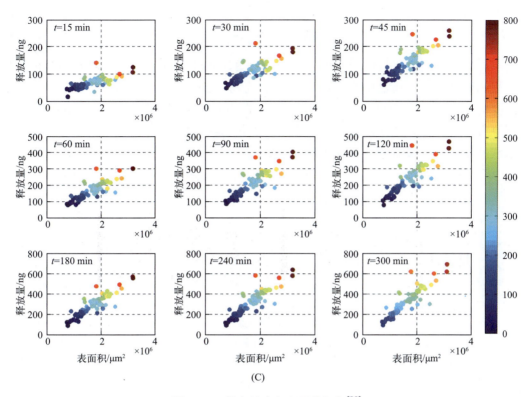

图6-11 微丸的表征和释放行为[90]

6.5.4.9 结构参数与药物释放之间的相关性

药物释放的累积量与微丸表面积密切相关，在45~120分钟的溶出时间段内观察到特别强的线性相关性。因此，微丸的表面积代表了一个关键的空间参数，它是药物释放曲线的主要决定因素。药物释放动力学也可能受到药物从微丸中扩散的影响。根据观察，含药微丸在药物释放测试期间保持其原始形状；没有观察到膨胀或崩解。单微丸的药物释放模式可以表示为T. Higuchi报道的众所周知的关系，并简化为公式（6-4）：

$$\frac{Q}{A} = \sqrt{\frac{DK}{\tau}(2-KC_s)C_s t} \tag{6-4}$$

释放速率由药物浓度、溶解速率以及溶解的药物在基质中扩散的速率控制。所研究颗粒的M_∞/V最大值为3.5 μg·mm^{-3}，该值远低于TSH的溶解度。因此，如果TSH在释放的第一阶段和中期容易溶解，则微丸中的药物浓度恒定且等于M_∞/V，因为微丸的表面积几乎没有变化，从而允许τ和表面积保持不变。对于D、K、C_s和τ恒定的情况，该方程可以简化为方程（6-5）：

$$\frac{Q}{A} = \sqrt{\omega t} \tag{6-5}$$

式中，ω是时间平方根的斜率；Q可以重写为dM/S；A可以重写为M/V，故方程（6-5）改写为式（6-6）：

$$dM = \frac{M}{V} S \sqrt{\omega t} \qquad (6\text{-}6)$$

式中，M 是微丸的载药量；V 和 S 分别是微丸的体积和表面积。药物释放的累积量是时间平方根的线性函数。通过研究 $M \times (S/V)$ 和药物释放动力学之间的相关性水平证实了它们的高度相关性。溶解开始时，只有外表面会被溶出介质渗透。颗粒充分水化后，空隙中也会充满溶出介质，内部空隙的表面积会影响溶解并加速扩散过程。然后，出于计算目的，将释放曲线的重要空间参数表面积调整为 S_a（S_a = 颗粒表面积 + 空隙表面积）。调整后的参数 $M \times (S_a/V)$ 与较高的 R^2 值产生了更好的相关性，表明空隙在药物释放过程中也发挥着重要作用。

6.6　展望

近年来，在固体给药系统的设计领域，越来越重视在分子水平上的计算机模拟和使用电子显微镜等仪器直接观察剂型的组成颗粒。在相关研究中，人们通常认为传统剂型的宏观结构及其单元成分（如片剂、胶囊剂、颗粒剂、粒剂和粉末）已经针对各种结构和形式进行了彻底和充分的研究。然而，一般考虑的是外部结构，而不是微观结构。也许是由于缺乏原位成像方法和难以量化三维特征，从纳米到毫米尺寸范围内的剂型微观结构似乎还没有得到很好的定量研究，并成为一个缺失的研究领域。虽然使用 SR-μCT 有一定的局限性，但上文重点介绍的研究示例证明了这种方法的潜力，并展示了此类研究如何揭示更多的内容。更重要的是，与传统的成像表征技术相比，SR-μCT 能以独特的视角观察药片的内部三维结构。因此，它可以为一系列固体制剂的设计提供依据，以满足特定的预期性能标准。利用这项技术重新审视剂型的整体结构，这将丰富我们的三维结构视野，并为创造和设计新的给药系统结构提供机会。

参考文献

[1] Shekunov B Y, Chattopadhyay P, Tong H H, et al. Particle size analysis in pharmaceutics: principles, methods and applications[J]. Pharmaceutical Research, 2007, 24(2): 203-227.

[2] Feng Y, Grant D J, Sun C C. Influence of crystal structure on the tableting properties of n-alkyl 4-hydroxybenzoate esters(parabens)[J]. Journal of Pharmaceutical Sciences, 2007, 96(12): 3324-3333.

[3] Rohrs B R, Amidon G E, Meury R H. et al. Particle size limits to meet USP content uniformity criteria for tablets and capsules[J]. Journal of Pharmaceutical Sciences, 2006, 95(5): 1049-1059.

[4] Jain S. Mechanical properties of powders for compaction and tableting: an overview[J]. Pharmaceutical Science & Technology today, 1999, 2(1): 20-31.

[5] Sun C, Grant D J. Influence of crystal structure on the tableting properties of sulfamerazine polymorphs[J]. Pharmaceutical Research, 2001, 18(3): 274-280.

[6] Zhang Q, Gladden L, Avalle P, et al. In vitro quantitative(1)H and(19)F nuclear magnetic resonance spectroscopy and imaging studies of fluvastatin ™ in Lescol® XL tablets in a USP-IV dissolution cell[J]. Journal of Controlled Release: Official Journal of the Controlled Release Society, 2011, 156(3): 345-354.

[7] Lyon R C, Lester D S, Lewis E N, et al. Near-infrared spectral imaging for quality assurance of pharmaceutical products:

[8] Xie Y L, Zhou H M, Liang X H, et al. Study on the morphology, particle size and thermal properties of vitamin A microencapsulated by starch octenylsucciniate[J]. Agricultural Sciences in China, 2010, 9(7): 1058-1064.

[9] Iryna A, Mauro G. 3D electron diffraction for structure determination of small-molecule nanocrystals: A possible breakthrough for the pharmaceutical industry[J]. Wiley Interdiscip Rev Nanomed Nanobiotechnol, 2022, 14(5): 1810.

[10] Cooper D M, Turinsky A L, Sensen C W, et al. Quantitative 3D analysis of the canal network in cortical bone by micro-computed tomography[J]. Anatomical Record. Part B, New anatomist, 2003, 274(1): 169-179.

[11] Stock S R. X-ray microtomography of materials[J]. International Materials Reviews, 1999, 44(4): 141-164.

[12] Redenbach C, Ohser-Wiedemann R, Loffler R, et al. Characterization of powders using micro computed tomography[J]. Particle and Particle Systems Characterization, 2012, 28(1-2): 3-12.

[13] Farber L, Tardos G, Michaels J N. Use of X-ray tomography to study the porosity and morphology of granules[J]. Powder Technology, 132(2): 57-63.

[14] Young P M, Nguyen K, Jones A S, et al. Microstructural analysis of porous composite materials: dynamic imaging of drug dissolution and diffusion through porous matrices[J]. American Association of Pharmaceutical Scientists, 2008, 10(4): 560-564.

[15] Fu X W, Dutt M, Bentham A C, et al. Investigation of particle packing in model pharmaceutical powders using X-ray microtomography and discrete element method[J]. Powder Technology, 2006, 167(3): 134-140.

[16] Wang D, Li N, Wang Z, et al. Three-dimensional study of poly(lactic coglycolic acid)micro-porous microspheres using hard X-ray nano-tomography[J]. Journal of Synchrotron Radiat, 2014, 21(5): 1175-1179.

[17] Huang X Z, Li N, Wang D, et al. Quantitative three-dimensional analysis of poly (lactic-co-glycolic acid) microsphere using hard X-ray nano-tomography revealed correlation between structural parameters and drug burst release[J]. Journal of Pharmaceutical and Biomedical Analysis, 2015, 112, 43-49.

[18] Guo Z, Yin X Z, Liu C B, et al. Microstructural investigation using synchrotron radiation X-ray microtomography reveals taste-masking mechanism of acetaminophen microspheres[J]. International Journal of Pharmaceutics, 2016, 499(1-2): 47-57.

[19] Qin W, He Y Z, Guo Z, et al. Optimization of taste-masking on ibuprofen microspheres with selected structure features[J]. Asian Journal of Pharmaceutical Science, 2019, 14(2): 174-182.

[20] Radon J, Parks P C. On the determination of functions from their integral values along certain manifolds[J]. IEEE Transactions on Medical Imaging, 1986, 5(4): 170-176.

[21] Elder A M, Langmuir R V, Pollock H C. Radiation from electrons in a synchrotron[J]. Physical Review, 1947, 71(11): 829-830.

[22] Wiedemann H. Synchrotron radiation[M]. In: Particle Accelerator Physics I, Springer Berlin Heidelberg, Berlin, 1999, 300-336.

[23] Wang Y M, Heng P A, Wahl F M. Image reconstructions from two orthogonal projections[J]. International Journal of Imaging Systems and Technology, 2003, 13(2): 141-145.

[24] Liu R H, Yin X Z, Li H Y, et al. Visualization and quantitative profiling of mixing and segregation of granules using synchrotron radiation X-ray microtomography and three dimensional reconstruction[J]. International Journal of Pharmaceutics, 2013, 445(1-2): 125-133.

[25] Karakosta E, Jenneson P M, Sear R P, et al. Observations of coarsening of air voids in a polymer-highly-soluble crystalline matrix during dissolution[J]. Physical Review E, 2007, 74(1): 011504.

[26] Chauve G, Raverielle F, Marchessault R H. Comparative imaging of a slow-release starch excipient tablet: Evidence of membrane formation[J]. Carbohydrate Polymers, 2007, 70(1): 61-67.

[27] Yin X Z, Li H Y, Guo Z, et al. Quantification of swelling and erosion in the controlled release of a poorly water-soluble drug using synchrotron X-ray computed microtomography[J]. American Association of Pharmaceutical Scientists, 2013, 15(4): 1025-1034.

[28] Appoloni C R, Macedo A, Fernandes C P, et al.Characterization of porous microstructure by X-ray microtomography[J]. X-Ray Spectrom, 2002, 31(2): 124-127.

[29] Shiny J, Ramchander T, Goverdhan P, et al. Development and evaluation of a novel biodegradable sustained release microsphere formulation of paclitaxel intended to treat breast cancer[J]. International Journal of Pharmaceutical Investigation, 2013, 3(3): 119-125.

[30] Lin Q, Pan J, Lin Q, et al. Microwave synthesis and adsorption performance of a novel crosslinked starch microsphere[J]. Journal of Hazardous Materials, 2013, 263(2): 517-524.

[31] Islan G A, Castro G R. Tailoring of alginate-gelatin microspheres properties for oral Ciprofloxacin-controlled release against Pseudomonas aeruginosa[J]. Drug Delivery, 2014, 21: 615-626.

[32] Caktü K, Baydemir G, Ergün B, et al. Cholesterol removal from various samples by cholesterol-imprinted monosize microsphere-embedded cryogels[J]. Artificial Cells, Nanomedicine, and Biotechnology, 2014, 42(6): 365-375.

[33] Gordon K C, McGoverin C M. Raman mapping of pharmaceuticals[J]. International Journal of Pharmaceutics, 2011, 417(1-2): 151-162.

[34] Broadbent A L, Fell R J, Codd S L, et al. Magnetic resonance imaging and relaxometry to study water transport mechanisms in a commercially available gastrointestinal therapeutic system(GITS)tablet[J]. International Journal of Pharmaceutics, 2010, 397(1-2): 27-35.

[35] Li H Y, Yin X Z, Ji J Q, et al. Microstructural investigation to the controlled release kinetics of monolith osmotic pump tablets via synchrotron radiation X-ray microtomography[J]. International Journal of Pharmaceutics, 2012, 427(2): 270-275.

[36] Crean B, Parker A, Le Roux D, et al. Elucidation of the internal physical and chemical microstructure of pharmaceutical granules using X-ray micro-computed tomography, Raman microscopy and infrared spectroscopy[J]. European Journal of Pharmaceutics and Biopharmaceutics, 2010, 76(3): 498-506.

[37] Yin X Z, Abi M, Fang L W, et al. Cavities spatial distribution confined by microcrystalline cellulose particles determines tablet disintegration patterns[J]. Powder Technology, 2018, 339: 717-727.

[38] Dasgupta S, Khakhar D V, Bhatia S K. Axial segregation of particles in a horizontal rotating cylinder[J]. Chemical Engineering Science, 1991, 46(5-6): 1513-1517.

[39] Savage S B, Lun C K K. Particle-size segregation in inclined chute flow of dry cohesionless granular solids[J]. Journal of Fluid Mechanics, 1988, 189: 311-335.

[40] Yalkowsky S H, Bolton S. Particle-size and content uniformity[J]. Pharmaceutical Research, 1990, 7(9): 962-966.

[41] Fan A, Parlerla S, Carlson G, et al. Effect of particle size distribution and flow property of powder blend on tablet weight variation[J]. Latin American Journal of Pharmacy, 2005, 8: 73-78.

[42] Heng P W, Chan L W, Easterbrook M G, et al. Investigation of the influence of mean HPMC particle size and number of polymer particles on the release of aspirin from swellable hydrophilic matrix tablets[J]. Journal of controlled release : official journal of the Controlled Release Society, 2001, 76(1-2): 39-49.

[43] Carless J R, Sheak A. Changes in the particle size distribution during tableting of sulphathiazole powder[J]. The Journal of Pharmacy and Pharmacology, 1976, 28(1): 17-22.

[44] Jillavenkatesa A, Kelly J, Dapkunas S J. Some issues in particle size and size distribution characterization of powders[J]. Latin American Journal of Pharmacy, 2002, 5: 98-105.

[45] Berman J, Planchard J A. Blend uniformity and unit dose sampling[J]. Drug Development and Industrial Pharmacy, 1995, 21(11): 1257-1283.

[46] El-Hagrasy A S, Morris H R, D'Amico F, et al. Near-infrared spectroscopy and imaging for the monitoring of powder bend homogeneity[J]. Journal of Pharmaceutical Sciences, 2001, 90(9): 1915-1915.

[47] Poutiainen S, Pajander J, Savolainen A, et al. Evolution of granule structure and drug content during fluidized bed granulation by X-Ray microtomography and confocal Raman spectroscopy[J]. Journal of Pharmaceutical Sciences, 2011, 100(12): 5254-5269.

[48] El-Hagrasy A S, Drennen J K. A process analytical technology approach to near-infrared process control of pharmaceutical powder blending. Part III: quantitative near-infrared calibration for prediction of blend homogeneity and characterization of powder mixing kinetics[J]. Journal of Pharmaceutical Sciences, 2006, 95(2): 422-434.

[49] Porion P. Dynamics of size segregation and mixing of granular materials in a 3D-blender by NMR imaging investigation[J]. Powder Technology, 2004, 141(1-2): 55-68.

[50] Nguyen T T M, Sederman A J, Mantle M D, et al. Segregation in horizontal rotating cylinders using magnetic resonance imaging[J]. Physical Review E, 2011, 84(1): 011304.

[51] Akseli I, Iyer S, Lee H P, et al. A quantitative correlation of the effect of density distributions in roller-compacted ribbons on the mechanical properties of tablets using ultrasonics and X-ray tomography[J]. AAPS Pharmaceutical SciencesTechnology, 2011, 12(3): 834-853.

[52] Fang L W, Yin X Z, Wu L, et al., Classification of microcrystalline celluloses via structures of individual particles measured by synchrotron radiation X-ray microcomputed tomography[J]. International Journal of Pharmaceutics, 2017, 531(2): 658-667.

[53] Sun, X, Wu, L, Abi M, et al., Static and dynamic structural features of single pellets determine the release behaviors of metoprolol succinate sustained-release tablets[J]. European Journal of Pharmaceutical Sciences, 2020, 149: 105324.

[54] Sun H Y, He S Y, Wu L, et al. Bridging the structure gap between pellets inartificial dissolution media and in gastrointestinal tract in rats[J]. Acta Pharmaceutica Sinica B, 2022, 12(1): 326-338.

[55] Zhang L, Wu L, Wang C, et al. Synchrotron radiation microcomputed tomography guided chromatographic analysis for displaying the material distribution in tablets[J]. Analytical Chemistry, 2018, 90(5): 3238-3244.

[56] Yin X, Li L, Gu X, et al. Dynamic structure model of polyelectrolyte complex based controlled-release matrix tablets visualized by synchrotron radiation micro-computed tomography[J]. Materials Science & Engineering C, 2020, 116: 111137.

[57] Abi M, Sun H Y, Cao Z Y, et al. Redefinition to bilayer osmotic pump tablets as subterranean river system within mini-earth via three-dimensional structure mechanism[J]. Acta Pharmaceutica Sinica B, 2022, 12(5): 2568-2577.

[58] Malaterre V, Ogorka J, Loggia N, et al. Oral osmotically driven systems: 30 years of development and clinical use[J]. European Journal of Pharmaceutics and Biopharmaceutics, 2009, 73(3): 311-323.

[59] Verma R K, Arora S, Garg S. Osmotic pumps in drug delivery[J]. Critical Reviews in Therapeutic Drug Carrier System, 2004, 21(6): 477-520.

[60] Kumar P, Mishra B. An overview of recent patents on oral osmotic drug delivery systems[J]. Recent patents on drug delivery & formulation, 2007, 1(3): 236-255.

[61] Verma R K, Krishna D M, Garg S. Formulation aspects in the development of osmotically controlled oral drug delivery systems[J]. Journal of Controlled Release: Official Journal of the Controlled Release Society, 2002, 79(1-3): 7-27.

[62] Sawada T, Sako K, Fukui M, et al. A new index, the core erosion ratio, of compression-coated timed-release tablets predicts the bioavailability of acetaminophen[J]. International Journal of Pharmaceutics, 2003, 265(1-2): 55-63.

[63] Sako K, Sawada T, Nakashima H, et al. Influence of water soluble fillers in hydroxypropyl methyl cellulose matrices on in vitro and in vivo drug release[J]. Journal of Controlled Release, 2002, 81(1-2): 165-172.

[64] Zeitler J A, Gladden L F. In-vitro tomography and non-destructive imaging at depth of pharmaceutical solid dosage forms[J]. European Journal of Pharmaceutics and Biopharmaceutics, 2009, 71(1): 2-22.

[65] Laity P R, Mantle M D, Gladden L F, et al. Magnetic resonance imaging and X-ray microtomography studies of a gel-forming tablet formulation[J]. European Journal of Pharmaceutics and Biopharmaceutics, 2010, 74(1): 109-119.

[66] Metz H, Mader K. Benchtop-NMR and MRI—a new analytical tool in drug delivery research[J]. International Journal of Pharmaceutics, 2008, 364(2): 170-175.

[67] Dorozynski P P, Kulinowski P, Młynarczyk A, et al. Foundation review: MRI as a tool for evaluation of oral controlled release dosage forms[J]. Drug Discovery Today, 2012, 17(3-4): 110-123.

[68] Zeitler J A, Shen Y, Baker C, et al. Analysis of coating structures and interfaces in solid oral dosage forms by three dimensional terahertz pulsed imaging[J]. Journal of Pharmaceutical Science, 2007, 96(2): 330-340.

[69] Mantle M D. Quantitative magnetic resonance micro-imaging methods for pharmaceutical research[J]. International Journal of Pharmaceutics, 2011, 417(1-2): 173-195.

[70] Mikac U, Kristl J, Baumgartner S. Using quantitative magnetic resonance methods to understand better the gel-layer formation on polymer-matrix tablets[J]. Expert Opinion on Drug Delivery, 2011, 8(5): 677-692.

[71] Kimber J A, Kazarian S G, Stepanek F. Microstructure-based mathematical modelling and spectroscopic imaging of tablet dissolution[J]. Computers & Chemical Engineering, 2011, 35(7): 1328-1339.

[72] Lopes R, Betrouni N. Fractal and multifractal analysis: a review[J]. Medical Image Analysis, 2009, 13(4): 634-649.

[73] Mandelbrot B B. Self-affine fractals and fractal dimension[J]. Physica Scripta, 1985, 32: 257-260.

[74] Mabilleau G, Baslé M F, Chappard D. Evaluation of surface roughness of hydrogels by fractal texture analysis during swelling[J]. Langmuir, 2006, 22(10): 4843-4845.

[75] Jelcic Z, Hauschild K, Ogiermann M, et al. Evaluation of tablet formation of different lactoses by 3D modeling and fractal analysis[J]. Drug Development and Industrial Pharmacy, 2007, 33(4): 353-372.

[76] Fini A, Ospitali F, Zoppetti G, et al. ATR/Raman and fractal haracterization of HPBCD/progesterone complex solid particles[J]. Pharmaceutical Research, , 2008, 25(9): 2030-2040.

[77] Cavallari C, Rodriguez L, Albertini B, et al. Thermal and fractal analysis microparticles obtained by of diclofenac/Gelucire 50/13 ultrasound-assisted atomization[J]. Journal of Pharmaceutical Sciences, 2005, 94(5): 1124-1134.

[78] Li T, Park K. Fractal analysis of pharmaceutical particles by atomic force microscopy[J]. Pharmaceutical Research, 1998, 15(8): 1222-1232.

[79] Tahara K, Yamamoto K, Nishihata T. Overall mechanism behind matrix sustained-release (Sr) tablets prepared with hydroxypropyl methylcellulose-2910[J]. Journal of Controlled Release, 1995, 35(1): 59-66.

[80] Efentakis M, Pagoni I, Vlachou M, et al. Dimensional changes, gel layer evolution and drug release studies in hydrophilic

matrices loaded with drugs of different solubility[J]. International Journal of Pharmaceutics, 2007, 339(1-2): 66-75.

[81] Yin X Z, Li H Y, Liu R H, et al. Fractal structure determines controlled release kinetics of monolithic osmotic pump tablets[J]. Journal of Pharmacy and Pharmacology, 2013, 65(7): 953-959.

[82] Hoffman A, Donbrow M, Benita S. Direct measurements on individual microcapsule dissolution as a tool for determination of release mechanism[J]. Journal of Pharmacy and Pharmacology, 1986, 38(10): 764-766.

[83] Hoffman A, Donbrow M, Gross S T, et al. Fundamentals of release mechanism interpretation in multiparticulate systems-determination of substrate release from single microcapsules and relation between individual and ensemble release kinetics[J]. International Journal of Pharmaceutics, 1986, 29(2-3): 195-211.

[84] Benita S, Babay D, Hoffman A et al. Relation between individual and ensemble release kinetics of indomethacin from microspheres[J]. Pharmaceutical Research, , 1988, 5(3): 178-182.

[85] Gross S T, Hoffman A, Donbrow M, et al. Fundamentals of release mechanism interpretation in multiparticulate systems-the prediction of the commonly observed release equations from statistical population-models for particle ensembles[J]. International Journal of Pharmaceutics, , 1986, 29(2-3): 213-222.

[86] Borgquist P, Zackrisson G, Nilsson B, et al. Simulation and parametric study of a film-coated controlled-release pharmaceutical[J]. Journal of Controlled Release, 2002, 80(1-3): 229-245.

[87] Borgquist P, Nevsten P, Nilsson B, et al. Simulation of the release from a multiparticulate system validated by single pellet and dose release experiments[J]. Journal of Controlled Release, 2004, 97(3): 453-465.

[88] Sirotti C, Colombo I, Grassi M. Modelling of drug-release from polydisperse microencapsulated spherical particles[J]. Journal of Microencapsulation, 2002, 19(5): 603-614.

[89] Sirotti C, Coceani N, Colombo I, et al. Modeling of drug release from microemulsions: a peculiar case[J]. Journal of Membrane Science, 2002, 204(1-2): 401-412.

[90] Yang S, Yin X Z, Wang C F, et al. Release behaviour of single pellets and internal fine 3D structural features co-define the in vitro drug release profile[J]. The AAPS Journal, 2014, 16(4): 860-871.

第7章

基于非平衡热力学模型研究药物及制剂的溶解机制

吉远辉　东南大学，中国
张　政　东南大学，中国
葛　凯　东南大学，中国
拉斐尔·波斯（Raphael Paus）　多特蒙德工业大学，德国
加布里埃莱·萨多夫斯基（Gabriele Sadowski）　多特蒙德工业大学，德国

7.1 引言

活性药物成分（API）的溶解特性直接关系到其生物利用度，因而对于API的开发至关重要[1-4]。然而，目前的研究表明，大多数现有及开发中的API是具有复杂溶解特性的难溶性药物[5,6]。这些药物的低溶解度通常导致其在胃肠液中缓慢溶解和较差的生物利用度[7-10]。因此，在药物开发中探究其溶解机制越来越重要。然而，现有研究表明，难溶性API的溶解过程是极其复杂和动态的，不仅难以使用模型完全描述，还受到pH和温度等条件的影响[11,12]。在过去的几十年里，研究人员根据Noyes和Whitney提出的方法[13-19]，建立了几种经验模型来总结溶解机制。值得一提的是，Costa和Lobo通过研究评估了这些模型[14]，经比较发现，API的溶解过程涉及多种物理化学现象的多个步骤，很难建立一种具有普遍适用性和较高的预测能力的理论模型来准确描述API的溶解行为，以及深入理解API的溶解机制。因此，难溶性API的溶解机制分析和准确预测在药物开发中仍然是巨大的挑战[20,21]。

为了应对溶解度和生物利用度的限制，在过去的几十年里，API的增溶技术取得了重大进展[22-25]。其中，固体分散技术是一种很有前景的提高溶解度的技术，通过将无定形API分散到聚合物赋形剂中，从而提高生物利用度和稳定性[26,27]。例如，聚乙二醇（PEG）、聚乙烯吡咯烷酮（PVP）、β-环糊精和糖类（如甘露醇）常被用作难溶性药物的赋形剂[28-34]。Kakran等[35]通过分别将β-环糊精、PVP和普朗尼克F127与槲皮素结合制备了纳米颗粒和固体分散体。研究发现，槲皮素在复合分散体和固体分散体中的溶解速率明显提高[35]。众所周知，多种因素均会影响API的溶解，例如赋形剂、介质组成、pH、温度和搅拌速率等[36-42]，对其溶解机制的探索和溶解曲线的预测是非常复杂的。迄今为止，详细的影响机制尚未得到充分解释。因此，尽管溶解机制对于设计具有可控溶解动力学的最佳制剂具有重要意义，但通过模型研究溶解机制仍是一件困难的事情[43-47]。至今，只有少数研究是关注固体分散体溶解的基本机制的阐释[48]。在大多数情况下，研究者们采用经验方法来描述API的溶解曲线[49-58]。例如，Mooney等[57,58]根据转盘法，分析了几种弱酸性的API在有无缓冲液条件下的溶解情况。随后，提出了一个基于菲克（Fick）第二定律的模型来描述初始稳态溶解速率。模型假设所研究的API溶解过程为扩散控制，API分子穿过假想的扩散层，认为达到一个简单瞬时的反应平衡。为了研究赋形剂对API溶解的影响，有必要将溶解模型与适当的热力学模型相结合以讨论API与水、API与赋形剂、赋形剂与水等的分子相互作用对溶解的影响。同时，对溶解度较差的API在无定形固体分散体中的溶解也进行了广泛的研究[9,59-63]。已报道的多种模型（Weibull模型[64]、Higuchi模型[65,66]、Hixson Crowell模型[67,68]、Baker Lonsdale模型[69]等）均已用于研究API的溶解机制[70]。

API产品开发应考虑更现实的因素，如许多赋形剂和现实的溶解方法。此外，通过测定API的本征溶解速率来合理评价API的溶解行为十分重要[71,72]。然而，API溶解动力学的实验测定既昂贵又耗时。使用合适的理论模型来描述和预测API的溶解曲线，有利于减少实验工作量，提高API产品设计的有效性[73]。因此，固体分散体的溶解曲线和理论模型的建立十分值得研究。例如，Craig等[74]研究了控制溶解理论，并提出了一种理论模型来研究API从固体分散体中的释放。Siepmann等[75]报道了一种基于菲克第二定律的模型以探讨水和API

的传质，其中考虑了API的扩散速率、基质膨胀和溶解。最近，Langham等[76]报道了一种通过结合颗粒溶解和生长过程的理论模型来研究非洛地平固体分散体的释放行为。

在过去的几十年里，包括固体分散体在内的API制剂为药物开发提供了有效的策略[77,78]。同时，API/聚合物制剂因其可减少使用频率和总剂量、减少副作用、提高患者依从性/便利性的独特优势而备受关注[79]。同时，API/聚合物制剂的溶解研究也因其广阔的发展前景而日益引起人们的关注。例如，Van der Veen等[80]在1994年讨论了对乙酰氨基酚在淀粉糊精片中的受控溶解。此外，共聚物作为一种制备API/聚合物制剂良好的候选物，可以将单体的多种优良性质结合。通常，这些共聚物由两个或两个以上的单体组成，可以促进不溶性API的溶解。例如，Eudragit®是一种具有不同侧基的甲基丙烯酸共聚物[81-85]，它结合了黏度和pH依赖性溶解特性[86]。受共聚物的启发，其他重要的API/聚合物制剂层出不穷，如聚合物微球[87]、聚合物微针[88]以及聚合物共混物[89]。值得一提的是，聚乳酸-羟基乙酸共聚物（PLGA）具有可生物降解性和较高的生物相容性，并且具有可调节的机械性能。美国和欧洲的API管理部门已批准其用于药物制剂。因此，PLGA在缓释和控释制剂设计中的应用越来越受到重视[90-95]。

为了设计具有适当API/聚合物组合的最佳API制剂，研究API/聚合物制剂中的API释放机制非常关键[96-100]。在过去的几十年里，研究人员提出了几种模型来描述各种固体制剂的API溶解曲线，如基质体系[101-103]、可蚀片剂[104,105]、微球[106]、水凝胶[107]、粉剂[108]和快速释放片剂[109-112]等。此外，研究人员也提出了多种数学模型用于描述溶解动力学，包括Baker-Lonsdale模型[113]和Korsmeyer-Peppas模型[114]。Shipmann等[115]回顾了描述固体制剂中API溶解曲线的经验模型、半经验模型和机械模型。根据研究，这些模型的预测能力难以令人满意，其中传统经验模型或半经验模型的预测能力较差[116-119]。尽管数学模型在分子尺度上提供了深入的理解，但由于其复杂性而通常难以应用[120]。例如，Siepmann等[121]应用Fick第二扩散定律模拟了PVAc/PVP基质片剂的API释放。然而，该研究没有考虑特定的分子间相互作用，并使用浓度差而不是化学势差作为溶解的驱动力。显然，这有一定的局限性和偏差。Zhang等[122]选择水不溶性的法莫替丁作为药物模型，建立一种释放行为的预测模型，并构建专家系统进行制剂设计。专家系统是人工智能研究的热点之一，但专家系统的完善仍有待进一步开展。最近，基于分子水平研究的化学势梯度模型，是在明确考虑API、聚合物和水之间的非理想性的相互作用基础上提出的一种较为全面和有效的模型。它被用来研究API的溶解机制和预测API的溶解动力学。此外，一些晶体API和聚合物也得到了进一步的研究[123-127]，如萘普生（NAP）和吲哚美辛（IND）由聚乙烯吡咯烷酮K25（PVP K25）、聚乳酸-羟基乙酸共聚物（PLGA）和丙烯酸树脂组成的制剂中的释放[128,129]等。

因此，本章将系统地综述化学势梯度模型、微扰-统计缔合流体理论（PC-SAFT）和统计速率理论等用于分析API的溶解机制和预测API溶解动力学的研究进展，具体包括纯API和API/聚合物制剂的溶解动力学和溶解机制分析，以及API负载、API类型和聚合物对其溶解动力学及溶解机制的影响。此外，本章还将介绍API溶解过程的模型预测。

7.2 理论基础和模型

7.2.1 相平衡和化学势

7.2.1.1 固-液平衡（SLE）

固-液平衡用于描述许多工业过程中的相形成和组成。例如，结晶是从液体混合物中分离纯固体物质的常用单元操作。结晶器的设计需要固体在液体中溶解度的可靠数据。根据SLE[130]，晶体API在固相（μ_{API}^{S}）中的化学势等于其在饱和溶液（μ_{API}^{L}）中的化学势，如式（7-1）所示。

$$\mu_{API}^{S} = \mu_{API}^{L} \tag{7-1}$$

这里，μ_{API}^{S}和μ_{API}^{L}可以根据式（7-2）计算得出。

$$\mu_{API}^{S} = \mu_{API}^{L} = \mu_{0API}^{L} + RT \ln a_{API}^{L} \tag{7-2}$$

对于晶体API，μ_{API}^{L}表示API在饱和溶液中的化学势；a_{API}^{L}表示API在饱和溶液中的活度；μ_{0API}^{L}表示API在标准状态下的化学势。

通过假设固相为纯组分，晶体API以摩尔分数表示的溶解度x_{API}^{L} [131, 132]，如式（7-3）所示：

$$x_{API}^{L} = \frac{1}{\gamma_{API}^{L}} \exp\left\{ -\frac{\Delta h_{0API}^{SL}}{RT}\left(1 - \frac{T}{T_{0API}^{SL}}\right) - \frac{\Delta C_{p,0API}^{SL}}{R}\left[\ln\left(\frac{T_{0API}^{SL}}{T}\right) - \frac{T_{0API}^{SL}}{T} + 1\right]\right\} \tag{7-3}$$

对于晶体API，Δh_{0API}^{SL}、T_{0API}^{SL}和$\Delta C_{p,0API}^{SL}$可以通过实验测量获得，分别表示熔化焓、熔化温度以及API固体和液体之间的等压热容差值。γ_{API}^{L}表示活度系数。这里，通过微扰-统计缔合流体理论（PC-SAFT）计算API的活度系数[133]。

7.2.1.2 液-液平衡（LLE）

当两种不同的纯液体不能全比例混合时，称为部分混溶。当这些液体彼此接触并达到热、机械和转移平衡时，就会形成两种不同组成的共存液体混合物。如式（7-4）和式（7-5）所示，根据LLE[134]，无定形API和水在富API相L1中的化学势分别等于其在富水相L2中的化学势：

$$\mu_{API}^{L1} = \mu_{API}^{L2} \tag{7-4}$$

$$\mu_{水}^{L1} = \mu_{水}^{L2} \tag{7-5}$$

式中，μ_{API}^{L1}和μ_{API}^{L2}分别表示无定形API在富API相L1和富水相L2中的化学势；$\mu_{水}^{L1}$和$\mu_{水}^{L2}$分别是水在富API相L1和富水相L2中的化学势。式（7-6）和式（7-7）可以从式（7-4）和式（7-5）中导出：

$$x_{API}^{L1} \cdot \gamma_{API}^{L1} = x_{API}^{L2} \cdot \gamma_{API}^{L2} \tag{7-6}$$

$$x_{水}^{L1} \cdot \gamma_{水}^{L1} = x_{水}^{L2} \cdot \gamma_{水}^{L2} \tag{7-7}$$

式中，x_{API}^{L1}，x_{API}^{L2}，$x_{水}^{L1}$和$x_{水}^{L2}$分别为 API 和水在液相 L1 和 L2 中的摩尔分数。因此x_{API}^{L2}可以认为是无定形 API 在水中的溶解度，γ_{API}^{L1}、γ_{API}^{L2}、$\gamma_{水}^{L1}$和$\gamma_{水}^{L2}$是通过 PC-SAFT 计算的活度系数。

7.2.2 化学势梯度模型

如图 7-1 所示，晶体 API 从旋转圆盘中溶解可以描述为两个步骤。第一步是"表面反应"，主要涉及崩解和水化。第二步可以认为是水合 API 分子从固液界面扩散到主体相的"扩散"过程[135-137]。因此，两步的驱动力可以认为是相与相之间的化学势梯度。

API 的溶解速率如式（7-8）所示：

$$J_{API} = V \frac{dc_{API}^B}{dt} \cdot \frac{1}{A} \tag{7-8}$$

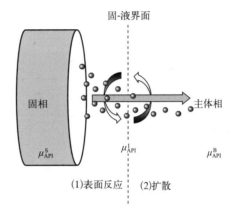

图 7-1 API 的溶解过程包括表面反应和扩散两个步骤；μ_{API}^S表示 API 在固相中的化学势；μ_{API}^I表示 API 在固-液界面的化学势；μ_{API}^B表示 API 在主体相中的化学势[137]

式（7-8）中，J_{API}和V分别表示 API 的溶解速率（$mol \cdot m^{-2} \cdot s^{-1}$）和溶解介质的体积（$m^3$）；$A$和$c_{API}^B$分别表示溶解的 API 与介质的有效接触表面积（$m^2$）和主体相中的 API 浓度（$mol \cdot m^{-3}$）。第一步以及第二步的速率可以分别由式（7-9）和式（7-10）来描述：

$$J_{API} = k_S \left(\frac{\mu_{API}^S}{RT} - \frac{\mu_{API}^I}{RT} \right) \tag{7-9}$$

$$J_{API} = k_D \left(\frac{\mu_{API}^I}{RT} - \frac{\mu_{API}^B}{RT} \right) \tag{7-10}$$

式（7-9）和式（7-10）中，化学势标记为μ_{API}^S、μ_{API}^I和μ_{API}^B，分别表示为 API 在固相、固-液界面和主体相中的化学势；k_S和k_D分别为表面反应速率常数和扩散速率常数。如果$k_S < k_D$，API 的溶解过程由表面反应控制。反过来，如果$k_D < k_S$，API 的溶解过程由扩散控制。此外，如果k_D接近或等于k_S，API 的溶解过程由表面反应和扩散共同控制。

在式（7-9）中，μ_{API}^S可以基于相平衡原理进行计算。饱和溶液中μ_{API}^S等于μ_{API}^L，如式（7-11）所示：

$$\mu_{API}^S = \mu_{API}^L = \mu_{0API}^L + RT \ln a_{API}^L \tag{7-11}$$

式中，对于晶体 API，饱和溶液中活度a_{API}^L通过 SLE 计算；对于无定形 API，则通过 LLE 计算。

μ_{API}^{B} 和 μ_{API}^{I} 通过式（7-12）和式（7-13）进行计算：

$$\mu_{API}^{B} = \mu_{0API}^{L} + RT \ln a_{API}^{B} \tag{7-12}$$

$$\mu_{API}^{I} = \mu_{0API}^{L} + RT \ln a_{API}^{I} \tag{7-13}$$

式中，API 在主体相中的活度 a_{API}^{B} 可以基于式（7-14）获得，并且API在固-液界面的活度 a_{API}^{I} 可以通过统计速率理论确定：

$$a_{API}^{B} = x_{API}^{B} \gamma_{API}^{B} \tag{7-14}$$

式中，x_{API}^{B} 表示与时间相关的摩尔分数；γ_{API}^{B} 表示活度系数。

接下来，将式（7-11）~式（7-13）代入式（7-9）和式（7-10），得到式（7-15）~式（7-16）。k_S 和 k_D 是根据式（7-15）~式（7-16）和统计速率理论确定。

$$J_{API} = k_S \left(\ln a_{API}^{L} - \ln a_{API}^{I} \right) \tag{7-15}$$

$$J_{API} = k_D \left(\ln a_{API}^{I} - \ln a_{API}^{B} \right) \tag{7-16}$$

7.2.3 统计速率理论

Dejmek 等和 Ward 等[138, 139]报道了统计速率理论用于研究固-液界面上的瞬时分子传递速率。API 在固-液界面的传输速率如式（7-17）所示。

$$J_{API} = k_e \left\{ \exp\left(\frac{\mu_{API}^{S} - \mu_{API}^{I}}{RT} \right) - \exp\left(\frac{\mu_{API}^{I} - \mu_{API}^{S}}{RT} \right) \right\} \tag{7-17}$$

式中，k_e 是每单位界面面积的固相和液相之间的平衡交换率。

J_{API} 和 k_e 之间的关系可以通过将式（7-11）和式（7-13）代入式（7-17）来获得，如式（7-18）所示。

$$J_{API} = k_e \left(\frac{a_{API}^{L}}{a_{API}^{I}} - \frac{a_{API}^{I}}{a_{API}^{L}} \right) \tag{7-18}$$

在式（7-17）和式（7-18）中，k_e 可由式（7-19）表示。

$$k_e = v_r \alpha_f + v_c \alpha_f \tag{7-19}$$

在式（7-19）中，v_c 表示因对流增强的平衡交换率，可以通过式（7-20）计算；α_f 表示固-液界面的面积分数；v_r 表示API分子的碰撞频率，通过API溶解度 x_{API}^{L}、温度 T 和比例常数 α_1 计算，如式（7-21）所示：

$$v_c = -x_{API}^{L} \alpha_2 \phi w(\delta) \tag{7-20}$$

$$v_r = x_{API}^{L} \alpha_1 \sqrt{T} \tag{7-21}$$

这里，α_2 和 ϕ 分别是比例常数（mol·m^{-3}）和与固体表面碰撞的分子分数。轴向流体速度 $w(\delta)$ 可通过式（7-22）计算[140, 141]：

$$w(\delta) = -0.51 \sqrt{\frac{\omega^3}{v}} \delta^2 \tag{7-22}$$

在式（7-22）中，ω、v 和 δ 分别表示搅拌速度、介质的运动黏度和扩散层的厚度。参考式（7-19）~式（7-22），k_e 最终可以通过式（7-23）获得：

$$k_e = x^L_{API}\alpha_1 a_f\sqrt{T} + x^L_{API}\alpha_2\phi a_f 0.51\sqrt{\frac{\omega^3}{v}}\delta^2 \tag{7-23}$$

$k_1 = \alpha_1 a_f$，$k_2 = \alpha_2\phi a_f\delta^2$，$k_D$ 和 k_S 根据式（7-9）、式（7-10）、式（7-18）拟合测量数据获得。

7.2.4 微扰-统计缔合流体理论（PC-SAFT）

PC-SAFT通常用于计算活度系数和化学势。如式（7-24）所示，剩余亥姆霍兹能 a^{res} 是分子排斥（a^{hc}）、范德华吸引（a^{disp}）、缔合（a^{assoc}）、离子相互作用（a^{elec}）等产生的各种贡献的总和。

$$a^{res} = a^{hc} + a^{disp} + a^{assoc} + a^{elec} \tag{7-24}$$

在PC-SAFT中，分子被视为由 m 个直径为 σ 的球形链节段组成的链。范德华相互作用在 a^{disp} 中是通过色散能参数 u_i/k_B 来考虑的。缔合能量参数 $\varepsilon^{A_iB_i}$ 和缔合体积参数 $\kappa^{A_iB_i}$ 被用来描述缔合分子。此外，可以根据每个分子的分子结构来指定可以形成氢键的结合位点的数量 N^{assoc}。为了描述混合物，不同组分 i 和 j 之间的相互作用由Bertrot-Lorentz混合规则描述：

$$\sigma_{ij} = \frac{1}{2}(\sigma_i + \sigma_j) \tag{7-25}$$

$$u_{ij} = (1 - k_{ij})\sqrt{u_i u_j} \tag{7-26}$$

式（7-26）中，k_{ij} 是温度相关的二元相互作用参数，如式（7-27）所示：

$$k_{ij} = k_{ij,slope}(T/K) + k_{ij,intercept} \tag{7-27}$$

可以使用式（7-28）和式（7-29）中的以下组合规则来计算两个不同缔合组分之间的交叉缔合相互作用[142]：

$$\varepsilon^{A_iB_j} = \frac{1}{2}\left(\varepsilon^{A_iB_i} + \varepsilon^{A_jB_j}\right) \tag{7-28}$$

$$\kappa^{A_iB_j} = \sqrt{\kappa^{A_iB_i}\kappa^{A_jB_j}}\left[\frac{\sqrt{\sigma_i\sigma_j}}{0.5\times(\sigma_i+\sigma_j)}\right]^3 \tag{7-29}$$

7.2.5 用PC-SAFT计算活度系数

剩余化学势 μ_i^{res} 可以根据系统的剩余亥姆霍兹能 a^{res} 计算得到，如式（7-30）所示：

$$\frac{\mu_i^{res}}{k_B T} = \frac{a^{res}}{k_B T} + Z - 1 + \left[\frac{\partial(a^{res}/k_B T)}{\partial x_i}\right] - \sum_{j=1}^{N}\left[x_j\left(\frac{\partial(a^{res}/k_B T)}{\partial x_j}\right)\right] \tag{7-30}$$

这里，压缩因子 Z 可以利用 a^{res} 计算，如式（7-31）所示：

$$Z = 1 + \rho \left[\frac{\partial \left(a^{\mathrm{res}} / k_{\mathrm{B}} T \right)}{\partial \rho} \right] \tag{7-31}$$

由 μ_i^{res} 确定组分 i 的逸度系数,如式(7-32)所述:[143]

$$\ln \varphi_i^{\mathrm{L}} = \frac{\mu_i^{\mathrm{res}}}{k_{\mathrm{B}} T} - \ln Z \tag{7-32}$$

可以根据式(7-33)来计算组分 i 的活度系数:

$$\gamma_i^{\mathrm{L}} = \frac{\varphi_i^{\mathrm{L}}}{\varphi_{0i}^{\mathrm{L}}} \tag{7-33}$$

这里,φ_i^{L} 和 $\varphi_{0i}^{\mathrm{L}}$ 分别是混合物中组分 i 的逸度系数和纯物质 i 的逸度系数。

7.2.6 溶解动力学的计算

为了计算和预测本征溶解动力学,通过结合式(7-9)、式(7-10)、式(7-15)和式(7-16)获得式(7-34):

$$J_{\mathrm{API}} = \frac{1}{A} \cdot V \cdot \frac{\mathrm{d} c_{\mathrm{API}}^{\mathrm{B}}}{\mathrm{d} t} = k_{\mathrm{T}} \left(\frac{\mu_{\mathrm{API}}^{\mathrm{S}}}{RT} - \frac{\mu_{\mathrm{API}}^{\mathrm{B}}}{RT} \right) = k_{\mathrm{T}} \left(\ln a_{\mathrm{API}}^{\mathrm{L}} - \ln a_{\mathrm{API}}^{\mathrm{B}} \right) \tag{7-34}$$

式(7-34)中,k_{T} 为 API 溶解的总速率常数,并由式(7-35)计算:

$$k_{\mathrm{T}} = \frac{1}{\frac{1}{k_{\mathrm{D}}} + \frac{1}{k_{\mathrm{S}}}} \tag{7-35}$$

7.3 实验方法

7.3.1 API 溶解度的测定

测定 API 的溶解度,目的是用化学势梯度模型计算晶体 API 在饱和溶液中的活度 $a_{\mathrm{API}}^{\mathrm{L}}$。为了测定纯 API 在不同温度下的溶解度,在带有加热装置的玻璃容器(100 mL)中加入过量的 API 以得到饱和 API 溶液。以每分钟 600 转的速率搅拌 48 小时后,检测溶液的温度和 pH。在 API 浓度一定的情况下,使用孔径 0.45 μm 的聚醚砜(PES)过滤器对介质进行过滤,去除未溶解的 API 颗粒。最后,利用紫外-可见分光光度计测定饱和溶液的 API 浓度。在进行三次测定后取其平均值。

7.3.2 量热性质的测定

如式(7-3)所示,为了通过 SLE 建模计算得到 API 的溶解度,API 的量热性质是必要的参数。此外,API 溶解度建模可以得到 API 与水之间的 PC-SAFT 二元相互作用参数,并通过

LLE进一步预测无定形API在水中的溶解度,从而在化学势梯度模型中计算无定形API在饱和溶液中的活度a_{API}^L。通常使用调制差示扫描量热法(DSC)分析API的热特性,如熔化温度T_{0API}^{SL}、熔化焓Δh_{0API}^{SL}和热容差ΔCp_{0API}^{SL}。首先,仪器用纯铟校准。然后,将API样品(6~15 mg)装入并加热(速率为2 K·min^{-1})。测量热容时,振荡正弦曲线的调制周期设为100秒。为保证升温速率恒定,将温度幅度调至0.531 K。此外,实验测定在氮气(50 mL·min^{-1})保护下进行。采用软件TA Universal Analysis 2000对测量结果进行进一步分析。在进行三次分析后,取平均值。

7.3.3 API/聚合物制剂的制备

API/聚合物制剂是通过带有惰性闭路循环的喷雾干燥器得到的。合成过程中,API与聚合物按一定比例溶解在有机溶剂中。此外,还设置了进口温度、吸入器、溶液进料速率和氮气流量。所有喷雾干燥产品干燥24小时以去除剩余的有机溶剂。

7.3.4 DSC、XRD和SEM表征

7.3.4.1 DSC表征

固体分散体使用纯铟校准的调制DSC测量。为了保持惰性气氛,氮气吹扫的流量为50 mL·min^{-1}。然后,将样品10~20 mg装入样品盘中称重。样品在283.15 K下平衡5 min后加热,加热速率为2 K·min^{-1}。调制幅度为±0.318 K,调制周期为60 s。每次测量至少进行两次。同时,利用TA Universal Analysis 2000软件对测量结果进行进一步分析。如果加热过程中样品发生熔化,则通过分析熔化峰来确定API的结晶度。API的结晶度β_{API}(%)由式(7-36)计算:

$$\beta_{API}(\%) = \frac{\Delta h_{SD,API}^{SL}}{\Delta h_{0API}^{SL} \times \omega_{API}} \times 100 \tag{7-36}$$

其中,Δh_{API}^{SL}和$\Delta h_{SD,API}^{SL}$分别为纯API和固体分散体中API的熔化焓。

7.3.4.2 XRD和SEM表征

用X射线粉末衍射仪对固体分散体的固体形态进行表征,采用0.05°的步长扫描并采集数据。此外,利用扫描电镜可观察原料和不同制剂的尺寸和形貌。

7.3.5 体外本征溶解动力学测定

将纯晶体API或固体分散体称重,并用2 kN压力压入挤压装置的圆盘模具中,得到圆柱状片剂(D=8 mm)。然后,将得到的圆柱形片剂插入溶解介质(500 mL)中。采用旋转圆盘系统(USPⅡ)测定其本征溶解动力学。由此研究各种因素对柱状片剂溶解行为的影响。值得注意的是,溶解实验所用的介质用氦气吹扫90 min。利用化学势梯度模型对溶解动力学进行建模,回归k_S和k_D参数,确定API的溶解机制。进一步用k_S和k_D计算k_T,并预测API的溶解动力学。

7.3.6 紫外-可见分光光度分析

每隔15 min用紫外-可见分光光度计对采集的样品进行测量。首先，通过测量相应波长下不同浓度的标准API溶液或赋形剂得到校准曲线。采用定量多组分分析方法获得API和赋形剂的同步释放曲线。然后，根据该方法测定的API在溶解过程中相应波长处的吸光度随时间的变化来确定API的浓度。根据API的浓度，在相应的赋形剂波长下计算每个样品的API吸光度。最后，根据测量的总吸光度计算赋形剂在相应波长下的吸光度。

7.4 机制分析与模型预测

7.4.1 晶体API的溶解动力学与溶解机制

7.4.1.1 分析和测量方法

通过引入化学势梯度模型研究晶体API的溶解机制[144]。另外，利用PC-SAFT理论和统计速率理论，可得到建模所需的溶解度、化学势和传质速率。具体来说，使用PC-SAFT理论计算API的溶解度和化学势，在分析过程中，应用统计速率理论研究API在固-液界面的传质速率。例如，如图7-2所示，采用旋转圆盘系统（USP Ⅱ）获得了包括吲哚美辛（IND）、萘普生（NAP）和格列本脲（GLIB）在内的晶体API的溶解动力学。然后，分析API的量热和解离性质以及PC-SAFT参数。此外，还分析了溶解机制，确定了不同晶体API溶解的速率控制步骤，并利用计算的速率常数对溶解动力学进行了建模。最后，将建模结果与实验数据进行对比，分析其预测结果的精度。

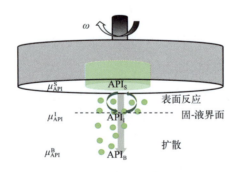

图7-2 通过旋转圆盘系统（USP Ⅱ）获得晶体API的溶解动力学[144]

7.4.1.2 API在水介质和缓冲介质中的溶解度

首先，测定IND、NAP和GLIB在水介质和pH为5.0、6.5和7.2的缓冲介质中的溶解度[144]。图7-3和表7-1为IND、NAP和GLIB在水中的溶解度，并根据式（7-3）用PC-SAFT建模。

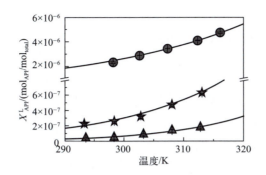

图7-3 实验测定的吲哚美辛(星号)、萘普生(圆形)和格列本脲(三角形)在水中的溶解度及相应的模型计算结果(曲线)[144]

表7-1 IND、NAP和GLIB饱和溶液中的pH测定值和计算值[144]

IND/水			NAP/水			GLIB/水	
T/K	pH测定	pH计算	T/K	pH测定	pH计算	T/K	pH计算
293.26	4.76	5.06	298.12	4.27	4.18	293.55	6.27
298.33	4.63	4.96	302.68	4.21	4.13	298.28	6.18
302.9	4.55	4.87	307.35	4.16	4.09	303.25	6.09
308.09	4.44	4.77	312.25	4.11	4.04	308.07	6.00
313.17	4.33	4.68	316.19	4.06	4.00	312.75	5.92

如式(7-37)和式(7-38)所示,平均相对偏差[ARD(%)]和平均绝对偏差(AAD)常用于分析溶解度计算的准确性。

$$\text{ARD}(\%) = 100 \frac{1}{n} \sum_{k=1}^{n} \left| 1 - \frac{x_{\text{API}}^{\text{L,计算}}}{x_{\text{API}}^{\text{L,实验}}} \right| \tag{7-37}$$

$$\text{AAD} = \frac{1}{n} \sum_{k=1}^{n} \left| x_{\text{API}}^{\text{L,计算}} - x_{\text{API}}^{\text{L,实验}} \right| \tag{7-38}$$

表7-2为ARD(%)和AAD的计算结果。从ARD和AAD结果可以看出,模型结果与实验测定结果吻合良好。此外,IND和GLIB的ARD均高于NAP。尽管如此,考虑到这些API的水溶解度非常低(<6×10⁻⁶ mol$_{\text{API}}$/mol$_{\text{total}}$),因此AAD仍然很小。

表7-2 API与水之间的二元相互作用参数k_{ij},计算数据与实验测定数据之间的ARD和AAD[144]

k_{ij}	$k_{ij, \text{slope}} \times 10^{-3}$	$k_{ij, \text{intercept}}$	ARD/%	AAD (mol$_{\text{API}}$/mol$_{\text{total}}$)
IND	0.1691	−0.1099	7.55	2.61 × 10⁻⁸
NAP	0.2269	−0.0612	2.38	6.32 × 10⁻⁸
GLIB	0.1299	−0.0833	9.26	8.18 × 10⁻⁹

IND、NAP和GLIB饱和溶液中的pH测定值和计算值见表7-1。根据Henderson-Hasselbalch方程计算了API的溶解度随pH的变化。表7-3总结了API溶解度的计算结果，并将其用于研究溶解机制和建立溶解动力学预测模型。

表7-3 计算IND、NAP和GLIB在310.15 K水中的溶解度[144]

物质	API溶解度（摩尔分数）		
	IND	NAP	GLIB
水	5.33×10^{-7}	3.77×10^{-6}	1.54×10^{-7}
pH 5.0	8.51×10^{-7}	1.60×10^{-5}	1.36×10^{-7}
pH 6.5	2.06×10^{-5}	4.38×10^{-4}	2.02×10^{-7}
pH 7.2	1.03×10^{-4}	2.18×10^{-3}	4.72×10^{-7}

7.4.1.3 溶解机制分析

实验测定和理论计算API的溶解度后，利用所提出的模型分析API的溶解机制，确定速率控制步骤。例如，根据式（7-38）研究了不同因素（介质组成和pH）对IND、NAP和GLIB的溶解机制的影响。如图7-4所示，IND、NAP和GLIB的k_S和k_D是通过实验溶解动力学并结合化学势梯度模型拟合得到的。此外，表7-4总结了k_S，k_D，k_1，k_2和ARD（%）。对于溶解分析来讲，有必要根据式（7-39）和式（7-40）求得310.15 K时的摩尔密度和介质运动黏度。

$$\rho/(\text{mol}\cdot\text{L}^{-1}) = -0.0003 \times (T/℃)^2 - 0.0008 \times (T/℃) + 55.525 \quad (7-39)$$

$$v/(\text{m}^2\cdot\text{s}^{-1}) = 2.248 \times 10^{-10} \times (T/℃)^2 - 3.195 \times 10^{-8} \times (T/℃) + 1.572 \times 10^{-6} \quad (7-40)$$

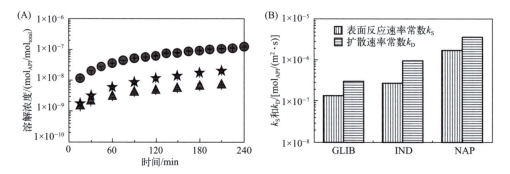

图7-4 310.15 K、50 r·min⁻¹下实验测定的IND（星形）、NAP（圆形）和GLIB（三角形）在水中的溶解动力学曲线（A）和这些药物在水中溶解过程的表面反应速率常数k_S和扩散速率常数k_D[144]（B）

表7-4 拟合参数k_S，k_D，k_1，k_2，k_T和ARD[144]

系统	k_D	$k_1=a_1a_f$	$k_2=a_2\phi a_f\delta^2$	k_S	k_T	ARD/%
IND/水	9.69×10^{-7}	1.35×10^{-3}	1.82×10^{-4}	2.80×10^{-7}	2.17×10^{-7}	17.52
IND/pH 5.0	9.59×10^{-7}	3.97×10^{-6}	2.20×10^{-6}	3.69×10^{-7}	2.67×10^{-7}	24.78

续表

系统	k_D	$k_1=a_1a_f$	$k_2=a_2\phi a_f \delta^2$	k_S	k_T	ARD/%
IND/pH 6.5	1.46×10^{-5}	1.98×10^{-4}	4.86×10^{-4}	2.95×10^{-6}	2.45×10^{-6}	5.43
IND/pH 7.2	1.56×10^{-5}	2.04×10^{-5}	1.65×10^{-5}	7.74×10^{-6}	5.17×10^{-6}	9.78
NAP/水	3.70×10^{-6}	8.99×10^{-4}	1.39×10^{-4}	1.73×10^{-6}	1.18×10^{-6}	16.35
NAP/pH 5.0	5.02×10^{-6}	1.28×10^{-5}	2.39×10^{-5}	1.92×10^{-6}	1.39×10^{-6}	11.42
NAP/pH 6.5	2.10×10^{-5}	4.68×10^{-5}	3.03×10^{-5}	1.77×10^{-4}	1.88×10^{-5}	10.83
NAP/pH 7.2	4.72×10^{-5}	1.62×10^{-4}	2.44×10^{-3}	7.51×10^{-4}	4.44×10^{-5}	12.09
GLIB/水	2.94×10^{-7}	5.43×10^{-3}	3.75×10^{-4}	1.35×10^{-7}	9.25×10^{-8}	15.18
GLIB/pH 5.0	1.16×10^{-7}	7.22×10^{-4}	3.08×10^{-5}	2.82×10^{-8}	2.27×10^{-8}	17.92
GLIB/pH 6.5	4.88×10^{-7}	3.17×10^{-3}	6.49×10^{-4}	8.89×10^{-8}	7.52×10^{-8}	19.52
GLIB/pH 7.2	1.04×10^{-6}	8.46×10^{-3}	5.90×10^{-4}	1.04×10^{-7}	9.45×10^{-8}	18.32

如图7-4（A）所示，IND、NAP和GLIB在水中的实验溶解动力学曲线表明，NAP的热力学驱动力$\mu_{API}^S - \mu_{API}^B$大于GLIB和IND的，因此GLIB和IND的溶解速率小于NAP。API在水中的溶解机制分析结果见图7-4（B）。结果表明，由于k_D比k_S大得多，API在水中的溶解过程受表面反应控制。API的缓慢崩解和水化限制了其溶解。GLIB的k_S和k_D仅为IND的1/2和近1/3，GLIB的k_S和k_D仅为NAP的近1/13和1/12。造成溶解动力学差异的原因主要有以下几个方面：①不同热力学驱动力$\mu_{API}^S - \mu_{API}^B$（GLIB<IND<NAP）；②不同$k_S$（GLIB<IND<NAP）；③不同$k_D$（GLIB<IND <NAP）。

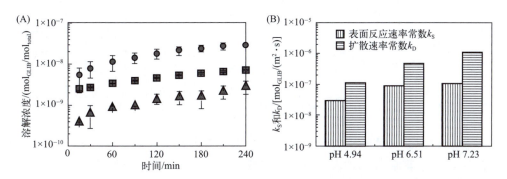

图7-5 在pH分别为7.23（圆形）、6.51（方形）和4.94（三角形）的缓冲溶液中，实验测定的GLIB的溶解动力学曲线（A）及其溶解过程中表面反应速率常数k_S和扩散速率常数k_D（B）[144]

接下来，测定IND、NAP和GLIB在不同pH下的溶解动力学曲线。此外，还分析了API在缓冲溶液中的溶解机制，结果如图7-5所示。由于热力学驱动力的增加，随着pH的升高，IND、NAP和GLIB的溶解速率明显提高。k_D和k_S，以及常数k_1（$k_1 = \alpha_1 a_f$）、k_2（$k_2=\alpha_2\phi a_f \delta_2$）和ARD的计算结果如表7-4所示。

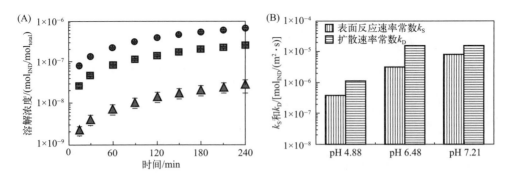

图7-6 在pH分别为7.21（圆形）、6.47（方形）和4.88（三角形）时，IND的溶解动力学曲线（A）及其溶解过程中表面反应速率常数k_S和扩散速率常数k_D（B）[144]

对于GLIB[图7-5（B）]，当pH从4.94增加到6.51时，k_S增加了约3倍，而k_D则要小得多，这说明溶解过程是由GLIB从固体到介质的缓慢崩解和水化作用决定。当pH增加到7.23时，k_S进一步增加[图7-5（B）]。如图7-6（B）所示，在pH为7.21时，由于k_S与k_D大小接近，IND的溶解受表面反应和扩散控制。然而，在pH为4.88和6.48时，IND溶解的k_S远小于k_D，说明溶解过程主要受表面反应控制。很明显，随着pH增加，k_S增加。这表明随着pH增加，IND的崩解和水化作用增强。同样，NAP的溶解（pH 4.97）被认为是表面反应控制的，而在更高的pH下则被认为是扩散控制。如图7-7（B）所示，IND和GLIB的k_S和k_D远小于NAP，这在一定程度上解释了NAP溶解更快的原因。另一个重要因素是NAP的溶解度较高，因此NAP的热力学驱动力高于IND和GLIB。因此，溶解速率的提高主要得益于溶解度和动力学部分k_S和k_D的提高。

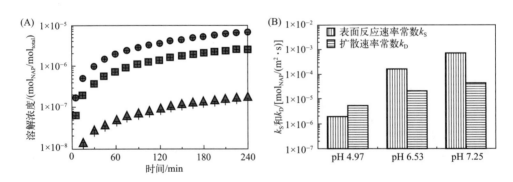

图7-7 在pH为7.25（圆形）、6.53（方形）和4.97（三角形）时，NAP的溶解动力学曲线（A）及其溶解过程中表面反应速率常数k_S和扩散速率常数k_D（B）[144]

7.4.1.4 API溶解动力学曲线的计算

对溶解机制进行分析，并计算表面反应速率常数k_S和扩散常数k_D后，根据式（7-38）和式（7-39）计算并预测总溶解速率常数k_T和溶解动力学曲线。在以下案例中比较IND和NAP的溶解模型。

案例1：用pH 5.0时的k_S和k_D以及pH 7.2时的API溶解度来预测pH 7.2时API的溶解动

力学曲线。

案例2：用pH 7.2时的k_S和k_D以及pH 5.0时的API溶解度来预测API的溶解动力学曲线。

案例3：用pH 7.2时的k_S和k_D以及pH 7.2时的API溶解度来预测API的溶解动力学曲线。在310.15 K和50 r·min^{-1}下，IND和NAP在不同缓冲溶液中的溶解动力学曲线分别如图7-8（A）和（B）所示。灰色虚线、点划线和黑色实线分别为案例1、案例2和案例3的建模结果。图7-8表明API的溶解度和溶解速率常数对API的溶解非常关键，因为案例1和案例2中的实验测定数据高于其预测的溶解动力学曲线。另外，从案例1和案例2可以看出，API速率常数对API溶解的影响大于API溶解度对其的影响。只有同时考虑了这两个因素（案例3），预测结果才与实测数据一致。API/水和GLIB/缓冲液体系的计算结果分别如图7-9（A）和图7-9（B）所示。结果表明，计算得到的API溶解动力学曲线与实测数据吻合良好，说明化学势梯度模型可以很好地描述API在水和缓冲介质中的溶解。

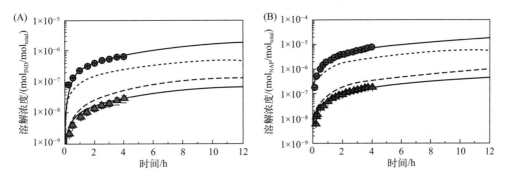

图7-8　在310.15 K和50 r·min^{-1}下，IND（A）和NAP（B）在不同缓冲溶液中的溶解动力学曲线[144]。深灰色圆圈分别表示pH 7.21时吲哚美辛和pH 7.25时萘普生的实测溶解动力学曲线。浅灰色三角形分别表示pH 4.88时吲哚美辛和pH 4.97时萘普生的实测溶解动力学曲线。灰色实线分别表示pH 5.0时计算得到的API溶解动力学曲线。灰色虚线、点划线和黑色实线分别表示案例1、案例2和案例3的建模结果

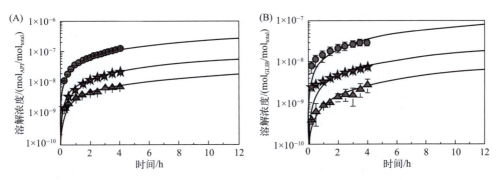

图7-9　IND（星形）、NAP（圆形）和GLIB（三角形）在水中的溶解动力学曲线（A）和GLIB在pH为4.94（三角形）、6.51（星形）和7.23（圆形）的溶解动力学曲线（B），其中实线为计算结果[144]

7.4.2　API/聚合物制剂的溶解动力学

本节将基于已有的关于API/聚合物制剂模型研究的文章[145-147]，通过与晶体API比较，

研究API/聚合物制剂中API的溶解动力学,以及API负载、API类型、聚合物类型、pH和共聚物组成等影响因素。此外,还将化学势梯度模型与PC-SAFT相结合,以研究API/聚合物制剂的API溶解机制。

首先,利用旋转圆盘系统(USP Ⅱ)测量聚乙酸乙烯酯(PVAc)和聚乙烯吡咯烷酮/乙酸乙烯64(PVPVA 64)制剂中IND和NAP的溶解动力学。然后,结合化学势梯度模型和PC-SAFT[145]分析这些制剂中难溶性IND和NAP的溶解机制,研究API负载和聚合物类型对API/聚合物制剂的溶解动力学和溶解机制的影响。

其次,使用旋转圆盘系统(USP Ⅱ)测定具有不同共聚物组成和分子量的API/PLGA制剂中IND和氢氯噻嗪(HCT)的溶解动力学[146]。利用化学势梯度模型和PC-SAFT分析API/PLGA制剂中IND和HCT的溶解机制,研究API类型、共聚物组成和分子量对API/聚合物制剂中API溶解的影响。

最后,采用喷雾干燥技术将四种Eudragit®(聚合物赋形剂)和对乙酰氨基酚(PARA)结合,制备出无定形的PARA/Eudragit®制剂[147]。采用旋转圆盘系统(USP Ⅱ)测定PARA和Eudragit®在制剂中的同步溶解动力学,并通过比较PARA和赋形剂的溶解速率分析PARA的溶解机制。此外,关于pH对API/聚合物制剂中API释放的影响也进行了研究,并模拟了API/聚合物制剂的溶解动力学。研究结果表明,结合PC-SAFT的化学势梯度模型是研究API/聚合物制剂中API溶解机制的有效方法,可以很好地关联和预测API的溶解动力学,并有助于研究者们节省时间和长期API溶解动力学测定的成本。

7.4.2.1 API/聚合物制剂中的API溶解动力学及溶解机制

在310.15 K和50 r·min^{-1}的搅拌速度下,对PVAc和PVPVA 64制剂中IND和NAP的溶解动力学进行测定[145]。通过与晶体API对比,研究API/聚合物制剂中API的溶解动力学,探讨API负载和聚合物种类等因素对API溶解动力学的影响。此外,将化学势梯度模型与PC-SAFT相结合,研究了API/聚合物制剂中API的溶解机制。在模型中,根据式(7-39)和式(7-40)计算了310.15 K时水的摩尔密度和运动黏度。

采用PC-SAFT法测定活度系数。对k_D和k_S,以及常数k_1($k_1 = \alpha_1 a_f$)和k_2($k_2 = \alpha_2 \phi a_f \delta_2$)进行了分析和总结,结果如表7-5所示。

表7-5 IND和NAP制剂的k_S、k_D、k_1、k_2和k_T参数

体系	API负载量	k_S	k_D	k_1	k_2	k_T
IND/PVAc制剂	w_{IND}=0.6	1.92×10^{-7}	1.28×10^{-6}	2.65×10^{-7}	5.33×10^{-7}	1.67×10^{-7}
	w_{IND} = 0.4	2.27×10^{-7}	1.37×10^{-6}	1.47×10^{-5}	4.81×10^{-7}	1.95×10^{-7}
IND/PVPVA 64制剂	w_{IND}=0.6	1.86×10^{-6}	3.14×10^{-6}	2.33×10^{-4}	5.23×10^{-5}	1.17×10^{-6}
	w_{IND} = 0.4	4.98×10^{-7}	7.66×10^{-7}	2.38×10^{-5}	9.55×10^{-7}	3.02×10^{-7}
NAP/PVAc制剂	w_{NAP} = 0.2	5.01×10^{-7}	4.64×10^{-6}	3.35×10^{-6}	2.24×10^{-6}	4.53×10^{-7}
NAP/PVPVA 64制剂	w_{NAP} = 0.6	2.05×10^{-6}	2.92×10^{-6}	2.48×10^{-6}	2.85×10^{-6}	1.20×10^{-6}
	w_{NAP} = 0.4	4.45×10^{-6}	7.32×10^{-6}	2.40×10^{-6}	2.91×10^{-6}	2.77×10^{-6}
	w_{NAP} = 0.2	3.63×10^{-5}	1.49×10^{-4}	4.53×10^{-4}	3.61×10^{-4}	2.92×10^{-5}

如式（7-41）所示，利用建模数据与测定数据之间的ARD（%）来评估建模准确性。ARD（%）结果列在表7-6中。

$$\text{ARD}(\%) = 100 \frac{1}{n_{\exp}} \sum_{m=1}^{n_{\exp}} \left| \frac{x_m^{\exp} - x_m^{\text{model}}}{x_m^{\exp}} \right| \tag{7-41}$$

表7-6 模拟和实测的溶解动力学之间的ARD（%）[145]

体系	条件	API负载量	ARD/%
IND/PVAc 制剂	50 r·min⁻¹，310.15 K	$w_{\text{IND}} = 0.6$	19.25
		$w_{\text{IND}} = 0.4$	13.15
IND/PVPVA 64 制剂	50 r·min⁻¹，310.15 K	$w_{\text{IND}} = 0.6$	5.96
		$w_{\text{IND}} = 0.4$	6.13
NAP/PVAc 制剂	50 r·min⁻¹，310.15 K	$w_{\text{NAP}} = 0.2$	13.74
NAP/PVPVA 64 制剂	50 r·min⁻¹，310.15 K	$w_{\text{NAP}} = 0.6$	2.67
		$w_{\text{NAP}} = 0.4$	8.26
		$w_{\text{NAP}} = 0.2$	8.26

7.4.2.2 API负载对API/聚合物制剂溶解动力学及溶解机制的影响

通过制备IND/PVAc和IND/PVPVA 64制剂，进一步研究IND负载的影响[145]，结果如图7-10和图7-11所示。与晶体IND相比，在310.15 K和50 r·min⁻¹时，两种制剂的溶解速率均有提高。通过DSC、XRD和SEM对IND进行表征，发现IND为无定形，因此提高的溶解速率可能得益于IND结晶状态的转变。此外，IND的溶解速率随IND的负载量减少而增加。如图7-10（B）所示，API负载量为0.4和0.6时，IND/PVAc制剂的溶解机制均受表面反应控制。此外，IND的k_D和k_S都随着IND负载量的减少而略有增加，导致IND负载量为0.4时从PVAc的溶解速率高于0.6时的溶解速率。

但与IND/PVAc制剂不同的是，PVPVA 64中IND的溶解速率随着IND负载量的增加而增加，如图7-11（A）所示。图7-11（B）表明，更高的IND负载量也提高了PVPVA 64制剂

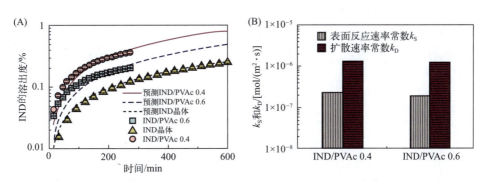

图7-10 IND/PVAc制剂和纯晶体IND在水中的溶解动力学曲线（A）以及k_D和k_S参数（B）[145]

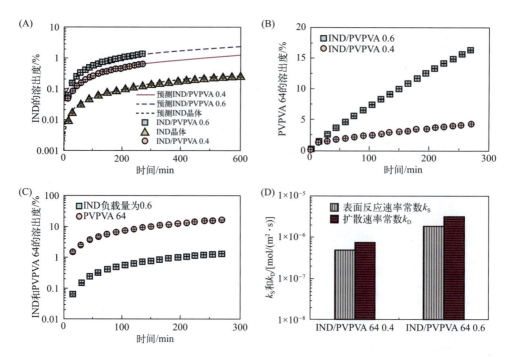

图7-11 IND（A）、PVPVA 64（B）以及IND和PVPVA 64（C）从制剂中同步溶解的动力学曲线；在水介质中，IND从PVPVA 64制剂中溶解的k_S和k_D（D）[145]

的溶解速率。图7-11（C）为API负载量为0.6时IND/PVPVA 64制剂在300 min内的同步溶解结果。结果表明，溶解受API和赋形剂共同控制。通过计算并比较k_D和k_S发现，API负载量为0.4和0.6时PVPVA 64制剂中的IND溶解决定于表面反应[图7-11（D）]。随着IND负载量的增加，k_S值也随之提高。

7.4.2.3　API类型对API/聚合物制剂中API溶解的影响

在研究了API的负载后，关于API类型对IND和HCT负载的PLGA制剂的影响也进行了进一步研究[146]。如图7-12（A）所示，RG 752 S和RG 750 S负载的IND溶解速率分别小于HCT和大于HCT。此外，IND/RESOMERVR RG 750 S制剂的IND溶解速率比IND高，因为IND在RG 750 S中呈无定形状态。然而，由于IND持续溶解，RG 752 S也很重要。对于HCT，与纯HCT相比，RG 752 S和RG 750 S的溶解速率均是关键的。上述结果证明IND/PLGA和HCT/PLGA制剂中API的溶解受API和赋形剂释放的控制。IND和HCT的溶解均受表面反应控制。如图7-12（B）所示，HCT的溶解速率高于IND，因为HCT的k_S和k_D都高于IND。对于IND和HCT，RG 750 S中HCT的溶解速率低于PLGA中的IND，因为RG 750 S中HCT的k_S低于IND。

7.4.2.4　聚合物种类对API/聚合物制剂溶解动力学和溶解机制的影响

在研究了API类型的影响后，关于聚合物种类的影响也进行了深入研究。如图7-13所示，与IND相比，PVP制剂、PVAc制剂和PVPVA 64制剂中的IND溶解速率有所提高[145]。此外，PVPVA 64制剂中的IND溶解速率高于PVAc制剂。PVP制剂中的IND溶解速率明显高于 PVPVA 64 制剂和 PVAc 制剂。对于 PVP 制剂、PVPVA 64 制剂和 PVAc 制剂 [图 7-13（C）]，当 IND 负载量为 0.4 时，IND 在水中的溶解仅由表面反应决定；表面反应受 IND 从聚合物中运输、水渗透到聚合物中以及 IND 与聚合物的水化作用的影响。随后，研究人员进一步研究了聚合物种类的影响。得益于无定形，当 NAP 负载量为 0.2 时，PVP 制剂、PVPVA 64 制剂和 PVAc 制剂中的 NAP 溶解速率明显高于 NAP[图 7-14（A）]。NAP 在制剂中的溶解速率由快到慢依次为 PVP 制剂、PVPVA64 制剂、PVAc 制剂，因为 PVP 的溶解速率高于 PVPVA64 和 PVAc。因此从制剂中溶解的 NAP 受到 API 和高分子赋形剂的共同控制。如图 7-14（B）所示，制剂的 k_D 和 k_S 从高到低依次为 PVP 制剂、PVPVA 64 制剂、PVAc 制剂。当 NAP 负载量为 0.2 时，表面反应对 NAP 的溶解起关键作用。

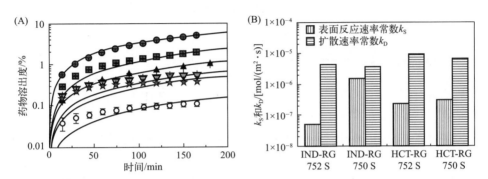

图 7-12 （A）RESOMERRG® 752 S（圆形）和 RG 750 S（方形）制剂中 IND 的溶解动力学曲线，以及 RG 752 S（星形）和 RG 750S（三角形）制剂中 HCT 的溶解动力学曲线。实线为模型关联的 IND 和 HCT 溶解动力学曲线，虚线为预测的 IND 溶解动力学曲线。（B）RG 752 S 和 RG 750 S 中 IND 和 HCT 溶解时的 k_S 和 k_D [146]

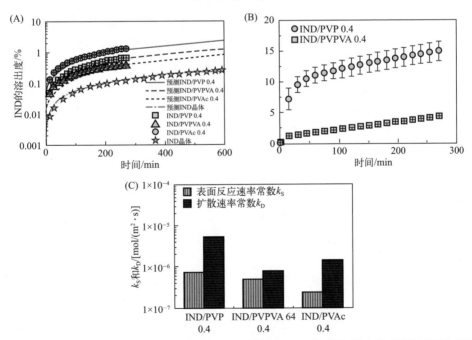

图 7-13 PVP K25 制剂、PVAc 制剂和 PVPVA 64 制剂中 IND（A）和聚合物（B）的同步溶解动力学曲线以及溶解时的 k_D 和 k_S（C）[145]

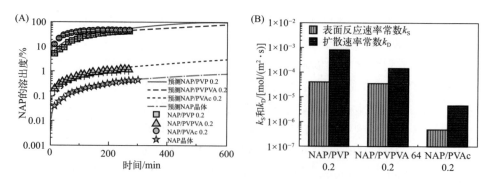

图7-14 在水中负载量为0.2的NAP从PVP制剂（圆圈）、PVPVA制剂（正方形）以及PVAc（三角形）制剂中溶解的动力学曲线以及纯NAP的溶解动力学曲线（A）；在水中NAP从PVP制剂、PVPVA制剂以及PVAc制剂中溶解的速率常数k_D和k_S（B）[145]

7.4.2.5 pH对API/聚合物制剂中API溶解的影响

通过制备含有四种Eudragit®的无定形对乙酰氨基酚（PARA）/Eudragit®制剂，进一步分析其溶解机制[147]。如图7-15（A）和图7-15（B）所示，在所有研究的pH（pH 4.97、6.53和7.25）下，制剂中的Eudragit®L 100-5和无定形PARA均受pH的影响较大，且溶解速率随pH的增加而增加。对于PARA/Eudragit®L 100-55制剂，PARA的溶解受控于PARA的溶解度。从图7-16（A）和图7-16（B）可以看出，PARA和Eudragit®L 100的溶解速率普遍随着pH的增加而增加，并且在pH为6.51和7.27时，PARA的溶解受Eudragit®L 100的溶解控制。然而，在pH为4.92的条件下，PARA和Eudragit®L 100对其均有控制作用。与PARA[图7-16（A）]相比，PARA从PARA/Eudragit®L 100制剂中持续溶解。对于PARA/Eudragit®S 100制剂（图7-17），pH为6.48时，PARA和Eudragit®S 100的溶解速率与pH为4.92时接近，均远低于pH为7.27时的溶解速率。通过图7-17（B）分析，PARA/Eudragit®S 100制剂的PARA溶解速率在pH为6.48和4.92时由PARA和Eudragit®S 100控制，在pH为7.27时仅由赋形剂控制。如图7-18所示，PARA和Eudragit®EPO的瞬时溶解动力学随pH的变化而变化。制剂中的PARA受pH的影响明显，其溶解速率随pH的增加而增加。此外，Eudragit®EPO的溶解速率随着pH的降低而提高[图7-18（B）]。在pH为4.89、6.51和7.26时，PARA的溶解速率与Eudragit®EPO相近。PARA的溶解由Eudragit®EPO控制。

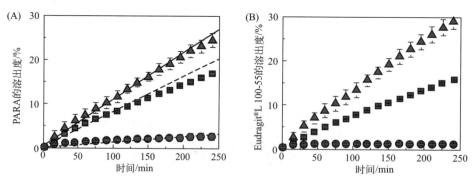

图7-15 在pH 4.97（圆形）、pH 6.53（方形）和pH 7.25（三角形）下，（A）PARA和（B）Eudragit®L 100-55从PARA/Eudragit®L 100-55制剂中溶解的同步溶解动力学曲线。曲线表示模型计算得到的PARA在pH 4.97（点划线）、pH 6.53（虚线）和pH 7.25（实线）下的溶解动力学[147]

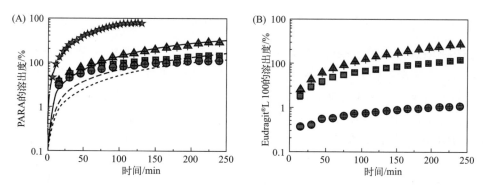

图7-16 在pH 4.92（圆形）、pH 6.51（方形）和pH 7.27（三角形）下，（A）PARA和（B）Eudragit®L 100从PARA/Eudragit®L 100制剂中溶解的同步溶解动力学曲线。曲线表示模型计算得到的PARA在水介质中的溶解动力学（星形）以及在pH 4.97（点划线）、pH 6.51（虚线）和pH 7.25（实线）时的溶解动力学[147]

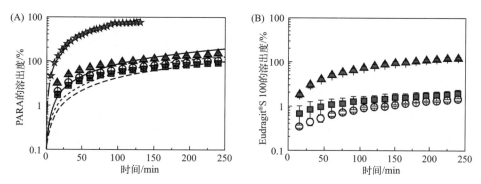

图7-17 在pH 4.92（圆形）、pH 6.48（方形）和pH 7.27（三角形）下，（A）PARA和（B）Eudragit®S 100从PARA/Eudragit®S 100制剂中溶解的同步溶解动力学曲线。曲线表示模型计算得到的PARA在水介质中的溶解动力学（星形）以及在pH 4.97（点划线）、pH 6.48（虚线）和pH 7.25（实线）时的溶解动力学[147]

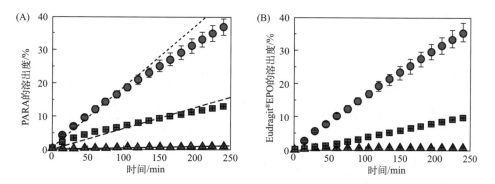

图7-18 在pH 4.89（圆形）、pH 6.51（方形）和pH 7.26（三角形）下，（A）PARA和（B）Eudragit®EPO从PARA/Eudragit®EPO制剂中溶解的同步溶解动力学曲线。曲线表示模型计算得到的PARA在pH 4.89（点划线）、pH 6.51（虚线）和pH 7.26（实线）时溶解动力学[147]

7.4.2.6 共聚物组成和分子量对API/聚合物制剂的影响

通过选择RESOMERVR RG 502和RG 752 S作为赋形剂，研究共聚物组成的影响[146]。如图7-19（A）所示，RG 502制剂中的IND溶解速率比RG 752 S高，这是因为RG 502（DLLA与GA的摩尔比为50∶50）的GA单体单元量大于RG 752 S（DLLA与GA的摩尔比为75∶25）。如图7-19（B），RG 502制剂中IND的k_S高于RG 752 S制剂中IND的k_S。RG 502制剂中IND的k_D与RG 752 S制剂中IND的k_D相近，这是因为RG 502的黏度几乎等于RG 752 S。RG 502制剂中的IND高溶解速率是由IND的高k_S导致的，这与RG 502制剂中IND的运输、水对RG 502的渗透以及IND与RG 502的水化作用有关。接下来，选择RESOMER® RG 752 S（M_w为13000 g·mol^{-1}）、RG 756 S（M_w为103000 g·mol^{-1}）和RG 750 S（M_w为128000 g·mol^{-1}）作为赋形剂，评估分子量对赋形剂的影响，因为它们满足不同分子量和相同组成的条件（DLLA与GA的摩尔比为75∶25）。一般来说，IND的溶解速率会随着PLGA分子量的增加而提高[图7-20（A）]。如图7-20（B）所示，这些PLGA制剂的IND溶出是由表面反应控制的。随着分子量的增加，PLGA制剂中IND的k_D减小。然而，由于表面反应

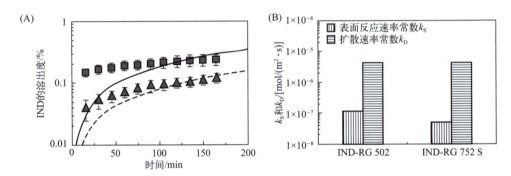

图7-19 在缓冲溶液（pH 6.5）中，IND从RESOMER®RG 502制剂（方形）和RG 752 S（三角形）制剂中溶解的溶解动力学曲线（A），以及IND从RG 502制剂（虚线）和RG 752 S制剂（实线）中溶解的速率常数k_S和k_D（B）[146]

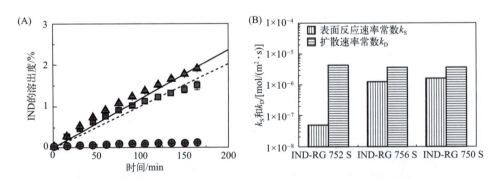

图7-20 在缓冲溶液（pH 6.5）中，IND从RESOMER®RG 752 S制剂（圆形）、RG 756 S制剂（方形）和RG 750 S制剂（三角形）中溶解的溶解动力学曲线（A），以及IND从RG 752 S制剂（点线）、RG 756 S制剂（虚线）和RG 750 S制剂（实线）中溶解的速率常数k_S和k_D[146]

速率的提高，IND的溶解速率仍然随着PLGA分子量的增加而提高。当IND在PLGA制剂中的溶解度较大时，其在水介质中的溶解速率较慢。从文中的水吸收实验（T=298.15 K，RH=75%）可以看出，随着分子量的增加，PLGA吸附的水越多（RG 750 S > RG 756 S > RG 752 S）[146]。此外，IND/PLGA制剂的玻璃化转变温度（T_g）随着PLGA分子量的增加而升高，而溶解温度低于RG 756 S和RG 750 S制剂的T_g。所有结果都表明，PLGA分子量的增加，增强了表面反应步骤，从而提高了IND的溶解速率。

7.4.2.7 API/PLGA制剂的API溶解动力学的关联及预测

将化学势梯度模型与PC-SAFT相结合，是关联和预测API/聚合物制剂溶解动力学的重要方法。显然，这种方法可以节省时间和成本。例如，根据预测的k_S和k_D，关联并预测了PLGA制剂中IND和HCT的溶解动力学[146]。结果与实测数据基本一致[图7-20（A）]。预测结果表明，RG 750 S在pH 6.5下的IND溶解动力学与实验数据一致（ARD=13.59%）。此外，对PVP制剂、PVPVA 64制剂和PVAc制剂中IND和NAP的溶解动力学进行了模拟[145]。根据ARD得知，模型数据与实测数据基本一致。其中，ARD<9%说明其溶解动力学模型与API/PVPVA 64制剂十分吻合。此外，对PARA的溶解动力学也进行了模拟[147]。结果经ARD验证，与实测数据基本一致。然而，对于pH 4.97时的Eudragit®L 100-55和pH 4.92时的Eudragit®L 100，模型结果与实测数据之间的ARD存在很大偏差（表7-7）。高偏差可能是由低溶解速率和浓度导致的。总体而言，将化学势梯度模型与PC-SAFT相结合来计算和预测溶解动力学是一种非常有价值的方法。

表7-7　PARA/Eudragit®制剂中的PARA溶解动力学拟合参数k_t[147]

体系	pH	k_t	ARD
PARA/Eudragit®L 100-55	4.9	1.08×10^{-6}	22.77%
	6.53	8.17×10^{-6}	11.09%
	7.25	1.23×10^{-5}	12.16%
PARA/Eudragit®L 100	4.92	4.89×10^{-6}	25.21%
	6.51	6.76×10^{-6}	21.33%
	7.27	1.43×10^{-5}	13.12%
PARA/Eudragit®S 100	4.92	5.34×10^{-6}	17.97%
	6.48	4.06×10^{-6}	21.08%
	7.27	8.40×10^{-6}	19.41%
PARA/Eudragit®EPO	4.89	1.81×10^{-5}	11.32%
	6.51	5.69×10^{-6}	15.20%
	7.26	4.17×10^{-7}	20.76%

7.5 总结

化学势梯度模型结合 PC-SAFT 在 API 溶解机制和溶解动力学预测方面具有良好的应用前景，有望为获取 API 和制剂的长时间溶解动力学节省实验时间和资源。溶解速率常数（k_S 和 k_D）本质上与 API、聚合物和溶剂之间的复杂相互作用有关。建立 API 释放速率与分子间相互作用参数之间的定量关系，有助于实现制剂的高通量筛选。随着现代计算机技术的发展，对难溶性药物溶解机制分析和模型预测的研究与人工智能深度融合可望在该领域取得更大的研究进展。结合现代数据处理和分析技术，研究人员将更深入、更全面地研究难溶性 API 的溶解行为和溶解机制，并有望实现药物在体外和体内溶解动力学相关性的定量构筑和定量预测。

参考文献

[1] Blagden N, De Matas M, Gavan P T, et al. Crystal engineering of active pharmaceutical ingredients to improve solubility and dissolution rates[J]. Adv Drug Deliv Rev, 2007, 59: 617-630.

[2] Garcia E, Veesler S, Boistelle R, et al. Crystallization and dissolution of pharmaceutical compounds: an experimental approach[J]. J Cryst Growth, 1999, 198: 1360-1364.

[3] Lawrence X Y. Pharmaceutical quality by design: product and process development, understanding, and control[J]. Pharm Res, 2008, 25: 781-791.

[4] Shefter E, Higuchi T. Dissolution behavior of crystalline solvated and non-solvated forms of some pharmaceuticals[J]. J Pharm Sci, 1963, 52: 781-791.

[5] Lipinski C A. Drug-like properties and the causes of poor solubility and poor permeability[J]. J Pharmacol Toxicol Methods, 2000, 44: 235-249.

[6] Lipinski C A, Lombardo F, Dominy B W, et al. Experimental and computational approaches to estimate solubility and permeability in drug discovery and development settings[J]. Adv Drug Deliv Rev, 2012, 64: 4-17.

[7] Ku M S, Dulin W. A biopharmaceutical classification-based right-first-time formulation approach to reduce human pharmacokinetic variability and project cycle time from first-in-human to clinical proof-of-concept[J]. Pharm Dev Technol, 2012, 17: 285-302.

[8] Newman A, Knipp G, Zografi G. Assessing the performance of amorphous solid dispersions[J]. J Pharm Sci, 2012, 101(4): 1355-1377.

[9] Sun D D, Ju T C, Lee P I. Enhanced kinetic solubility profiles of indomethacin amorphous solid dispersions in poly(2-hydroxyethyl methacrylate)hydrogels[J]. Eur J Pharm Biopharm, 2012, 81(1): 149-158.

[10] Hancock B C, Parks M. What is the true solubility advantage for amorphous pharmaceuticals?[J]. Pharm Res, 2000, 17(4): 397-404.

[11] de Almeida L P, Simões S, Brito P, et al. Modeling dissolution of sparingly soluble multisized powders[J]. J Pharm Sci, 1997, 86: 726-732.

[12] Lu X H, Ji Y H, Liu H L. Non-equilibrium thermodynamics analysis and its application in interfacial mass transfer[J]. Sci China: Chem, 2011, 54: 1659-1666.

[13] de Almeida L P, Simões S, Brito P, et al. Modeling dissolution of sparingly soluble multisized powders[J]. J Pharm Sci, 1997, 86: 726-732.

[14] Costa P, Lobo J M S. Modeling and comparison of dissolution profiles[J]. Eur J Pharm Sci, 2001, 13: 123-133.

[15] Gibaldi M, Feldman S. Establishment of sink conditions in dissolution rate determinations theoretical considerations and application to nondisintegrating dosage Forms[J]. J Pharm Sci, 1967, 56: 1238-1242.

[16] Higuchi T. Rate of release of medicaments from ointment bases containing drugs in suspension[J]. J Pharm Sci, 1961, 50: 874-875.

[17] Higuchi T. Mechanism of sustained-action medication theoretical analysis of rate of release of solid drugs dispersed in solid matrices[J]. J Pharm Sci, 1963, 52: 1145-1149.

[18] Korsmeyer RW, Gurny R, Doelker E, et al. Mechanisms of solute release from porous hydrophilic polymers[J]. Int J Pharm, 1983, 15: 25-35.

[19] Hopfenberg H B. Controlled release from erodible slabs, cylinders, and spheres[J]. ACS Symp Ser, 1976, 33: 26-32.

[20] DeAlmeida L P, Simoes S, Brito P, et al. Modeling dissolution of sparingly soluble multisized powders[J]. J Pharm Sci, 1997, 86: 726-732.

[21] Lu X H, Ji Y H, Liu H L. Non-equilibrium thermodynamics analysis and its application in interfacial mass transfer[J]. Sci China Chem, 2011, 54: 1659-1666.

[22] Dash S, Murthy P N, Nath L, et al. Kinetic modeling on drug release from controlled drug delivery systems[J]. Acta Pol Pharm, 2010, 67: 217-223.

[23] Gibson M. Pharmaceutical preformulation and formulation: a practical guide from candidate drug selection to commercial dosage form[M]. Informa Healthcare USA, Inc, New York, USA, 2009.

[24] Lewis G A, Mathieu D, Phan-Tan-Luu R. Pharmaceutical experimental design[M]. CRC Press, Marcel Dekker, Inc, New York, Basel, 1998.

[25] Stella V J, Nti-Addae K W. Prodrug strategies to overcome poor water solubility[J]. Adv Drug Deliv Rev, 2007, 59: 677-694.

[26] Vasconcelos T, Sarmento B, Costa P. Solid dispersions as strategy to improve oral bioavailability of poor water soluble drugs[J]. Drug Discov Today, 2007, 12(23-24): 1068-1075.

[27] Sivert A, Bérard V, Andrès C. New binary solid dispersion of indomethacin with surfactant polymer: from physical characterization to in vitro dissolution enhancement[J]. J Pharm Sci, 2010, 99(3): 1399-1413.

[28] Caron V, Bhugra C, Pikal M J. Prediction of onset of crystallization in amorphous pharmaceutical systems: phenobarbital, nifedipine/PVP, and phenobarbital/PVP[J]. J Pharm Sci, 2010, 99: 3887-3900.

[29] Joshi H N, Tejwani R W, Davidovich M, et al. Bioavailability enhancement of a poorly water-soluble drug by solid dispersion in polyethylene glycol-polysorbate 80 mixture[J]. Int J Pharm, 2004, 269: 251-258.

[30] Kochling J D, Miao H, Young C R, et al. Understanding the degradation pathway of a poorly water-soluble drug formulated in PEG-400[J]. J Pharm Biomed Anal, 2007, 43: 1638-1646.

[31] Lakshman J P, Cao Y, Kowalski J, et al. Application of meltextrusion in the development of a physically and chemically stable high-energy amorphous solid dispersion of a poorly water-soluble drug[J]. Mol Pharm, 2008, 5: 994-1002.

[32] Papadimitriou S A, Barmpalexis P, Karavas E, et al. Optimizing the ability of PVP/PEG mixtures to be used as appropriate carriers for the preparation of drug solid dispersions by melt mixing technique using artificial neural networks: I[J]. Eur J Pharm Biopharm, 2012, 82: 175-186.

[33] Windbergs M, Strachan C J, Kleinebudde P. Tailor-made dissolution profiles by extruded matrices based on lipid polyethylene glycol mixtures[J]. J Control Release, 2009, 137: 211-216.

[34] Liao X, Krishnamurthy R, Suryanarayanan R. Influence of the active pharmaceutical ingredient concentration on the physical state of mannitol-implications in freeze-drying[J]. Pharm Res, 2005, 22: 1978-1985.

[35] Kakran M, Sahoo N G, Li L. Dissolution enhancement of quercetin through nanofabrication, complexation, and solid dispersion[J]. Colloids Surf B, 2011, 88: 121-130.

[36] Amidon G L, Lennernäs H, Shah V P, et al. A theoretical basis for a biopharmaceutic drug classification: the correlation of in vitro drug product dissolution and in vivo bioavailability[J]. Pharm Res, 1995, 12: 413-420.

[37] Dressman J B, Amidon G L, Reppas C, et al. Dissolution testing as a prognostic tool for oral drug absorption: immediate release dosage forms[J]. Pharm Res, 1998, 15: 11-22.

[38] Ei-Arini S K, Leuenberger H. Modelling of drug release from polymer matrices: effect of drug loading[J]. Int J Pharm, 1995, 121: 141-148.

[39] Kostewicz E S, Wunderlich M, Brauns U, et al. Predicting the precipitation of poorly soluble weak bases upon entry in the small intestine[J]. J Pharm Pharmacol, 2004, 56: 43-51.

[40] Rao K R, Devi K P, Buri P. Influence of molecular size and water solubility of the solute on its release from swelling and erosion controlled polymeric matrices[J]. J Control Release, 1990, 12: 133-141.

[41] Snyder R C, Doherty M F. Faceted crystal shape evolution during dissolution or growth[J]. AIChE J, 2007, 53: 1337-1348.

[42] Tsinman K, Avdeef A, Tsinman O, et al. Powder dissolution method for estimating rotating disk intrinsic dissolution rates of low solubility drugs[J]. Pharm Res, 2009, 26: 2093-2100.

[43] de Almeida L P, Simões S, Brito P, et al. Modeling dissolution of sparingly soluble multisized powders[J]. J Pharm Sci,

1997, 86(6): 726-32.

[44] Craig D Q M. The mechanisms of drug release from solid dispersions in water-soluble polymers[J]. Int J Pharm, 2002, 231(2): 131-144.

[45] Langham Z A, Booth J, Hughes L P, et al. Mechanistic insights into the dissolution of spray-dried amorphous solid dispersions[J]. J Pharm Sci, 2012, 101(8): 2798-2810.

[46] Alonzo D E, Zhang G G, Zhou D, et al. Understanding the behavior of amorphous pharmaceutical systems during dissolution[J]. Pharm Res, 2010, 27(4): 608-618.

[47] Shi Q, Moinuddin S M, Wang Y, et al. Physical stability and dissolution behaviors of amorphous pharmaceutical solids: Role of surface and interface effects[J]. Int J Pharm, 2022, 625: 122098.

[48] Langham Z A, Booth J, Hughes L P, et al. Mechanistic insights into the dissolution of spray-dried amorphous solid dispersions[J]. J Pharm Sci, 2012, 101(8): 2798-2810.

[49] Costa P, Manuel J, Lobo S. Modeling and comparison of dissolution profiles[J]. Eur J Pharm Sci, 2001, 13: 123-133.

[50] DeAlmeida L P, Simoes S, Brito P, et al. Modeling dissolution of sparingly soluble multisized powders[J]. J Pharm Sci, 1997, 86: 726-732.

[51] Gibaldi M, Feldman S. Establishment of sink conditions in dissolution rate determinations-theoretical considerations and application to nondisintegrating dosage forms[J]. J Pharm Sci, 1967, 56: 1238-1242.

[52] Higuchi T. Rate of release of medicaments from ointment bases containing drugs in suspension[J]. J Pharm Sci, 1961, 50: 874-875.

[53] Higuchi T. Mechanism of sustained-action medication-theoretical analysis of rate of release of solid drugs dispersed in solid matrices[J]. J Pharm Sci, 1963, 52: 1145-1149.

[54] Higuchi W, Parrott E L, Wurster D E, et al. Investigation of drug release from solids II Theoretical and experimental study of influences of bases and buffers on rates of dissolution of acidic solids[J]. J Am Pharm Assoc, 1958, 47: 376-383.

[55] Hopfenberg H B. Controlled release from erodible slabs, cylinders, and spheres[M]. In: Controlled Release Polymeric Formulations；Paul D, et al. ACS Symposium Series；American Chemical Society: Washington, DC, 1976, 62.

[56] Korsmeyer R W, Gurny R, Doelker E, et al. Mechanisms of solute release from porous hydrophilic polymers[J]. Int J Pharm, 1983, 15: 25-35.

[57] Mooney K, Mintun M, Himmelstein K, et al. Dissolution kinetics of carboxylic acids I: effect of pH under unbuffered conditions[J]. J Pharm Sci, 1981, 70: 13-22.

[58] Mooney K, Mintun M, Himmelstein K, et al. Dissolution kinetics of carboxylic acids II: effect of buffers[J]. J Pharm Sci, 1981, 70: 22-32.

[59] Mura P, Faucci M T, Manderioli A, et al. Thermal behavior and dissolution properties of naproxen from binary and ternary solid dispersions[J]. Drug Dev Ind Pharm, 1999, 25(3): 257-264.

[60] Kogermann K, Penkina A, Predbannikova K, et al. Dissolution testing of amorphous solid dispersions[J]. Int J Pharm, 2013, 444(1-2): 40-46.

[61] Alonzo D E, Gao Y, Zhou D, et al. Dissolution and precipitation behavior of amorphous solid dispersions[J]. J Pharm Sci, 2011, 100(8): 3316-3331.

[62] Arthur A N, Willis R W. The rate of solution of solid substances in their own solutions[J]. J Am Chem Soc, 1897, 19(12): 930-934.

[63] Lu A T, Frisella M E, Johnson K C. Dissolution modeling: factors affecting the dissolution rates of polydisperse powders[J]. Pharm Res, 1993, 10(9): 1308-1314.

[64] Vudathala G K, Rogers J A. Dissolution of fludrocortisone from phospholipid coprecipitates[J]. J Pharm Sci, 1992, 81(3): 282-286.

[65] Higuchi T. Rate of release of medicaments from ointment bases containing drugs in suspension[J]. J Pharm Sci, 1961, 50(10): 874-875.

[66] Higuchi T. Mechanism of sustained-action medication Theoretical analysis of rate of release of solid drugs dispersed in solid matrices[J]. J Pharm Sci, 1963, 52(12): 1145-1149.

[67] Hixson A W, Crowell J H. Dependence of reaction velocity upon surface and agitation[J]. Ind Eng Chem, 1931, 23(8): 923-931.

[68] de Almeida L P, Simöes S, Brito P, et al. Modeling dissolution of sparingly soluble multisized powders[J]. J Pharm Sci, 1997, 86(6): 726-732.

[69] Baker R W, Lonsdale H K. Controlled release: mechanisms and rates In: Tanquary A C, Lacey R E, editors Controlled release of biologically active agents. Advances in experimental medicine and biology[M]. New York: Plenum, 1974: 15-72.

[70] Korsmeyer R W, Gurny R, Doelker E, et al. Mechanisms of solute release from porous hydrophilic polymers[J]. Int J Pharm, 1983, 15(1): 25-35.

[71] Costa P, Sousa Lobo J M. Modeling and comparison of dissolution profiles[J]. Eur J Pharm Sci, 2001, 13(2): 123-133.

[72] Alonzo D E, Zhang G G, Zhou D, et al. Understanding the behavior of amorphous pharmaceutical systems during dissolution[J]. Pharm Res, 2010, 27(4): 608-618.

[73] Alonzo D E, Gao Y, Zhou D, et al. Dissolution and precipitation behavior of amorphous solid dispersions[J]. J Pharm Sci, 2011, 100(8): 3316-31.

[74] Craig D Q M. The mechanisms of drug release from solid dispersions in water-soluble polymers[J]. Int J Pharm, 2002, 231(2): 131-144.

[75] Siepmann J, Kranz H, Bodmeier R, et al. HPMC-matrices for controlled drug delivery: a new model combining diffusion, swelling, and dissolution mechanisms and predicting the release kinetics[J]. Pharm Res, 1999, 16(11): 1748-1756.

[76] Langham Z A, Booth J, Hughes L P, et al. Mechanistic insights into the dissolution of spray-dried amorphous solid dispersions[J]. J Pharm Sci, 2012, 101(8): 2798-2810.

[77] Giri T K, Kumar K, Alexander A, et al. A novel and alternative approach to controlled dissolution drug delivery system based on solid dispersion technique[M]. Bulletin of Faculty of Pharmacy, Cairo University, 2012, 50.

[78] Tran P H, Tran T T, Park J B, et al. Controlled formulations containing solid dispersions: strategies and mechanisms[J]. Pharm Res, 2011, 28: 2353-2378.

[79] De Haan P, Lerk C F. Oral controlled dissolution dosage forms A review[J]. Pharm Weekbl Sci, 1984, 6: 57-67.

[80] van der Veen J, Eissens A C, Lerk C F. Controlled dissolution of paracetamol from amylodextrin tablets: in vitro and in vivo results[J]. Pharm Res, 1994, 11: 384-387.

[81] Aceves J M, Cruz R, Hernandez E. Preparation and characterization of furosemide-Eudragit controlled formulations[J]. Int J Pharm, 2000, 195: 45-53.

[82] Higashi K, Hayashi H, Yamamoto K, et al. The effect of drug and EUDRAGIT®S 100 miscibility in solid dispersions on the drug and polymer dissolution rate[J]. Int J Pharm, 2015, 494: 9-16.

[83] Mehta K A, Kislalioglu M S, Phuapradit W, et al. Dissolution performance of a poorly soluble drug from a novel, Eudragit®-based multi-unit erosion matrix[J]. Int J Pharm, 2001, 213: 7-12.

[84] Wu P C, Huang Y B, Chang J S, et al. Design and evaluation of sustained dissolution microspheres of potassium chloride prepared by Eudragit[J]. Eur J Pharm Sci, 2003, 19: 115-122.

[85] Barea M J, Jenkins M J, Lee Y S, et al. Encapsulation of liposomes within pH responsive microspheres for oral colonic drug delivery[J]. Int J Biomater, 2012, 458712.

[86] Hua S. Orally administered liposomal formulations for colon targeted drug delivery[J]. Front Pharmacol, 2014, 5: 1-8.

[87] Freiberg S, Zhu X X. Polymer microspheres for controlled drug dissolution[J]. Int J Pharm, 2004, 282: 1-18.

[88] Park J H, Allen M G, Prausnitz M R. Polymer microneedles for controlled-dissolution drug delivery[J]. Pharm Res, 2006, 23: 1008-1019.

[89] Siepmann F, Siepmann J, Walther M, et al. Polymer blends for controlled dissolution coatings[J]. J Control Dissolution, 2008, 125: 1-15.

[90] Corrigan O I, Li X. Quantifying drug release from PLGA nanoparticulates[J]. Eur J Pharm Sci, 2009, 37: 477-485.

[91] Zhang Y, Schwendeman S P. Minimizing acylation of peptides in PLGA microspheres[J]. J Control Release, 2012, 162: 119-126.

[92] Gasmi H, Danede F, Siepmann J, et al. Does PLGA microparticle swelling control drug release? New insight based on single particle swelling studies[J]. J Control Release, 2015, 213: 120-127.

[93] Feng S B, Nie L, Zou P, et al. Effects of drug and polymer molecular weight on drug release from PLGA-mPEG microspheres[J]. J Appl Polym Sci, 2015, 132: 41431-41438.

[94] Martın-Sabroso C, Fraquas-Sanchez A I, Aparicio-Blanco J, et al. Critical attributes of formulation and of elaboration process of PLGA-protein microparticles[J]. Int J Pharm, 2015, 480: 27-36.

[95] Sanna V, Roqqio A M, Pala N, et al. Effect of chitosan concentration on PLGA microcapsules for controlled release and stability of resveratrol[J]. Int J Biol Macromol, 2015, 72: 531-536.

[96] Vudathala G K, Rogers J A. Dissolution of fludrocortisone from phospholipid coprecipitates[J]. J Pharm Sci, 1992, 81: 282-286.

[97] Higuchi T. Rate of dissolution of medicaments from ointment bases containing drugs in suspension[J]. J Pharm Sci, 1961, 50: 874-875.

[98] Higuchi T. Mechanism of sustained-action medication: theoretical analysis of rate of dissolution of solid drugs dispersed in

[99] de Almeida L P, Simões S, Brito P, et al. Modeling dissolution of sparingly soluble multisized powders[J]. J Pharm Sci, 1997, 86: 726-732.

[100] Hixson A W, Crowell J H. Dependence of reaction velocity upon surface and agitation[J]. Ind Eng Chem, 1931, 23: 923-931.

[101] Korsmeyer R W, Gurny R, Doelker E, et al. Mechanisms of solute release from porous hydrophilic polymers[J]. Int J Pharm, 1983, 15: 25-35.

[102] Higuchi T. Mechanism of sustained-action medication. Theoretical analysis of rate of release of solid drugs dispersed in solid matrices[J]. J Pharm Sci, 1963, 52: 1145-1149.

[103] Siepmann J, Peppas N. Hydrophilic matrices for controlled drug delivery: an improved mathematical model to predict the resulting drug release kinetics(the "sequential layer" model)[J]. Pharm Res, 2000, 17: 1290-1298.

[104] Hopfenberg H. Controlled release from erodible slabs, cylinders, and spheres[J]. Controlled Release Polym Formul, 1976, 33: 26-32.

[105] Siepmann J, Göpferich A. Mathematical modeling of bioerodible, polymeric drug delivery systems[J]. Adv Drug Delivery Rev, 2001, 48: 229-247.

[106] Arifin D Y, Lee L Y, Wang, C H. Mathematical modeling and simulation of drug release from microspheres: implications to drug delivery systems[J]. Adv Drug Delivery Rev, 2006, 58: 1274-1325.

[107] Lin C C, Metters A T. Hydrogels in controlled release formulations: network design and mathematical modeling[J]. Adv Drug Delivery Rev, 2006, 58: 1379-1408.

[108] De Almeida L P, Simões S, Brito P, et al. Modeling dissolution of sparingly soluble multisized powders[J]. J Pharm Sci, 1997, 86: 726-732.

[109] Higuchi W, Parrott E L, Wurster D E, et al. Investigation of drug release from solids II Theoretical and experimental study of influences of bases and buffers on rates of dissolution of acidic solids[J]. J Am Pharm Assoc, 1958, 47: 376-383.

[110] Parrott E L, Wurster D E, Higuchi T. Investigation of drug release from solids I Some factors influencing the dissolution rate[J]. J Am Pharm Assoc, 1955, 44: 269-273.

[111] Mooney K, Mintun M, Himmelstein K, et al. Dissolution kinetics of carboxylic acids I: effect of pH under unbuffered conditions[J]. J Pharm Sci, 1981, 70: 13-22.

[112] Mooney K, Mintun M, Himmelstein K, et al. Dissolution kinetics of carboxylic acids II: effect of buffers[J]. J Pharm Sci, 1981, 70: 22-32.

[113] Baker R W, Lonsdale H K. Controlled dissolution: mechanisms and rates In controlled dissolution of biologically active agents[M]. Springer, 1974: 15-71.

[114] Korsmeyer R W, Gurny R, Doelker E, et al. Mechanisms of solute dissolution from porous hydrophilic polymers[J]. Int J Pharm, 1983, 15: 25-35.

[115] Siepmann J, Siepmann F, Mathematical modeling of drug delivery[J]. Int J Pharm, 2008, 364: 328-343.

[116] Korsmeyer R W, Gurny R, Doelker E, et al. Mechanisms of solute release from porous hydrophilic polymers[J]. Int J Pharm, 1983, 15(1): 25-35.

[117] Siepmann J, Siepmann F. Mathematical modeling of drug delivery[J]. Int J Pharm, 2008, 364(2): 328-343.

[118] Hixson A W, Crowell J H. Dependence of reaction velocity upon surface and agitation I: theoretical consideration[J]. Ind Eng Chem, 1931, 23: 923-931.

[119] Higuchi T. Mechanism of sustained-action medication: theoretical analysis of rate of release of solid drugs dispersed in solid matrices[J]. J Pharm Sci, 1963, 52(12): 1145-1149.

[120] Siepmann J, Göpferich A. Mathematical modeling of bioerodible, polymeric drug delivery systems[J]. Adv Drug Delivery Rev, 2001, 48: 229-247.

[121] Siepmann F, Eckart K, Maschke A, et al. Modeling drug release from PVAc/PVP matrix tablets[J]. J Control Release, 2010, 141(2): 216-222.

[122] Zhang Z H, Dong H Y, Peng B, et al. Design of an expert system for the development and formulation of push-pull osmotic pump tablets containing poorly water-soluble drugs. Int. J. Pharm., 2011, 410, 41-47.

[123] Ji Y H, Lemberg M, Prudic A, et al. Modeling and analysis of dissolution of paracetamol/Eudragit® formulations[J]. Chem Eng Res Des, 2017, 121: 22-31.

[124] Ji Y H, Lesniak A K, Prudic A, et al. Drug release kinetics and mechanism from PLGA formulations[J]. AIChE J, 2016, 62(11): 4055-4065.

[125] Prudic A, Lesniak A K, Ji Y H, et al. Thermodynamic phase behaviour of indomethacin/PLGA formulations[J]. Eur J Pharm Biopharm, 2015, 93: 88-94.

[126] Prudic A, Ji Y H, Luebbert C, et al. Influence of humidity on the phase behavior of API/polymer formulations[J]. Eur J Pharm Biopharm, 2015, 94: 352-362.

[127] Prudic A, Kleetz T, Korf M, et al. Influence of copolymer composition on the phase behavior of solid dispersions[J]. Mol Pharm, 2014, 11(11): 4189-4198.

[128] Prudic A, Ji Y H, Sadowski G. Thermodynamic phase behavior of API/-polymer solid dispersions[J]. Mol Pharm, 2014, 11(7): 2294-2304.

[129] Reschke T, Naeem S, Sadowski G. Osmotic coefficients of aqueous weak electrolyte solutions: influence of dissociation on data reduction and modeling[J]. J Phys Chem B, 2012, 116(25): 7479-7491.

[130] Prausnitz J M, Lichtenthaler R N, de Azevedo E G. Molecular thermodynamics of fluid-phase equilibria[M] Pearson Education. Prentice-Hall, Inc. Upper Saddle River, New Jersey, 1998.

[131] Ruether F, Sadowski G. Modeling the solubility of pharmaceuticals in pure solvents and solvent mixtures for drug process design[J]. J Pharm Sci, 2009, 98(11): 4205-4215.

[132] Prausnitz J M, Lichtenthaler R N, de Azevedo E G. Molecular thermodynamics of fluid-phase equilibria[M]. Upper Saddle River: Prentice Hall PTR, 1999.

[133] Gross J, Sadowski G. Perturbed-chain SAFT: an equation of state based on a perturbation theory for chain molecules[J]. Ind Eng Chem Res, 2001, 40(4): 1244-1260.

[134] Prudic A, Ji Y H, Sadowski G. Thermodynamic phase behavior of API/polymer solid dispersions[J]. Mol Pharm, 2014, 11(7): 2294-2304.

[135] Lu X H, Ji Y H, Liu H L. Non-equilibrium thermodynamics analysis and its application in interfacial mass transfer[J]. Sci China Chem, 2011, 54(10): 1659-1666.

[136] Dokoumetzidis A, Papadopoulou V, Valsami G, et al. Development of a reaction-limited model of dissolution: application to official dissolution tests experiments[J]. Int J Pharm, 2008, 355: 114-125.

[137] Raphael P, Yuanhui J. Modeling and predicting the influence of variable factors on dissolution of crystalline pharmaceuticals[J]. Chem Eng Sci, 2016, 145: 10-20.

[138] Dejmek M, Ward C A. A statistical rate theory study of interface concentration during crystal growth or dissolution[J]. J Chem Phys, 1998, 108: 8698-8704.

[139] Ward C A, Findlay R D, Rizk M. Statistical rate theory of interfacial transport 0.1. theoretical development[J]. J Chem Phys, 1982, 76: 5599-5605.

[140] Cochrane W G. The flow due to a rotating disc[J]. Proc Cambridge Philos. Soc, 1934, 30: 365-375.

[141] Von Karman T. Über laminare und turbulente reibung[J]. Z Angew Math Mech, 1921, 1: 233-252.

[142] Wolbach J P, Sandler S I. Using molecular orbital calculations to describe the phase behavior of cross-associating mixtures[J]. Ind Eng Chem Res, 1998, 37: 2917-2928.

[143] Ruether F, Sadowski G. Modeling the solubility of pharmaceuticals in pure solvents and solvent mixtures for drug process design[J]. J Pharm Sci, 2009, 98: 4205-4215.

[144] Raphael P, Yuanhui J, Florian B, et al. Dissolution of crystalline pharmaceuticals: experimental investigation and thermodynamic modeling[J]. Ind Eng Chem Res, 2015, 54: 731-742.

[145] Yuanhui J, Dule H, Christian L, et al. Insights into influence mechanism of polymeric excipients on dissolution of drug formulations: A molecular interaction-based theoretical model analysis and prediction[J]. AIChE J, 2021, 67: e17372.

[146] Yuanhui J, Anna Katharina L, Anke P, et al. Drug release kinetics and mechanism from PLGA formulations[J]. AIChE J, 2016, 62: 4055-4065.

[147] Yuanhui J, Max L, Anke P, et al. Modeling and analysis of dissolution of paracetamol/Eudragit® formulations[J]. Chem Eng Res Des, 2017, 121: 22-31.

第8章

PBPK建模在制剂开发中的应用

刘 波 武汉工程大学,中国
李 学 英翰医药科技(上海)有限公司,中国

8.1 引言

新药的开发过程包括临床前、Ⅰ期、Ⅱ期、Ⅲ期和上市后评价。Ⅰ期和Ⅱa期被认为是早期临床研究,它们侧重于临床药理学的研究。这是临床研究初始的和关键的阶段。Ⅱb期和Ⅲ期侧重于对治疗效果的确认。在实际操作中,虚拟药物开发始终领先于实际药物的开发,如图8-1所示。

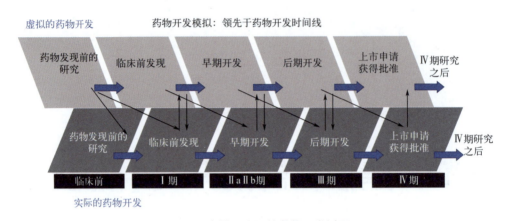

图8-1 虚拟和实际的药物开发过程

虚拟药物开发包括所有的基于计算机的建模和模拟,例如群体药代动力学(popPK)模型和基于生理的药代动力学(PBPK)模型。模拟可用于药物发现之前的研究,模拟结果可以用于指导实际药物开发。当实际开发结果与虚拟模拟一致时,开发可以进入临床发现阶段;不一致时,将使用观测数据优化模型。在临床前发现阶段,该模型还可用于指导实际的临床前研究。如果实际临床前研究和模拟结果一致,则可以进入开发过程的下一阶段。如果没有,观测数据将用于优化模型。随后的过程是对这个循环进行的重复。这是一项在整个制药行业推广的工作,模型开发的过程是一个不断完善的过程,而且过程不是固定的。一些制药公司,如Pfizer、JSK和Big Pharma,连续模拟研究前的发现工作、临床前工作和早期开发,然后进入实际工作并对模型进行验证。实际的药物开发通过虚拟世界中利用经验构建起来的模型加速临床研究,并获得可预测和可靠的结果。

8.2 用于建模的药代动力学软件

8.2.1 定量构效/构性关系(QSAR/QSPR)建模

基于计算机的模拟技术已经广泛应用于药物开发的每一个步骤。从药物发现开始,基于配体的定量构效/构性关系(QSAR/QSPR)建模被用来预测药物生物活性和药代动力学参数，如吸收、分布、代谢、排泄和毒性（ADME）。该模型使用人工智能（AI）技术将官能团等结构特征转换为机器可读的数字，以发现化学结构与其生物活动之间的定性关系。它的原理是结构相似的化学物质可能具有相似的物理化学和生物学特性。如今，QSAR/QSPR方法已经从线性回归等经典模型过渡到现代机器学习技术，旨在解释化学结果与其物理化学/生物学特性之间更复杂的和潜在的非线性关系。应用QSAR模型最方便、最一致的方法是在软件中实现该模型。

已有很多软件工具可用于预测药物的物理化学特性、毒理学终点和生物效应。例如，评估程序接口（EPI）Suit™软件包可估算一系列物理化学特性、环境参数和生态毒性，它是由美国环境保护署（US EPA）与锡拉丘兹研发公司（SRC）合作开发，可从美国环境保护署网站免费下载，并已被政府和行业组织广泛用于对新的和现有的工业化学品的评估。OncoLogic™是一个可下载的软件工具，由美国EPA与美国国家癌症研究所（NCI）合作开发。它通过应用构效关系（SAR）分析规则，结合相关作用机制和人类流行病学研究，预测化学品的致癌潜力。这个系统由四个子系统组成，分别评估纤维、金属、聚合物和具有不同化学结构的有机化学物质。Toxtree将化学物质分类，并通过应用决策树方法预测各种毒性作用。该系统包含一种系统毒理分类方案，这是一种广泛应用于构建化学物质以估算毒理学相关阈值（TTC）的方法。新版本（v2.1.0，2010年6月）还应用了SMARTCyp，这是一种预测细胞色素P450介导代谢的二维方法[1]，用于研究药物相互作用时的有用信息。经济合作与发展组织（OECD）的定量构效关系（QSAR）应用工具箱是一个可下载的研究工具，用于解释（生态）毒性数据以评估化学品的危害性。工具箱通过遵循灵活的工作流程来填充数据，通过应用本地的QSAR来预测缺失的数据。工具箱包含一个广泛的数据库，其中包含实验研究结果，以支持趋势分析。它还包括一系列分析仪，用于快速评估常见化学品的机理或者作用方式。局部惰性构效关系（Lazar）也是欧盟OpenTox项目中正在开发的Web可访问的和开源的工具。它用人工智能机器学习的方法预测毒理学终点，如致突变性、人类肝脏毒性、啮齿动物和仓鼠的致癌性以及每日最大推荐剂量。Lazar处理的不是化学相似性的绝对值，而是研究与所研究的毒性终点相关的那些片段。根据符合规定的化学物质（CAESAR）进行计算机辅助评估是另一个与预测毒理学相关的项目。该预测侧重于五个终点，包括致突变性（Ames）、致癌性、发育毒性、皮肤致敏性和生物富集因子。物质活性谱预测（PASS）由俄罗斯莫斯科医学科学院生物医学化学研究所开发。它可预测毒性，如致突变性、致癌性、致畸性和胚胎毒性，以及作用机制和药理作用。该系统通过估计新物质与具有已知生物活性的物质的相似性/不同性来预测新化合物生物活性的概率（P_a）。以上所有有关常用免费软件工具的信息都总结和更新自一篇名为"毒性预测软件工具评价"的评论文章[2]。该综述还总结了常用的商业软件工具，比如用于预测吸收、分布、代谢、排泄和毒性特性的建模软件ADMET Predictor（由Simulations Plus开发），以及用于预测毒性的各种其他的软件。

8.2.2 药物从头设计（*de novo*）和合成计划

'*de novo*'是一个拉丁短语，意思是"从头开始"。从头药物设计是指用计算方法从头开始设计新的药物分子，也就是说设计基于的不是已知药物的结构。根据可参考的信息，相应的方法可以是基于配体的、基于结构的，或者是基于两者的混合[3]。由于新型的神经网络的计算方法快速发展，基于配体的设计的数量急剧增加。在过去的几年中，已经开发的新模型有40多种[4]。分子设计完成后，还可以用AI辅助设计合成的过程。人工智能在有机化学合成中的复兴是计算能力提高、大数据的出现以及对深度学习和优化的新算法的开发的结果[3]。

当化学结构被确定后，可以使用化学信息学和生物信息学软件，如Chemaxon来预测药物的理化性质，例如$\log P$、溶解度、pK_a和极性表面积。这个免费下载的软件还可以计算分子中的特定原子作为氢键供体或者受体的可能性[5]。

8.2.3 使用分子动力学模拟进行药物制剂设计

分子动力学（MD）模拟是辅助药物处方设计的计算方法之一。在药学中，MD模拟已经逐渐成为帮助研究人员了解药物递送机制中的溶出度、控释和靶向递送的重要工具[6]。Gao和欧阳教授的课题组在2021年报告的研究中，收集了4495个自乳化给药系统（SEDDS）制剂的数据，并利用机器学习方法预测了伪三元相图。伪三元相图和三元相图类似，但是其中一个轴代表两个组分的混合物，有效地将四组分系统简化为一个类似三组分的系统。伪三元相图用于理解不同相，比如油、表面活性剂、共乳化剂和水稳定的组成区域，以帮助设计处方，预测可以形成稳定乳化剂的浓度区域。同一研究组在过去实验中研究了多种剂型，包括固体分散体的制备和溶解行为的预测[7-10]、药物与环糊精之间的相互作用[11]、脂质体[12]、药物-磷脂复合物[13]和自组装铂前药[14]。

8.2.4 基于生理的药代动力学模型的制剂开发设计

基于生理的药代动力学（PBPK）建模可用于优化药物的配制过程。在为口服固体制剂建立的通用的PBPK模型中，需要输入的相关参数包括药物的物理化学性质、ADME相关参数以及体外实验获得的口服固体制剂的溶出度。连续流动技术（图8-2）与美国药典设备4（USP 4）相结合用于测量口服固体的体外溶解度。制剂放置于圆锥形释放池中。缓冲液以恒定的流速穿过释放池，被释放的药物随着缓冲液进入检测装置进行浓度测定。

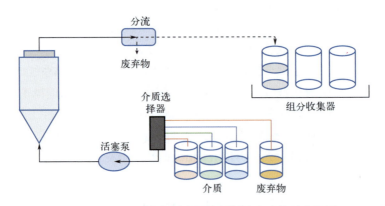

图8-2 连续流动技术测定固体制剂溶出度的基本原理

当所有药物的理化参数、ADME参数、溶出度数据以及人体物理特征参数和临床试验设计参数一起输入到一个成熟且经过验证的PBPK模型中时，该模型将能够预测体内药物在血浆中的浓度。同时，可以用风险评估来确定对药代动力学（PK）结果影响最大的关键参数。这样通过调整从临床前研究获得的关键参数，就可以获得所需的PK结果。

作为向制药行业提供药物开发建模和模拟软件支持的全球领导者，Simcyp模拟器已经成功地支持了各种药物开发和监管决策过程。所提供的信息主要集中在有关临床药物相互作用（DDI）和剂量调整的信息上。Simcyp模型有三个关键组成部分，分别是人体生理参数、药物数据和实验设计信息。对于人体参数这一部分，除了健康的志愿者之外，还可以选择孕妇、儿童等群体建立子模型进行研究。这些人群在生理参数上的变化可能会影响体内药物的暴露结果。对于每个人群，还考虑了CYP酶的活性，从而可以评估虚拟受试者的暴露及其与酶的活性关系。模拟器还可以模拟药物在身体不同器官中的浓度，辅助评估和毒性相关的问题。模拟器中还包含其他的复杂的机制化模型，例如皮肤、脑、肺和肿瘤模型。模拟结束后，结果被输出到Excel表格中，结果中总结了实验设计、化合物参数和模拟结果。结合个体间的变异性，模拟结果还显示每个虚拟受试者的模拟细节，以帮助了解药物的分布和风险。

GastroPlus是一个基于机制化的模型软件包，可模拟人体和动物中药物通过不同途径进入，包括静脉内、口腔、眼部、吸入、皮肤、皮下和肌肉内的吸收，以及药代动力和药效特征。GastroPlus使用不同的文件类型来管理其数据和模拟，如数据库和记录。该数据库包含所有用户的项目信息，可以在软件的"文件"菜单中访问。在数据库中，可以创建多个记录。打开软件时，默认加载数据库，可以在复合界面中调用。其他的界面包括肠道生理特性、药代动力学、模拟和图形。在肠道生理特性界面中，可以在人体或者动物中定义肠道生理学参数；在药代动力学界面中，可以定义模型的结构来描述API的分布和消除。

8.3 不同类型制剂的建模机制

不同类型的药物剂型，比如口服药物、鼻腔喷雾剂、外敷治疗和注射剂，每种剂型都是针对特定的给药途径而设计的，以确保药物在体内运输后发挥最佳效果。药代动力学使用数学模型来描述药物在体内的动力学过程。最初的模型是将身体部位分为几个隔室，大致描述了ADME的过程。当简单的隔室模型不足以为复杂机制提供详细信息时，基于生理的药代动力学模型被推导了出来。模型的建立基于人体生理学、生物化学和解剖学知识，将药物在不同器官中的分布体积和流速与生理参数联系起来。例如，图8-3所示是一个全身PBPK模型的结构，用来解释芬太尼和去甲芬太尼的消除过程[15]。连接一旦建立，就可以使用数学模型根据已知生理参数来预测药物的PK结果。

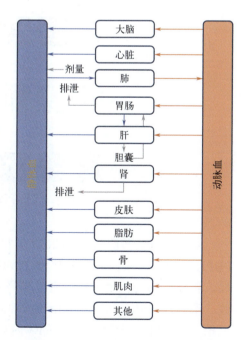

图8-3 全身PBPK模型的结构图

8.3.1 针对口服固体制剂的模型

当只研究口服药物时，可以将全身的PBPK模型简化，只专注于药物在肝脏中的吸收和代谢。这种情况下的模型可以称为mini-PBPK模型（图8-4），它只描述肝脏的相关信息。

为了了解不同药物在胃肠道（GI）中的性能，胃肠道被进一步细化。Agoram及其同事[16]开发了吸收、隔室分布和转运模型（ACAT）来描述口服固体制剂在胃肠道中的吸收。基于该ACAT模型，B^2O软件中固体制剂的PBPK模型结构如图8-5所示。在这个模型中，肠壁分为十二指肠、空肠、回肠和结肠等隔室。空肠进一步分为两部分，回肠进一步分为四部分。该模型中的药物被分开成固体状态和液体状态。模型同时还考虑了药物的溶解，这样就将药物体外溶出的实验数据和体内的药代动力学结果相关联起来。模型中还加入了溶液中药物通过肠壁的运动以及溶解物质通过每个隔室最终被吸收到血液中的运动。用户可以直接使用平台上的PBPK模型来预测药物在体内的药代动力学结果。

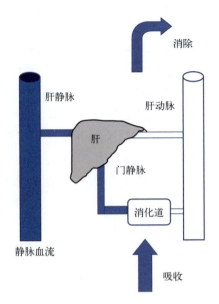

图8-4 包含肝脏相关信息的mini-PBPK模型

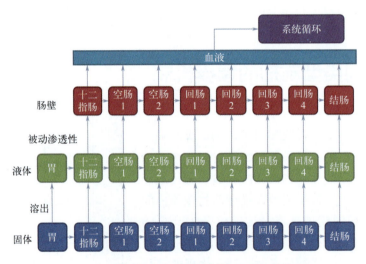

图8-5 B^2O软件中固体制剂的PBPK结构图

Kushwah及其团队[17]在2021年报告的研究中，使用GastroPlus中的ACAT模型开发了PBPK模型，用来评估食物对利伐沙班吸收的影响。输入参数分为三类：第一类是制剂特性，包括药物的粒度分布、密度和释放曲线；第二类是药物的物理化学性质，包括扩散系数、亲脂性、pK_a、溶解度和渗透性；第三类是药代动力学参数，包括清除率、分布体积和沉积。经过用口服溶液和片剂的体内数据验证以后，用该模型预测了高剂量强度片剂在体内的性能。片剂溶出度是使用美国药典（USP）流通池方法进行测量的[17]。

8.3.2 针对吸入制剂的模型

根据生理上的差异，药物在呼吸道中的沉积从上到下分为五个部分[18]。这个针对呼吸道的分割是 Gastroplus、B^2O 软件和其他软件中 PBPK 模型的基础。这五部分是鼻腔、口腔/咽部、包括气管和支气管在内的大气道、包括细支气管和终末支气管在内的小气道以及肺泡（图8-6）。

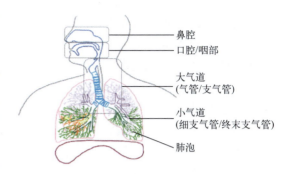

图8-6 呼吸系统被分为五个部分

通过这五个生理片段，可以将体外测量的沉积速率与体内沉积位置相关联。颗粒的沉积速率很大程度上取决于颗粒的空气动力学，颗粒大小≤5 μm 时在细支气管沉积的概率很高，颗粒大小≤2 μm 时更有可能沉积在肺泡区域[19]。具体的沉积比还要取决于制剂的类型和特征。例如，当使用 B^2O 模拟软件研究异丙托溴铵（IB）吸入气溶胶的 PK 特性时[20]，PBPK

在咽部，药物被吞咽并最终进入胃肠道，然后以类似于口服制剂的形式被吸收。对于口服气雾剂或者粉末喷雾剂，这部分药物的沉积会超过通过鼻子吸收的制剂的沉积，并且大部分药物血浆浓度是由药物通过口腔进入胃肠道系统引起的

模型将人体呼吸道分为四个部分：口咽、支气管（大气道）、细支气管（小气道）和肺泡区。作为口服吸入制剂，鼻段被省略了。在递送剂量下，由于惯性的冲击效应，那些>9.0 μm 的颗粒直接沉积在口咽中，然后通过吞咽进入胃肠道吸收系统中；大小介于5.8～9.0 μm 的颗粒沉积在支气管区域，大部分溶解在支气管上皮衬液（ELF）中，并且由于黏膜腺状清除（MCC），未溶解的药物颗粒从肺部排出到口咽部；大小在2.1～5.8 μm 的颗粒大部分溶解在细支气管 ELF 中，一小部分通过 MCC 排出到支气管和支气管 ELF 中；大小≤2.1 μm 的颗粒进入肺泡区域后溶解在肺泡液中，不受消除的影响。溶解在各个肺部区域的药物颗粒随后被吸收到循环系统中。图8-7是一个双室模型，用来描述药物在全身的沉积。

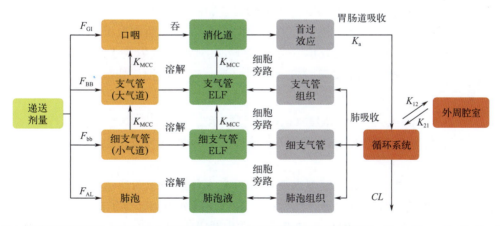

图8-7 描述异丙托溴铵（IB）吸入气溶胶的浓度-时间曲线的 PBPK 模型。F_{GI}、F_{BB}、F_{bb} 和 F_{AL} 分别是沉积在口咽、支气管、细支气管和肺泡中的药物的百分比；K_{MCC} 是黏液纤毛清除率常数；K_a 是吸收速率常数；K_{12} 和 K_{21} 是隔室模型中的一阶分布速率常数；CL 是系统清除率。该模型应用于在 B^2O 模拟软件中[20]

在最近发表的另外一项研究中，研究组用 GastroPlus 建立了一个 PBPK 模型，其中包括对奈米拉利西布（nemiralisib）的肺部吸收、全身分布和口服吸收的完整机制的描述，以预测药物在组织和血浆中的浓度[21]。该模型用五个隔室描述了药物在肺部的吸收，分别是：鼻子（包含鼻前通道）、胸外（鼻咽和口咽以及喉）、胸腔（气管和支气管）、细支气管（细支气管和末端支气管）和肺泡间质（呼吸细支气管、肺泡管和囊以及间质结缔组织）[21]。一旦药物沉积，其在肺部的分布由下面几个过程控制：通过黏液纤毛运输，从胸部外区域摄入，在黏液中溶解，摄取到肺细胞中，并最终进入全身血液。研究最后用临床数据验证了给药部位的药物浓度，并使用大鼠的静脉输入数据验证了对组织浓度的预测[21]。

8.3.3 皮肤模型

皮肤是一个复杂的器官，由充满亲脂性的物质和富含蛋白质的堆叠层组成。作为哺乳动物中最大的器官，皮肤约占体重的百分之十[22]，是人体抵抗外界环境的重要屏障。皮肤的外层称为角质层。角质层由源自表皮深处的死细胞组成，是防止化学吸收的最有效屏障，特别是对亲水性化学物质[23]。活表皮在角质层下，作为哺乳动物皮肤的活层，活表皮由各种细胞组成，最终成为角质层的细胞[24]。表皮下较厚的皮肤层是真皮，其中包含毛细血管、毛囊根和汗腺[25]。血管仅限于真皮，但是位于表皮下方的毛细血管为活表皮提供营养[24]。药物在皮肤中的渗透取决于其在身体上的位置、湿度、温度和皮肤的健康[26]，还取决于不同的皮肤的结构、厚度、毛囊密度和汗腺[27]。这些结构差异在开发皮肤模型的时候都应该考虑进来。用于皮肤的 PBPK 模型是根据皮肤独特的生理和结构在身体的其他部位的模型基础上专门定制的。该模型最初是为了描述吸入制剂吸入和吸入之后药物的吸收、分布、代谢和消除而开发的，后来被修改为仅包括皮肤并且是在药物暴露下的皮肤模型[24]。这样这个模型在未来可以同时研究皮肤和吸入情况下的药物暴露。

Kwon 及其团队[28-30]在 2021 年报告的研究中，开发了 2-苯氧基乙醇（2-phenoxyethanol）对大鼠的全身 PBPK 模型，并对先前报告的模型进行了修改。2-苯氧基乙醇在化妆品中被广泛用作防腐剂。该模型涵盖 14 个隔室，包括肠道、脂肪、大脑、心脏、骨骼、肾脏、肝脏、肺、肌肉、脾脏、动脉、静脉、皮肤和其他身体部位。隔室通过血流连接，假定血流在各个隔室之间分布良好。药物在血液和组织之间分布的速率主要取决于流向该组织的血流量。隔室的常微分方程改编自已经发表的方程[29, 31, 32, 33]。对于吸收，外敷治疗后的渗透率由式（8-1）决定[30, 34]。

$$渗透率（\mu g \cdot h^{-1}）= PE\ 浓度（\mu g \cdot cm^{-3}）\times K_{per}（cm \cdot h^{-1}）\times SA（cm^2） \tag{8-1}$$

式中，K_{per} 是穿过皮肤的渗透系数；SA 是 PE 处方应用在皮肤上的表面积。该模型用观测数据进行了验证。

另一项研究则开发了 PBPK 模型来研究林丹在人体皮肤上的渗透性。林丹是一种用于治疗皮肤上存在的虱子和疥疮的神经性物质[35]。这项研究使用菲克扩散定律（Fick's law of diffusion）和与蛋白质和脂质的化学结合来确定皮肤吸收的各项参数，然后将其纳入 PBPK 模型中以描述体内动力学特征[35]。

8.3.4 长效注射剂模型

目前市场上的大多数长效缓释注射液都是围绕三种处方设计的：聚合物微球悬浮液、脂质体悬浮液或者是纳米晶悬浮液。这些处方被设计成在较长时间内缓慢释放活性成分，目的是最大限度地减少注射频率并延长作用持续的时间。制剂的选择取决于药物的具体特性和所需的释放曲线。

8.3.4.1 聚合物微球和体内-体外相关性（IVIVC）

在聚合物微球中，活性药物被包裹在可降解聚合物中，进入人体后，药物随着聚合物的降解而释放。例如，聚乳酸-羟基乙酸共聚物（PLGA）是一种用于药物递送和组织工程的聚合物。作为一种可生物降解并且生物相容的聚合物，PLGA由丙交酯和乙交酯聚合而成。进入人体以后，聚合物通过乳酸和乙醇酸之间的酯键水解而裂解，聚合物降解形成乳酸单体和乙醇酸单体，最终以二氧化碳和水的形式排出体外。发生降解所需的唯一条件是存在于水性环境中。通过控制丙交酯与乙交酯的比例，可以控制聚合物的降解速率，从而调节包裹的活性药物在体内释放的时间。PLGA已经被用于包裹多种药物，包括蛋白质、肽和小分子。这仅代表一种用于药物递送的聚合物。还有许多其他聚合物用作药物载体，例如壳聚糖和透明质酸等天然聚合物。图8-8所示是扫描电子显微镜（SEM）下的PLGA纳米颗粒。

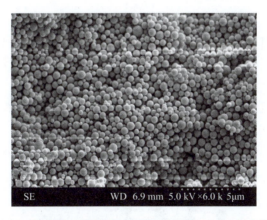

图8-8　扫描电子显微镜（SEM）下的PLGA纳米颗粒

被包裹的药物从聚合物中释放的过程可以分为两个或者三个阶段：初始爆发释放、稳态释放和最终释放[36]。后面两个阶段可以是合二为一。初始爆发释放是药物从聚合物中释放的第一阶段，释放的主要部分是聚合物表面上存在的药物分子。在这个阶段药物的释放主要由扩散控制。稳态释放是药物释放速率相对恒定的时期。在最终释放时，药物释放速率降低或增加，直到所有的药物从聚合物基质中释放。药物释放的最后两个阶段与聚合物的降解有关。

体内-体外相关性（IVIVC）是一种用于预测的数学模型，描述了体外特性（如药物溶解）与体内反应（如药物血浆浓度或药物吸收量）之间的关系。它是一种工具，即用体外实验室的测量结果预测药物在人体内的作用。一个成功的IVIVC可以提供许多的用途。该方法可以验证用体外溶出度的测试结果替代药物之间生物等效性研究的可行性，从而减少对人体实验的依赖。它还可以用于支持药品的开发和监管批准，确保产品质量的一致，并协助生产。

美国食品药品管理局（FDA）在1997年发表的工业指南中，提供了建立IVIVC和在缓释剂型中应用的框架。A级相关性是点对点关系，是IVIVC信息量最大的水平，因为它可以帮助了解药物在体内的溶解，还可以支持生物豁免[37]。尽管FDA指南提供了开发和建立IVIVC的框架，但是目前它仅适用于缓释口服制剂，不适用于非口服的剂型，如经皮吸收或者长效注射剂。一些已经发表的文章报告了对长效注射液建立IVIVC的几个尝试[13, 38, 39, 40]。

通过评估体内吸收的药物分数与体外药物溶出之间的点对点相关性，A级IVIVC的一般形式被开发出来[41]。模型中包含一个时间缩放函数，以解释体外和体内过程中潜在的时间差。建立的IVIVC模型用式（8-2）表示：

$$r_{vivo}(t) = a_1 + a_2 r_{vito}(tt)$$
$$tt = b_1 + b_1 \cdot t^{b_3} \tag{8-2}$$

在r_{vivo}和r_{vitro}之间没有时间缩放的情况下：$a_1 = 0$，$a_2 = 1$，$b_1 = 0$，$b_2 = 1$，$b_3 = 1$。否则，可以通过估计a_1、a_2、b_1、b_2、b_3的参数值来定义时间缩放。式（8-1）包含一个线性分量（截距a_1和斜率a_2）和一个描述时间位移（b_1）、时间尺度（b_2）和时间形状因子（b_3）的非线性分量[41]。

8.3.4.2 脂质体

脂质体由磷脂双层组成，磷脂由疏水（防水）的尾部和亲水（吸水）的头部组成。这些磷脂双层形成球形结构，疏水尾部朝内，亲水头部朝外（图8-9）。脂质体内的空间被这些双层结构包围，成为水隔室，可用于封装药物或其他分子。脂质体的磷脂双层在结构上与细胞膜相似。这使得脂质体很容易与细胞膜合并，直接将其封装的药物输送到细胞中。

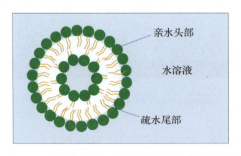

图8-9 脂质体具有亲水性头部和疏水性尾部

脂质体大小和尺寸分布是其体内应用的两个重要因素，因为脂质体大小会影响药物的负载能力、体内的生物分布、药物清除率、针对特定器官的功效和整体治疗效率等方面[42]。用于药物输送时，所需囊泡的尺寸限制在50~150 nm[43]。脂质体可以使用水合法或者批量方法制备。水合法是将脂质体引入水性环境中，通常是对干脂质膜进行水合，或者是对脂质悬浮液进行超声处理。批量法是在一定的温度和搅拌条件下将脂质体与水溶液混合。最终方法的选择取决于具体的应用和最终脂质体产品所需的特性。

药物从脂质体中的扩散主要由三个机制控制：以扩散介导的释放，以孔介导的释放和以膜扰动介导的释放，或者是这三个机制的组合[44, 45]。为了建立更好的体内-体外相关性，研究人员不断利用释放动力学模型来预测药物释放曲线。通常，药物从脂质体中释放受动力学因素（如药物渗透性）和热力学因素（如药物在双层表面上的分布方式）的影响。

然而，还没有一个模型可以恰当地描述胶束或者脂质体的所有的释放行为，因为释放取决于载体的大小和组成、药物类型和上载的工艺[45]。因此，根据药物的性质和脂质体的组成，不同的脂质体模型被提出，以探索更好的体内-体外相关性。探索脂质体的数学模型包括：Peppas模型、Higuchi模型、一阶动力学（First-order kinetics）模型、零阶释放动力学（Zero-order release kinetics）模型、Weibull释放动力学模型、两层胶片理论（two-film theory）数学模型等。各模型的详细信息详见2016年发表的一篇综述[44]。

8.3.4.3 纳米晶体

纳米晶体是另一种用于药物递送的处方设计，它将药物制备成小颗粒，来增加难溶性药物的表面积和曲率[46, 47]。这样可以提高药物的溶解度和生物利用度，从而实现更有效的治疗。纳米晶体的制备可以使用自上而下或者自下而上的方法。自上而下的方法是从散装材料开始，然后将其分解成更小的结构或颗粒，通常达到纳米级。这种方法可以通过机械研磨等来实现。在这个过程中，较大的材料被机械研磨以产生较小的颗粒。而自下而上的方法是从溶液中生长纳米晶体[48]。相比之下，自上而下的方法比自下而上的方法对生产规模更加具有适应性和灵活性[49]。总之，配制纳米晶体是为了保持药物的结晶状态，同时保持小粒径。

难溶性药物的溶解度可以通过纳米化而显著增强[47]。但是，体内环境和体外实验环境是不相同的。在体外实验时，纳米晶体接触的是有限体积的生理液，并且搅动条件不同。因此，依靠体外测试可能无法准确或充分地了解纳米晶体在体内的运动，甚至可能具有误导性[49]。

现在还不清楚纳米晶体在静脉注射以后是立刻溶解还是在一定时间段内先保持完整。假设纳米晶体在注射以后迅速溶解在血液中，并且作为药物释放到体循环中[49]。在纳米晶体表面用亲水聚合物修饰，可以让晶体在体内避免被吞噬，从而延长药物在体内的循环时间[47]。这种时间上的延长可以促进它们在肿瘤组织中的积累。

以棕榈酸酯注射液为例，棕榈酸帕潘立酮被配制成具有微小粒径的水悬浮液，让药物能够缓慢释出。这种配制可以让药物达到每月给药一次。因为它具有极低的水溶性，帕潘立酮棕榈酸酯在肌内注射以后在注射部位缓慢溶解，然后水解形成帕潘立酮。一旦在肌肉内水解，帕潘立酮就进入体循环。Samtani和团队在2009年对组合数据使用NONMEM软件进行了称为非线性混合效应建模的复杂统计分析。目的是了解药物帕潘立酮在作为长效注射剂在体内的行为。这种注射剂由帕潘立酮的棕榈酸酯形式制成，在不同的剂量下给药，并在不同的位点注射。模型用NONMEM软件中一阶条件估计（FOCE）的方法建模，同时对数据进行了对数转换。选择具有一级吸收和消除的最简单的开室药代动力学模型进行拟合。肌内注射棕榈酸酯后的帕潘立酮的浓度-时间数据，最适合采用具有一级消除的单室模型进行拟合。该模型的吸收成分允许一小部分剂量（f_2）通过零阶过程相对快速地进入中央隔室。经过一个滞后时间后，剩余的部分通过一阶过程进入体循环[50]。

长效缓释注射剂也可以使用其他技术配制，例如水凝胶、聚乙二醇化制剂、前药制剂等。这些不同的处方可以改变药物释放的速度和在体内持续的时间，从而提供更广泛的靶向和有效治疗的选择。如前所述，每种制剂都有自己的优点和缺点，需要根据药物的特定性质和所需的释放曲线进行选择。

8.3.5 不足与改进

虽然PBPK模型的建模和预测功能在制药业有很多有价值的应用，但是也有一些局限性。首先，构建和验证PBPK模型需要对药代动力学、生理学和数学有深入的了解，需要操作人员具备很专业的知识。然后，PBPK模型预测的准确性在很大程度上取决于输入数据的质量和完整性。比如药物的物理化学性质、体外数据，以及特定酶/转运蛋白等相关数据的缺失或者不准确，都会导致对结果的错误预测。另外，很重要的是，与所有模型一样，PBPK模型的建立基于有关生理学、药物特性及其相互作用的一些假设。其中一些假设可能不适用于所有药物或者所有条件。例如，通常假设每个隔室内的血液和组织混合均匀，这就意味着药物在每个隔室内的浓度是均匀的。另外，假设血流在各个隔室之间分布均匀，但这是基于人体的平均生理值。血流速率可能存在个体差异，这些差异会影响药物的分布，在一个标准的PBPK模型中，这些个体差异通常无法获得。其他的可能还包括关于新陈代谢和机制的假设、血液和组织蛋白性质的假设，以及化学物质穿过细胞膜的能力等。这些假设都可能给模型带来误差。所以在应用前去了解模型的局限性和它所基于的假设是非常重要的。其他挑战包括是否能够准确预测特殊人群的个体间变异性，是否能够获得用于验证的体内数据，是否能够准确预测长期影响，以及纳入由于疾病或其他病理变化引起的生理变化。

在未来，有很多可以改进的地方。例如，可以为药物特征、酶/转运蛋白动力学和其他相关数据建立标准化数据库；也可以进一步改进体外实验方法，以生成一致且稳定的体外数据，为模型提供信息；还可以结合使用机器学习和人工智能技术来优化模型参数，并预测个体间的变异性。在辅助制剂开发的过程中，使用"学习并确认"的迭代方法，根据新的实验数据和临床观察，不断细化模型。利用来自上市后监测的真实数据来完善和验证PBPK模型，确保它们能够继续反映实际的临床结果。同时，加强对操作人员的培训，针对特殊人群如孩子、老人和患者的生理变化做进一步的研究，加强合作，包括与监管部门的合作。这些都可以增加PBPK模型帮助药物开发和临床决策的潜力。

8.4 总结

PBPK建模用数学方法提供了一个强大的框架，来帮助大家理解和预测药物在体内的行为。当应用于制剂开发和对药代动力学结果预测试时，它可以提供有价值的指导，促进具有最佳治疗性能的药物产品的设计。作为数学模型之一，在无须进行广泛的体内研究的情况下，PBPK模型可以预测各种制剂药物在全身和组织的暴露，还有助于评估同一药物不同处方的生物等效性。这在开发现有药物的仿制药或者缓释药时特别有用。此外，PBPK模型还可以帮助研究食物对药物吸收的影响、药物剂量的调整、与其他药物的相互作用，以及各种生理因素对药物吸收的影响，如pH、胃排空率、肠道转运时间等。在开发针对特殊人群如儿童、老人或者器官损伤患者的处方时，可以定制PBPK模型以代表特定人群。模型将体外溶出度或者渗透性数据集成到模型中，实现了从体外实验转变为体内性能的预测。总之，PBPK 建模在制剂开发过程中提供了对影响药代动力学的各种因素（包括生理因素）的全面理解。这种理解可以对制剂的设计进行合理的指导，从而简化开发过程，最终提高临床试验的成功率。

参考文献

[1] Rydberg P, Gloriam D E, Zaretzki J, et al. SMARTCyp: a 2D method for prediction of cytochrome P450-medicated drug metabolism[J]. ACS Medicinal Chemistry Letters 1, 2010, 1(3): 96-100.

[2] Worth A, Fuart G M. Review of software tools for toxicity prediction. Joint Research Centre, Institute of Health and Consumer Protection, Publications Office, 2010.

[3] Jiménez-Luna J, Grisoni F, Weskamp N, Schneider G. Artificial intelligence in drug discovery: recent advances and future perspectives[J]. Expert Opinion Drug Discovery, 2021, 16(9): 949-959.

[4] Elton D C, Boubouvalas Z, Fuge M D, et al. Deep learning for molecular design: a review of the state of the art[J]. Molecular Systems Design and Engineering, 2019, 4(4): 828-849.

[5] Toure O, Dussap C G, Lebert A. Comparison of predicted pKa values for some amion-acids, dipeptides and tripeptides, using COSMO-RS, ChemAxon and ACD/Labs methods[J]. Oil & Gas Science and Technology-Revue d'IFP Energies Nouvelles, 2013, 68(2): 281-297.

[6] Bunker A, Róg T. Mechanistic understanding from molecular dynamics simulation in pharmaceutical research 1: drug delivery[J]. Frontiers in Molecular Biosciences, 2020, 7: 604770.

[7] Ouyang D F. Investigating the molecular structures of solid dispersions by the simulated annealing method[J]. Chemical Physics Letters, 2012, 554: 177-184.

[8] Gao H, Jia H, Dong J, et al. Integrated in silico formulation design of self-emulsifying drug delivery systems[J]. Acta Pharmaceutica Sinica B, 2021, 11(11): 3585-3594.

[9] Gao H L, Wang W, Dong J, et al. An integrated computational methodology with data-driven machine learning, molecular modeling and PBPK modeling to accelerate solid dispersion formulation design[J]. European Journal of Pharmaceutics and Biopharmaceutics, 2021, 158: 336-346.

[10] Gao G F, Ashtikar M, Kojima R, et al. Predicting drug release and degradation kinetics of long-acting microsphere formulations of tacrolimus for subcutaneous injection[J]. Journal of Controlled Release, 2021, 329: 372-384.

[11] Zhao Q Q, Miriyala N, Su Y, et al. Computer-aided formulation design for a highly soluble lutein-cyclodextrin multiple-component delivery system[J]. Molecular Pharmaceutics, 2018, 15(4): 1664-1673.

[12] Wilkhu J S, Ouyang D F, Kirchmeier M H, et al. Investigating the role of cholesterol in the formation of non-ionic surfactant based bilayer vesicles: thermal analysis and molecular dynamics[J]. International Journal of Pharmaceutics, 2014, 461: 331-341.

[13] Gao H S, Ye Z Y F, Dong J, et al. Predicting drug/phospholipid complexation by the lightGBM method[J]. Chemical Physics Letters, 2020, 747: 137354.

[14] Yang C L, Tu K, Gao H L, et al. The novel platinum (Ⅳ) prodrug with self-assembly property and structure-transformable character against triple-negative breast cancer[J]. Biomaterials, 2020, 232: 119751.

[15] Kovar L, Weber A, Zemlin M, et al. Physiologically-based pharmacokinetic (PBPK) modelling providing insights into fentanyl pharmacokinetics in adults and paediatric patients[J]. Pharmaceutics, 2020, 12: 908.

[16] Agoram B, Woltosz W S, Bolger M B. Predicting the impact of physiological and biochemical processes on oral drug bioavailability[J]. Advanced Drug Delivery Reviews, 2001, 50: S41-S67.

[17] Kushwah V, Arora S, Tamás Katona M, et al. On absorption modeling and food effect prediction of rivaroxaban, a BCS II drug orally administered as an immediate-release tablet[J]. Pharmaceutics, 2021, 13(2): 283.

[18] ICRP Publication 66. Human respiratory tract model for radiological protection[J]. Annals of the ICRP, 1994, 24(1-3): 1-482.

[19] Perry J, Brian Trautman, Takher-Smith J, et al. Particle size and gastrointestinal absorption influence tiotropium pharmacokinetics: a pilot bioequivalence study of PUR0200 and Spiriva HandiHaler[J]. British Journal of Clinical Pharmacology, 2019, 85(3): 580-589.

[20] Zhang J, Wu K, Liu B, et al. Bioequivalence study of ipratropium bromide inhalation aerosol using PBPK modelling[J].

Frontiers in Medicine(Lausanne), 2023, 10: 1056318.

[21] Miller N A, Graves R H, Edwards C D, et al. Physiologically based pharmacokinetic modelling of inhaled nemiralisib: mechanistic components for pulmonary absorption, systemic distribution, and oral absorption[J]. Clinical Pharmacokinetics, 2022, 61(2): 281-293.

[22] Montagna W, Parakkal P F. The structure and function of the skin[M]. Academic Press, New York, third edition, 1974: 1-17.

[23] Scheuplein R J, Blank I H. Permeability of the skin[J]. Physiological Reviews, 1971, 51: 702-744.

[24] Bookout R L, McDaniel C R, Quinn D W, et al. Multilayered dermal subcompartments for modelling chemical absorption[J]. SAR and QSAR in Environmental Research, 1996, 5(3): 133-150.

[25] Schaefer H, Zesch A, Stuttgen G. Skin permeability[M]. Springer-Verlag, Berlin, 1982: 545-550.

[26] Bartek M J, LaBudde J A, Maibach H I. Skin permeability in vivo: comparison in rat, rabbit, pig, and man[J]. The Journal of Investigative Dermatology, 1972, 54: 114-123.

[27] Wester R C, Maibach H I. Regional variation in percutaneous absorption[M]. In: Mechanisms-Methodology-Drug Delivery(R.L. Bronaugh and H.I. Maibach, Eds.). Marcel Dekker, New York, 1989: 111-119.

[28] Kwon M, Park J B, Kwon M, et al. Pharmacokinetics of 2-phenoxyethanol and its major metabolite, phenoxyacetic acid, after dermal and inhaled routes of exposure: application to development PBPK model in rats[J]. Archives of Toxicology, 2021, 95: 2019-2036.

[29] Elmokadem A, Riggs M M, Baron K T. Quantitative systems pharmacology and physiologically-based pharmacokinetic modelling with mrgsolve: a hands-on tutorial[J]. CPT Pharmacometrics & Systems Pharmacology, 2019, 8(12): 883-893.

[30] Troutman J A, Rick D L, Stuard S B, et al. Development of a physiologically-based pharmacokinetic model of 2-phenoxyethanol and its metabolite phenoxyacetic acid in rats and humans to address toxicokinetic uncertainty in risk assessment[J]. Regulatory Toxicology and Pharmacology, 2015, 73(2): 530-543.

[31] Jones H, Rowland-Yeo K. Basic concepts in physiologically based pharmacokinetic modelling in drug discovery and development[J]. CPT Pharmacometrics & Systems Pharmacology, 2013, 2: e63.

[32] Pawaskar D K, Straubinger R M, Fetterly G J, et al. Physiologically based pharmacokinetic models for everolimus and sorafenib in mice[J]. Cancer Chemotherapy and Pharmacology, 2013, 71(5): 1219-1229.

[33] Thompson M D, Beard D A. Development of appropriate equations for physiologically based pharmacokinetic modelling of permeability-limited and flow-limited transport[J]. Journal of Pharmacokinetics and Pharmacodynamics, 2011, 38(4): 405-421.

[34] Wong B A. Inhalation exposure systems: design, methods and operation[J]. Toxicologic Pathology, 2007, 35(1): 3-14.

[35] Sawyer M E, Evans M V, Wilson C A, et al. Development of a human physiologically based pharmacokinetic (PBPK) model for dermal permeability for lindane[J]. Toxicology Letters, 2016, 245: 106-109.

[36] Corrigan O I, Li X. Quantifying drug release from PLGA nanoparticulates[J]. European Journal of Pharmaceutical Sciences, 2009；37(3-4): 477-85. doi: 10.1016/j.ejps.2009.04.004.

[37] Food and Drug Administration(1997). Guidance for industry: extended release oral dosage forms: development, evaluation, and application of in vitro/in vivo correlations.

[38] D'Souza S, Faraj J A, Giovagnoli S, et al. IVIVC from Long Acting Olanzapine Microspheres[J]. International Journal of Biomaterials, 2014: 407065.

[39] D'Souza S, Faraj J A, Giovagnoli S, et al. In vitro-in vivo correlation from lactide-co-glycolide polymeric dosage forms[J]. Progress in Biomaterials, 2014, 3(2-4): 131-142.

[40] Dubey V, Saini T R. Formulation development and pharmacokinetic studies of long acting in situ depot injection of risperidone[J]. Brazilian Journal of Pharmaceutical Sciences, 2022, 58: e18809.

[41] Gomeni R, Fang L L, Bressolle-Gomeni F, et al. A general framework for assessing in vitro/in vivo correlation as a tool for maximizing the benefit-risk ratio of a treatment using a convolution-based modelling approach[J]. CPT Pharmacometrics Syst Pharmacol, 2019, 8(2): 97-106.

[42] Has C, Sunthar P. A comprehensive review on recent preparation techniques of liposomes[J]. Journal of Liposome Research 2020, 30(4): 336-365.

[43] Dhand C, Prabhakara M P, Beuerman R W, et al. Role of size of drug delivery carriers for pulmonary and intraveneous administration with emphasis on cancer therapeutics and lung-targeted drug delivery[J]. RSC Advances, 2014, 4(62): 32673-32689.

[44] Jain A, Jain S K. In vitro release kinetics model fitting of liposomes: an insight[J]. Chemistry and Physics of Lipids, 2016, 201: 28-40.

[45] Sawaftah N A, Paul V, Awad N, Husseini G A. Modelling of anti-cancer drug release kinetics from liposomes and micelles:

a review[J]. IEEE Transactions on Nanobioscience, 2021, 20(4): 565-576.

[46] Merisko-Liversidge E M, Liversidge G G. Drug nanparticles: formulating poorly water-soluble compounds[J]. Toxicologic Pathology, 2008, 36(1): 43-48.

[47] Muller R H, Gohla S, Keck C M. State of the art of nanocrystals-special features, production, nanotoxicology aspects and intracellular delivery[J]. European Journal of Pharmaceutics and Biopharmaceutics, 2011, 78(1): 1-9.

[48] Sinha B, Muller R H, Moschwitzer J P. Bottom-up approaches for preparing drug nanocrystals: formulations and factors affecting particle size[J]. International Journal of Pharmaceutics, 2013, 453(1): 126-141.

[49] Lu Y, Lv Y, Li T. Hybrid drug nanocrystals[J]. Advanced Drug Delivery Reviews, 2019, 143: 115-133.

[50] Samtani M N, Vermeulen A, Stuyckens K. Population pharmacokinetics of intramuscular paliperidone palmitate in patients with schizophrenia: a novel once-monthly, long-acting formulation of an atypical antipsychotic[J]. Clinical Pharmacokinetics, 2009, 48(9): 585-600.

第9章

药物递送中的分子建模

王佳文　澳门科技大学，澳门，中国；苏州大学，中国
于　怡　苏州大学，中国
李有勇　澳门科技大学，澳门，中国；苏州大学，中国

9.1 引言

疾病一直是人类的头号杀手。因此，研究疾病的病因、致病机制以及治愈方法是人类医学的永恒追求。药物研发是帮助患者恢复健康、减轻疼痛、缓解或消除病因、预防疾病的有效途径。目前，药物的种类和数量正在迅速增加。而传统的经皮、口服和注射等给药途径，存在吸收不良、作用时间短、分布不理想、化学稳定性差、水溶性差、脂溶性差、口感和气味不佳以及存在副作用等缺点[1]。此外，一些新型药物，如前药、蛋白质和核酸生物制剂等，需要新的递送载体来实现其有效传递[2]。因此，寻找更合适的药物载体也是当前药物研发的重要任务之一。

通常，理想的药物载体应具备以下优点：①限制药物在目标区域、器官、组织、细胞和隔室的分布；②可在毛细血管水平上实现均匀分布；③延长药物的局部化控制时间；④将大部分药物递送到靶细胞，例如肿瘤细胞；⑤控制药物释放速率；⑥释放药物时不会显著降低药物的生物活性；⑦在所需的分子靶标处达到治疗浓度；⑧在血液中转运时最小化游离药物泄漏；⑨保护药物免受血浆酶的破坏；⑩具备生物降解性，能够在体内被分解和排出，以减少潜在的毒性；⑪可以应用于多种物质（诊断和治疗）；⑫易制备。

在20世纪60年代左右，科学家们首次提出药物递送系统（drug delivery system，DDS）的概念[3]。DDS是一个综合的技术系统，旨在全面调节体内药物的空间、时间和剂量分布，并具有合理的分布、小剂量和少副作用等优点[4]。通常情况下，DDS可以划分为持续释放递送系统、靶向递送系统、纳米颗粒递送系统、经皮递送系统、黏附递送系统、无针粉末注射递送系统和其他新型递送系统[5]。因此，DDS综合了药理学、生物学、化学、纳米科学、材料科学、计算机科学等多个跨学科领域的知识和技术。

随着纳米技术的飞速发展，纳米颗粒递送系统也取得了一些进展[6]。这种系统利用纳米颗粒作为载体，通过共价或非共价键与药物分子结合，最终形成纳米级的颗粒。经过纳米晶化处理后，药物分子的物理性质、化学性质和生物学性质发生改变，从而影响药物的吸收、分布、代谢和排泄，进而显著增强治疗效果以及降低不良反应[7]。

根据不同类型的纳米颗粒，纳米颗粒递送系统又可分为以下类型：①固体无机；②胶束；③囊泡；④脂质；⑤脂质聚合物结构；⑥碳纳米粒；⑦树状分子；⑧蛋白质/肽；⑨纳米晶体；⑩金属和金属氧化物；⑪非金属氧化物等[8]。按照元素类别，纳米颗粒递送系统也可以进一步分为碳基纳米材料、硅基纳米材料、金属基纳米材料和其他纳米材料[9]。接下来，本章将探讨这些纳米颗粒在药物递送系统中的应用策略。

碳基纳米材料是纳米材料的一个庞大分支，主要包括石墨烯量子点（GQD）、富勒烯、碳纳米管（CNT）、石墨烯、纳米金刚石和其他衍生物[10-14]。碳基纳米材料具有稳定的理化性质、易于功能化和修饰、良好的生物相容性以及强大的穿透能力，因此在能源存储、生物医学等诸多领域被广泛应用和研究[15]。

GQD是理想的药物载体，具有小尺寸、良好的生物相容性、稳定的荧光特性、水稳定性和易于化学修饰等优点。它们既保留了石墨烯的出色特性，又展现出独特的理化性质，如量子局域效应和边界效应等。其中最令人兴奋的是，GQD具有稳定的荧光特性，可应用于生物成像和细胞定位等。如图9-1所示，Ding等[16]利用GQD的固有荧光特性来监测抗肿瘤药物的装载、递送和释放过程。

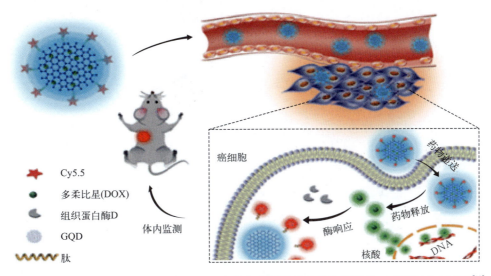

图9-1　基于GQD的治疗诊断剂：用于程序化监测抗肿瘤药物的装载、递送和响应过程[16]

富勒烯是一类碳同素异构体，具有多种形式和结构。其中C_{60}是最常见的富勒烯，其宽度为7.1 Å，由12个五元环和20个六元环。这些五元环和六元环为共价衍生物提供了反应位点，为非共价相互作用提供了锚定位点。由于其小尺寸和易于修饰，富勒烯正在成为药物递送的有效候选者之一。例如，伊立替康（irinotecan）是一种很有前景的抗肿瘤药物，已被FDA批准单独或联合静脉注射用于结肠癌治疗。然而，它对肿瘤细胞缺乏选择性和特异性，从而导致全身毒性。为此，Dhiman等[17]研制出一种富勒烯功能化生物素给药系统，将伊立替康吸附在功能化富勒烯-生物素复合物表面。研究结果表明，这种复合系统具有药物控释的特性，并对重要器官产生的毒性较低以及对结肠癌肿瘤细胞具有较好的疗效。

CNT是另一种重要的碳纳米材料。其能够被细胞迅速高效地吸收，因此它们被广泛应用于高度靶向的药物递送。Datir等[18]合成了一种新型的多壁碳纳米管（MWCNT）-透明质酸偶联物，并通过π-π堆积作用将这种偶联物与多柔比星（doxorubicin）结合。与游离的多柔比星相比，负载了多柔比星的MWCNT-透明质酸偶联物表现出更高的细胞毒性和凋亡活性，这表明这种新型MWCNT-透明质酸偶联物有望成为针对肿瘤治疗的智能递送平台候选者。

石墨烯是一种由sp^2杂化碳原子按六角形排列形成的二维碳纳米材料。这种材料具有巨大的比表面积、出色的稳定性和易于修饰等特点，且可通过改变其结构、氧化、氟化及引入缺陷、杂原子和功能基团等方法来制备各种石墨烯相关材料（GRM）[19-21]。这些方法极大地扩展了石墨烯在DDS中的应用。例如，某些芳香族药物因其不溶性而受到应用限制。为解决这一问题，Liu等[22]使用分支聚乙二醇（PEG）功能化纳米氧化石墨烯（NGO），最终获得一种生物相容性优异的NGO-PEG偶联化合物[22]。该化合物在各种生物溶液中具有良好的稳定性，并进一步与疏水性芳香族药物分子（SN38）连接。NGO-PEG-SN38复合物展现出优异的水溶性，同时拥有高癌细胞杀伤能力（图9-2）。

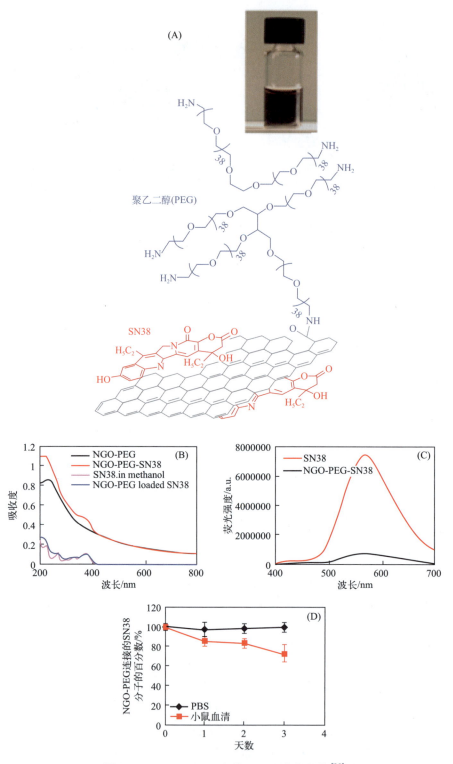

图9-2　NGO-PEG上的SN38药物负载[22]

类似地，Yang等[23]使用PEG功能化纳米还原氧化石墨烯（RGO）-铁氧化物纳米颗粒（IONP）复合物，成功获得了具有出色生理稳定性、强近红外吸收和超顺磁性的RGO-IONP-PEG复合物。该复合物被用于有效光热消融小鼠肿瘤[23]。此外，氟化石墨烯（FG）在药物装载和递送领域显示出具有巨大优势。2020年，Jahanshahi等[24]开发了一种高效绿色合成FG的方法。结果表明，FG作为姜黄素的载体具有较高的载药率（78.43%）和良好的体外抗癌效果。

硅基纳米材料同样引起了人们的广泛关注。除了具备传统无机纳米材料的卓越特性外，硅基纳米材料还具备出色的生物相容性、丰富的储备量、低毒性和独特的光电性能等优点。因此，硅基纳米材料在DDS领域展现出广泛的应用前景。最近，Sun等[25]利用可穿过血脑屏障的荧光硅纳米颗粒开发了一种高效的DDS（图9-3），通过将一种葡萄糖摄取聚合物与吲哚菁绿修饰的荧光硅纳米颗粒结合，成功构建了特洛伊细菌载药体系。这种DDS可以携带药物穿过血脑屏障并靶向渗透到胶质母细胞瘤组织中。在808 nm激光照射下，吲哚菁绿产生的光热效应可裂解细菌并破坏肿瘤细胞。

介孔二氧化硅（SiO_2）是另一种具有药物递送潜力的硅基纳米材料。基于介孔SiO_2的氧化还原、温度和酶协同效应，Wu等[26]成功地将介孔SiO_2和多柔比星结合，构建了一种用于肿瘤治疗的DDS。结果表明，该系统可以精确地靶向肝癌细胞，在具有较高安全性的同时，也在抗肿瘤治疗潜力方面表现出良好的效果。

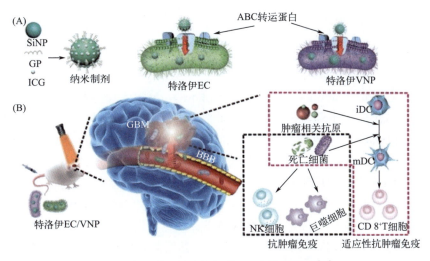

图9-3 基于特洛伊细菌DDS的示意图[25]

SiNP—硅纳米颗粒；GP—葡萄糖聚合物；ICG—吲哚菁绿；EC—大肠埃希菌；VNP—减毒鼠伤寒沙门氏菌；GBM—胶质母细胞瘤；BBB—血脑屏障；iDC—未成熟树突状细胞；mDC—成熟树突状细胞

除了碳基和硅基纳米材料外，金属基纳米材料在药物负载、成像、标记和癌症治疗等方面也得到广泛应用。金属基纳米材料包括纯金属纳米材料、金属氧化物/硫化物/碳化物/氮化物以及合金等。其中，金纳米颗粒（Au nanoparticle，AuNP）已被证明在DDS中非常高效，并展现出用于肿瘤治疗的良好潜力。如图9-4所示，Chen等[27]开发了一种通用方法，用含有透明质酸（hyaluronic acid，HA）靶向基团和双氯芬酸（diclofenac，DC）的小分子Glut1抑制剂修饰等离子金纳米棒（gold nanorod，GNR），获得了GNR/HA-DC该复合体系通过抑制厌氧糖酵解，选择性敏感化肿瘤细胞，展现出光热疗法的优越性。除此之外，其他金属基纳米材料也在DDS中展现出良好的应用。例如，Bai等[28]通过热分解法合成了超小的铁掺杂二氧化钛纳米点，这种材料可作为一种增强声动力治疗的声敏剂。Song等[29]合成了具有pH依赖性氧化降解特性的钼氧化物纳米片，这些纳米片可用作可降解的光热剂和药物载体。

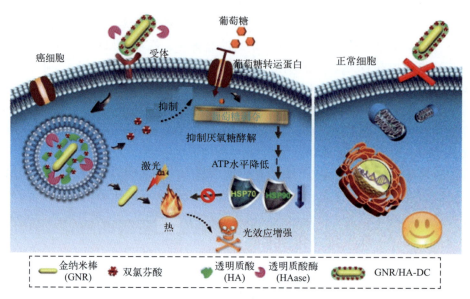

图9-4 GNR/HA-DC通过干扰厌氧糖酵解代谢使肿瘤细胞对光热治疗选择性增敏的示意图[27]

近年来，单层黑磷（monolayer black phosphorus，MBP）、氮化硼和硼碳纳米片等新型纳米材料也已被广泛应用于药物递送领域。此外，基于多种纳米材料的DDS也是未来研究的重点。例如，Molaei等[30]成功合成了可以同时实现成像和药物传递功能的$Fe_3O_4@SiO_2$超磁性纳米粒。

纳米材料在DDS中的应用引起了广泛的关注和研究。与传统实验方法相比，虚拟筛选、分子对接、密度泛函理论计算、分子动力学（MD）模拟等方法在DDS的设计中变得愈发重要。这些方法不仅可以加速药物分子的筛选与设计，也可用于探索DDS各组分的互作机制。特别地，基于统计力学的MD可以提供有关系统内各组分互作过程的关键信息，从而促进和验证DDS的设计[31]。由于纳米材料与生物分子之间的互作机制对于DDS设计至关重要，接下来本章将重点介绍MD模拟的基本原理、分子建模过程和不同纳米材料的传递策略，最后简单介绍MD模拟在DDS中的其他应用。

9.2 分子动力学模拟的基本原理和分子建模方法

本章重点关注DDS中常见纳米材料的应用，并介绍一些采用经典分子力学范式进行MD建模的研究工作。本节将着重介绍MD模拟的基本原理（基于统计力学）以及分子建模方法。

9.2.1 分子动力学模拟的基本原理

实验通常揭示宏观现象，而宏观现象背后的微观机制则可借助MD模拟来阐明。随着计算机科学的快速发展和计算能力的不断增强，模拟微观粒子在宏观物质中的运动变得愈发便利，这使得MD模拟成为一种重要且不可或缺的研究工具。MD模拟的主要优点在于快速、可扩展、代价小、受约束条件少。此外，其还能够为微观粒子的热力学和动力学行为提供直观解释。

MD模拟分为基于量子力学原理的量子化学模拟和基于统计力学原理的分子模拟。本章所介绍的工作主要为基于统计力学原理的分子模拟，即：通过给定体系特定的力场以及一个初始状态，则可根据牛顿第二定律精确求解体系内所有粒子的运动轨迹。模拟结束后，通过提取所有粒子的运动状态并分析它们的热力学和动力学数据以获得有关宏观行为的信息。MD模拟能够处理大量的粒子，从而特别适用于生物大体系。

在1950年代，Alder等[32]进行了最早的MD模拟，研究了一个仅由32个原子组成的凝聚态系统。接下来，Rahman等[33]引入了时间步长的概念，极大地推进了MD模拟的发展，这种方法仍然广泛应用于如今的模拟研究中。另一个里程碑事件是引入Verlet积分算法，这种算法极大地提高了计算效率[34]。McCammon等[35]的研究是将MD模拟应用于生物大分子系统的第一个例子，他们研究了牛胰蛋白酶的运动，模拟时长为9.2皮秒。在20世纪80年代，科学家们又引入了"系综"的概念，进一步发展了MD模拟方法[36]。接下来，将简要介绍运动方程、力场、系综、周期边界条件等MD模拟中的基本知识。

在由n个原子组成的模拟体系中，所有原子的运动必须通过运动方程求解。根据这些方程，当确定原子i的初始位置和速度时，在时间间隔δt后获取原子i下一时刻的位置和速度。以此类推，在循环中可以获取模拟体系中所有原子的热力学和动力学属性。然而，MD体系中的原子数相对较多，只能通过特定的数值积分算法来获得势能函数的数值解。因此，有限差分法在MD模拟中被广泛使用。该方法被细分为Verlet算法、Leap-frog算法、Rahman算法、Beeman算法、Gear算法等[37-39]。在这些算法中，Verlet算法具有最快的计算速度和最低的内存消耗，使其成为解决问题最合适的算法。然而，由于计算过程中可能会出现较大的数值，Verlet算法会导致计算精度降低。Leap-frog算法具有克服Verlet算法局限性的能力，其通过在时间上交替更新位置和速度来模拟系统的演化。具体而言，它使用离散化的时间步长，在每个时间步长中，先更新速度，然后根据更新后的速度更新位置。因此，Leap-frog算法具有更高的收敛速度、稳定性和精度，是目前最广泛使用的算法之一。

在MD模拟中，所有原子的计算都依赖于分子力场（势函数）。力场用于描述体系中所有原子的力和运动，包括化学键长、键角、二面角、原子范德华半径和原子电荷等。如果力场能够准确描述体系中每个原子的运动情况，模拟结果将更加可靠和准确。力场的参数化可以通过实验数据或量子化学计算得到，且不同的力场具有不同的参数和适用范围，因此没有适用于所有模拟体系的力场。目前生物体系常用的力场有CHARMM力场、COMPASS力场、Dreiding力场、AMBER力场、OPLS力场等[40-44]。需要强调的是，在选择力场时，需要注意所选择的力场是否受商业版权保护。此外，可利用Sobtop、Antechamber和CGenFF等工具构建分子力场[45-47]。

系综是统计力学中的一个关键概念，用于描述热力学系统中观察到的统计模式。在进行

MD模拟时，选择适当的系综是至关重要的。系综主要包括以下几个要素：原子数量（N）、体积（V）、温度（T）、能量（E）和压力（P）。因此，常见的集合包括正则系综（NVT）、微正则系综（NVE）、等温等压系综（NPT）、巨正则系综、半巨正则系综等。在MD模拟中，最常用的系综是NPT和NVT。

由于计算能力的限制，通常使用周期性边界条件减少边界效应。周期性边界条件意味着模拟盒子在三个方向上具有相同的镜像盒子，形成一个周期性镜像系统。换句话说，当一个粒子离开模拟盒子的一侧边界时，它会通过相应的边界进入盒子的另一侧，仿佛进入了一个相同的镜像粒子，从而保持盒子中的总粒子数恒定。在设置模拟参数时，需要考虑模拟盒子的大小与分子间相互作用的最长范围之间的关系。也就是，盒子的大小应该大于分子相互作用的最长范围，否则镜像系统的存在将导致分子间相互作用的重复计算。

9.2.2 分子建模

蛋白质的晶体结构可以从蛋白质数据库（Protein Data Bank）和AlphaFold蛋白质结构数据库中获得，也可以通过同源建模的方法构建。蛋白质的晶体结构可通过Schrödinger和Discovery Studio等软件进行初步处理，包括残基修复、去除结晶水、添加氢原子、能量最小化等[48, 49]。通常使用Discovery Studio、H++和PropKa等工具预测组氨酸和其他残基的质子化状态和pK_a值[49-51]。

DNA的构建可使用Amber、Discovery Studio和3D-DART等软件完成[49, 52, 53]。细胞膜的基本框架为脂质双分子层，其中镶嵌了蛋白质、糖类和其他大分子。因此，为了构建膜蛋白，通常需要先分别构建细胞膜和所需的蛋白质、糖类等，然后将这些组分插入细胞膜中。常用于构建细胞膜和膜蛋白的软件包括VMD、Schrödinger、Packmol和CHARMM GUI[48, 54-56]。配体的电荷可以通过一些软件进行计算，例如Amber、Multiwfn和Gaussian[52, 57, 58]。

纳米材料的结构可以从Materials Studio和Materials Project等软件中获取，这些软件可以为模拟提供有效的初始结构[59, 60]。另外，也可以使用Atomic Simulation Environment（ASE）软件构建特殊的纳米材料[61]。这些结构可以通过Materials Studio进行优化，使用Forcite模块进行结构优化，并使用Dreiding力场和Gasteiger进行能量计算[42, 62]。优化后的结构作为后续模拟的初始结构。

9.2.3 分子动力学模拟

在得到纳米材料和生物分子的初始结构后，可以使用VMD、PyMOL等软件构建模拟体系[54, 63]。为了确保模拟的平稳启动并避免任何不利的直接相互作用，建议将纳米材料和生物分子之间的初始最小距离保持在1.6 nm。然后，将纳米材料-生物分子复合物插入一个合适大小的水溶液中，并移除距离复合物4~6 Å范围内的水分子[64]。

在进行正式的MD模拟采样之前，模拟体系需要经历能量最小化和平衡过程。最小化过程通常需要5000步以上，而平衡过程通常包括以下步骤：首先，将纳米材料-生物分子复合物固定，对水分子进行3~5 ns的平衡；然后取消对生物分子的约束，同时水分子和生物分子进行3~5 ns平衡。最后取消对纳米材料的约束，再进行3~5 ns的平衡。值得一提的是，最小化和平衡过程所需的时间并不固定，要视具体情况决定。一般可通过监测体系并分析模拟软件生成的日志文件，以确定模拟体系是否充分平衡。正式的MD模拟采样过程通常需要至少100 ns，且同一体系应该进行至少三组独立的采样以确保结果的准确性。MD模拟可以使用GROMACS、AMBER、NAMD、CHARMM和OpenMM等软件进行[52, 65-68]。轨迹分析可以使用VMD、GROMACS、PyMOL等软件进行[54, 63, 65]。同样的，Schrödinger、Material Studio和Discovery Studio等软件是商业产品，需要购买许可证，而PyMOL、AMBER22、VMD等软件可供学术（非商业）使用。在使用这些软件之前，用户应仔细阅读软件使用协议。

9.3 纳米颗粒给药策略中的分子动力学模拟

9.3.1 碳基纳米材料

最近，在DDS领域中，研究人员对碳基纳米材料进行了大量的MD模拟研究，现按类别分别介绍它们。

石墨烯量子点（GQD）是一种新型的准零维纳米材料，其具有稳定的荧光强度、优异的生物相容性和较小的副作用等优点，这使得其在生物医学领域具有广泛应用[69]。Ren等[70]通过MD模拟了GQD与细胞膜以及抗肿瘤药物在不同条件下的相互作用，这一研究有望推动GQD在药物递送领域的应用[70]。这些研究主要包括：GQD和氧化石墨烯量子点（GOQD）与四种模型药物在水溶液中的吸附行为和强度；不同pH对壳聚糖（CHS）-GQD复合物负载和释放多柔比星的影响；不同尺寸和分子比例对GQD辅助药物穿过细胞膜的影响。研究表明，5-氟尿嘧啶无法正常地与GQD和GOQD吸附，而多柔比星可以迅速与GQD和GOQD吸附。此外，相比于阿糖胞苷，脱氧腺苷可以更快地吸附到GQD表面上；而相比于脱氧腺苷，阿糖胞苷与GOQD之间展现出更强的相互作用。随着浓度进一步增加，可以观察到脱氧腺苷、阿糖胞苷与GQD、GOQD之间的相互作用差异逐渐减小。这项工作对于深入理解两种GQD作为模型药物载体的机制提供了帮助[70]。此外，对于碳点（和GQD类似，为一类具有显著荧光性能的零维碳纳米材料）的靶向递送所涉及的穿越脂质双层膜的过程机制仍不清楚。为此，Erimban等[71]通过全原子MD模拟研究了羟基化碳点直接穿过POPC脂质双层膜的过程。结果显示，碳点需要较高的能垒高度（170 kJ·mol^{-1}）才能穿越脂质双层膜，因此它几乎无法直接穿过脂质双层膜。这一结果对科学家们设计基于碳点的DDS具有重要意义。

富勒烯是一种较早发现的碳同素异构体，包含六元环、五元环，并偶尔包含七元环。由于其尺寸小且易于修饰，富勒烯正成为有效的药物递送候选者。例如，在设计针对COVID-19的DDS时，脂溶性DDS可能会被脂肪组织所隔离，导致其难以排泄和释放药物。为此，如图9-5所示，Giannopoulos等[72]提出了一种基于高度水溶性C_{60}衍生物（树状[C_{60}]富勒烯）的DDS新思路，通过简单的N—N键将莫卢匹韦（molnupiravir）分子连接到亲水的树状[C_{60}]富勒烯上。当受到刺激时，N—N键往往会断裂，从而实现药物向靶器官的有效释放。通过MD模拟，计算了该DDS的溶剂化自由能，为纳米载体的有效性提供了证据。这项研究工作通过利用C_{60}衍生物，为针对COVID-19的药物递送提出了创新性的概念。此外，富勒烯及其衍生物代表了一种新型纳米颗粒并被设计用于有效地穿透人体皮肤，实现药物的经皮途径输送。为此，Gupta等[73]通过MD模拟调查了原始富勒烯C_{60}通过皮肤脂质层的渗透机制。有趣的是，在低浓度下，富勒烯在水相中形成小团簇（由3或5个分子组成），这些团簇进一步自发地穿透双层膜的内部，并在双层膜内部分散而不引起显著的结构变化。在较高浓度下，富勒烯会在水层中积累，并以这种形式穿透到双层膜内，并保持其浓度。此外，可以观察到结构的波动。换句话说，富勒烯分子的渗透性取决于其浓度。未来，研究人员可以根据富勒烯的聚集和分散情况确定用于药物递送的最佳富勒烯浓度。

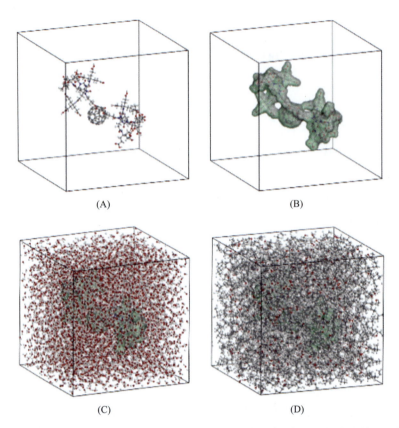

图9-5　树状[C_{60}]富勒烯/莫卢匹韦DDS作为溶质的单元格：（A）溶质的中心位置，（B）溶质的Connolly表面，（C）水溶剂中的溶质，（D）正辛醇溶剂中的溶质[72]

一维CNT拥有出色的理化性质、高的比表面积、高热导功能和电子传输等特性。CNT可以被看作是沿着其平面的晶格矢量（n, m）卷曲成空心结构的石墨烯，这也直接决定了CNT的直径和手性。CNT被认为是生物传感器、药物递送载体、体内成像和癌症治疗等生物医学领域中最有前景的材料之一[74]。CNT优先与两亲性磷脂分子或蛋白质中的疏水结合位点结合，为其作为药物递送载体奠定了基础。例如，由于CNT的高疏水性，它们在水溶性环境中容易发生不受控制的聚集。为此，如图9-6所示，Xue等和Yu等[75, 76]分别通过实验和MD模拟证明，聚集的CNT在药物成瘾治疗中可有效抑制酪氨酸羟化酶活性。此外，传统的抗癌疗法由于非选择性的生物分布，无法实现理想的效果。然而，CNT已经被开发成为针对特定癌细胞的药物载体。为此，von Ranke等[77]研究了CNT与三种抗癌药物（多柔比星、苯达莫司汀、卡莫司汀）之间的相互作用。三种药物代表了生理pH下不同的电离形式：

多柔比星（质子化）、苯达莫司汀（负性）和卡莫司汀（中性）。研究发现，配体的物理化学特性可能会影响它们与CNT的相互作用。具体来说，带正电的阳离子，如质子化氮，会增强它们与CNT的亲和力，而羧基和其他阴离子的存在会降低它们与CNT的亲和力。且在设计DDS时，还应考虑CNT的直径。总之，这项研究对于理解和设计装载药物的CNT具有重要意义。

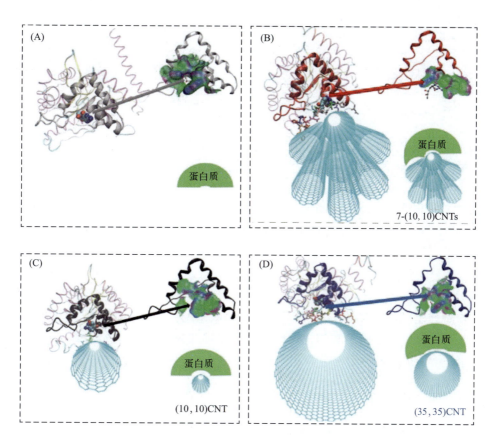

图9-6　TyrOH的活性位点在（A）晶体结构（灰色）、（B）吸附在（10，10）CNT（黑色）、（C）吸附在7-（10，10）CNT（红色）和（D）吸附在（35，35）CNT（蓝色）中的比较。活性口袋的表面由氢键区域（紫色）、疏水区域（绿色）和极性区域（蓝色）显示[76]

自从成功合成石墨烯以来，其已成为最广泛研究的材料之一。石墨烯的主要特性包括较大的比表面积、良好的稳定性和功能化特性，使其适用于多种应用，如药物递送、细胞成像、生物传感器开发以及抗菌和抗病毒药物研发等。例如，Luo等[78]发现PEG修饰的NGO优先吸附并部分插入细胞膜中，从而触发强大的细胞因子反应。随后，Chen等[79]通过MD模拟揭示了石墨烯诱导整合素αVβ8（一种在免疫细胞中表达的重要膜受体）从内而外激活的潜在机制。CS修饰的碳基纳米材料可用于药物递送，但药物递送过程受到官能团质子化状态等影响[80]。因此，Shen等[81]构建了由不同电荷状态的单元组成的CHS链，并将其用于创建一个石墨烯-多柔比星的模拟系统。MD模拟用于研究多柔比星与CHS修饰的石墨烯之间的相互作用（图9-7）。结果表明，通过调整溶液的pH（CHS的质子化状态）以及多柔比星和CHS分子的浓度，可实现对CHS修饰的石墨烯中多柔比星的可控装载和释放。

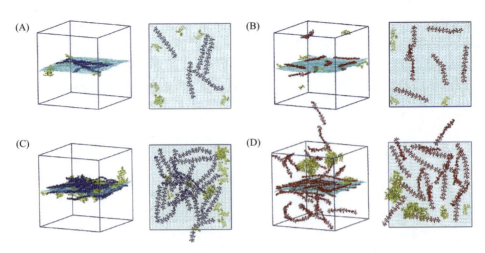

图9-7 石墨烯与多柔比星（DOX）之间的分子模拟。（A）石墨烯和DOX的初始构象。（B）在pH=7.4的生理条件下，DOX进入石墨烯的过程。（C）在pH=5.3的酸性条件下，DOX从石墨烯中释放的过程[80]

新型冠状病毒感染是最致命的传染病之一。根据约翰·霍普金斯大学的数据库，截至2023年3月初，全球已有约6.7亿确诊病例，其中近700万人死亡[82]。各款疫苗在降低病毒的发病率和死亡率方面非常成功。但是，由于病毒的高变异性，仅通过接种疫苗难以为人类提供持久且充分的保护[83, 84]。GRM被寄望用于抗病毒研究。如图9-8所示，Wang等[85]通过MD模拟研究了石墨烯、NGO和缺陷石墨烯与M^{pro}（SARS-COV-2的重要靶蛋白）之间的相互作用。该研究发现，NGO和缺陷石墨烯更容易吸附M^{pro}，并使其活性口袋更加灵活，从而适应来自不同位置和方向的底物，因此缺陷石墨烯和NGO可能更适合作为有效的小分子抑制剂载体并用于抗病毒药物递送。

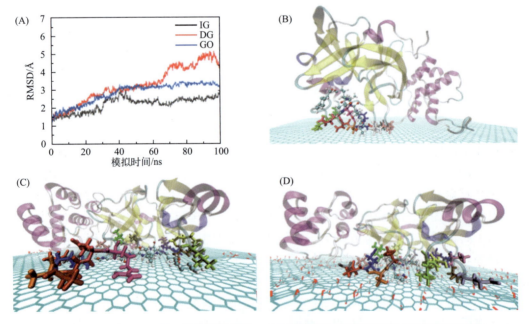

图9-8 三种GRM用于药物递送策略。NGO和缺陷石墨烯吸附M^{pro}使活性口袋更加灵活，有助于抗病毒药物的联合使用[85]

氟化石墨烯（FG）和氟化氧化石墨烯（FGO）是另一类重要的GRM，这类材料通过将氟原子连接到石墨烯以及NGO的碳原子上而制成[86]。为了探索这类材料在生物医学中的应用，Gu等[87]通过MD模拟详细阐述了FG与磷脂双分子层在分子水平上的相互作用，为FG作为药物递送平台提供了理论基础。此外，Romero-Aburto等[88]合成了FGO，该材料不仅具有磁性，还具有多样的化学官能团和出色的负载能力。换言之，FGO可以用作靶向药物载体和近红外激光诱导的热材料，用于消融热敏癌细胞。如将FGO与多柔比星等药物连接起来，有助于实现对肿瘤环境或特定组织的选择性靶向。总之，他们认为，通过改进FGO并搭配不同的尺寸，以及在体内外试验高温疗法和靶向FGO释放药物的协同作用，将使FGO成为治疗各种疾病的更具吸引力的选择。

碳基材料的杂原子（BC_3、NC_3、C_2N、C_3N_4等）替代可以扩展碳基材料的生物医学应用。先于实验，科学家已通过MD模拟研究了这些材料与生物分子之间的相互作用机制，以评估它们的应用潜力。例如，Deng等[89]研究了dsDNA与BC_3和C_3N的结合模式、结构稳定性和扩散动力学。通过研究发现，与石墨烯相比，BC_3和NC_3对dsDNA的结构破坏并不明显，从而表现出较好的生物相容性。且由于dsDNA与基底具有不同的结合亲和力，BC_3/石墨烯和NC_3/石墨烯平面异质结能够有效引导高度定向的dsDNA输运。这种定向输运为设计DDS提供了新思路。Jia等[90]研究了BC_3、NC_3与YAP65WW结构域（一种模型蛋白）之间的相互作用，研究结果表明，异元素掺杂能够有效调节YAP65WW与这两种纳米材料之间的结合特性，为开发和生产具有所需功能的先进纳米材料提供了理论基础。Gu等[91, 92]通过MD模拟研究了C_3N_4和C_3N的生物相容性，结果表明C_3N_4可以作为蛋白质药物输送平台。如图9-9所示，C_3N对HP_{35}蛋白（一种广泛用于折叠研究的模型蛋白质）具有潜在的变性能力。Shariatinia等[93]评估了一种CHS纳米复合材料的传递效率，该材料由氮或磷掺杂的石墨烯纳米颗粒组成，并以环磷酰胺作为模型药物，该研究为寻找最佳的DDS提供了宝贵的见解。

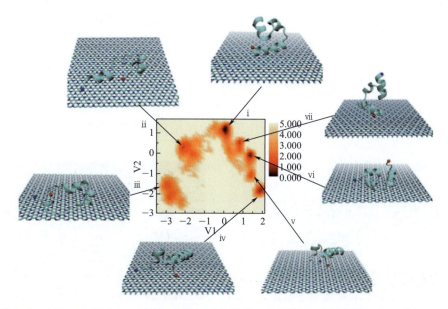

图9-9 HP_{35}的dPCA。对来自6组独立轨迹的dPCA的两个最低特征向量进行投影，得到了HP_{35}与C_3N纳米片之间相互作用的自由能表面[92]

9.3.2 硅基纳米材料

除了碳基纳米材料外，硅基纳米材料如介孔 SiO_2 和硅纳米颗粒也因其优良的生物安全性和独特的性质而受到了广泛的关注。介孔 SiO_2 具有高比表面积、显著的孔隙、巨大的药物载荷能力、优异的生物相容性以及易于化学修饰等特点，被认为是一种理想的药物载体[94]。CHS 作为第二大天然多糖，具备生物相容性、无毒性和可降解性等一系列有价值的特性。在体内，它被分解为无害的产物，因此成为生物医学应用中的理想材料。如图9-10所示，Shariatinia 等[95]通过 MD 模拟研究了三种基于 CHS、聚乳酸（polylactic acid，PLA）和 PEG 的 SiO_2 填充的聚合物纳米复合材料对抗癌药物氯氨丁胺（chlorambucil）药物的传递。研究结果表明，基于 CHS 的 DDS 具有最佳的药物递送和扩散性能，表明其在三种 DDS 中的优越性。

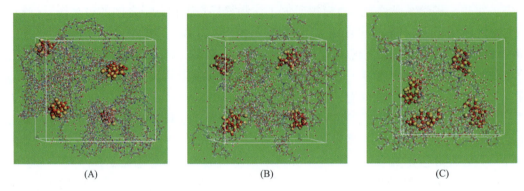

图9-10 MD 模拟运行后得到的（A）CHS、（B）PLA 和（C）PEG-SiO_2 聚合物的 DDS 快照[95]

对于每种 DDS，确定包裹在球形纳米颗粒周围的单层蛋白质的最大数量是非常重要的。为了解决这个问题，Soloviev 等[96]开发了一种几何模型，用于确定可以作为单层包裹球形纳米颗粒的理论上的最大蛋白质数量，并通过 MD 模拟验证了 SARS-CoV-2 刺突蛋白受体结合域（receptor binding domain，RBD）与 SiO_2 纳米颗粒之间的吸附作用（图9-11）。这项研究工作为 RBD 与 SiO_2 纳米颗粒的结合程度、可能的定向性和结构完整性损失提供了新的见解。此外，在生物材料中控制药物的释放非常重要，尤其是在药物通过生物屏障进行扩散时。因此，Raffaini 等[97]通过 MD 模拟研究了无定形 SiO_2 表面与抗炎药物酮洛芬（ketoprofen）之间的潜在相互作用。考虑到药物浓度的影响，将模拟结果与实验数据进行比较发现，当药物浓

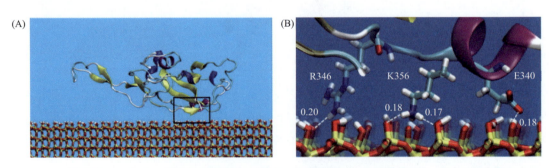

图9-11 RBD 与 SiO_2 相互作用的 MD 模拟。（A）模拟结束时，RBD 吸附在 SiO_2 表面的代表性构型。（B）与 SiO_2 密切接触的三个氨基酸残基[96]

度较高时，药物分子之间会发生疏水相互作用，使得这些药物分子可良好地分散在无定形SiO_2表面上（图9-12）。这一发现再次强调了生物材料的外表面的重要性，并为利用硅纳米载体用于药物释放提供了新的见解。

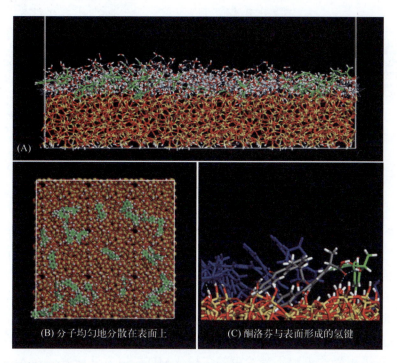

图9-12　MD模拟结束后，14个酮洛芬药物分子吸附在水合无定形SiO_2表面上的几何结构[97]

9.3.3　金属基纳米材料

一些金属基纳米材料也被应用于药物递送研究领域。例如，金（Au）、银（Ag）和钯（Pd）等纯金属纳米颗粒。

AuNP具有良好的生物相容性、体内相容性、光学性质和表面化学修饰等特点，其在生物医学领域得到了广泛的研究。根据先前的研究，AuNP能够穿过细胞核、细胞质、肿瘤血管等，这一特性为开发Au基DDS提供了良好的理论基础。此外，AuNP可以通过多糖、蛋白质、肽、脂肪酸、质粒或寡核苷酸进行功能化，但是不同的功能化对AuNP的生物学影响还需要进一步阐明。也就是说，AuNP的表面功能化对于设计DDS至关重要。计算模拟可以系统且直观地探索不同表面性质的AuNP与生物大分子之间的相互作用。例如，Maity等[98]通过实验和MD模拟研究了不同相态（室温下的凝胶相和液晶相）下，苯丙氨酸功能化的AuNP（Au-Phe NP）与不同的两性离子脂质囊泡之间的相互作用。研究结果表明，Au-Phe NP与不同脂质双层的相互作用会导致脂质诱导的聚集或冠状物的形成，这具体取决于相态、每个脂质头基的面积以及缓冲介质等。DPPC、DMPC、DLPC和DOPC的高脂质浓度导致了冠状物的形成，为纳米颗粒提供了额外的稳定性。此外，如图9-13所示，Farcas等[99]对巯基修饰的AuNP进行了MD模拟，为共轭纳米颗粒的设计提供了洞察力。该项研究成功地证明了AuNP的大小和巯基修饰的表面覆盖度是控制这些巯基修饰纳米颗粒性能的关键因素，这个结论有助于研究人员设计基于AuNP的递送载体。

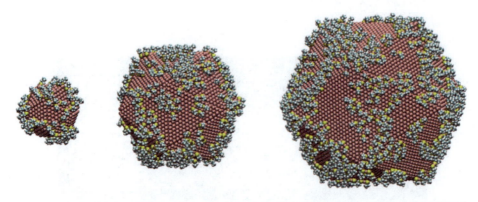

图9-13 巯基修饰的AuNP。5 nm（左）、10 nm（中）和15 nm（右）AuNP的图像，每个AuNP表面的巯基覆盖度为25%[99]

当然，MD模拟也常被用于探索AuNP与生物分子之间的互作机制。在生理条件下控制生物医学纳米颗粒的聚集至关重要。Lavagna等[100]通过MD模拟直观地展示了由阴离子、两亲性壳功能化的AuNP在两性离子脂质双层中的自发组装。另外，皮肤递送作为局部或全身分布途径，与口服、静脉注射、肌内注射和其他传统途径相比具有许多优势。然而，由于生物分子（如蛋白质）的大小和结构特征，通过皮肤递送它们是具有一定挑战性的。因此，了解它们在分子水平上穿越皮肤屏障的转运方式对于成功设计DDS来说是必不可少的。为此，Gupta等[101]采用受约束和不受约束的粗粒化MD模拟方法研究了在AuNP存在和不存在的情况下，辣根过氧化物酶（horseradish peroxidase，HRP）蛋白渗透到皮肤中的分子机制[101]。当HRP单独存在时，在皮肤脂质层中存在自由能壁垒，阻止HRP突破皮肤屏障。而在AuNP存在的情况下，HRP首先与AuNP结合，然后突破屏障。基于分子建模，该研究为经皮递送特定蛋白质的载体设计提供了见解。此外，Tavanti等[102]通过多尺度MD模拟探讨了血红蛋白、肌红蛋白和胰蛋白酶在柠檬酸修饰的AuNP表面的吸附信息，并详细描述了以下内容：①识别过程；②参与早期冠状物形成的蛋白质数量；③被AuNP吸附的蛋白质之间的竞争；④AuNP与蛋白质结合位点之间的相互作用模式，以及⑤蛋白质结构的保持和变化。这项工作展示了MD模拟的优势：可以直观地展示吸附过程，并解释分子水平上的吸附机制。

银纳米颗粒（silver nanoparticles，AgNP）也因其在抗癌、抗菌和抗病毒剂的显著潜力而在生物医学中得到了应用[103]。AgNP对硫和磷具有很高的亲和力，因此会影响细胞的存活能力。也就是说，AgNP易与细菌细胞膜中含硫的蛋白质以及DNA中含有磷的部分结合，以此破坏细胞膜以及抑制DNA活性[104]。此外，在诸如血清、血浆或黏液等生物流体中，纳米材料与蛋白质的相互作用会进一步导致不同聚集体的形成，并引起各种生物化学和生物物理反应。这些反应可能导致蛋白质和纳米材料之间形成生物冠，而这种生物冠为纳米材料提供了一种"新的身份"，帮助它们逃避免疫监视，使其能够穿过细胞膜并与细胞内的各种成分相互作用，包括细胞器、脂质双分子层、蛋白质、DNA和其他生物分子等。而药物分子可以与这些纳米材料结合，形成靶向递送的DDS。因此，不同类型、形状、尺寸、表面性质的纳米颗粒与不同类型的生物分子之间的相互作用机制对于设计 DDS 至关重要。通过分子建模，可以预先筛选和设计安全、最佳的"药物载体/偶合剂/纳米复合材料"。Subbotina 等[105]使用 UnitedAtom 多尺度方法对各种生物分子和 AgNP 之间的相互作用进行了系统的研究。结合实验数据并通过计算一组血浆和膳食蛋白质来评估 UnitedAtom 多尺度方法的性能，最后测试了一组界面描述符（$\log P^{NM}$、吸附亲和力和吸附亲和力排序），用以表征 AgNP 的相对疏水性/亲水性/亲脂性以及它们形成生物冠的能力。这项工作对于纳米材料的发展、纳米颗粒的蛋白质冠层成分以及 DDS 的预筛选具有重要意义。类似地，Sarker 等[106]采用多尺度模拟研究 AgNP 的尺寸和表面亲水性对肽冠形成动力学和结构的影响。结果显示，单个肽在 AgNP 表面的附着倾向性取决于 AgNP 的曲率、大小等因素，且在较大的表面观察到更强的附着倾向性。如图 9-14 所示，尽管肽可以吸附在直径为 3.2 nm 的 AgNP 表面上，但仍可能发生脱附现象。相比之下，在直径为 10 nm 的 AgNP 表面上，这种吸附-脱附-再吸附现象明显较少。由于具有充足的表面积和表面相互作用位点，可供多个肽同时吸附以及作用，大部分吸附的肽可牢固附着在其表面，这也表明尺寸在设计基于 AgNP 的 DDS 中至关重要。

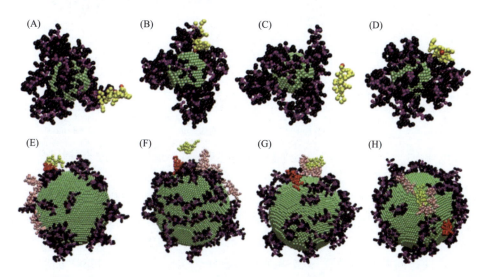

图 9-14　肽的吸附-脱附-再吸附循环。肽（黄色球体）（A）首先吸附在蛋白质聚集体上，（B）然后短暂地附着在 3.2 nm AgNP 表面上，（C）该肽脱附以及（D）再吸附。（E）~（H）为肽在 10 nm 表面上的吸附-脱附-再吸附模式[106]

钯纳米颗粒（palladium nanoparticle，PdNP）在有机催化和生物医学领域也受到了广泛关注。Palem 等[107]强调环境友好的 PdNP 具有普遍的抗氧化、化疗和抗菌活性，这使得 PdNP 在生物医学领域具有巨大的应用前景。同样，PdNP 的实际应用受其尺寸、形状、稳定性和其他因素的影响。如图 9-15 所示，Cao 等[108]通过实验和 MD 模拟研究了 *Candida antarctic* 脂肪酶 B 与 PdNP 之间的界面对于酶结构的调节作用、动力学特征和催化作用。结果表明，他们之间的相互作用遵循形状匹配机制，且随着 PdNP 的尺寸增加，它们之间的结合从饱和向不饱和转变。这项工作有助于研究人员理解生物纳米界面的作用以及合理设计先进生物纳米复合材料。

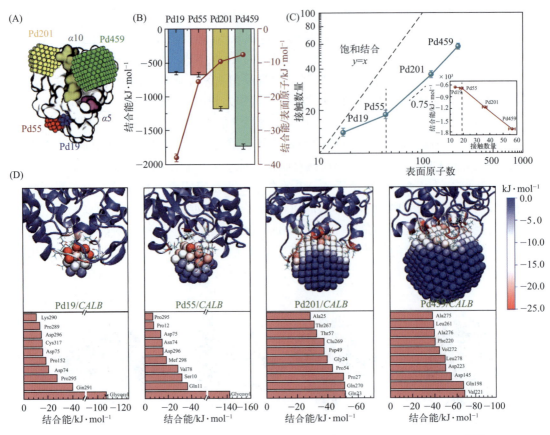

图9-15 *Candida antarctic* 脂肪酶B与不同尺寸PdNP之间的结合行为[108]

除了纯金属纳米颗粒外，科学家还深入研究了金属氧化物/硫化物等纳米颗粒。在各种金属氧化物中，IONP表现出超顺磁性、良好的生物相容性和分散性，因而被认为在生物医学领域具有潜在的应用价值。例如，氧化铁纳米颗粒（IONP）可用作核磁共振成像的对比剂，以及特异性靶向药物递送载体和基因治疗载体。实际上，磁性IONP的实际应用也取决于它们（尤其是表面）与生物分子的相互作用。众所周知，淀粉样蛋白的错误折叠和聚集可能是阿尔茨海默病和帕金森病的主要原因。而随着全球范围内老龄化现象的显著增加，这些疾病患者的数量也在不断增加，这对人类健康构成了重大威胁。为此，Andrikopoulos等[109]合成了一种多功能的淀粉样蛋白聚集抑制剂β-酪蛋白-IONP，通过实验和MD模拟研究了β-酪蛋白-IONP对β淀粉样蛋白（β-amyloid protein，Aβ）、α-突触核蛋白（α-synaptic nucleoprotein，αS）和人胰岛淀粉样多肽（human islet amyloid polypeptide，IAPP）聚集的抑制作用。该研究发现β-酪蛋白-IONP在体外有效抑制了Aβ、αS和IAPP的积累。MD模拟结果表明，β-酪蛋白的吸附是由IONP表面的疏水聚集体驱动的，导致构象扩展并使更多的疏水性残基暴露出来，从而有效地结合淀粉样肽。

与常规涂层的IONP相比，新型的裸露表面活性磁赤铁矿纳米颗粒（naked surface active maghemite nanoparticles，SAMN）可以共价结合DNA。例如带有GFP编码基因的质粒（pDNA）被直接化学吸附到SAMN上，从而产生了新的DNA纳米载体（SAMN@pDNA）。Magro等[110]通过实验和MD模拟计算了SAMN@pDNA的相关性质，并认为SAMN可以被视为高效细胞转染的新型智能DNA纳米载体。还有一些其他金属氧化物纳米颗粒的MD模拟研究。例如，Hosseinali等[111]研究了氧化镍纳米颗粒（nickel oxide nanoparticle，NiONP）对tau蛋白结构的影响。该研究证实NiONP可能对神经系统产生不良影响，这对基于NiONP的DDS的设计具有重要意义。

在众多金属硫化物纳米材料中，二硫化钼（MoS_2）是一种受到广泛关注并具有潜在应用前景的二维材料。MoS_2的物理化学性质类似于石墨烯，其高近红外吸收和广泛的表面积使其成为新型光热响应药物递送的理想平台[112]。为了解MoS_2与各种生物分子之间的详细互作机制，Gu等[113]通过MD模拟研究了MoS_2与HP_{35}之间的相互作用（图9-16），研究结果表明，MoS_2对HP_{35}具有显著的破坏作用，可能会带来严重的纳米毒性风险。有趣的是，随后Gu等[114]对用于描述MoS_2和HP_{35}之间相互作用的力场进行了修正，进一步的MD模拟结果显示，MoS_2对HP_{35}的破坏作用并没有之前报道的那么显著。这项研究间接强调了力场在MD模拟中的重要性。

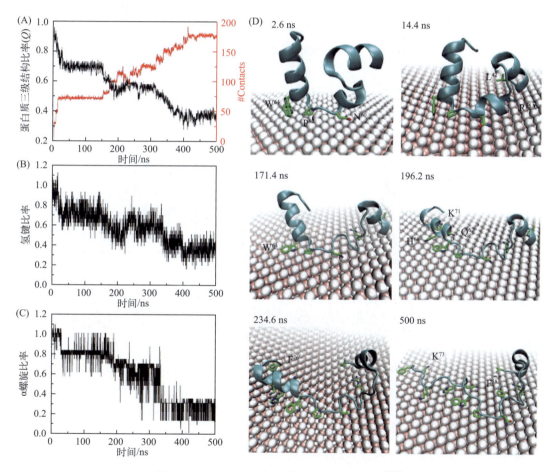

图9-16　HP_{35}在MoS_2表面的结构动力学[113]

9.3.4　其他纳米材料

近年来，大量新型纳米材料涌现，尽管它们在生物医学领域的应用仍相对有限。然而，这些新兴纳米材料具有为DDS的开发提供有价值见解的潜力。氮化硼纳米管（boron nitride nanotube，BNT）与CNT结构相似，它的机械、热学、电学、磁学和其他物理化学性质已被广泛研究。在生物医学领域，Luo等[115]通过将紧束缚密度泛函理论（tight-binding density functional theory，DFTB）与MD模拟相结合，系统地探讨和描述了BNT曲率对蛋白质结构的影响（图9-17）。结果表明，随着BNT曲率的降低，稳定吸附的氨基酸数量和结合强度显著增加。这项研究证明了BNT的曲率不仅影响吸附氨基酸的类型和结合强度，而且间接影响蛋白质的吸附。这项研究为BNT在药物递送中的应用提供了微观视角。

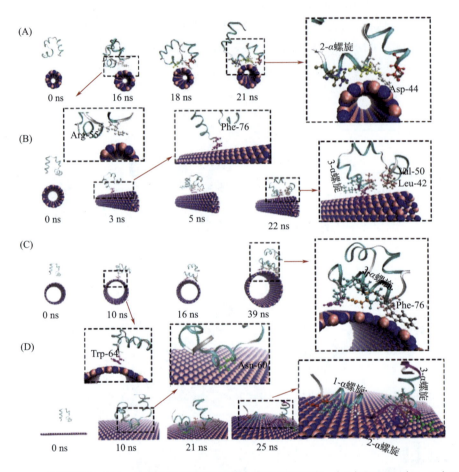

图9-17　50 ns模拟期间，HP$_{35}$与不同曲率的氮化硼之间的关键构象：（A）HP$_{35}$-（5，5）BNT，（B）HP$_{35}$-（10，10）BNT，（C）HP$_{35}$-（20，20）BNT，和（D）HP$_{35}$-BN[115]

此外，MBP引起了广泛关注。在结构上，MBP由两个磷原子层组成，每个磷原子与三个相邻原子形成共价键。因此，这种排列导致了沿着纵向方向的褶皱结构。同时通过第一原理计算，研究人员理论预测了一种新的二维材料α相磷碳化合物（α-phase phosphorus carbide，α-PC）。α-PC可以看作是在MBP的脊线上引入碳原子。因此，α-PC保持了折叠结构和各向异性，这使得其在生物医学研究中备受期待。为此，Liu等[116]通过MD模拟研究了α-PC和MBP与HP$_{35}$之间的结合动力学、结构稳定性和生物相容性。结果表明，α-PC和MBP具有良好的生物相容性，形成了增强蛋白质横向扩散的异质结构。然而，蛋白质似乎被禁止穿过α-PC凹槽。换句话说，α-PC可有效引导蛋白质扩散。这一发现对利用各向异性纳米结构开发靶向DDS具有重要意义。

9.3.5 分子动力学在药物递送系统中的其他应用

分子动力学（MD）在药物设计与开发过程中变得越来越重要。在前面的章节中，深入介绍了如何利用MD研究不同纳米颗粒的递送策略。除此之外，MD在DDS领域有着广泛的应用，例如探索纳米颗粒和药物靶标的结构和功能特征、药物的装载和控制释放、药物的溶解和溶解度等[117, 118]。本节将简要介绍MD在这些领域的一些应用。

了解纳米颗粒的固有属性可以为基于纳米颗粒的DDS设计提供有价值的理论指导。例如，Zojaji等[119]通过MD模拟研究了GO和SiO$_2$纳米颗粒的形状和尺寸对流体剪切增稠行为的影响。结果表明，将锯齿形状的GO和立方体形状的SiO$_2$纳米颗粒添加到原始流体中将最大限度地增加该原子结构的黏度。聚己内酯（polycaprolactone，PCL）是一种常见的聚（羟基酸）型生物聚合物。Ezquerro等[120]利用MD模拟预测了PCL的界面区域以及纳米复合系统的结构和机械性能，并探索了羟基（未接枝）和PEG（接枝或PEG化）功能化的SiO$_2$两种类型的纳米颗粒。结果表明，PEG化纳米颗粒增强了SiO$_2$纳米颗粒和PCL基质之间的亲和力，从而改善了分散性能，但似乎并未进一步提高复合材料的力学性能。通常，GRM对生物体系的毒性与其分散状态密切相关，使得了解GRM在溶液中的聚集对于设计DDS非常关键[121]。因此，Tang等[122]通过MD模拟研究了GRM的聚集过程以及离子功能团、溶液pH、金属阳离子、天然有机物、尺寸和密度对该过程的影响。这项工作提供了对不同溶液化学条件下GRM聚集过程的分子水平上的理解。此外，润湿性梯度因其在纳米和微米尺度上改善单向液体传输的潜力而受到关注，特别是在快速药物递送和高效热传输领域[123, 124]。如图9-18所示，Papadopoulou等[125]发现图案化的石墨烯表面可以实现极快的水传输速度，超出了宏观尺度的预期。通过MD模拟发现，增加的传输速度归因于移动液滴的前进和后退接触角的变化，这种接触角滞后和随后的传输取决于表面图案和液滴尺寸。最后，研究者提出了一个关于具有不同润湿性的石墨烯表面上水的归一化摩擦系数的标度定律和模型。这项工作对于指导有效、快速和精确的药物递送具有重要意义。

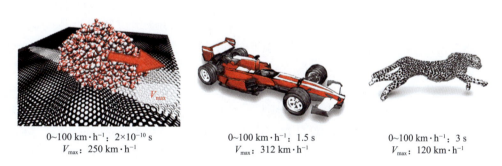

0~100 km·h^{-1}；2×10^{-10} s
V_{max}：250 km·h^{-1}

0~100 km·h^{-1}；1.5 s
V_{max}：312 km·h^{-1}

0~100 km·h^{-1}；3 s
V_{max}：120 km·h^{-1}

图9-18　图案化石墨烯表面上水纳米液滴的超快推进[125]

MD模拟可以为药物靶标的设计提供重要见解，例如探索药物靶标的结构特征，并研究突变和pH等因素对靶标功能的影响。例如，Kneller等[126]研究了M^{pro}活性位点的灵活性，这有助于其抑制剂的设计。Barazorda-Ccahuana等[127]通过MD模拟研究了pH对M^{pro}结构的影响，结果表明 M^{pro} 在中性 pH 条件下最稳定，在碱性 pH 条件下不稳定。Amamuddy 等[128]研究了 M^{pro} 突变体的结构特征。其次，MD 模拟可以探索药物靶标与配体之间的结合关系。Baig 等[129]结合分子对接、虚拟筛选和 MD 模拟研究了抑制剂分子对 M^{pro} 及其突变体的抑制效果，发现 PF-00835231 不仅对野生型有效，对突变体也具有较高亲和力。类似地，Bharadwaj 等[130]结合虚拟筛选、分子对接、量子化学计算、ADMET 分析、MD 模拟和量子力学/分子力学（quantum mechanics，QM/molecular mechanics，MM）计算，成功地发现了可以抑制 M^{pro} 活性的化合物。这项工作对设计针对 SARS-CoV-2 的药物具有重要意义[130]。

MD 也适用于研究不同纳米颗粒的药物装载和释放能力。Mousavi 等[131]研究了壳聚糖纳米颗粒（CHS-NP）对多奈哌齐（donepezil）和利他林（rivastigmine）药物分子的吸附能力。与多奈哌齐系统相比，利他林系统中 CHS-NP 的药物装载能力有所降低。Monti 等[132]采用 MD 和反应力场（ReaxFF）方法研究了功能化 CHS 修饰、多柔比星负载的 AuNP 的结构、动力学和药物释放行为。研究结果显示，药物载荷能力受载体的大小、CHS 聚合物链的长度以及纳米颗粒合成技术的影响。此外，以一定比例和顺序沉积 CHS 和多柔比星层能更有效地调控药物的释放和维持。

MD 模拟在 DDS 中的另一个应用是深入了解溶解和溶剂化的过程机制。Lehto 等[133]结合实验和 MD 模拟研究揭示了有机分子在水溶液中与 C_{60} 共聚合的容易性。有机溶剂从外部覆盖 C_{60}，只有少量有机分子存在于团簇内部[133]。提高不溶性药物的溶解度在制药行业中至关重要，而与环糊精（cyclodextrin，CD）络合常用于提高不溶性药物的溶解度。为此，Zhao 等[134]通过 MD 模拟和实验方法成功开发了一种叶黄素-环糊精多组分递送系统（lutein-CD-MCDS），该系统显著提高了药物的溶解度和生物利用度[134]。

9.4 总结

无疑，MD 模拟方法为设计 DDS 提供了快速和高效的解决方案，几乎不受时间和空间的限制。这些方法既简化了实验，又提供了理论探索，且进一步减少了对复杂实验的需求，为 DDS 提供了有力支持。本章全面回顾了纳米颗粒在 DDS 中的应用进展，并进一步讨论了各种分子建模方法。具体而言，我们专注于利用经典牛顿力学基于 MD 模拟的不同纳米颗粒递送策略。需要注意的是，基于量子化学的 MD 模拟可能不适用于生物体系。

随着计算能力的提高和算法的优化，可以使用 MD 模拟更大规模的体系以及更长的时间尺度。其次，多尺度模拟研究变得愈发重要，包括 MD 模拟、第一性原理计算、蒙特卡洛（Monte Carlo，MC）模拟、QM/MM 计算、有限元分析（finite element analysis，FEA）等。结合多尺度方法研究基于纳米颗粒的 DDS 变得愈发可行，这代表了未来的研究趋势。

未来，MD 模拟、计算辅助药物设计（computer-aided drug design，CADD）和人工智能（artificial intelligence，AI）的联合使用有望加速药物研发。机器学习可以显著加快药物筛选与设计的速度，使得 CADD 正加速演变为人工智能辅助药物设计（AI drug design，AIDD）。与传统方法相比，AIDD 可以更快速、更准确地识别潜在的药物候选物，使其正成为药物研发中强有力的工具。因此，进一步将 AIDD 和 MD 模拟整合也是未来的研究趋势之一。

此外，MD的准确性与经验力场有关。有趣的是，类似于DeePMD，机器学习也用于开发和训练MD模拟所需的力场。然而，受限于目前算法和计算能力，将DeePMD应用于生物体系仍存在挑战。解决这些限制也是其未来的研究趋势。

参考文献

[1] Wang D, Dong H, Li M, et al. Hyaluronic acid encapsulated CuS gel-mediated near-infrared laser-induced controllable transdermal drug delivery for sustained therapy[J]. ACS Sustainable Chemistry & Engineering, 2017, 5(8): 6786-6794.

[2] Delahousse J, Skarbek C, Paci A. Prodrugs as drug delivery system in oncology[J]. Cancer Chemotherapy and Pharmacology, 2019, 84(5): 937-958.

[3] Peppas N A. Historical perspective on advanced drug delivery: How engineering design and mathematical modeling helped the field mature[J]. Advanced Drug Delivery Reviews, 2013, 65(1): 5-9.

[4] Zhu M, Whittaker A K, Han F Y, et al. Journey to the market: The evolution of biodegradable drug delivery systems[J]. Applied Sciences, 2022, 12(2): 935.

[5] Bácskay I, Ujhelyi Z, Fehér P, et al. The evolution of the 3D-printed drug delivery systems: A review[J]. Pharmaceutics, 2022, 14(7): 1312.

[6] Wang T, Zhang D, Sun D, et al. Current status of in vivo bioanalysis of nano drug delivery systems[J]. Journal of Pharmaceutical Analysis, 2020, 10(3): 221-232.

[7] Lombardo D, Kiselev M A, Caccamo M T. Smart nanoparticles for drug delivery application: Development of versatile nanocarrier platforms in biotechnology and nanomedicine[J]. Journal of Nanomaterials, 2019, 2019: 3702518.

[8] Shariatinia Z. Big family of nano-and microscale drug delivery systems ranging from inorganic materials to polymeric and stimuli-responsive carriers as well as drug-conjugates[J]. Journal of Drug Delivery Science and Technology, 2021, 66: 102790.

[9] Jain P K, El-Sayed I H, El-Sayed M A. Au nanoparticles target cancer[J]. Nano Today, 2007, 2(1): 18-29.

[10] van Dam B, Nie H, Ju B, et al. Carbon dots: Excitation-dependent photoluminescence from single-carbon dots[J]. Small, 2017, 13(48): 1770251.

[11] Krätschmer W, Lamb L D, Fostiropoulos K, et al. Solid C_{60}: a new form of carbon[J]. Nature, 1990, 347(6291): 354-358.

[12] Dresselhaus M S, Dresselhaus G, Saito R. Physics of carbon nanotubes[J]. Carbon, 1995, 33(7): 883-891.

[13] Novoselov K S, Fal' ko V I, Colombo L, et al. A roadmap for graphene[J]. Nature, 2012, 490(7419): 192-200.

[14] Bagheri S, Muhd Julkapli N. Nano-diamond based photocatalysis for solar hydrogen production[J]. International Journal of Hydrogen Energy, 2020, 45(56): 31538-31554.

[15] Feng L, Liu Z. Graphene in biomedicine: opportunities and challenges[J]. Nanomedicine, 2011, 6(2): 317-324.

[16] Ding H, Zhang F, Zhao C, et al. Beyond a carrier: graphene quantum dots as a probe for programmatically monitoring anti-cancer drug delivery, release, and response[J]. ACS Applied Materials & Interfaces, 2017, 9(33): 27396-27401.

[17] Dhiman S, Kaur A, Gupta, G. L, et al. Development and evaluation of biotin functionalized fullerenes for the delivery of Irinotecan to colon tumors[J]. Current Drug Delivery, 2023, 7(20): 978-991.

[18] Datir S R, Das M, Singh R P, et al. Hyaluronate tethered, "smart" multiwalled carbon nanotubes for tumor-targeted delivery of doxorubicin[J]. Bioconjugate Chemistry, 2012, 23(11): 2201-2213.

[19] Banerjee A N. Graphene and its derivatives as biomedical materials: future prospects and challenges[J]. Interface Focus, 2018, 8(3): 20170056.

[20] Pei S, Cheng, H M. The reduction of graphene oxide[J]. Carbon, 2012, 50(9): 3210-3228.

[21] Qu L, Liu Y, Baek J B, et al. Nitrogen-doped graphene as efficient metal-free electrocatalyst for oxygen reduction in fuel cells[J]. ACS Nano, 2010, 4(3): 1321-1326.

[22] Liu Z, Robinson J T, Sun X, et al. PEGylated nanographene oxide for delivery of water-insoluble cancer drugs[J]. Journal of the American Chemical Society, 2008, 130(33): 10876-10877.

[23] Yang K, Hu L, Ma X, et al. Multimodal imaging guided photothermal therapy using functionalized graphene nanosheets anchored with magnetic nanoparticles[J]. Advanced Materials, 2012, 24(14): 1868-1872.

[24] Jahanshahi M, Kowsari E, Haddadi-Asl V, et al. An innovative and eco-friendly modality for synthesis of highly fluorinated graphene by an acidic ionic liquid: Making of an efficacious vehicle for anti-cancer drug delivery[J]. Applied Surface Science, 2020, 515: 146071.

[25] Sun R, Liu M, Lu J, et al. Bacteria loaded with glucose polymer and photosensitive ICG silicon-nanoparticles for glioblastoma photothermal immunotherapy[J]. Nature Communications, 2022, 13(1): 5127.

[26] Wu Y J, Sun Z Q, Song J F, et al. Preparation of multifunctional mesoporous SiO_2 nanoparticles and anti-tumor action[J]. Nanotechnology, 2023, 34(5): 055101.

[27] Chen, W H, Luo G F, Lei Q, et al. Overcoming the heat endurance of tumor cells by interfering with the anaerobic glycolysis metabolism for improved photothermal therapy[J]. ACS Nano, 2017, 11(2): 1419-1431.

[28] Bai S, Yang N, Wang X, et al. Ultrasmall iron-doped titanium oxide nanodots for enhanced sonodynamic and chemodynamic cancer therapy[J]. ACS Nano, 2020, 14(11): 15119-15130.

[29] Song G, Hao J, Liang C, et al. Degradable molybdenum oxide nanosheets with rapid clearance and efficient tumor homing capabilities as a therapeutic nanoplatform[J]. Angewandte Chemie International Edition, 2016, 55(6): 2122-2126.

[30] Molaei M J, Salimi E. Magneto-fluorescent superparamagnetic Fe_3O_4@SiO_2@alginate/carbon quantum dots nanohybrid for drug delivery[J]. Materials Chemistry and Physics, 2022, 288: 126361.

[31] Mollazadeh S, Sahebkar A, Shahlaei M, et al. Nano drug delivery systems: Molecular dynamic simulation[J]. Journal of Molecular Liquids, 2021, 332: 115823.

[32] Alder B J, Wainwright T E. Phase transition for a hard sphere system[J]. The Journal of Chemical Physics, 2004, 27(5): 1208-1209.

[33] Rahman A. Correlations in the motion of atoms in liquid argon[J]. Physical Review, 1964, 136(2A): A405-A411.

[34] Verlet L. Computer "Experiments" on Classical Fluids. I. Thermodynamical properties of Lennard-Jones molecules[J]. Physical Review, 1967, 159(1): 98-103.

[35] McCammon J A, Gelin B R, Karplus M. Dynamics of folded proteins[J]. Nature, 1977, 267(5612): 585-590.

[36] Andersen H C. Molecular dynamics simulations at constant pressure and/or temperature[J]. The Journal of Chemical Physics, 2008, 72(4): 2384-2393.

[37] Min B J. Critically damped verlet algorithm for the study of the structural properties of condensed matter systems[J]. Journal of the Korean Physical Society, 2005, 46(4): 872-874.

[38] Rahman A, Stillinger F H. Molecular dynamics study of liquid water[J]. Journal of Chemical Physics, 1971, 55(7): 3336.

[39] Beeman D. Some multistep methods for use in molecular-dynamics calculations[J]. Journal of Computational Physics, 1976, 20(2): 130-139.

[40] MacKerell A D. Bashford D, Bellott M, et al. All-atom empirical potential for molecular modeling and dynamics studies of proteins[J]. The Journal of Physical Chemistry B, 1998, 102(18): 3586-3616.

[41] Sun H. COMPASS: An ab initio force-field optimized for condensed-phase applications overview with details on alkane and benzene compounds[J]. The Journal of Physical Chemistry B, 1998, 102(38): 7338-7364.

[42] Mayo S L, Olafson B D, Goddard W A. DREIDING: a generic force field for molecular simulations[J]. The Journal of Physical Chemistry, 1990, 94(26): 8897-8909.

[43] Case D A, Cheatham III T E, Darden T, et al. The amber biomolecular simulation programs[J]. Journal of Computational Chemistry, 2005, 26(16): 1668-1688.

[44] Jorgensen W L, Tirado-Rives J. The OPLS [optimized potentials for liquid simulations] potential functions for proteins, energy minimizations for crystals of cyclic peptides and crambin[J]. Journal of the American Chemical Society, 1988, 110(6): 1657-1666.

[45] Lu T. Sobtop. Version 1.0(dev3.1)http://sobereva.com/soft/Sobtop.

[46] Vanommeslaeghe K, Raman E P, MacKerell A D. Automation of the CHARMM General Force Field(CGenFF) II: Assignment of bonded parameters and partial atomic charges[J]. Journal of Chemical Information and Modeling, 2012, 52(12): 3155-3168.

[47] Wang J, Wang W, Kollman P A, et al. Automatic atom type and bond type perception in molecular mechanical calculations[J]. Journal of Molecular Graphics and Modelling, 2006, 25(2): 247-260.

[48] Schrödinger Release 2021-3: FEP+. Schrödinger, LLC: New York, 2021.

[49] Dassault Systèmes BIOVIA. Discovery Studio Modeling Environment, Release 2016, San Diego: Dassault Systèmes, 2015.

[50] Anandakrishnan R, Aguilar B, Onufriev A V. H++3.0: automating pK prediction and the preparation of biomolecular structures for atomistic molecular modeling and simulations[J]. Nucleic Acids Research, 2012, 40(W1): W537-W541.

[51] Olsson M H M, Søndergaard C R, Rostkowski M, et al. PROPKA3: Consistent treatment of internal and surface residues in empirical pK_a predictions[J]. Journal of Chemical Theory and Computation, 2011, 7(2): 525-537.

[52] Pearlman D A, Case D A, Caldwell J W, et al. AMBER, a package of computer-programs for applying molecular

mechanics, normal-mode analysis, molecular-dynamics and free-energy calculations to simulate the structural and energetic properties of molecules.[J] Computer Physics Communications, 1995, 91(1-3): 1-41.

[53] van Dijk M, Bonvin, A M J J, 3D-DART: a DNA structure modelling server[J]. Nucleic Acids Research, 2009, 37: W235-W239.

[54] Humphrey W, Dalke A, Schulten K. VMD: Visual molecular dynamics[J]. Journal of Molecular Graphics & Modelling, 1996, 14(1): 33-38.

[55] Martinez L, Andrade R, Birgin E G, et al. PACKMOL: A package for building initial configurations for molecular dynamics simulations[J]. Journal of Computational Chemistry, 2009, 30(13): 2157-2164.

[56] Jo S, Kim T, Iyer V G, et al. CHARMM-GUI: A web-based graphical user interface for CHARMM[J]. Journal of Computational Chemistry, 2008, 29(11): 1859-1865.

[57] Lu T, Chen F W. Multiwfn: A multifunctional wavefunction analyzer[J]. Journal of Computational Chemistry, 2012, 33(5): 580-592.

[58] Frisch M T G, Schlegel H, Scuseria G, et al. Gaussian 09, Revision D.01. Wallingford, CT: Gaussian Inc, 2013.

[59] Accelrys Materials Studio. National Computational Infrastructure National Facility.

[60] Jain A, Ong S P, Hautier G, et al. Commentary: The Materials Project: A materials genome approach to accelerating materials innovation[J]. APL Materials, 2013, 1(1): 011002.

[61] Larsen A H, Mortensen J J, Blomqvist J, et al. The atomic simulation environment-a Python library for working with atoms[J]. Journal of Physics-Condensed Matter, 2017, 29: 273002.

[62] Gasteiger J, Marsili M. Iterative partial equalization of orbital electronegativity-a rapid access to atomic charges[J]. Tetrahedron 1980, 36(22): 3219-3228.

[63] DeLano W L. Use of PYMOL as a communications tool for molecular science[J]. Abstracts of Papers of the American Chemical Society, 2004, 228: U313-U314.

[64] Jorgensen W L, Chandrasekhar J, Madura J D, et al. Comparison of simple potential functions for simulating liquid water[J]. Journal of Chemical Physics 1983, 79(2): 926-935.

[65] Hess B, Kutzner C, van der Spoel D, et al. GROMACS 4: Algorithms for highly efficient, load-balanced, and scalable molecular simulation[J]. Journal of Chemical Theory and Computation, 2008, 4(3): 435-447.

[66] Phillips J C, Braun R, Wang W, et al. Scalable molecular dynamics with NAMD[J]. Journal of Computational Chemistry, 2005, 26(16): 1781-1802.

[67] Eastman P, Swails J, Chodera J D, et al. OpenMM 7: Rapid development of high performance algorithms for molecular dynamics[J]. PLOS Computational Biology, 2017, 13(7): e1005659.

[68] Brooks B R, Brooks Ⅲ C L, Mackerell Jr. A D, et al. CHARMM: The biomolecular simulation program[J]. Journal of Computational Chemistry, 2009, 30(10): 1545-1614.

[69] Perini G, Palmieri V, Ciasca G, et al. Unravelling the potential of graphene quantum dots in biomedicine and neuroscience[J]. International Journal of Molecular Sciences, 2020, 21(10): 3712.

[70] Ren H. Molecular simulation of graphene quantum dots as carrier materials for anticancer drugs[D]. Hangzhou Normal University, 2021.

[71] Erimban S, Daschakraborty S. Translocation of a hydroxyl functionalized carbon dot across a lipid bilayer: an all-atom molecular dynamics simulation study[J]. Physical Chemistry Chemical Physics, 2020, 22(11): 6335-6350.

[72] Giannopoulos G I. Fullerene derivatives for drug delivery against COVID-19: A molecular dynamics investigation of dendro[60]fullerene as nanocarrier of molnupiravir[J]. Nanomaterials, 2022, 12(15): 2711.

[73] Gupta R, Rai B. Molecular dynamics simulation study of translocation of fullerene C_{60} through skin bilayer: effect of concentration on barrier properties[J]. Nanoscale, 2017, 9(12): 4114-4127.

[74] Cui X, Xu S, Wang X, et al. The nano-bio interaction and biomedical applications of carbon nanomaterials[J]. Carbon, 2018, 138: 436-450.

[75] Xue X, Yang J Y, He Y, et al. Aggregated single-walled carbon nanotubes attenuate the behavioural and neurochemical effects of methamphetamine in mice[J]. Nature Nanotechnology, 2016, 11(7): 613-620.

[76] Yu Y, Sun H, Gilmore K, et al. Aggregated single-walled carbon nanotubes absorb and deform dopamine-related proteins based on molecular dynamics simulations[J]. ACS Applied Materials & Interfaces, 2017, 9(38): 32452-32462.

[77] von Ranke N L, Castro H C, Rodrigues C R. Molecular modelling and dynamics simulations of single-wall carbon nanotube as a drug carrier: New insights into the drug-loading process[J]. Journal of Molecular Graphics and Modelling, 2022, 113: 108145.

[78] Luo N, Weber J K, Wang S, et al. PEGylated graphene oxide elicits strong immunological responses despite surface

passivation[J]. Nature Communications , 2017, 8(1): 14537.

[79] Chen S H, Perez-Aguilar J M, Zhou R. Graphene-extracted membrane lipids facilitate the activation of integrin αvβ8[J]. Nanoscale , 2020, 12(14): 7939-7949.

[80] Shen J W, Li J. Zhao Z. et al. Molecular dynamics study on the mechanism of polynucleotide encapsulation by chitosan[J]. Scientific Reports, , 2017, 7(1): 5050.

[81] Shen, J W.; Li J, Dai J, et al. Molecular dynamics study on the adsorption and release of doxorubicin by chitosan-decorated graphene[J]. Carbohydrate Polymers , 2020, 248: 116809.

[82] Dong E, Ratcliff J, Goyea T D, et al. The Johns Hopkins University Center for Systems Science and Engineering COVID-19 Dashboard: data collection process, challenges faced, and lessons learned[J]. The Lancet Infectious Diseases , 2022, 22(12): e370-e376.

[83] Krammer F. SARS-CoV-2 vaccines in development[J]. Nature , 2020, 586(7830): 516-527.

[84] Zhao F, Zai X, Zhang Z, et al. Challenges and developments in universal vaccine design against SARS-CoV-2 variants[J]. npj Vaccines , 2022, 7(1): 167.

[85] Wang J, Yu Y, Leng T, et al. The inhibition of SARS-CoV-2 3CL Mpro by graphene and its derivatives from molecular dynamics simulations[J]. ACS Applied Materials & Interfaces , 2022, 14(1): 191-200.

[86] Cheng L, Jandhyala S, Mordi G, et al. Partially fluorinated graphene: Structural and electrical characterization[J]. ACS Applied Materials & Interfaces , 2016, 8(7): 5002-5008.

[87] Gu Z, Xie G, Perez-Aguilar J M. Fluorinated graphene nanomaterial causes potential mechanical perturbations to a biomembrane[J]. Journal of Molecular Modeling , 2022, 28(2): 49.

[88] Romero-Aburto R, Narayanan T N, Nagaoka Y, et al. Fluorinated graphene oxide: a new multimodal material for biological applications[J]. Advanced Materials , 2013, 25(39): 5632-5637.

[89] Deng Y, Wang F, Liu Y, et al. Orientational DNA binding and directed transport on nanomaterial heterojunctions[J]. Nanoscale , 2020, 12(8): 5217-5226.

[90] Jia X, Yang Y, Liu Y, et al. Tuning the binding behaviors of a protein YAP65WW domain on graphenic nano-sheets with boron or nitrogen atom doping[J]. Nanoscale Advances , 2020, 2(10): 4539-4546.

[91] Gu Z, Perez-Aguilar J M, Shao Q. Restricted binding of a model protein on C_3N_4 nanosheets suggests an adequate biocompatibility of the nanomaterial[J]. RSC Advances , 2021, 11(13): 7417-7425.

[92] Gu Z, Perez-Aguilar J M, Meng L, et al. Partial denaturation of villin headpiece upon binding to a carbon nitride polyaniline(C_3N)nanosheet[J]. The Journal of Physical Chemistry B , 2020, 124(35): 7557-7563.

[93] Shariatinia Z, Mazloom-Jalali A. Chitosan nanocomposite drug delivery systems designed for the ifosfamide anticancer drug using molecular dynamics simulations[J]. Journal of Molecular Liquids , 2019, 273: 346-367.

[94] Luo Z, Ding X, Hu Y, et al. Engineering a hollow nanocontainer platform with multifunctional molecular machines for tumor-targeted therapy in vitro and in vivo[J]. ACS Nano , 2013, 7(11): 10271-10284.

[95] Shariatinia Z, Jalali A M. Chitosan-based hydrogels: Preparation, properties and applications[J]. International Journal of Biological Macromolecules , 2018, 115: 194-220.

[96] Soloviev M, Siligardi G, Roccatano D, et al. Modelling the adsorption of proteins to nanoparticles at the solid-liquid interface[J]. Journal of Colloid and Interface Science , 2022, 605: 286-295.

[97] Raffaini G, Catauro M. Surface interactions between ketoprofen and silica-based biomaterials as drug delivery system synthesized via sol-gel: A molecular dynamics study[J]. Materials , 2022, 15(8): 2759.

[98] Maity A, De S K, Bagchi D, et al. Mechanistic pathway of lipid phase-dependent lipid corona formation on phenylalanine-functionalized gold nanoparticles: A combined experimental and molecular dynamics simulation study[J]. Journal of Physical Chemistry B , 2022, 126(11): 2241-2255.

[99] Farcas A, Janosi L, Astilean S. Size and surface coverage density are major factors in determining thiol modified gold nanoparticles characteristics[J]. Computational and Theoretical Chemistry , 2022, 1209: 113581.

[100] Lavagna E, Bochicchio D, De Marco A L, et al. Ion-bridges and lipids drive aggregation of same-charge nanoparticles on lipid membranes[J]. Nanoscale , 2022, 14: 6912-6921.

[101] Gupta R, Kashyap N, Rai B. Transdermal cellular membrane penetration of proteins with gold nanoparticles: a molecular dynamics study[J]. Physical Chemistry Chemical Physics , 2017, 19(11): 7537-7545.

[102] Tavanti F, Pedone A, Menziani M C. Multiscale molecular dynamics simulation of multiple protein adsorption on gold nanoparticles[J]. International Journal of Molecular Sciences , 2019, 20(14): 3539.

[103] Ghiuță I, Cristea D. Silver nanoparticles for delivery purposes[M]. In *Nanoengineered Biomaterials for Advanced Drug Delivery*, 2020, 347-371.

[104] Praphakar R A, Jeyaraj M, Ahmed M, et al. Silver nanoparticle functionalized CS-g-(CA-MA-PZA)carrier for sustainable anti-tuberculosis drug delivery[J]. International Journal of Biological Macromolecules, 2018, 118: 1627-1638.

[105] Subbotina J, Lobaskin V. Multiscale modeling of bio-nano interactions of zero-valent silver nanoparticles[J]. Journal of Physical Chemistry B, 2022, 126(6): 1301-1314.

[106] Sarker P, Sajib M S J, Tao X P, et al. Multiscale simulation of protein corona formation on silver nanoparticles: Study of ovispirin-1 peptide adsorption[J]. Journal of Physical Chemistry B, 2022, 126(3): 601-608.

[107] Palem R R, Shimoga G, Kim S Y, et al. Biogenic palladium nanoparticles: An effectual environmental benign catalyst for organic coupling reactions[J]. Journal of Industrial and Engineering Chemistry, 2022, 106: 52-68.

[108] Cao Y, Qiao Y, Cui S, et al. Origin of metal cluster tuning enzyme activity at the bio-nano interface[J]. JACS Au, 2022, 2(4): 961-971.

[109] Andrikopoulos N, Song Z Y, Wan X L, et al. Inhibition of amyloid aggregation and toxicity with janus iron oxide nanoparticles[J]. Chemistry of Materials, 2021, 33(16): 6484-6500.

[110] Magro M, Martinello T, Bonaiuto E, et al. Covalently bound DNA on naked iron oxide nanoparticles: Intelligent colloidal nano-vector for cell transfection[J]. Biochimica Et Biophysica Acta-General Subjects, 2017, 1861(11): 2802-2810.

[111] Hosseinali S H, Boushehri Z P, Rasti B, et al. Biophysical, molecular dynamics and cellular studies on the interaction of nickel oxide nanoparticles with tau proteins and neuron-like cells[J]. International Journal of Biological Macromolecules, 2019, 125: 778-784.

[112] Wang L, Wang Y, Wong J I, et al. Functionalized MoS_2 nanosheet-based field-effect biosensor for label-free sensitive detection of cancer marker proteins in solution[J]. Small, 2014, 10(6): 1101-1105.

[113] Gu Z L, Yang Z X, Kang S G, et al. Robust denaturation of villin headpiece by MoS_2 nanosheet: Potential molecular origin of the nanotoxicity[J]. Scientific Reports, 2016, 6: 28252.

[114] Gu Z L, De Luna P, Yang Z X, Zhou R H. Structural influence of proteins upon adsorption to MoS_2 nanomaterials: comparison of MoS_2 force field parameters[J]. Physical Chemistry Chemical Physics, 2017, 19(4): 3039-3045.

[115] Luo M, Yu Y, Jin Z, et al. Multi-scale simulations on biocompatibility of boron nitride nanomaterials with different curvatures: A comparative study[J]. Applied Surface Science, 2020, 517: 146181.

[116] Liu Y, Song X H, Yang Y M, et al. Anisotropic protein diffusion on nanosurface[J]. Nanoscale, 2020, 12(8): 5209-5216.

[117] Salo-Ahen, O M H, Alanko I, Bhadane R, et al. Molecular dynamics simulations in drug discovery and pharmaceutical development[J]. Processes, 2021, 9(1): 71.

[118] Bunker A, Rog T. Mechanistic understanding from molecular dynamics simulation in pharmaceutical research 1: Drug delivery[J]. Frontiers in Molecular Biosciences, 2020, 7.

[119] Zojaji M, Hydarinasab A, Hashemabadi S H, et al. Rheological study of the effects of size/shape of graphene oxide and SiO_2 nanoparticles on shear thickening behaviour of polyethylene glycol 400-based fluid: molecular dynamics simulation[J]. Molecular Simulation, 2022, 48(2): 120-130.

[120] Ezquerro C S, Aznar, J M G, Laspalas M. Prediction of the structure and mechanical properties of polycaprolactone-silica nanocomposites and the interphase region by molecular dynamics simulations: the effect of PEGylation[J]. Soft Matter, 2022, 18(14): 2800-2813.

[121] Chowdhury I, Duch M C, Mansukhani N D, et al. Colloidal Properties and Stability of Graphene Oxide Nanomaterials in the Aquatic Environment[J]. Environmental Science & Technology, 2013, 47(12): 6288-6296.

[122] Tang H, Zhao Y, Yang X N, et al. Understanding the roles of solution chemistries and functionalization on the aggregation of graphene-based nanomaterials using molecular dynamic simulations[J]. Journal of Physical Chemistry C, 2017, 121(25): 13888-13897.

[123] Zhang G Y, Zhang X, Li M, et al. A surface with superoleophilic-to-superoleophobic wettability gradient[J]. ACS Applied Materials & Interfaces, 2014, 6(3): 1729-1733.

[124] Brochard F. Motions of droplets on solid-surfaces induced by chemical or thermal-gradients[J]. Langmuir 1989, 5(2): 432-438.

[125] Papadopoulou E, Megaridis C M, Walther J H, et al. Ultrafast propulsion of water nanodroplets on patterned graphene[J]. ACS Nano, 2019, 13(5): 5465-5472.

[126] Kneller D W, Phillips G, O'Neill H M, et al. Structural plasticity of SARS-CoV-2 3CL M-pro active site cavity revealed by room temperature X-ray crystallography[J]. Nature Communications, 2020, 11(1): 3202.

[127] Barazorda-Ccahuana H L, Nedyalkova M, Mas F, et al. Unveiling the effect of low pH on the SARS-CoV-2 main protease by molecular dynamics simulations[J]. Polymers, 2021, 13(21): 3823.

[128] Amamuddy O S, Verkhivker G M, Bishop O T. Impact of early pandemic stage mutations on molecular dynamics of SARS-

CoV-2 M-pro[J]. Journal of Chemical Information and Modeling, 2020, 60(10): 5080-5102.

[129] Baig M H, Sharma T, Ahmad I, et al. Is PF-00835231 a Pan-SARS-CoV-2 Mpro inhibitor? A comparative study[J]. Molecules, 2021, 26(6): 1678.

[130] Bharadwaj S, Dubey A, Yadava U, et al. Exploration of natural compounds with anti-SARS-CoV-2 activity via inhibition of SARS-CoV-2 M-pro[J]. Briefings in Bioinformatics, 2021, 22(2): 1361-1377.

[131] Mousavi S V, Hashemianzadeh S M. Molecular dynamics approach for behavior assessment of chitosan nanoparticles in carrying of donepezil and rivastigmine drug molecules[J]. Materials Research Express, 2019, 6(4): 045069.

[132] Monti S, Jose J, Sahajan A, et al. Structure and dynamics of gold nanoparticles decorated with chitosan-gentamicin conjugates: ReaxFF molecular dynamics simulations to disclose drug delivery[J]. Physical Chemistry Chemical Physics, 2019, 21(24): 13099-13108.

[133] Lehto M, Karilainen T, Rog T, et al. Co-exposure with fullerene may strengthen health effects of organic industrial chemicals[J]. PLOS ONE, 2014, 9(12): e114490.

[134] Zhao Q Q, Miriyala N, Su Y, et al. Computer-aided formulation design for a highly soluble lutein-cyclodextrin multiple-component delivery system[J]. Molecular Pharmaceutics, 2018, 15(4): 1664-1673.

第 10 章

基于树枝状聚合物的递送技术与计算药剂学的结合及其在纳米医学时代的潜力

卡纳克·R. 图帕利（Karnaker R. Tupally） 昆士兰大学，澳大利亚

普拉桑吉特·西尔（Prasenjit Seal） 坦佩雷大学，芬兰

普里蒂·潘迪（Preeti Pandey） 昆士兰大学，澳大利亚

林克－扬·洛曼（Rink-Jan Lohman） 昆士兰大学，澳大利亚

肖恩·史密斯（Sean Smith） 澳大利亚国立大学，澳大利亚

欧阳德方 澳门大学，澳门，中国

哈伦德拉·帕雷克（Harendra Parekh） 昆士兰大学，澳大利亚

10.1 引言

新型冠状病毒感染为健康研究和药物研发带来了巨大的飞跃，推动了新的药物递送方式的出现，并且让人们意识到其在应对疫情和其他未满足的医疗需求方面的重要性。目前，基于大量临床证据，脂质纳米颗粒（lipid nanoparticle，LNP）已被广泛接受并普遍使用。这些基于脂质的制剂，特别是RNA疗法，现已出现在新冠疫苗中。为了应对新型冠状病毒感染并且尽快开发出疫苗，使用现有的脂质纳米颗粒进行肌内注射[1]。对于这种COVID-19 mRNA疫苗来说，脂质纳米颗粒的物理化学性质使其可以与RNA形成复合物，从而成为临床治疗的有效递送系统。然而，由于缺乏理化稳定性，特别是要求冷链储存条件和运输，脂质纳米颗粒系统仍然面临挑战[2, 3]。从长远来看，必须研究更适合环境条件的药物和基因系统的替代策略[2, 3]。树枝状聚合物是一种已被用于各种药物和基因递送应用的系统，它们似乎有很大的潜力获得临床使用批准[4, 5]。本章将回顾树枝状聚合物的现有知识，并且探讨其多样化的临床应用潜力。

树枝状聚合物是合成的有机大分子，具有对称和非对称分支树状结构且具有多种功能特征，这使其在药剂学领域具有多种应用。它不仅可以通过共价偶联、静电作用和络合作用与药物分子结合从而促进药物溶解，保护药物免受酸、酶攻击或活性氧等环境的影响，还可以加强膜相互作用从而促进生物屏障渗透。这些关键的物理化学优势使树枝状聚合物成为靶向给药的理想多功能载体系统[3, 4, 6, 7]。用树枝状聚合物递送的潜在疗法包括但不限于小分子、肽、遗传物质（核酸，如mRNA）和生物制剂（酶或抗体）。图10-1总结了树枝状聚合物的一般结构特征和不同的递送应用[6]。

用于药物递送的合成树枝状聚合物的理化性质的合理演变促进了树枝状、超支化、线性、星形和超分子树枝状聚合物结构的发展——图10-1也总结了树枝状聚合物的物理、化学、结构和表面功能化的多样性[6]。树枝状聚合物的化学多功能性使得具有多种性质的治疗分子通过静电或共价键（优先选择可裂解的键）连接，不同的核心化学成分可以通过各种封装、复合、胶束化和静电相互作用技术装载治疗药物。

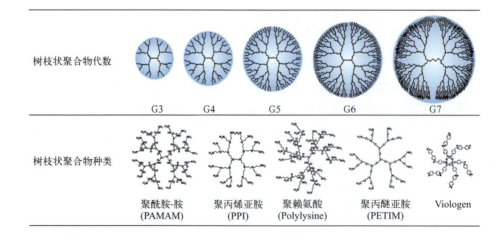

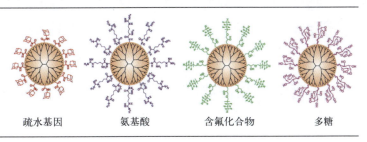

图10-1 树枝状聚合物及其典型类别、化学多样性、结构和表面功能化[6]

树枝状聚合物作为非病毒载体具有优势,通常通过表面官能团带有正电荷,使其能够与带负电荷的阴离子核酸结合,形成树枝复合物,从而有助于将遗传物质转染到细胞中。树枝状聚合物作为载体系统,还可以保护核酸免受酶促或化学降解,从而保持生物流体中和维持跨膜屏障的有效负载稳定性。总体而言,树枝状聚合物是高效的基因和药物递送系统;目前,一些国家已对携带药物分子或遗传物质的树枝状聚合物制剂进行了临床试验或监管审批。表10-1概述了已获批准和处于临床阶段的基于树枝状聚合物的产品。

表10-1 临床阶段和已上市的基于树枝状聚合物的产品

基于树枝状聚合物的产品	应用	树枝状聚合物类型	状态	参考文献
OP-101	减少严重新型冠状病毒感染中的炎症和神经损伤	羟基PAMAM树枝状聚合物	临床Ⅱ期	[7]
D-4517.2	新生血管性(湿性)年龄相关性黄斑变性(AMD)	羟基PAMAM树枝状聚合物	临床Ⅱ期	[4]
siCoV/KK46	减少COVID-19感染中的肺部炎症	基于聚赖氨酸	临床Ⅰ期	[5]
VIRALEZE™ Nasal Spray	预防COVID-19感染	基于赖氨酸的树枝状聚合物	已上市	[8]
Vivagel®BV	预防细菌性阴道病	基于赖氨酸的树枝状聚合物	已上市	[9]
Stratus®	心脏生物标志物的测量	基于PAMAM的树枝状聚合物	*已上市	[10]
Superfect®	转染剂	基于PAMAM的树枝状聚合物	*已上市	[11]
Priostar®	转染剂	基于赖氨酸的树枝状聚合物	*已上市	[12]
DEP™ docetaxel	抗癌剂	基于赖氨酸的树枝状聚合物	临床Ⅱ期	[13]

*销售用于实验室和其他用途,但不用于临床用途。

大多数药物递送系统通常是多组分的。同时，每个成分与治疗部分相互作用。然而，树枝状聚合物是具有多种优点的单一成分。计算建模、模拟和动态研究方面的技术发展极大地促进了对树枝状聚合物和药物的复合过程和潜在给药机制的理解。这些技术将有助于进一步改进树枝状聚合物的设计。与其他载体系统不同，树枝状聚合物化学结构的明确性质使其可以进行精确的建模，有助于创建理想的树枝状聚合物药物递送系统。这种计算方法及其重要性将有助于提高树枝状聚合物（如用于递送药物和其他物质的载体系统）的研究质量。

10.2　树枝状聚合物作为药物/基因递送系统及其制药应用

10.2.1　多功能载体系统

随着新型疗法和个性化医疗方面未得到满足的临床需求的日益增长，基于纳米颗粒的载体的潜力不断提高，这些纳米载体可以递送核酸（siRNA、mRNA）、蛋白质以及简单和复杂的药物分子[14, 15]。值得一提的是，纳米颗粒在合成上的多样性带来了连接化学的进步，使其能够结合多种治疗分子、靶向配体，实现隐形效果，并通过表面功能化结合成像剂，同时组装成纳米颗粒的核心结构也得到了优化[16, 17]。

众所周知，树枝状聚合物具有多样化的应用适应性和化学反应性，这使其成为多功能载体系统。值得注意的是，在治疗癌症时，最好避免有毒药物与正常组织接触，而目前的化疗药物往往会导致机体衰弱、剂量限制和不可接受的副作用。理想情况下，缓释机制可以延长药物释放情况，从而避免多次给药。树枝状聚合物有可能通过靶向递送（例如只递送到肿瘤细胞）来解决这些问题，并在到达靶标后提供缓释库，从而减少给药剂量、临床就诊次数和治疗成本。尽管临床上可用的树枝状聚合物载体系统并不多，但已经取得了重大进展和显著贡献。本节将讨论树枝状聚合物作为多功能载体系统的最新进展及其对于不同疾病治疗的优势。这些研究例证了树枝状聚合物系统作为多功能载体系统用于治疗一系列疾病的多样性[6, 17, 18]。

树枝状聚合物的多样性对于它们成功地应用于各种临床研究或治疗中至关重要。肽类树枝状聚合物就是其中一种，肽化学的优势和"绿色"化学应用领域的不断发展，合成的简易性、多样性，以及天然和非天然氨基酸的存在，为基于肽的树枝状聚合物提供了广泛的探索空间。例如，使用碱性氨基酸（赖氨酸、精氨酸和组氨酸）与基于聚集诱导发射（aggregation-Induced Emission，AIE）的光敏剂四苯基乙烯噻吩修饰氰基丙烯酸酯（tetraphenyl ethene thiophene modified cyanoacrylate，TTC）结合，设计并开发出来一类肽类树枝状聚合物[19]。

使用此类方法，一种与二亚油酰磷脂酰乙醇胺（dioleoyl phosphatidyle thanolamine，DOPE）结合形成脂质体的纳米制剂已被联合用于转录因子（p53）-基因疗法（gene therapy，GT）和光动力疗法（photodynamic therapy，PDT）[19]，如图10-2所示。

图10-3[20]通过介绍（+/-PEG）-H3/H6-AuNP的化学合成和制剂（+/-PEG）-H3H6-AuNP/AuNS的制备过程阐明了细胞内的药物递送机制。这些树枝状聚合物在末端用阳离子氨基酸进行功能化从而提供许多特性，例如细胞渗透（精氨酸）、与带负电的遗传物质（赖

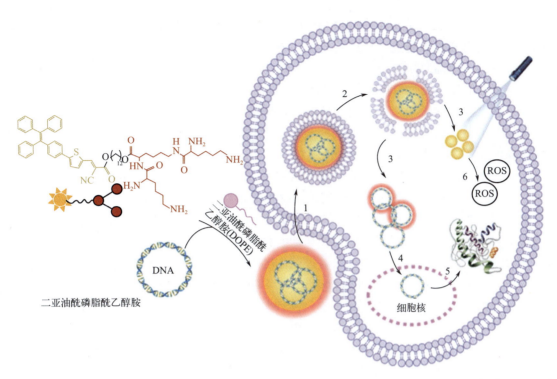

图10-2　p53介导的基因和光动力疗法协同治疗的示意图。（1）细胞摄取,（2）内体逃逸,（3）DNA释放,（4）DNA释放,（5）DNA表达和（6）LED照射下产生活性氧（reactive oxygen species，ROS）[19]

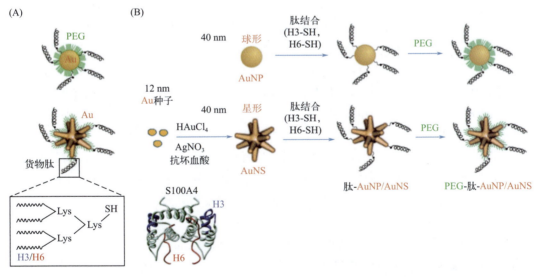

图10-3　（+/-PEG）-H3/H6-结合金纳米颗粒结构的合成。（A）PEG和肽结合的球形和星形金纳米颗粒结构的示意图。（B）（+/-PEG）-H3/H6-AuNP/AuNS的制备方案以及每一步的合成结构示意图[20]

氨酸）的强烈缩合以及质子海绵效应（组氨酸）。这本质上将基因治疗剂容纳在树枝状聚合物内，保护其免受细胞内溶酶体的降解。此外，赖氨酸功能化的树枝状聚合物在基于荧光的转染测定中比精氨酸和组氨酸树枝状聚合物表现更好。据报道，该制剂的总体转染效率比市售的脂质纳米颗粒Lipo2000®高5.7倍[19]。最重要的是，这些树枝状聚合物系统显示出成功的细胞内递送和内体逃逸，然后将完整的核酸药物释放到细胞核[19]，为成功的靶向药物递送系统提供了明确的功能证据。所开发的制剂在约575 nm处显示荧光，斯托克斯位移为150 nm，可用于荧光成像和肽树枝状聚合物的定位。

树枝状聚合物的最新应用主要是研究与药物治疗相结合的诊断。相比之下，通过共价结合和物理捕获，带有树枝状聚合物的金纳米颗粒可以在目标位点进行扫描。它们有望作为载体系统发挥多功能作用。另一种肽树枝状大分子H3/H6，与神经营养性S100A4蛋白结合，随后包裹星形金纳米颗粒并进一步用PEG修饰，可成功穿过高达40%的血脑屏障，延长循环时间，并可能避免暴露于其他组织。这种复合材料可减少氧化应激，并具有S100A4蛋白神经保护机制，可防止β淀粉样蛋白斑块的形成[20]。环糊精是众所周知的疏水性药物的药用辅料。环糊精具有高生物相容性和低毒性，已被用于许多医药产品中。环糊精具有许多固有特性，使其适合作为许多水溶性差的药物的递送系统。环糊精阳离子树枝状大分子（cyclodextrin-appended cationic dendrimer，CDE）是一种新型多靶标治疗药物，通过分别靶向转甲状腺素蛋白和β淀粉样蛋白，对全身性转甲状腺素蛋白淀粉样变性（transthyretin-mediated amyloidosis，ATTR）和局部淀粉样变性具有治疗作用。这种树枝状聚合物-shRNA（short hairpin RNA）复合物对淀粉样蛋白的产生具有抑制作用，能抑制淀粉样蛋白的形成，并能破坏现有的淀粉样蛋白原纤维[21]。

聚酰胺-胺（polyamidoamine，PAMAM）树枝状聚合物因其良好的生物相容性而经常被使用。PAMAM（G2和G3）树枝状聚合物涂有链霉亲和素（dendronized streptavidin，DSA）可模拟基于蛋白质的疗法。生物素结合的树枝状聚合物覆盖在链霉亲和素上并组装成纳米颗粒。这些特制的树枝状聚合物纳米颗粒已被研究用于治疗神经系统疾病的脑部递送。最有前景的纳米树枝状聚合物由于其纳米尺寸较为适合，可通过小窝介导的内吞作用成功地通过血脑屏障，同时在体外和体内也能逃脱溶酶体降解。纳米颗粒（NP）到达血脑屏障（blood-brain barrier，BBB）以外的脑星形胶质细胞和神经元，且没有毒性作用。因此，DSA模型表明，这种树枝状聚合物系统可以通过穿过BBB递送大分子，例如，可以给予肽/蛋白质等神经生长因子来治疗多种神经系统疾病[22]。

类似地，当PAMAM树状聚合物与荧光共振能量转移（FRET）探针结合时，使用7-二乙基氨基-4-羟甲基香豆素作为受体，罗丹明作为供体，然后与蛋白质结合，由此形成纳米颗粒，通过荧光的变化来确认药物释放速率[23]。因此，多功能PAMAM树枝状聚合物与具有两种荧光团（对甲基红、异硫氰酸荧光素）的MMP-2可裂解肽缀合作为FRET探针，可用于淋巴结肿瘤细胞成像[24]。

T细胞监测和跟踪是基于T细胞的免疫疗法的重要方面。多功能PAMAM（G5）树枝状聚合物被金纳米颗粒偶联物包裹以实现这一目标，从而实现双模式计算机断层扫描（computed tomography，CT）和荧光成像。其表面用聚乙二醇部分功能化以捕获金纳米颗粒，其他游离氨基被乙酰化中和电荷以防止毒性。这种多功能树枝状聚合物纳米探针具有高度水溶性。它表现出高X射线衰减系数，可通过CT进行检测，并且荧光成像可用于各种应用[25]。

另有研究将代谢稳定的焦谷氨酸螺旋B表面肽（pyroglutamate helix B surface peptide，pHBSP）与聚乙二醇化树枝状聚合物G2缀合，进一步用$^{99m}TcO_4^-$标记以检测缺血的心肌。

这种靶向和标记的树枝状聚合物与缺氧细胞的结合力是正常氧细胞的3倍。靶向传递和传递效率已被单光子发射计算机断层扫描（SPECT）成像证实[26]。类似的掺杂钆的树枝状聚合物用于MRI/CT[27]，以及掺有锝-99 m（^{99m}Tc）的树枝状聚合物用于SPECT/CT[28]，这些聚合物可与或不与抗癌剂同时进行双重成像，已被开发用于各种癌症治疗。其他几项研究表明，两种PAMAM树枝状聚合物都选择性地与靶向配体如RGD、肽、叶酸、生物素、转铁蛋白、肝素检测剂[例如荧光团（吲哚菁绿，IR820）]和药物（如双硫仑、紫杉醇、雷帕霉素、多柔比星）结合[29-36]，因此研究者们都将此类树枝状聚合物用作多功能和组织靶向的药物递送系统。

天麻素（gastrodin，GAS）是一种天然中药酚苷，用于治疗某些中枢神经系统疾病，这项研究旨在提高GAS的脑靶向性/通透性，同时改善成像。研究人员按比例使用含有乙酰化游离胺基团的1,3-丙烷砜（1,3-PS）功能化PAMAM（G5）树枝状聚合物，并载入了金纳米颗粒和GAS。所得纳米颗粒显示出非细胞毒性作用，具有更高的GAS负载效率，在脑缺血再灌注损伤临床前模型中具有抗炎作用，并且可进行CT成像[37]。

树状聚合物-金纳米颗粒还与抗氧化剂α-生育酚琥珀酸酯（α-TOS）结合，将基因药物直接递送至巨噬细胞，作为治疗关节炎的潜在疗法。图10-4为树枝状聚合物的化学组成和递送TNF-α siRNA的应用。该产品在体外抑制RAW264.7巨噬细胞样细胞中的TNF-α和ROS，并且其在体内胶原诱导的关节炎小鼠模型中显示出优异的结果。该研究显示出多种治疗效果：通过明显抑制炎性巨噬细胞，减少关节炎病变中的巨噬细胞细胞因子表达，降低了

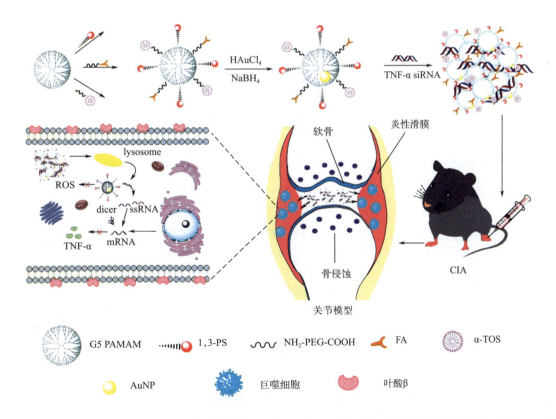

图10-4 用TNF-α siRNA递送的多功能树枝状大分子包埋金纳米颗粒用于治疗类风湿性关节炎（RA）[38]

临床评分，减少血清中的TNF-α水平，并对骨骼产生影响，减少了骨侵蚀，且由于生育酚的抗氧化特性ROS的生成减少。且抗关节炎结果经CT证实[38, 39]。这项研究表明，使用负载树枝状聚合物的抗氧化和抗炎组合治疗是可行的，且在体内表现出与体外试验数据高度相关的效果，验证了纳米颗粒的假设功能。

所有这些研究都提供了有趣的证据，即表面具有功能化物质的树枝状聚合物可以实现组织靶向。类似地，一旦进入靶细胞，应用靶向药物释放机制（例如酸敏感、光动力治疗）可以从树枝状聚合物载体提供靶向药物递送。最重要的是，添加第三个官能团，例如金、钆、锗或荧光团，可以利用各种相关的成像扫描（MRI、CT）技术确认树枝状聚合物的组织靶向性。在这种情况下，显然金纳米颗粒被广泛使用[20]。这种药物递送技术对于用于积极治疗的高毒性药物（例如化疗）或因长期、频繁剂量的全身暴露而导致不可接受的脱靶副作用的药物非常有用。

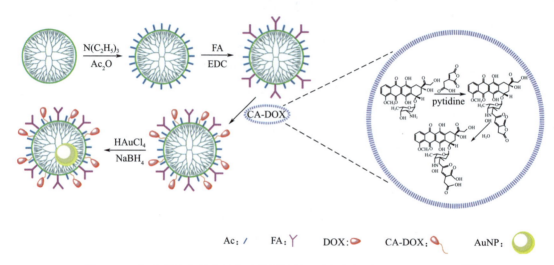

图10-5　与多柔比星结合的多功能树枝状聚合物包埋金纳米颗粒的合成[40]

采用癌症靶向治疗策略：用叶酸功能化树枝状聚合物，并使用可酸裂解的顺乌头基连接体来结合化疗抗肿瘤药物多柔比星（DOX）。如图10-5所示，这些药物还进一步掺入了金纳米颗粒。据推测，增殖性癌症组织高度利用的叶酸可能会促进癌细胞摄取树枝状聚合物。同一组织的低pH环境会促进DOX有效负载的释放。金纳米颗粒可以同时进行CT成像应用，从而确认纳米颗粒是否已递送至肿瘤部位[40]。这种树枝状药物递送复合物模型可用于各种应用，其中表面的功能化化合物（例如叶酸）可用于组织/细胞靶向，以及分子连接开关（如酸感应顺乌头基）具有对原位类型选择性的特性，可以调节释放药物。在这种情况下，金可能被认为具有格外的优势，可以通过CT检测树枝状聚合物对组织的靶向作用[40]。

与多柔比星一样，甲氨蝶呤（methotrexate，MTX）是一种化疗药物和缓解疾病的抗自身免疫药物。除其他作用外，MTX还可强烈抑制产生四氢叶酸的二氢叶酸还原酶（dihydrofolate reductase，DHFR）。该药物具有一系列与叶酸缺乏相关的显著生物毒性，特别是在肝脏、黏膜、肾脏和白细胞等肿瘤组织中，会引起严重的副作用。致畸性是一个主要问题。金纳米颗粒已被用作具有硫醇-金化学相互作用的核心，以羟基封端的硫醇化树枝状体对核心进行表面包覆。这种纳米金核心多功能树枝状聚合物的核心内含有MTX，并在分支中负载光热染料IR780，从而在近红外诱导下进一步发挥药物的药理作用。同时，金纳米颗粒还有利于成像。它被认为是一种用于温度敏感和光动力疗法的多功能树枝状聚合物[41]。在其他研究中，采用类似的多功能方法。相同的药物与软骨素硫酸盐一起使用，受益于协同效应，用PAMAM树状聚合物结合抗TNF-α抗体传递，以用于治疗类风湿性关节炎（rheumatoid arthritis，RA）[42]。

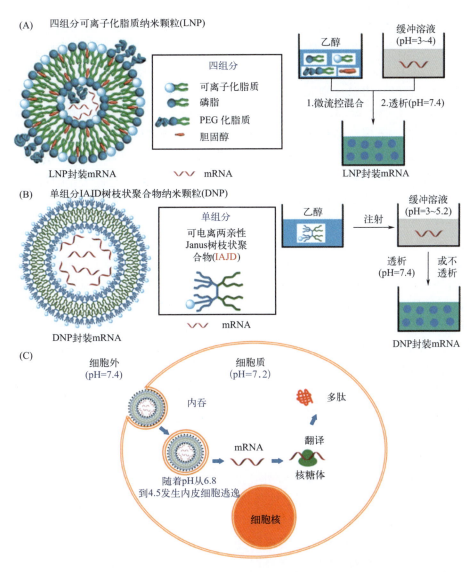

图10-6 （A）四组分LNP和（B）单组分DNP用于封装基因物质；以及（C）两种载体系统的细胞内传递和释放功能示意[43]

用于基因治疗的传统脂质纳米颗粒（LNP）包含可电离脂质、磷脂、用于机械特性的胆固醇或PEG化脂质。尽管此类组合物显示出用于基因治疗、疫苗递送和药物产品递送的前景，但它们的稳定性有限并且在较低温度（即5℃）下就开始降解。一项研究报告了使用化学策略和加速模块化正交方法的多功能可电离两亲性Janus树枝状聚合物（ionisable amphiphilic Janus dendrimer，IAJD）递送系统。研究者设计并开发了包含54个序列的文库，这使得与mRNA络合形成树枝状聚合物。该系统的体外转染率超过81%，体内转染率超过57%；有些体系在5℃下表现出稳定性[43]。所有这些研究都表明，表面具有功能化物质的树枝状聚合物可以实现组织靶向。

10.2.2 增溶剂

根据与活性相关的理化性质，目前大多数已获批准的药物和处于临床试验中的药物属于生物制药分类中的①低溶解、高渗透性和②高溶解、低渗透性药物。这些类别的分子对药物科学家开发合适的递送系统和制剂以改善药物的药代动力学行为带来了重大挑战。具有不同核心和外围物质的树枝状聚合物有助于提高药物溶解度和潜在渗透性。表10-2重点介绍了利用各种树枝状聚合物系统递送多种药物分子的几项研究。以下将讨论其他一些研究成果。树枝状聚合物核心、末端功能性与药物疏水性是评估药物溶解度的关键因素。因此，与所有制剂一样，树枝状聚合物并不是一种"放之四海而皆准"的方法，药物化学家在选择组合时，需要多加注意药物的理化性质，以及树枝状聚合物最合适的核心的化学性质。

例如，使用四环素和地塞米松作为模型药物，进行PAMAM和聚亚甲基聚苯基异氰酸酯（polymethylene polyphenylene isocyanate，PPI）树枝状聚合物的溶解度比较研究。PAMAM结合将四环素的溶解度从0.3 mg·mL^{-1}增加到9.5 mg·mL^{-1}，而PPI树枝状聚合物仅增加到0.5 mg·mL^{-1}。有趣的是，PAMAM树枝状聚合物并未增加地塞米松的溶解度，而PPI树枝状聚合物将溶解度从0.12 mg·mL^{-1}增加至1.0 mg·mL^{-1}。地塞米松的疏水性与四环素不同，可以利用PPI树枝状聚合物内部腔的疏水性质。因此，PAMAM树枝状聚合物更适合四环素，而PPI树枝状聚合物更适合地塞米松。

类似地，阳离子PAMAM树枝状聚合物使抗肿瘤药物苯嗪N, N'-二氧化物的溶解度增加了15倍（而中性PAMAM树枝状聚合物仅使溶解度增加了5倍）。

鞣花酸（EA）是一种具有抗氧化特性的天然多酚化合物。然而，由于其溶解度和生物利用度的较低，并未在临床研究中取得成功。为了提高鞣花酸（EA）的溶解度，分别对聚酯基树枝状聚合物、氨基酸亲水性第4代树枝状聚合物、氨基酸修饰（由精氨酸、赖氨酸、肌氨酸组成）的异质树枝状聚合物进行了测试，结果发现亲水性树枝状聚合物使EA的溶解度提高了1000倍，两亲性树枝状聚合物则增加了330倍。

各种研究充分证实了可通过将疏水性药物络合或封装到树枝状聚合物核心中来增加溶解度。然而，更先进的树枝状聚合物被开发为两亲性树枝状聚合物、亲脂性尾部结合树枝状聚合物，它们可被设计为自组装成"胶束"。因此，胶束可以增强溶解水溶性差的药物，从而改善个体药代动力学行为。与基于聚合物/表面活性剂的胶束不同，树枝状聚合物由于其高度适应性和易于修饰的表面化学性质，总是有更好的机会，这使它们成为更具吸引力的药物递送系统。Janus树枝状聚合物（如图10-7所示）以双面罗马神命名，是典型的两亲性树枝状聚合物，由亲水性和疏水性树枝状聚合物结构域组成。因此，它们的行为类似于表面活性剂。将Janus树枝状聚合物有机溶液掺入水溶液中稀释，会引起胶束、双层颗粒的自组装，能够通过内吞机制进入细胞。与溶液制剂相比，吲哚美辛的Janus树枝状聚合物制剂显示出更高的溶解度和稳定性[44]。

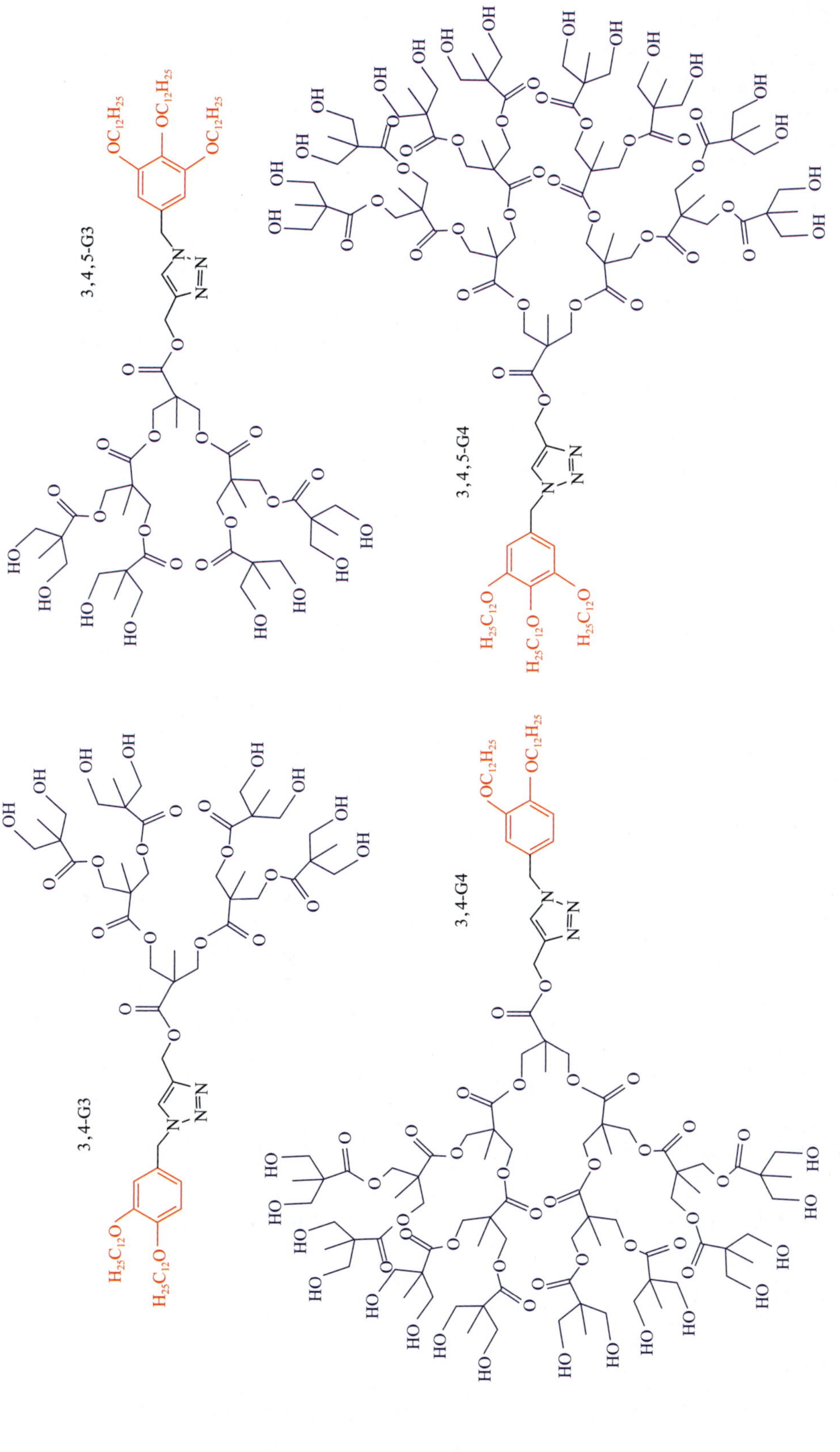

图10-7 G3和G4代Janus树枝状聚合物的化学和结构[44]

表10-2 树枝状聚合物的载体系统及其增强溶解度的应用

树枝状聚合物类型	药物	结果	参考
辛烯基琥珀酸酯羟丙基植物糖原（octenylsuccinate hydroxypropyl phytoglycogen，OHPP）是一种两亲性树枝状生物聚合物	紫杉醇[a]，氯硝柳胺[b]	[a] 联合 PTX-OHPP SD 的 PTX 是单独 PTX 的溶解度的 14000 倍以上 [b] 氯硝柳胺 OHPP 的溶解度约为单独氯硝柳胺的 11914 倍	[45, 46]
PAMAM 树枝状聚合物	3,4-二氟亚苄基二苯甲酰甲烷（CFD）	超过 20% 的包封率，改善了溶解度	[47]
树枝状 β-环糊精衍生物	阿苯达唑	使用 mβCD[1G] OH，溶解度为 27.1 mg·mL^{-1}；使用 mβCD[2G] OH，溶解度为 75.6 mg·mL^{-1}；使用 mβCD[3G]OH，溶解度为 119.4 mg·mL^{-1}	[48]
聚乙二醇化 PAMAM 树枝状聚合物	SN38	水溶解度从 11~38 μg·mL^{-1} 增加到 211 μg·mL^{-1} 和 477 μg·mL^{-1}	[49]
PAMAM-NH$_2$（4G）和 -PPI-NH$_2$（5G）树枝状聚合物	硼替佐米	使用 PPI 树枝状聚合物，溶解度提高了 1150 倍；使用 PAMAM 树枝状聚合物，溶解度提高了 730 倍	[50]
两亲性 Janus 树枝状聚合物	吲哚美辛	使用约 0.3 mg 的树枝状聚合物，溶解度达到 590 μg·mL^{-1}	[44]
氨基改性聚酯树枝状聚合物（G4）-OHG4K-树枝状聚合物	熊果酸	溶解度从 0.005 mg·mL^{-1} 增加到 10.2 mg·mL^{-1}	[51]
聚酯树枝状聚合物	依托泊苷	溶解度从 0.012~0.029 mg·mL^{-1} 提高到 162.1~391.7 mg·mL^{-1}	[52]
含糖玉米树枝状葡聚糖（SMDG）	辅酶 Q10	高达 189 倍	[53]
PAMAM 树枝状聚合物	卡马西平	可达 3 倍	[54]
肽树枝状聚合物-酮洛芬络合物	酮洛芬	G-K-(G-Keto)$_2$ 提高了溶解度 9.6 倍以上；G-K-(Keto)-K-(K)$_2$ 提高了溶解度 6.7 倍以上；G-K-(Keto)-K-(R)$_2$ 提高了溶解度 5.4 倍以上；G-K-(R-Keto)$_2$ 提高了溶解度 4.5 倍以上	[55]
氨基酸改性双（羟甲基）丙酸聚酯树枝状聚合物	*C-TCs 和 O-TCs	超过 50 mg·mL^{-1} 的水溶解度	[56]
α-生育酚琥珀酸酯锚定聚乙二醇化 PAMAM 树枝状聚合物	紫杉醇	PTX 在 G4-PEG 和 G4-TOS-PEG 溶解度分别是（521.5 ± 3.4）mg·mL^{-1} 和（742.3 ± 2.8）mg·mL^{-1}	[39]
基于 PEG 的阴离子线性球状树枝状聚合物（ALGD）	两性霉素 B	取决于制剂种类，溶解度在 478 和 840 mg·mL^{-1} 之间	[57]
阴离子线性球状树枝状聚合物（ALGD）	两性霉素（AD）桦木酸（BD）	AD（两性霉素 B）的溶解度提高了 478 倍；BD（桦木酸）的溶解度提高了 790 倍	[58]
葡萄糖庚酰胺修饰的 PAMAM 树枝状聚合物	5-氨基乙酰丙酸	溶解度增加 2 倍	[59]
聚甘油树枝状聚合物	紫杉醇	溶解度达到 0.6 mg·mL^{-1}	[60]

* O-（2-邻苯二甲酰亚氨基乙基）-N-芳基硫代氨基甲酸酯（C-TCs）及其酰亚胺开环同系物（O-TCs）。

如图10-8所示，使用二硫键与亲水性聚磷酸盐将两亲性超支化聚酯核基共聚物/树枝状聚合物（H40-star-PLA-SS-PEP）进行功能化，随后加载BCS Ⅲ类药物多柔比星（DOX），结果显示，这些胶束可自组装成70 nm的胶束，可以在水环境中穿过细胞膜直径。

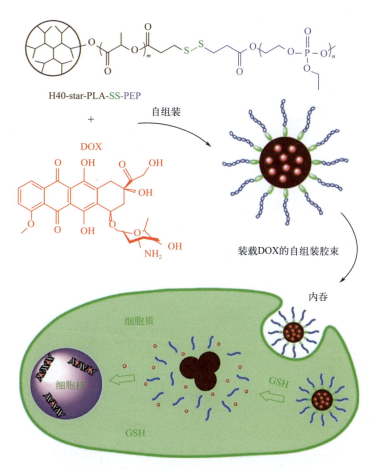

图10-8 用于细胞质药物传递的由亲水性多支共聚物构成的谷胱甘肽响应性胶束[61]

树枝状聚合物含有二硫键，因此胞质谷胱甘肽可以促进DOX的释放。这种氧化还原响应系统在谷胱甘肽单酯预处理的HeLa细胞和未用谷胱甘肽处理的细胞中成功释放药物并抑制细胞增殖[61]，表明在内源性谷胱甘肽还原酶和引入的谷胱甘肽单酯的促进下，DOX成功递送到HeLa细胞中。

如图10-9所示，与苯并硼氧共轭的多臂聚（乙二醇）两亲性树枝状聚合物很容易表现为两亲性，并自组装成胶束。这种载体系统显示出葡萄糖和pH介导的释放。当使用水介质将胰岛素组装成胶束时，胶束可保护胰岛素免受低pH和酶降解的影响。在胃等高酸环境中，胰岛素仍被胶束包裹，但在生理pH和高葡萄糖水平下，苯并硼氧释放胰岛素。因此，当口服胰岛素时，树枝状聚合物在体内包裹着胰岛素，当胰岛素在生理pH和高血糖环境下进入血液循环时，树枝状聚合物释放胰岛素，降低血糖。因此，葡萄糖和pH可调节胰岛素从胶束中的分解，并稳定血糖水平。这种"智能递送载体处方"在口服胰岛素树枝状聚合物制剂中有效地显示了按需释放葡萄糖的机制[62]。这种可口服的胰岛素递送载体为治疗目前需要每天注射胰岛素的 1 型糖尿病提供了卓越的临床价值。

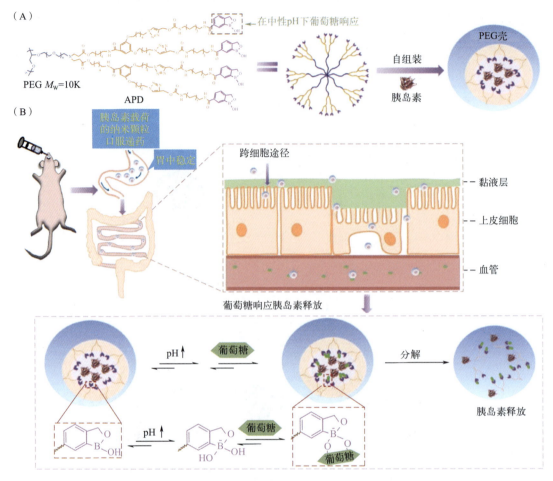

图 10-9　对 pH 和葡萄糖响应的蛋白传递载体的示意图：（A）亲水性树枝状聚合物的结构和自组装机制；（B）胰岛素载荷胶束的口服传递过程[62]

与脂肪酸结合的 PAMAM 的不对称树枝状分子可形成胶束。这些载入吉西他滨原药的胶束显示出约 33% 的载药效率，而选择性 pH 响应行为使药物能够在细胞和动物模型中释放，同时还降低了与游离药物相关的细胞毒性，并具有更出色的生物相容性[63]。总之，不管树枝状聚合物的化学结构如何，无论是 PAMAM、PEG、聚酯还是基于肽类树枝状聚合物，以及相对较新的两亲性和脂质化树枝状聚合物，通过其胶束机制能够提高多种药物分子的溶解度，从而获得更好的治疗特性。

10.2.3　渗透促进剂

大多数药物必须完好无损地通过至少一个生物膜屏障，才能到达靶标并产生预期效果。药物设计的一个主要重点是提高通过生物膜屏障的渗透性，从而改变其 BCS 分类。为促进渗透性而对母体分子进行的物理化学改变（比如改变 $\log P$、电荷、HBD/HBA），往往会通过改变溶解度、代谢过程或降低/消除作用于靶标的效力来改变分子的治疗潜力。开发前药、脂质化、添加肽和聚合物偶联物通常是为了在不严重破坏母体分子理化性质的情况下增强渗透性。然而，尽管药物具有药效和治疗作用，但一些药物往往无法通过皮肤层、血脑屏障和其他黏膜及组织屏障等屏障膜。这对实现药物分子的有效递送系统提出了巨大挑战。另外，表面活性剂、溶剂、脂肪酸、温和的毒素和萜烯类物质容易与膜蛋白和脂质发生作用，导致暂时性的开放或结构变化，从而有助于穿透膜屏障。超声波、离子渗透和微针等物理技术也会刺激这些过程。然而，只有少数药物通过上述技术进入市场，部分原因是破坏生物屏障系统会带来巨大风险，使本来不应穿越膜的其他潜在有害化合物也有机会穿越膜，从而暴露于通常加速排除的毒素，这在肠道和脑屏障的情况下尤为明显。

替代方法可能需要侧重于处方和药物递送载体的护航功能，而不是通过大幅改变药物性质来促进其通过细胞膜。大幅改变药物性质通常会影响药物原本有用的特性。正如所讨论的，树枝状聚合物可以通过合理设计核心和表面功能来增强药物溶解度，从而对生物膜的性质具有显著的适应性，甚至对于皮肤和血脑屏障等高度限制性屏障也是如此。

树枝状聚合物已被研究用于皮肤渗透和局部药物递送平台。PAMAM（G3）树枝状聚合物可递送二葡萄糖酸氯己定（chlorhexidine digluconate，CHG），它是一种阳离子双胍。在这项研究中，4%CHG和0.5%胶凝剂的1 mmol·L^{-1} PAMAM树枝状聚合物，与市售Hibiscrub® 局部凝胶相比，含有树枝状聚合物的凝胶渗透更深，改善了制剂的抗菌性能[64]。Venganti等[65]使用抗癌药物5-氟尿嘧啶（5-fluorouracil，5FU）作为模型药物，负载到PAMAM树枝状聚合物中，局部应用于皮肤进行透皮递送。在不同的电荷、分支复杂性（代数）和树枝状聚合物的浓度下，较低代（G2）阳离子树枝状聚合物比较高代（G4和G6）树枝状聚合物表现出更好的渗透性。表面乙酰化和羧化也使亲脂性树枝状聚合物囊泡通过跨细胞途径具有更好的屏障渗透性。这种渗透性增强被认为是脂质屏障的改变降低了皮肤的阻力，增加了药物在皮肤中的分布。然而，该研究还观察到经皮水分流失，表明屏障变化可能导致水分流失、水肿、红斑、皮肤刺激和潜在有害物质（例如皮肤传播的化合物、毒素、细菌、酵母或病毒）的阻隔问题，这些有害物质穿过本应起到保护作用的皮肤屏障，可能导致严重感染或其他并发症。因此，这引发了人们对通过渗透促进剂改变膜完整性的担忧。

肽类树枝状聚合物的毒性低于基于PAMAM、PPI树枝状聚合物。它们还会被酶降解，因此被认为是可生物降解的[66]。Mutalik等[67]也使用5-FU作为模型药物；然而，该研究将其加载到不对称树枝状聚合物/肽类树枝状聚合物作为载体系统。该研究调查了低分子量/非球状不对称树枝状聚合物。具有末端精氨酸的甘氨酸和赖氨酸支链显示出4$^+$、8$^+$和16$^+$电荷（分别为R4、R8、R16）的阳离子功能。研究表明，与普通药物相比，5-FU的肽类树枝状聚合物制剂增加了油/水分配系数并改善了5-FU的皮肤渗透性。有趣的是，与低电荷和高电荷树枝状聚合物相比，8$^+$树枝状聚合物在皮肤渗透方面表现出最高的功效。此外，研究者还注意到皮肤超微结构的变化，认为这是由于肽类树枝状聚合物引起的"脂质软化"。因此，尽管上述两项独立研究均表明树枝状大分子制剂中5-FU的皮肤分配得到改善，但两项研究也表明皮肤屏障结构发生变化，这可能不利于将树枝状聚合物用作局部治疗。尽管如此，仍需证明这些对皮肤结构或屏障完整性的改变是否是暂时的，并且是否仅在与局部使用的树枝状聚合物接触时发生，且只有在结合树枝状聚合物制剂时才允许药物穿透。另一方面，也有可能这些改变会带来长期风险，导致皮肤重要屏障功能的持久性破坏。当然，离体/体外测定在回答和确定此类问题方面的用途可能有限。

通过脂质膜的计算机动态分子模拟，将R8树枝状聚合物与线性阳离子肽进行进一步比较。实验结果表明，带电的肽类树枝状聚合物在与皮肤/细胞膜表面的高度疏水环境相互作用时，可能利用了脂质膜中磷脂头基的质子链传递机制。因此，推测这种质子转移相互作用使树枝状聚合物与疏水性膜环境相容，并允许直接通过膜双层到达胞质侧。这种相互作用被比作"变色龙"机制，并且被认为不涉及内吞途径[68]。

甲氧沙林是一种临床使用的口服疏水性光敏药物，适用于各种皮肤病，包括银屑病、湿疹、白癜风和皮肤淋巴瘤。它与紫外线A疗法（补骨脂素紫外线A疗法，psoralen-ultraviolet A therapy，PUVA）一起使用，其中裸露皮肤暴露于紫外线会激活该化合物，以剂量依赖性方式选择性抑制DNA、RNA和蛋白质合成。当与G3和G4 PAMAM树枝状聚合物复合时，该药物被证明可以渗透到皮肤更深层，提高PUVA疗法的效果[54]，将更多的药物递送至皮肤。这些结果与之前在树枝状聚合物制剂中递送疏水性药物（例如吲哚美辛[69]和坦索罗辛[70]）的报道一致。然而，从内部（循环）深入渗透到真皮的机制尚不清楚。增加溶解度可能有助于跨膜被动扩散[69-71]。更有可能的是，如前所述，树枝状聚合物上的阳离子胺基团可能与膜上带负电的成分相互作用，从而有助于膜相互作用和成功穿膜。然而，皮肤结构的变化无疑也会产生影响。研究人员对与疏水性酮洛芬复合的精氨酸功能化肽类树枝状聚合物（带有4^+、8^+、16^+）进行了皮肤渗透性研究[72]。研究发现，与单独药物相比，肽类树枝状聚合物将酮洛芬的透皮渗透性提高了3倍以上，其中最高的是16^+树枝状聚合物。当超声波与酮洛芬-16^+树枝状大分子复合物联合应用时，在细胞和动物模型观察到酮洛芬的透皮分配显著增加（>1300倍），未发现明显的皮肤损伤[72]。球状PAMAM和不对称肽类树枝状聚合物均显示出跨皮肤膜的渗透性[67, 70, 73, 74]。

药物递送策略的组合也是一种常用方法。例如：通过利用脂质体和无机纳米颗粒，多个载体系统来协同作用的药物递送机制，其中8^+带电树枝状聚合物被C_{18}脂肪酸链脂化。然后将该复合物与脂质体结合，通过负载马来酸阿塞那平来修饰表面。结果显示，通过皮肤给药途径的离体皮肤渗透性研究表明，与不含树枝状聚合物的制剂相比，树枝状聚合物制剂具有更高的药物渗透性，提供了优异的药代动力学特征，同时保留了中枢神经系统中的药理作用。图10-10展示了一个递送系统及其应用[75]。这种类型的树枝状聚合物可能为基因递送带来更多的优势。理论上，阳离子肽类树枝状聚合物可以与带负电荷的遗传物质形成复合物。脂质体/脂质纳米颗粒系统稳定了肽类树枝状聚合物并促进了其通过生物膜屏障。

再如，胶原Ⅰ（Col-Ⅰ）肽共轭树枝状聚合物（G5，PAMAM）被包覆在金纳米颗粒（G5，AuNP）上，并装载了5-氟尿嘧啶（5-FU）。这个肽类似于基质金属蛋白酶的底物，并且基于酶的降解允许药物释放。与单独使用5-FU相比，它在抗癌活性方面也表现出更好的性能[76]。另一种类型的树枝状聚合物，例如基于PEG的树枝状聚合物，也针对透皮递送应用进行了研究。这种树枝状聚合物类型具有PEG链和脂肪酸外围，在非极性溶剂中形成反胶束，与线性聚合物相比，渗透增强了6倍[77]。树枝状聚合物的理化性质和多样性使其在细胞水平上与皮肤膜相互作用充当渗透增强剂，无论是在皮肤层保留药物还是允许治疗成分穿过膜，都有可能使治疗成分通过非侵入性途径传递到其他靶组织，避免了口服降解。

基于树枝状聚合物的药物递送系统已用于中枢神经系统（central nervous system，CNS），其中树枝状聚合物表现出有效的BBB穿透机制。胞二磷胆碱（一种内源性膜成分）作为补充剂给予时，似乎可以通过保留心磷脂、鞘磷脂、花生四烯酸和磷脂酰胆碱（PC）等膜

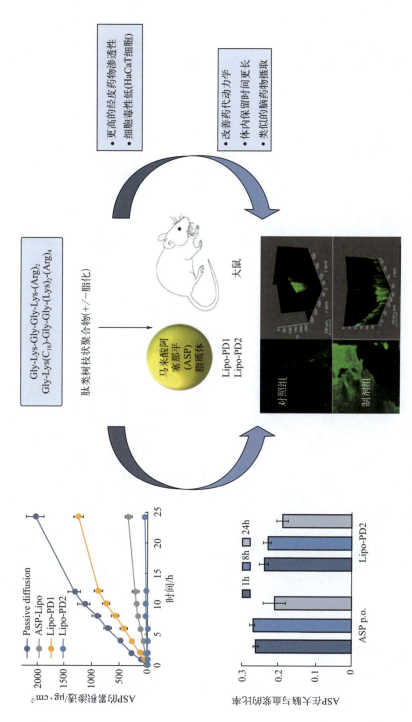

图10-10 脂质结合不对称肽类树枝状聚合物的图示及其细胞和小鼠模型应用[75]

成分来保护神经元免受脑卒中后损伤，从而促进膜修复和细胞再生。例如，一种杂交PAMAM（G2）树枝状聚合物与负载胞二磷胆碱的扩增白蛋白在BBB体外模型中测试渗透性。与仅装载白蛋白的药物相比，所得纳米制剂的跨膜渗透性提高了3倍以上[78]。此外，与上述构建体类似，胞二磷胆碱释放机制也受pH影响。另一种使用PAMAM树状聚合物/普鲁士蓝/血管内皮-2多肽的混合纳米颗粒系统（图10-11）已被开发并在体外使用。在体内，模型结果表明，增强的BBB通透性可恢复小胶质细胞的线粒体功能，而ROS清除作用可产生出色的神经保护作用，可用于治疗阿尔茨海默病等疾病[79]。

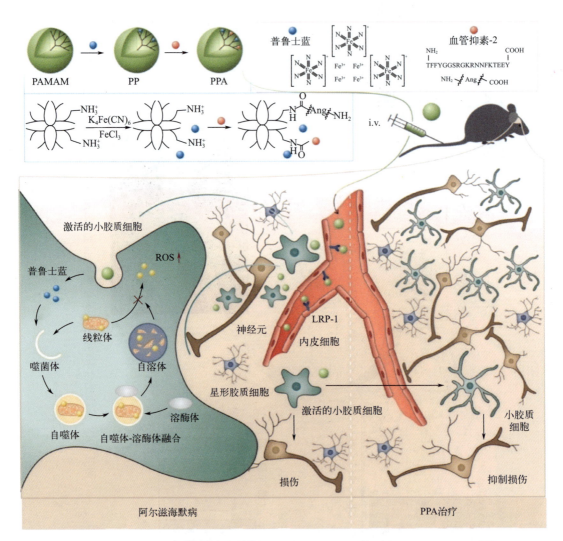

图10-11 一种可穿越血脑屏障的树枝状聚合物系统，用于治疗阿尔茨海默病[79]

其他几项研究表明，基于树枝状聚合物的技术可用于从鼻腔递送到大脑，避免血脑屏障，并显示黏膜渗透和大脑渗透能力。通过鼻腔途径给予不同浓度（3～15 μg）的PAMAM（G4）树枝状聚合物，并评估对神经元组织的相对毒性。结果显示，它们没有表现出毒性迹象，证实树枝状聚合物可以安全直接地在鼻内滴注诱导有益的神经效应[80]。有趣的是，另一项使用异硫氰酸荧光素标记葡聚糖（FD4，4400 Da）的PAMAM树枝状聚合物（G0至

G3）通过鼻黏膜屏障的渗透性研究显示，渗透性呈现浓度依赖性（G3 > G2 > G1 > G0），并且与高达2%的G3树枝状聚合物的对照相比，在LDH测定中未显示出相对毒性。随后，其他几种大分子药物，包括FD10、FD70、胰岛素和降钙素，也显示出成功的跨鼻膜递送[81]。这些结果也证实了之前的研究，其中PAMAM树枝状聚合物通过松弛紧密连接来降低跨上皮电阻（transepithelial electrical resistance，TEER）值，从而允许药物通过细胞旁途径递送[82]。另一种理论也支持PAMAM树枝状聚合物可以通过内吞途径内化并穿过鼻上皮细胞[81, 83, 84]。然而，这些结果都是基于细胞研究，可能需要进一步的动物研究加强其通过鼻内给药成功递送的有力论据。

4-苯基丁酸（4-phenylbutyrate，4-PBA）是FDA批准的治疗X连锁肾上腺脑白质营养不良（adrenoleukodystrophy，ALD）的药物。ALD是一种遗传性疾病，是过氧化物酶体转运蛋白2（ABCD2）的有效激活剂，由于其半衰期短，需要更高的剂量进行治疗。当4-PBA通过酯键连接至羟基PAMAM树枝状聚合物时，与单独的游离药物相比，显示出持续释放机制，从而导致持续吸收和生物暴露。这使得每周一次的给药成为可能，直接反映出所需剂量浓度降低为原来的1/20。

PAMAM树枝状聚合物也可用于药物的眼部递送；眼部解剖学和生理学上的屏障导致难以将药物递送至眼后段。例如，一种与新型环状RGD肽和渗透素共轭的PEG化PAMAM树状聚合物，已被验证用于抗血管生成。结果显示，其渗透性提高了1.5倍，药物可分布到角膜和视网膜，保留时间长达12 h，表明持续递送的可能性[85]。

为了治疗与青光眼或眼内高压相关的眼内压（intra-ocular pressure，IOP）升高，用PEG链间隔基（DenTimol）修饰的PAMAM树枝状聚合物（G3）制备了β受体阻滞剂噻吗洛尔，以实现直接的眼科治疗应用，用于离体角膜渗透测定。该产品显示8%的DenTimol在4 h内渗透到角膜，并且经组织学检查证实，即使每天使用一周后也没有表现出任何刺激或组织学细胞损伤。另一方面，它降低了相对于基线30%的眼压，显示出所期望的药理作用[86]。

上述研究证实，使用多种树枝状大分子作为载体系统来增强药物的渗透特性，特别是皮肤和血脑屏障，已经受到重视。有趣的是，PAMAM树枝状聚合物（低代≥4G）被发现是一种有吸引力的载体系统，无论是否具有表面功能化，通常与靶向部分结合可提高性能。然而，从使用基于肽的树枝状聚合物进行的研究中也发现了与PAMAM类似的结果；因此，这两种形式都可能作为安全有效的药物载体和递送系统。

10.2.4 药物递送系统

典型的药品主要由药物/活性药物成分（active pharmaceutical ingredient，API）和辅料（非活性成分）组成，通过溶解、吸收并递送到靶组织发挥作用。辅料在实现或维持药物的药理作用方面发挥着至关重要的作用，通常通过提高生物利用度和减少对生物屏障的阻碍来改善其药理特性，从而达到治疗疾病的药理作用。在临床和产品开发阶段，超过90%的药物失败，其中超过40%的药物缺乏临床疗效，30%有毒性，约15%的药物具有较差的药物特性[87-89]。然而，经典的聚合物树枝状聚合物并未被批准作为人体用非活性辅料。唯一的例外是基于聚赖氨酸的树枝状聚合物已被批准用于某些抗微生物产品。树枝状聚合物的其他独特性质，包括溶解度、渗透性和多功能性，已在其他部分中讨论，这里重点介绍使用树枝状聚合物递送目标药物的最新研究成果。

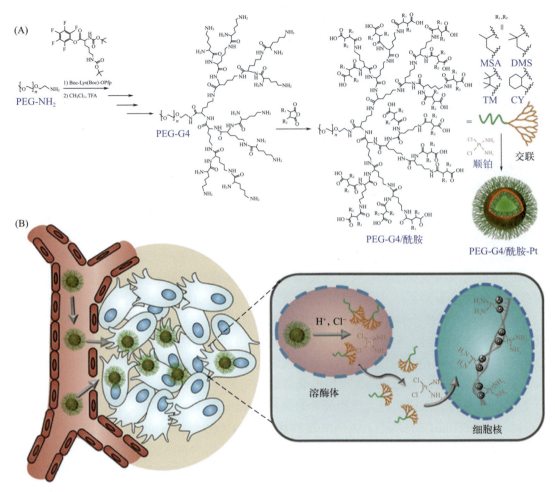

图10-12 （A）PEG-树枝状聚赖氨酸嵌段共聚物的合成和纳米胶囊的形成；（B）药物在酸性肿瘤环境下释放的图示[90]

PEG-聚赖氨酸嵌段共聚物被合成后，对树枝状聚赖氨酸进行酰胺化处理，与顺式二氨二氯合铂（Ⅱ，CDDP）进行复合，形成纳米胶囊。与单独药物相比，这种纳米胶囊在细胞和动物模型中均证明具有抗肿瘤活性。图10-12说明了CDDP在细胞和细胞核中的合成和释放机制。纳米胶囊具有多种优点，如稳定的复合物显示出更长的循环时间，而且酰胺键在低pH肿瘤环境下降解并促进解离和铂释放，因此该聚合物仅在细胞内、低pH肿瘤环境中释放药物[90]。

对于非小细胞肺癌（non-small cell lung cancer，NSCLC）的治疗，常常受到内在EGFR突变的限制，导致药物耐药。联合治疗和化疗可能是长期给药方案的临床上更可行的选择。通过将PAMAM树枝状聚合物进行氟化修饰，并结合适配体，成功开发了一种封装吉非替尼（Gef）和血卟啉（HP）的高效递送系统。树枝状聚合物的特点是可以携带氧气，而适体靶标可以将药物递送到EGFR阳性的NSCLC细胞上。因此，激光照射改善了缺氧条件的肿瘤微环境，药物的细胞内递送允许在NSCLC细胞上通过光动力疗法/分子靶向治疗产生协同作用[91]。

曲安奈德（triamcinolone acetonide，TA）是一种皮质类固醇药物，其副作用阻碍了其在黄斑水肿、白内障和青光眼等眼部疾病中的应用。例如，研究人员开发了基于PAMAM-OH（G4）树枝状聚合物的载体系统，通过将TA缀合至树枝状聚合物表面来递送TA。该药物制剂提供了局部和持续的递送，可抑制氧诱导的视网膜病变小鼠模型中炎症细胞因子的产生、微胶质细胞活化和视网膜新血管形成，进一步有助于改善氧诱导性视网膜病变引起的神经视网膜和视觉功能障碍[92]。再如，另有研究开发了胆固醇结合、组氨酸和精氨酸表面修饰的PAMAM（PamHR）树枝状聚合物，可与甘草酸（glycyrrhizic acid，GA）形成自组装胶束。此外，将GA固定在外围阳离子表面的树枝状聚合物核心已用于基因递送应用。胶束的形成带来了显著的优势，如改善转染性能并增强与细胞膜的相互作用，从而通过其破坏膜的效应有助于逃逸至内体溶酶体。当这些携带血红素氧合酶-1（HO-1）基因的胶束在急性肺损伤（ALI）小鼠模型上进行测试时，它们通过其抗炎特性降低了TNF-α水平，与经典的PEI 25 kDa聚合物相比，展现出了双重优势[93]。

随着树枝状聚合物生成的增加，核心体积和表面氨基官能团的数量将相应增加。然而，这并不一定能有效改善药物的溶解度，反而可能限制药物进入树枝状聚合物内部核心空腔的能力，从而带来一定的限制。同时，表面功能性在药物和树枝状聚合物之间建立相互作用方面也起着关键作用。但是，很少有研究强调这些因素的重要性。例如，使用PAMAM G4和G6树枝状聚合物，负载模型药物5-FU。有趣的是，G4树枝状聚合物可容纳25个5-FU分子，相当于16%的载药量，而G6树枝状聚合物可容纳20个5-FU分子，相当于5%。对多种癌细胞系进行细胞毒性测定，细胞毒性水平直接反映了理化性质，G4树枝状聚合物的负载效率较高，对癌细胞的毒性更大[94]。通常，这表现为对5-FU呈现剂量依赖性反应；更高的载药效率导致了更高效的药物递送。

在另一项研究中，通过用各种以羟基和半胱氨酸为核心的部分和组合表面胺改变表面官能度，用各种参数来控制表面官能度。所得的树枝状聚合物可以用姜黄素封装，并针对小鼠、大鼠和人源性胶质母细胞瘤细胞系进行测试。在所有测试的变体中，90%羟基修饰的树枝状聚合物表现出更好的细胞活力，同时药物组合的毒性增加。未改性的PAMAM-NH$_2$树枝状聚合物对正常细胞和癌细胞都显示毒性，而游离的姜黄素的存在对这些树枝状聚合物并没有带来任何优势[95]。

细胞内外谷胱甘肽浓度的差异约为1000倍，而在细胞的细胞质环境中更高。例如，研究者开发了一种基于谷氨酸的树枝状聚合物，其中一个羧基末端用于与半胱氨酸结合，另一个羧基末端用于与谷氨酸分支结合。一旦实现了所需的代数，树枝状聚合物的核心就与海藻酸钠结合，并通过氢键、半胱氨酸巯基和羟基PEG进一步交联，形成3D网络结构。内部巯基在氧化时，导致树枝状聚合物的自组装，从而实现高载药量。在这种情况下，多柔比星可以与这种复合物在水性介质中形成水凝胶。载药水凝胶制剂表现出控释特性，并且在细胞内还原剂谷胱甘肽存在的情况下释放了超过75%的药物。细胞毒性测试表明，制备的负载DOX的树枝状水凝胶对HepG-2细胞具有与阳性对照相当的抗肿瘤活性[96]。此前，已有多篇综述论文讨论了基于树枝状聚合物的药物输送应用[97-99]。表10-3提供了最近研究工作中用于递送不同药物分子的树枝状聚合物系统，及其各自的应用，展示了树枝状聚合物的多样性。

表10-3 用于药物递送应用的基于树枝状聚合物的载体系统

树枝状聚合物	药物	载药机制	应用	参考文献
'DEP®' G5 聚-L-赖氨酸树枝状聚合物	AZD4320	共轭	循环时间延长8倍，缓释，优先淋巴运输	[100]
基于三(2-氨基乙基)胺（TAEA）核心的肽类树枝状聚合物（Lys, Arg, 2,3-二甲基马来酸酐）	多柔比星和吉西他滨	封装/络合	平均肿瘤体积和肿瘤重量分别减少至13.5%和12.9%，渗透到更深的肿瘤组织	[101]
羟基-PAMAM 树枝状聚合物	2,6-二甲氧基-4-(5-苯基-4-噻吩-2-基-1H-咪唑-2-基)苯酚（DPTIP）	共轭	显著降低纹状体内 IL-1β 诱导的 Tau 蛋白血浆 EV 增加	[102]
聚甘油树枝状聚合物（PGD）e	紫杉醇	封装	水凝胶形成，溶解的 PTX 受控释放，无任何沉淀	[60]
L-丝氨酸和 D-丝氨酸修饰的 PAMAM 树枝状聚合物	五羰基溴化锰（CORM）	封装	AKI 小鼠可以使用 H_2O_2 荧光探针有效诊断 AKI	[103]
多面体低聚倍半硅氧烷（POSS）核 PLL 树枝状聚合物	SN38	封装	对多种癌细胞的增强杀伤力，同时具有持续释放 SN38 的特性	[104]
泊洛沙姆连接的树枝状聚合物 G4	香豆素	封装	低水平的溶血和细胞毒性，同时能够持续递送香豆素，并对耐甲氧西林金黄色葡萄球菌（MRSA）展现出增强的抗菌效果	[105]
PAMAM 树枝状聚合物	54 个 NO 释放基团 54 个 UDCA 单元	共轭	抗炎活性，通过抑制 76.1% IL-8 分泌达到 0.25 nmol·L^{-1}	[106]
基于细胞穿透肽的树枝状聚合物	喜树碱	共轭	针对一组癌细胞的最高活性，IC_{50} 在纳摩尔范围内（31~747 nmol·L^{-1}）	[107]
C_{18} 共轭 G2 PAMAM	达拉非尼和维莫非尼	封装	负载 DAB 和 VEM 的 NM 在 4 种不同的黑色素瘤细胞系中均引发了对游离药物治疗的增强反应	[108]
PAMAM（G5）	利塞膦酸钠/维生素 D3	共轭	这种治疗方法在 21 天内帮助恢复了钙、磷和骨密度（BMD）至正常水平	[109]
使用六氯环三磷腈（HCCP）的 PAMAM（PAD）	姜黄素	共轭	对破骨细胞的抑制和对成骨细胞的促进。治疗的双重效应通过 pH 响应性溶酶体释放实现	[110]
基于树枝状聚肌氨酸星形聚合物	SN38	共轭	长时间循环，与伊立替康相比具有相对更高的抗癌效果，且体重减轻较少	[111]
PAMAM（G4）树枝状聚合物-棕榈酸核壳纳米颗粒	姜黄素	封装	控制释放曲线，提高口服生物利用度，并在动物模型中具有更好的抗应激效果	[112]
聚磷腈（PPH）树枝状聚合物	氮杂二膦酸盐	共轭	减轻银屑病的炎症状况，在小鼠模型中局部应用时显示出更好的耐受性和安全性	[113]
乙二胺核 PAMAM（G4）树枝状聚合物	雷公藤甲素	共轭	引发细胞内释放，特异性靶向神经胶质母细胞瘤，与单独使用雷公藤甲素相比，更高程度减少肿瘤负担，减少非特异性副作用	[114]
超支化（PAMAM）树枝状聚合物（5G）	pan-HLA-DR-binding epitope（PADRE）aKXVAAWTLKAAaZC	共轭	与非树枝状结构的对照物相比，树枝状结构共轭物展出 3 倍的抗可卡因抗体反应	[115]

续表

树枝状聚合物	药物	载药机制	应用	参考文献
羟基 PAMAM（4G）树枝状聚合物	青藤碱	共轭	与单独使用青藤碱相比，改善了细胞内摄取，早期阻止了炎症，并以更高速度减少氧化应激	[116]
羟基-PAMAM 树枝状聚合物	BLZ945	共轭	渗透实体肿瘤并在与肿瘤相关的巨噬细胞中定位，调节免疫反应，树状聚合物选择性递送	[117]
Gc PAMAM 树枝状聚合物	曲妥珠单抗（TZ）、来那替尼	共轭封装	该药物受益于持续释放、高度选择性以及在 SKBR-3 细胞中的抗癌活性，这是通过药物-树枝状结构体系统实现的	[118]
羟基 PAMAM 树枝状聚合物	JHU29	共轭	增强水溶性，减少过量谷氨酸释放，上调 GLS 活性	[119]
天冬氨酸（Asp）修饰的 PAMAM（Asp-PAMAM-胶束）	紫杉醇（PTX）	封装	溶解度比游离药物高 3.5 倍，在下肢骨骼中积累的人获得了类似的治疗效益，同时保持低剂量的给药	[120]

10.2.5 治疗剂

树枝状聚合物结构不仅用于药物和基因递送应用，还用于研究不同类型树枝状聚合物的功能特性。通过对分支单体或表面基团进行轻微的修饰，树枝状聚合物本身就能展现出多种治疗特性，主要包括抗菌、抗癌和抗炎等作用[121-123]。这些特性可以与药物和其他治疗部分结合产生协同效应[123]。以下几个应用提供了基于树枝状聚合物的治疗剂的进展。

由于病原体对旧抗生素的耐药性日益增加，以及缺乏新获监管审批的抗菌药物，多重耐药性仍然是病原体对抗菌治疗的重大挑战。树枝状聚合物结构具有独特的特性，可能使其能够充当新型抗菌剂。其中一个开发成果是 Vivagel®，它是一种基于聚赖氨酸的树枝状聚合物，末端为 1-(羧基甲氧基)萘-3, 6-二磺酸钠[124]。树枝状聚合物已在各国获得批准，这为基于树枝状分子的新型抗生素开发技术赋予了重要意义，以应对挑战[124]。例如，利用赖氨酸（K）和亮氨酸（L）的组合模板（KL)$_8$-(KKL)$_4$-(KKLL)$_2$-KKKL 开发出了抗菌肽树枝状聚合物（AMPD）库，对革兰氏阴性菌 MDR 菌株显示出卓越的活性特征，并具有良好的血清稳定性[125]。此外，这些 AMPD 通过硫醇-马来酰亚胺化学结合在类壳聚糖天然聚合物上。然而，当这种 AMPD 与透明质酸和羧甲基壳聚糖等生物聚合物物理混合时，它就会失去功效。当它与壳聚糖共价结合并成功破坏内膜和外膜时，它被革兰氏阴性细菌细胞膜摄入，这表明其在急性和慢性细菌感染中的潜在应用[126]。在另一项研究中，研究者设计并合成了阳离子两亲性树枝状聚合物，其中基于 PEG 的核心具有胺官能化，随后与胆汁酸（胆酸）的二价、多价模板共价结合，并且各自的胆酸-OH 基团被修饰为季铵，带有正电荷。这两种树枝状聚合物都可以自组装成胶束，对金黄色葡萄球菌和大肠埃希菌的最小抑菌浓度（minimum inhibitory concentration，MIC）分别为 7.5 μmol·L^{-1} 和 7.8 μmol·L^{-1}，即使在 MIC 浓度的 16 倍时，溶血和细胞毒性也可以忽略不计[127]。此外，基于赖氨酸的 G2 树枝状聚合物在药用化妆品中应用研究令人兴奋，该研究能够改变膜的流动性，同时还显示对痤疮丙酸杆菌痤疮菌株（RT5）生物膜形成的影响，但对痤疮丙酸杆菌非痤疮菌株（RT6）的生物膜形成没有影响。树枝状聚合物还减少了炎症反应（IL-1α和TLR-2）并改善皮肤脱屑。在与安慰剂霜比较的体内研究中，这些结果也得到了验证。

基于PAMAM的不对称树枝状分子（树枝状分子）的制备是使其一端带电（如伯胺、季铵、叔胺、胍或羧基），而另一端则与长链脂肪酸结合。这使得树枝状聚合物能够自组装成胶束，同时显示出对革兰氏阳性和阴性细菌以及生物膜的形成的影响。这些结果支持计算建模研究中提出的作用机制，表明阳离子官能团有助于静电相互作用。脂肪酸尾部被埋入细菌膜中，导致细胞裂解[128]。一系列具有不同表面功能的硼酸修饰聚酰胺-胺（PAMAM）树枝状聚合物对革兰氏阳性细菌产生了选择性抗菌作用。

相反，在微生物浊度发生变化的20分钟内就能看到结果。其作用机制是与细菌表面的脂壁酸相互作用。苯硼酸不能识别脂多糖层最外层的O抗原。因此，伪离子性质有助于产生特异性和选择性抗菌剂，可进一步应用于临床[129]。

一种基于多肽树枝状聚合物的构建物，其序列为$(KKWK)_4$-K_2-K-G，末端Lys上的伯胺基团与不同的脂质基团官能化。荧光甲基氧羰基-4-KKWK通过阻断病毒与细胞膜的相互作用，靶向血凝素三聚体的HA2亚基，对甲型流感病毒显示出纳摩尔级的效力。这种树枝状聚合物对一系列流感亚型也有活性。有趣的是，发现这些树枝状结构分子能够减少与感染有关的炎症标志物[130]。用这些药物治疗的病毒（PR8）感染小鼠受到了一定程度的保护，并注意到肺部病毒负荷较少。

巨噬细胞在艾滋病毒感染中发挥着关键作用，它们将病毒颗粒传递给T细胞，从而建立病毒库[131]。碳硅烷树枝状聚合物（G2-S16树枝状聚合物）是一种具有磺酸盐末端和硅核心的聚阴离子树枝状聚合物。这些树枝状结构分子可以通过仅在巨噬细胞内阻止病毒的感染性，防止感染巨噬细胞将病毒传递到健康的T淋巴细胞。因此，巨噬细胞不会将病毒颗粒转运到身体的其他部位。此外，组织学的人类阴道外体外组织未显示上皮损伤、腺囊性扩张、炎症浸润、出血、血管增生、水肿或纤维化、坏死或钙化的迹象。这些树枝状聚合物对HSV-2感染动物模型也有疗效。其潜在应用可作为抗微生物剂局部用药，可用于预防HSV和HIV感染[132]。

设计甘露糖装饰的赖氨酸球状树枝状聚合物是为了实现显著的抗炎特性。在对小鼠骨髓衍生巨噬细胞（bone marrow-derived macrophage，BMDM）进行测试时，发现这些树枝状聚合物具有生物相容性和具有抗炎M2表型。这表明这类树枝状聚合物具有一些潜在的优势。因此，树枝状结构分子降低了M1巨噬细胞样细胞因子IL-1β、IL-6、TNF-α的分泌，并提高了成纤维细胞的增殖，同时也增加了M2表型的转化生长因子β1、IL-4和IL-10的产生。这些树枝状聚合物通过M2巨噬细胞极化，在2型糖尿病伤口局部给药后进行了体内测试。树枝状聚合物通过多种机制显示了其潜力，如提高伤口闭合率、胶原沉积、降低了促炎细胞因子的水平，同时增加TGF-β1的产生[133]。

醋酸格拉替雷是多发性硬化症（MS）的一线治疗药物，这是一种慢性神经退行性疾病。为了保留醋酸格拉替雷的大小和结构，并测试其在多种修饰（如阳离子化、乙酰化、硫醇反应性转换和酰化）下的疗效，人们研究开发了一个树枝状聚合物库。在这些修饰中，图10-13所示的树枝状聚合物表现出令人兴奋的效果，因为它能够诱导IL-1Ra（一种由纯化的人单核细胞或循环抗原呈递细胞释放的细胞因子）的产生。这些树枝状聚合物还下调了一般免疫抑制前体先天免疫反应受体CD14、CD16和CD68受体以及人类白细胞抗原Ⅱ类[134]。

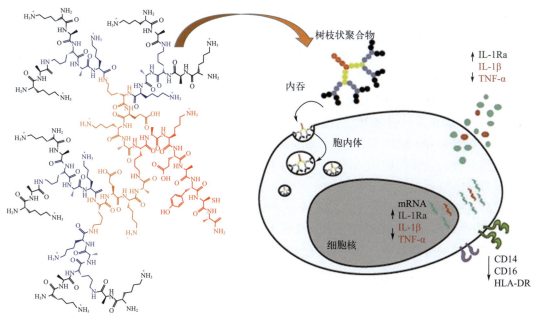

图10-13 树枝化醋酸格拉替雷及其作用机制[134]

具有胺表面的树枝状聚合物可以利用简单的多肽化学工具转换多价治疗肽，因此许多基于肽的化合物在各种疾病中显示出治疗潜力。然而，要获得理想的药理作用，必须具备靶向性、稳定性和有效性。四肽短序列AaTs-1（IWKS）在$500\ \mu mol\cdot L^{-1}$浓度下具有抗胶质母细胞瘤的作用。为了增强该肽的效果，将其转化为二分支（AaTs-1-2B）、四分支（AaTs-1-4B）和八分支（AaTs-1-8B）树枝状聚合物，结果显示，通过增强p53的表达和改变细胞膜钙浓度，该肽的效力提高了10~25倍。此外，还增加了ERK1/2和AKT的磷酸化形式[135]。

有机铁树枝状聚合物的开发旨在提高阿司匹林的生物利用度和抗癌活性，并降低其毒性。合成的树枝状聚合物的抗感染活性结果表明，其对革兰氏阴性菌的活性与庆大霉素相当。研究人员还测试了这些树枝状聚合物对不同癌细胞株的抗癌活性，同时，还比较了这些树枝状聚合物与标准抗癌药物多柔比星的效力。序列中的几种树枝状聚合物表现出明显的抗癌活性，比单独使用药物更有效。此外，这种显著的抗炎活性在动物模型中也得到了确认[136]。

10.2.6 基因递送系统

最近，新型冠状病毒感染和相关疫苗开发获得了监管部门的批准，激起了非病毒基因传递及其应用的浪潮。针对癌症、病毒和其他微生物感染的各种遗传疾病和疫苗浮出水面，其中许多正在积极进行临床研究。在非病毒载体中，除了脂质纳米颗粒外，树状聚合物也是一个经过大量的临床前研究和较少的早期临床试验而受到高度关注的载体，已有至少20年的研究历史。在此，将重点介绍该领域的最新进展。PEI、PAMAM和PPI是众所周知的阳离子树枝状分子，在早期开发阶段就已进行了研究[137-139]。在各种体外实验和动物模型试验中，人们发现一般高代树枝状聚合物具有毒性。该领域的不断发展可以开发出具有各种功能的更新低代树枝状聚合物，从而减少高阳离子电荷引起的毒性，同时保护遗传物质在生理环境中不被降解。本节也将介绍树枝状聚合物的发展趋势，尽管经过各种改良的 PAMAM 树枝状聚合物被认为是一种潜在的递送系统。然而，其他一些树枝状聚合物，如肽类树枝状聚合物、碳硅烷树枝状聚合物、聚酯树枝状聚合物和聚甘油树枝状聚合物，也吸引了制药研究人员对药物输送系统进行研究[133, 140-142]。

使用羟基 PAMAM 树枝状聚合物（G6）将 siRNA 递送到大脑，树枝状聚合物可保护 siGFP 免受酶降解和蛋白质吸附。细胞和临床前研究显示，siGFP 的基因敲除率为 30%~40%，同时保留了市售 RNAi Max 和 Lipofectamine 的效力。体内研究显示，D-siGFP 能定位到肿瘤实质内的肿瘤相关巨噬细胞中，减少了其他副作用，实现了细胞内递送[137]。

利用 PAMAM 树枝状分子可设计一种非病毒载体，并在树枝状分子上结合 Tat 肽（TA）和透明质酸（hyaluronic acid，HA）或两者（PA-TA-HA）。然后，将这些树枝状聚合物与脂质体（Lipo）结合，以研究 eGFP 质粒 DNA 的递送。在对结直肠癌细胞进行测试时，所得复合物显示出不同的转染效率。与单独的 PAMAM 复合物相比，含有所有成分 PA-TA-HA-Lipo 的复合物的转染效率提高了 10 倍，与 PA-TA 和 PA-TA-HA 相比，分别提高了 6 倍和 2 倍。体内研究也反映了同样的结果[140]。在 PAMAM 树枝状分子上结合了胆固醇二肽（HR），以改善树枝状分子的转染和内体逃逸特性。6% 和 23% 终端氨基与胆固醇-二肽（HR）官能团不同比例的结合，显示出与 PEI 25 kDa 相媲美的转染性能，并且具有较低的细胞毒性[143]。4, 4'-二硫代丁二酸对 PAMAM（G3）树枝状聚合物进行了表面官能化，形成了纳米团簇。这种简单的修饰就能使未修饰的 G3 和 G5 PAMAM 树枝状聚合物的性能提高 2 倍。此外，当这种树枝状结构分子与 pDNA-p53 进行测试时，通过上调 p53、p21 mRNA 和蛋白表达，从而使癌细胞停滞在 G1 期，这些载体系统的效能也在临床前模型中得到了确认[144]。

如上所述，经脂质修饰的树枝状聚合物或其他阳离子聚合物比其原生形态具有更好的转染效果和更低的毒性。然而，这些修饰会导致其他因素，如血清蛋白结合和与膜脂的相互作用，往往会限制其应用：部分氟化或氟共轭会导致亲脂性增强，稳定性提高和遗传物质的胞浆递送。使用含氟配体对 PAMAM 和其他树枝状结构分子进行修饰，以增加树枝状结构分子的亲脂性。G5 PAMAM 树枝状聚合物通过与含氟酸酐进行简单的氨解反应，产生了一种名为 G5-F768 PAMAM 的先导树枝状聚合物，在不同的细胞系、更高的非氟化和商业转染剂 Lipofectamine®2000 上进行测试时，显示出 90% 的转染效率。这些结果是在最小 N/P 比（1.5:1）的条件下取得的。理想的比例通常为 8:1 或更高。最值得注意的是，即使在含 50% 血清的培养基中，这些转染能力也可实现。树枝状分子的氟化引起了广泛关注，具有许多不同的优势，如更好的转染、更高的稳定性以及更好的凝结和细胞质基因传递，伴随着连续的内体逃逸[145, 146]。

另一项研究采用低代（G1 和 G2）PAMAM 树枝状分子与七氟丁酸酐（heptafluor obutyric anhydride，HFA）开发了具有可变氟功能化的树枝状分子候选物。初步研究了自组装情况，氟化程度低的呈现多孔纳米结构，氟化程度高的呈现坚固纳米结构—表面的氟化程度决定了各自的 N/P 比率和转染效率。与市售的 SuperFect® 和 jetPEI® 相比，大多数氟化树枝状分子都显示出更好的转染效果，可与 Lipo2000® 相媲美。用选定的氟化树枝状分子 G2-F7$_{11.3}$ 进行了进一步的剂量响应转染，与 20 ng 和 50 ng DNA 相比，足以显示荧光，而商用和 jet PEI® 和 Lipo2000®（0.2 μg）更像病毒载体。同样，这些树枝状聚合物显示出很高的血清稳定性。在效率测试中，使用 3D 球体结构和带肿瘤的小鼠模型。在 3D 球体组织中，与氟化树枝状分子相比，转染效果明显优于Lipo2000®。体内研究显示，2个氟化树枝状聚合物都有转染作用，而未氟化的树枝状聚合物则没有[147]。PAMAM树枝状聚合物的安全性常常得到提高。树枝状聚合物带有高阳离子电荷，因此可与脂质类[148]和白蛋白[149]等其他载体系统结合使用，以提高树枝状聚合物的生物相容性。进一步的糖基化[150]或靶向获取肽序列cRGD[149]、CVSR6G2R4[151]、RRILH[152]、DDDDDDVKRKKKP[153]和RHF[154]可以帮助到达靶组织和细胞内环境，并在细胞内递送遗传物质。PAMAM（G3）树枝状分子转化为异质树枝状分子G3-乙缩醛胺。这导致树枝状聚合物在弱酸性条件下因乙缩醛基的裂解而转化为羟基。再与pMAX-GFP质粒复合后，转染能力比PAMAM（G4-NH$_2$）树枝状聚合物提高了5倍。Kim等开发了精氨酸功能化的聚（胱胺双丙烯酰胺-二氨基己烷）（ABP）共轭PAMAM树枝状分子，测试了其生物可还原机制，以改善转染性能，同时递送pDNA、siRNA，并与非可还原的对照物或基于PEI的经典转染剂进行了比较。结果表明，生物还原系统的性能更优越[155-157]。

二氨基丁酸PPI树枝状聚合物与带有乳铁蛋白的金纳米笼结合，然后与质粒DNA（AuNC-DAB-Lf-DNA）复合。与细胞毒性最小的DAB树枝状复合物相比，编码TNF-α的AuNC-DAB-Lf-DNA的抗增殖活性提高了9倍[140]。

不同代的树枝状超支化聚合物（DHP）与聚酯或聚酯胺开发为基因传递的载体系统。[158]。图10-14说明了树枝状聚合物的化学结构。使用2种遗传物质pGFP和siGFP评估了效率。在

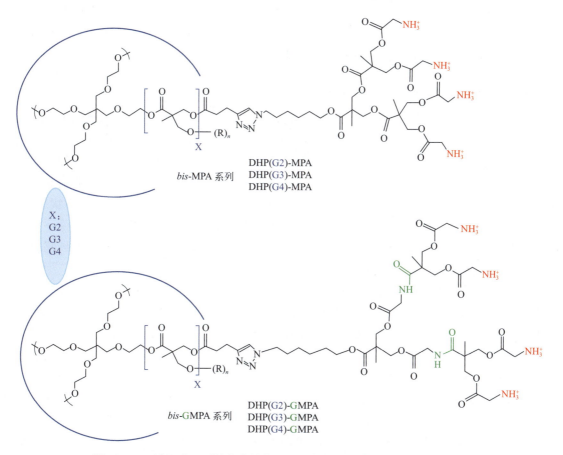

图10-14 这两个系列的化学结构是具有氨基末端树枝状超支化聚合物（G2、G3或G4）的超支化聚酯或聚酯酰胺[158]

该研究中，具有 bis-MPA 的树枝状聚合物在 pGFP 和 siGFP 中均具有优于 bis-GMPA 的转染特性。它显示出比商用基于树枝状聚合物的转染剂 SuperFect® 和 Lipofectamine ® 3000 更高的转染率。由于 N/P 比率在转染性能中起到关键作用，较高的百分比在同一时间表现更佳，但只有 60% 的细胞存活率。内化研究表明，基于双 GMPA 的树枝状聚合物仅结合细胞表面。同时，bis-GMPA 内化到细胞质环境和细胞核其他周围，表明 bis-GMPA 的转染能力较差[158]。在另一项研究中，PPI 树枝状聚合物经过 C_{18} 脂质和聚乙二醇化修饰，并将生物可还原成分纳入系统中。该系统在 PC-3 细胞中将转染增强了 16 倍，在 DU145 细胞中增强了约 27 倍。功能性树枝状聚合物在递送治疗性物质同时没有产生任何毒副作用[159]。

碳硅烷树枝状聚合物是一种以无机 Si 为核心、以碳氢化合物为分支的混合树枝状聚合物，其表面功能化既有阳离子也有阴离子，以满足其应用需求[142]。与其他树枝状聚合物相比，它们更具疏水性，并且更具有热稳定性[142, 160]。例如，研究人员开发了胍基末端碳硅烷树枝状聚合物（BDLS002），用于传递 siNrf2（一种靶向 Nrf2 基因的特定 siRNA），以克服膀胱癌治疗中的顺铂化疗耐药性。这导致 siRNA-树枝状聚合物复合物在选定的细胞系孵育 48 h 内释放并抑制 Nrf2，对正常细胞具有良好的安全性，降低了对顺铂耐药癌细胞的迁移，提高了对促氧化剂细胞毒药物的敏感性。

不对称肽树枝状聚合物在用作非病毒基因递送载体方面前景广阔。由于其氨基酸组成，它们可以模拟细胞穿膜肽、强烈缩合阴离子核酸、具有内体逃逸效应，且可以自然降解，可作为基因递送载体持续应用。例如，研究人员开发了名为 D3K2 和 D3G2 的多肽树枝状聚合物来递送 pcDNA3-EGFP。转染结果表明，D3K2 在癌细胞和正常细胞中的转染效果与商用 Lipo2000® 相当。然而，有趣的是，这些树枝状聚合物显示出对癌细胞具有细胞毒性，或许可用于具有协同机制的抗癌药物递送[161]。再如，以二硬脂酰基磷脂酰乙醇胺（DSPE）为疏水尾部，以树枝状 L-赖氨酸为亲水头部，开发出了两亲磷脂肽树枝状聚合物 DSPE-KK2 和 DSPE-KK2K4。当 N/P 比率≥5 时，与这两种树枝状分子形成稳定的复合物可保护 siRNA 不被降解。有趣的是，小树枝形分子 DSPE-KK2 在细胞和动物研究中都显示出更好的转染和基因敲除效果。树枝状聚合物成分中亲水性和亲油性的平衡有助于更好地进行细胞内递送和释放 siRNA[141]。此外，还有研究人员利用"鸟氨酸"开发了阳离子 G2 和 G3 肽树枝状聚合物。将相应的树枝状聚合物与 pDNA 复合，并通过与 PEI 25 kDa 比较来测试其转染特性，结果显示转染效率比 PEI 25 kDa 高 7 倍。当使用人体皮肤外植体进行 siRNA 递送时，发现鸟氨酸树枝状聚合物产生的蛋白质从 2% 增加到 12%[162]。

当前有一种令人兴奋的树枝状脂质纳米颗粒（LNP）组合被开发用于递送遗传物质。如图 10-15（A）所示，使用具有不同烷基链的各种胺核心来创建可电离的树枝状聚合物。最初筛选该树枝状聚合物是因为其与遗传物质络合的能力、稳定性以及针对不同细胞系的各自的细胞毒性。将选定的树枝状聚合物（4A3-SC8）与特定比例的其他成分树枝状聚合物-胆固醇-DOPE-PEG-DMG（38.5∶30∶30∶1.5）配制为脂质纳米粒，并用不同比例的 mRNA∶修饰的 sgRNA∶ssDNA 进行测试，1∶1∶3 和 2∶1∶3 的 HDR 校正率约为 56%。通过肿瘤内注射对异种移植肿瘤注入无胸腺裸 Foxn1 nu 小鼠进行进一步测试，结果显示 >20% HDR 介导的基因校正。图 10-15 显示了 LNP 的形成及其在动物模型中的递送。这可能是进一步开发基于 pDNA、siRNA 和 mRNA 等遗传物质传递的疫苗 LNP 的理想系统[163]。

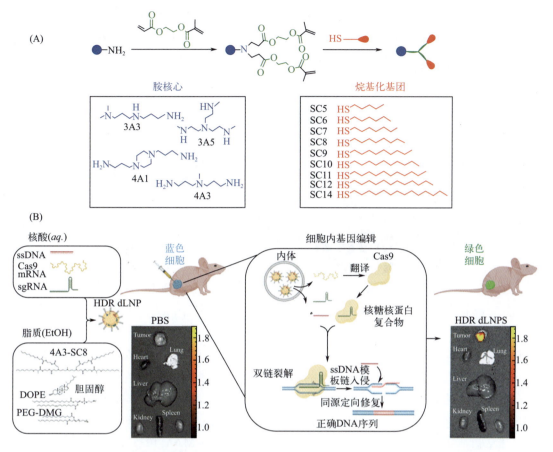

图10-15 （A）不同可电离树枝状聚合物的化学结构；（B）用Cas9 mRNA配制脂质纳米颗粒和体内递送效率[163]

10.2.7 树枝状大分子在新型冠状病毒感染中的应用

随着我们进入新型冠状病毒感染的不同阶段，越来越多的人正遭受着新型冠状病毒感染后期和长期问题的困扰。世卫组织报告称，超过200种症状与长期新型冠状病毒有关，这给医疗专业人员诊断和提供治疗造成了复杂的情况。一项基于800名志愿者及其新型冠状病毒感染前后（轻度感染）的大脑图像分析的研究结果表明，他们的大脑（主要是灰质）萎缩，并且新型冠状病毒对与主要嗅觉皮层相连的区域的组织造成更严重的损害。脑脊液量增加直接反映了长期新冠的认知、嗅觉和味觉、头痛和记忆问题。这主要是由身体各个区域、肺部和大脑的过度炎症所致[164]。

OP-101是一种基于树枝状聚合物的产品，由第4代PAMAM树枝状聚合物（约4 nm）和N-乙酰半胱氨酸共价键合而成，它可以在巨噬细胞胞浆内通过谷胱甘肽的还原机制迅速释放，从而产生显著的抗炎和抗氧化效果。随后的2 a临床试验展示了这种新型共轭物的耐受性，其在炎症性脑损伤标志物中的作用，以及在重症病例中的感染率和死亡人数方面的影响[7]。Viraleze™是一种抗病毒鼻喷雾剂——由Star Pharma开发的基于树枝状聚合物的治疗剂，已用于治疗细菌性阴道病，商品名为Vivagel™。核心树枝状聚合物由赖氨酸单体（第4

代）制成，其胺末端装饰有32个1-（羧基甲氧基）萘-3, 6-二磺酸钠，用于抗菌和抗病毒作用。该产品现在以不同的名称出售，用于治疗细菌性阴道病和避孕套润滑剂。其他实验室研究显示针对HIV、单纯疱疹病毒（HSV）和人乳头瘤病毒（HPV）的显示疗效[165]。

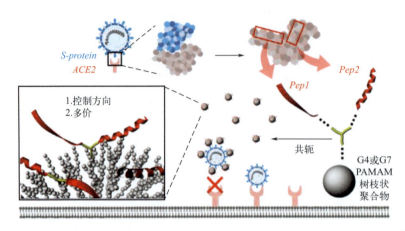

图10-16　使用多肽和树枝状聚合物共轭物抑制SARS-COV2-ACE2结合[78]

其他几项研究也显示了潜在的抗病毒应用，这些应用并非专门针对新型冠状病毒，而是探索树枝状聚合物作为多功能载体系统的优势和潜力。例如，一项研究发表了阳离子和阴离子树枝状聚合物的抗病毒治疗效果，研究发现阴离子树枝状聚合物（G1.5 COONa）在减少MERS-CoV斑块的形成中优于阳离子树枝状聚合物40%，这个低代树枝状聚合物无毒，同时可以递送抗病毒药物，提高了治疗效果[166]。G4和G7 PAMAM树状聚合物可与一些ACE2拮抗剂肽序列连接。这种基于亲和力的SARS-CoV-2拮抗剂根据代数在结合刺突蛋白上表现出差异，G7 PAMAM树枝状分子的SARS-CoV-2亲和力明显高于单独的肽。当用体外SAR-COV模拟微珠进行测试时，G4树枝状聚合物共轭物与表达ACE2的MCF-7细胞的结合率为39.5%，G7树枝状聚合物共轭物与表达ACE2的MCF-7细胞的结合率为51.4%[167]。

另有一项关于MIR 19®吸入器基因产品的临床试验，该产品是siRNA与生物相容性KK-46肽树枝状聚合物的复合物。虽然预防性疫苗SARS-CoV-2已被批准使用，但在空间抗病毒治疗方面的临床成功率却很有限，特别是对感染SARS-CoV-2的患者的治疗。因此，开发了这种siRNA疗法，以满足尚未得到满足的临床需求。到目前为止，初步结果表明，与随机对照试验中的标准疗法相比，MIR 19®是安全的，并改善了COVID-19患者的临床结果[168]。树枝状聚合物及其应用的多个方面已被用于开发新型COVID-19治疗方法，这些成果可能为未来基于树枝状聚合物的新疗法铺平道路。

10.3　树枝状聚合物给药的计算问题与挑战

近年来，人们对药物和基因传递系统表现出前所未有的兴趣，通过将强效治疗分子传递到身体中的特定组织，以治疗危及生命的疾病[68, 169-172]。通过控制给定药物的精确水平和位置，可以设计新的疗法，从而减少副作用并降低剂量。因此，从计算的角度来看，需要估计药物与其载体之间的结合和动力学，以更好地理解其作用机制[172]。在载体中，树枝状聚合物已成为众多分子动力学研究的主题，特别是探索药物相互作用[68,171]。

树枝状聚合物领域的计算应用主要用于药物和遗传物质的合成、结合和封装，与生物膜的相互作用，以及了解药理和临床使用的药代动力学行为。图10-17展示了计算药剂学在树枝状聚合物领域的应用[173]。例如，为了测量PAMAM（G0）树枝状分子与抗癌药物美法仑的化学反应性，研究人员进行了基于NHS/EDC的共价化学连接剂的几何优化和量子化学计算研究，其中包括分子轨道、自然键轨道、拓扑结构和其他物理化学分子参数的分析。化学反应性在气体和溶剂两相中都进行了测量。对这些理论计算和相应研究结果的分析表明，美法仑与树枝状聚合物的纯共价结合在气相和溶剂相中都没有显示出任何其他类型的相互作用，而药物与树枝状聚合物之间的结合能则从 -18.045 eV 降至 -43.134 eV[174]。由于这项研究只使用了PAMAM（G0）树枝状聚合物，因此结合下一代树枝状聚合物、表面功能和核心化学进一步扩展这些计算，可用于揭示药物与树枝状聚合物的化学反应性化学结合和任何其他相互作用，这对于高效的化学合成和各自的纯化策略以及临床使用的药物产品质量至关重要。

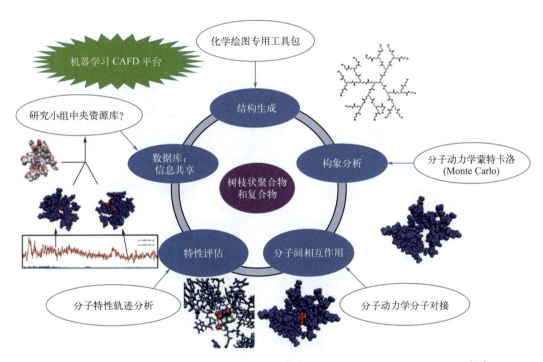

图10-17　计算药物学在树枝状聚合物的发现、开发和递送应用中的应用概述[173]

最近的一项研究[68]利用分子动力学模拟结合量子化学计算研究了5-氟尿嘧啶（5-FU）与不对称多肽树枝状载体系统之间的相互作用。使用NAMD 2.10代码进行了分子动力学（MD）计算[175]，使用CHARMM进行了针对不对称树枝状分子和5-FU的CGENFF通用力场计算[176]，优化与CHARMM力场兼容的5-FU，以与其他研究工作保持一致[177]。这些研究旨在更好地理解混合的5-FU和水系统[178]。这些量子数据被用于动力学模拟。

通过研究观察到，这些治疗分子与树枝状分子的相互作用与以往的研究不同，以往的研究中预期药物将保留在载体的疏水核心内。然而，5-FU 的溶解度较低，这导致其通过氢键和相关的接触事件，与肽树枝状分子之间发生了弱、瞬时的相互作用。这种相互作用随着高代数树枝状分子的增加而增加。图 10-18 展示了药物 5-FU 与中性和带电肽树枝状分子的相互作用快照。尽管树枝状分子的表面电荷对于它们与药物的相互作用有着与其反离子效应相反的影响，但带有中性电荷的树枝状分子具有形成簇状或聚集体的倾向。电荷排斥对于在溶液中保持独立是至关重要的。这个过程有助于选择合适的载体系统[178]。

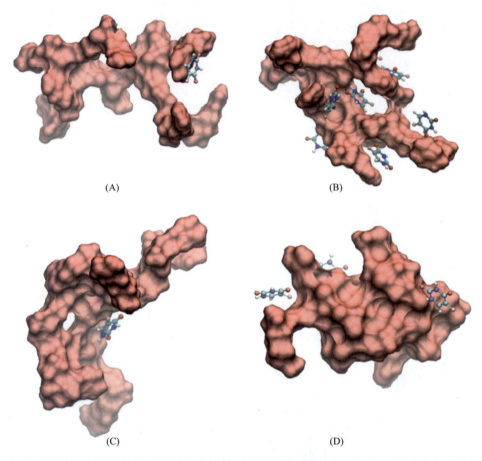

图 10-18　代表性快照（A）药物与带电肽树枝状聚合物末端氨基的相互作用；（B）药物与带电肽树枝状聚合物的相互作用；（C）药物与带电肽树枝状聚合物在 PMF 最小值处的相互作用；以及（D）药物与中性肽树枝状聚合物的相互作用[171]

多年来，计算方法还使研究人员能够更深入地探索已发展的分子过程，并使科学家能够深入探究那些无法通过当前实验技术实现的分子过程。其中一个必要的过程就是细胞膜穿透。这个屏障是与外部环境建立连接并调节外部成分进入细胞的通道。尽管生物膜的结构和成分已经被充分了解和研究，但物质进入机制以及穿越细胞膜屏障所需的运输过程仍然相当不清楚。需要进一步的研究来探索这个领域，以设计更好的载体系统。细胞膜由一层薄薄的脂质双分子层组成，其中的疏水屏障将亲水的内部和外部环境隔开。这种排列限制了极性分子在膜上的扩散。教科书上对物质如何通过膜进行交换的解释依赖于孔隙和通道的存在。虽然从许多实验和理论研究中可以推断出孔隙和通道的形成，但对这些孔隙的直接观察却一直难以实现。一些实验为膜的渗透提供了新的证据，但这些证据与孔隙形成的概念并不相符，这让人怀疑我们是否完全理解了这个问题。澄清膜渗透等分子过程需要一些工具，这些工具可以探测时间和空间尺度，超出目前的实验技术所能轻易实现的范围。这正是我们的计算方法发挥作用的地方。通过使用分子动力学和量子力学计算，研究人员从根本上对膜动力学有了新的认识，这对药物递送等应用具有变革潜力[68]。在这项工作中，研究者提出了一个多肽（线性和树枝状）转运模型，该模型不需要孔隙的存在，而且可能与此类实验相吻合。带电肽在膜的疏水性内部会遇到很高的障碍，这在意料之中，但实验告诉我们，这种细胞穿透肽穿过膜的速度相当快。实验发现，细胞穿透肽可以通过脱落部分正电荷来适应膜内的疏水环境。为此，它将部分质子通过质子线（基本上是水分子的线性链）传送回膜的表皮或靠近表皮区域的一些带负电荷的簇。质子从高电位的内部区域通过水链移动到低电位的表皮区域，就像金属线在电位差中连接电荷一样。这样就有效地留下了中性肽，它可以更快地通过膜扩散，而所需的能量成本只是阳离子肽的一小部分。这表明肽具有变色龙般的行为，通过这种行为，肽可以伪装自己，以应对疏水-亲水条件的变化：肽会失去质子，然后根据需要重新获得质子，以尽量减少其在环境中的自由能。

这项研究的另一个发现是，桥式结构（即多肽横跨两片膜片）似乎很稳定，在膜的两侧都有明确的锚点。如图10-19所示，这为小分子在膜上自如移动创造了迁移通道，这种现象通过抗癌药物 5-FU 得到了证实。实时 MD 捕捉到了多肽介导的药物分子的膜转移。这是一个惊人的观察结果，以前从未有过直接分子模拟的报道。这些关于多肽如何穿透膜的新的机制见解非常深刻。它们为肽如何在截然不同的环境中进行化学适应提供了新的基本认识，在化学和生物科学领域有着深远的应用前景[68]。除药物递送外，欧阳等[179, 180]还利用其他 MD 研究解释了遗传物质与树枝状聚合物的复合过程、不同 pH 条件下的释放机制，详细说明了复合体的主要力学情况，这有助于设计和优化高功能树枝状聚合物载体系统。

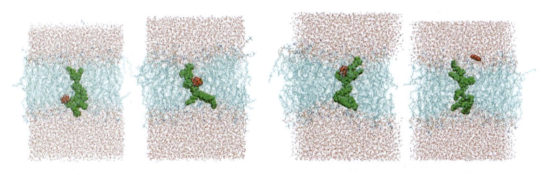

图10-19　药物5-FU（红色）穿过DOPC膜（青色），膜周围有水。多肽树枝状聚合物为绿色[68]

进一步可采用全原子分子动力学（AA-MD）研究来探讨 PAMAM 作为模型树枝状分子的封装效率和不同药物的释放情况，如利福平[181]、伊红 Y[182]、烟酸[183]、硼替佐米[50]等。例如，有一项研究使用了与呋塞米复合的低代 PAMAM，结合体内药代动力学与 AA-MD 进行了平行研究。结果表明，胺基团与药物分子之间的相互作用不仅能包裹药物，还能防止药物团聚，从而提高药物在溶液中的可用性，改善药代动力学[184]。这类模拟研究有助于预测药物的药代动力学行为。另一种不同的MD研究称为离散MD模拟，用于研究树枝状聚合物如何与血清蛋白和免疫球蛋白相互作用，同时使用不同的表面电荷和功能化中性磷酰胆碱、聚乙二醇和羟基。模拟数据有助于设计一种隐形纳米颗粒系统，减少与血清蛋白的结合[185]。为研究不同温度下规则和液晶树枝状聚合物的结构特性，如尺寸、粒子分布、中心到末端的距离，开发了一种粗粒度蒙特卡洛模拟研究。单分子模拟的结果有助于对各代数值聚合物的大小、分布、中心到末端的距离和堆积分数进行比较，从而调整树枝状聚合物的体积及其与相应治疗药物的分子水平关联[186]。

其他一些平台，如dendPoint，提供了有关不同树枝状聚合物及其药代动力学性能的综合信息[187]。该数据库有助于提供简明信息，以了解树枝状聚合物在药理条件下的行为。可以利用它来开发和改进树枝状聚合物的理化特性，从而推进临床应用。机器学习工具和人工智能的最新进展有望简化这一过程。已有多项研究利用人工智能将树枝状聚合物用于诊断淀粉样β纤维和疾病进展状态[188]。同样，在另一项研究中，ML工具被用于预测树枝状分子的细胞毒性[189]。计算药物学领域的技术进步和人工智能/ML工具的整合可大幅提高树枝状聚合物载体系统和纳米技术的临床性能。

10.4 总结

树枝状聚合物是高度确定的合成大分子，与纳米颗粒一样，可广泛应用于各个领域，包括环境和农业应用[190-192]，反映了树枝状聚合物的多样性。不过，生物医学和制药应用是人们最感兴趣的领域，如上所述，树枝状聚合物可用作载体系统，向靶组织递送更广泛的治疗分子。树枝状聚合物是一种多功能系统，对于开发治疗复杂疾病（如癌症）的新型治疗模式至关重要，可通过与单克隆抗体和抗癌药物结合，结合现有的治疗方案，精确地递送到癌症部位。同样，树枝状聚合物和各自的表面功能化可作为抗原产品进行开发，这有助于针对新型和现有的传染病和危及生命的疾病开发现代疫苗，进一步促进精准医学的研究与发展。与其他载体系统不同，树枝状聚合物及其多功能性递送模式降低了使用多种辅料组合的复杂性。例如，用于基因/疫苗递送的常用阳离子脂质纳米颗粒至少需要4种辅料组合才能用作载体系统。树枝状聚合物为复杂的基因载体提供了阳离子特性，其靶向性在保护治疗载体的酶降解和环境降解的同时，还提供了佐剂特性，是理想的载体平台。然而，许多树枝状聚合物已在细胞研究和临床前应用中进行了评估。只有通过稳健的设计、实验计划以及药代动力学和毒理学研究，才能取得临床成功，从而提高树枝状聚合物的能力。此外，复杂的合成和纯化策略以及降解机制对于扩大工艺规模以实现实际目标和临床疗效仍具有挑战性。

此外，先进的人工智能和机器学习应用可用于快速评估树枝状聚合物与药物和基因材料的物理化学相互作用，并评估其在不出现任何副作用的情况下用于递送载体的影响[193-195]。由于一些基于树枝状聚合物的载体系统和治疗剂已经进入临床阶段，监管批准为研究和开发基于树枝状聚合物的新系统和临床应用提供了机会。

参考文献

[1] Pilkington E H, Suys E J A, Trevaskis N L, et al. From influenza to COVID-19: Lipid nanoparticle mRNA vaccines at the frontiers of infectious diseases[J]. Acta biomater, 2021, 131: 16-40.

[2] Uddin M N, Roni M A. Challenges of storage and stability of mRNA-based COVID-19 vaccines[J]. Vaccines, 2021, 9(9): 1033.

[3] Rele S. COVID-19 vaccine development during pandemic: gap analysis, opportunities, and impact on future emerging infectious disease development strategies[J]. Human Vaccines Immunother, 2021, 17(4): 1122-1127.

[4] Ashvattha Therapeutics, I., A Study to Evaluate the Safety, Tolerability and Pharmacokinetics of D-4517.2 After Subcutaneous Administration in Subjects With Neovascular(Wet)Age-Related Macular Degeneration(AMD)or Subjects With Diabetic Macular Edema(DME)(Tejas). 2023.

[5] Russia, N.R.C.-I.o.I.F.M.-B.A.o. The siCoV/KK46 Drug Open-safety Study.

[6] Hu J, Hu K, Cheng Y. Tailoring the dendrimer core for efficient gene delivery[J]. Acta biomater, 2016, 35: 1-11.

[7] Gusdon A M, Faraday N, Aita J S, et al. Dendrimer nanotherapy for severe COVID-19 attenuates inflammation and neurological injury markers and improves outcomes in a phase 2a clinical trial[J]. Sci Transl Med, 2022, 14(654): eabo2652.

[8] Starpharma. VIRALEZE™ Nasal Spray Approved in Malaysia [cited 2023]

[9] Pharma, s. VivaGel® BV launched in Europe, 2019.

[10] Bénéteau‐Burnat B, Baudin B, Vaubourdolle M. Evaluation of stratus® CS Stat fluorimetric analyser for measurement of cardiac markers Troponin I(cTnI), creatine kinase MB(CK‐MB), and myoglobin[J]. J Clin Lab Anal, 2001, 15(6): 314-318.

[11] Akhtar S, Chandrasekhar B, Attur S, et al. On the nanotoxicity of PAMAM dendrimers: Superfect® stimulates the EGFR-ERK1/2 signal transduction pathway via an oxidative stress-dependent mechanism in HEK 293 cells[J]. Int J Pharm, 2013, 448(1): 239-246.

[12] Carpenter S. A star performer – Priostar® dendrimers, 2016.

[13] Starpharma. DEP® docetaxel clinical status.

[14] Mitchell M J, Billingsley M M, Haley R M, et al. Engineering precision nanoparticles for drug delivery[J]. Nat Rev Drug Discov, 2021, 20(2): 101-124.

[15] Zu H, Gao D. Non-viral vectors in gene therapy: Recent development, challenges, and prospects[J]. AAPS J, 2021, 23(4): 78.

[16] Wang J, Li B, Qiu L, et al. Dendrimer-based drug delivery systems: history, challenges, and latest developments[J]. J Biol Eng, 2022, 16(1): 1-12.

[17] Huang Y T, Kao C, Selvaraj A, et al. Solid-phase dendrimer synthesis: a promising approach to transform dendrimer construction[J]. Mater Today Chem, 2023, 27: 101285.

[18] Chauhan A S, Kulhari H. Pharmaceutical applications of dendrimers[M].Elsevier, 2019.

[19] Liu X Y, Zhang X, Yang J, et al. Multifunctional amphiphilic peptide dendrimer as nonviral gene vectors for effective cancer therapy via combined gene/photodynamic therapies[J]. Colloids Surf B: Biointerfaces, 2022, 217: 112651.

[20] Morfill C, Pankratova S, Machado P, et al. Nanostars carrying multifunctional neurotrophic dendrimers protect neurons in preclinical in vitro models of neurodegenerative disorders[J]. ACS Appl Mater Interfaces, 2022, 14(42): 47445-47460.

[21] Inoue M, Higashi T, Hayashi Y, et al. Multifunctional therapeutic cyclodextrin-appended dendrimer complex for treatment of systemic and localized amyloidosis[J]. ACS Appl Mater Interfaces, 2022, 14(36): 40599-40611.

[22] Moscariello P, Ng D Y W, Jansen M, et al. Brain delivery of multifunctional dendrimer protein bioconjugates[J]. Adv Sci, 2018, 5(5): 1700897.

[23] Li Y, Zhou Y, Wang T, et al. Photoenhanced cytosolic protein delivery based on a photocleavable group-modified dendrimer[J]. Nanoscale, 2021, 13(42): 17784-17792.

[24] Nagai K, Sato T, Kojima C. Design of a dendrimer with a matrix metalloproteinase-responsive fluorescence probe and a tumor-homing peptide for metastatic tumor cell imaging in the lymph node[J]. Bioorg Med Chem Lett, 2021, 33: 127726.

[25] Chen M, Betzer O, Fan Y, et al. Multifunctional dendrimer-entrapped gold nanoparticles for labeling and tracking T cells via dual-modal computed tomography and fluorescence imaging[J]. Biomacromolecules, 2020, 21(4): 1587-1595.

[26] Mohtavinejad N, Amanlou M, Bitarafan-Rajabi A, et al. Technetium-99 m-PEGylated dendrimer-G2-(Dabcyle-Lys6, Phe7)-pHBSP: A novel Nano-Radiotracer for molecular and early detecting of cardiac ischemic region[J]. Bioorg Chem, 2020, 98: 103731.

[27] Liu J, Xiong Z, Zhang J, et al. Zwitterionic gadolinium(Ⅲ)-complexed dendrimer-entrapped gold nanoparticles for

enhanced computed tomography/magnetic resonance imaging of lung cancer metastasis[J]. ACS Appl Mater Interfaces, 2019, 11(17): 15212-15221.

[28] Xing Y, Zhu J, Zhao L, et al. SPECT/CT imaging of chemotherapy-induced tumor apoptosis using 99 mTc-labeled dendrimer-entrapped gold nanoparticles[J]. Drug Deliv, 2018, 25(1): 1384-1393.

[29] Liu H, Wang J. Loading IR820 using multifunctional dendrimers with enhanced stability and specificity[J]. Pharmaceutics, 2018, 10(3): 77.

[30] Grześkowiak B F, Maziukiewicz D, Kozłowska A, et al., Polyamidoamine dendrimers decorated multifunctional polydopamine nanoparticles for targeted chemo-and photothermal therapy of liver cancer model[J]. Int J Mol Sci, 2021, 22(2): 738.

[31] Rompicharla S V K, Kumari P, Bhatt H, et al. Biotin functionalized PEGylated poly(amidoamine)dendrimer conjugate for active targeting of paclitaxel in cancer[J]. Int J Pharm, 2019, 557: 329-341.

[32] Hill E E, Kim J K, Jung Y, et al. Integrin alpha V beta 3 targeted dendrimer‐rapamycin conjugate reduces fibroblast‐mediated prostate tumor progression and metastasis[J]. J Cell Biochem, 2018, 119(10): 8074-8083.

[33] Hu Q, Wang Y, Xu L, et al. Transferrin conjugated pH-and redox-responsive poly(amidoamine)dendrimer conjugate as an efficient drug delivery carrier for cancer therapy[J]. Int J Nanomedicine, 2020: 2751-2764.

[34] Xia C, Yin S, Xu S, et al. Low molecular weight heparin-coated and dendrimer-based core-shell nanoplatform with enhanced immune activation and multiple anti-metastatic effects for melanoma treatment[J]. Theranostics, 2019, 9(2): 337-354.

[35] Zhang M, Zhu J, Zheng Y, et al. Doxorubicin-conjugated PAMAM dendrimers for pH-responsive drug release and folic acid-targeted cancer therapy[J]. Pharmaceutics, 2018, 10(3): 162.

[36] Wu P Y, Shen Z C, Jiang J L, et al. A multifunctional theranostics nanosystem featuring self-assembly of alcohol-abuse drug and photosensitizers for synergistic cancer therapy[J]. Biomater Sci, 2022, 10(21): 6267-6281.

[37] Huang W, Wang L, Zou Y, et al. Preparation of gastrodin‐modified dendrimer‐entrapped gold nanoparticles as a drug delivery system for cerebral ischemia-reperfusion injury[J]. Brain Behav, 2022, 12(12): e2810.

[38] Li J, Chen L, Xu X, et al. Targeted combination of antioxidative and anti‐inflammatory therapy of rheumatoid arthritis using multifunctional Dendrimer‐Entrapped gold nanoparticles as a platform[J]. Small, 2020, 16(49): 2005661.

[39] Bhatt H, Kiran Rompicharla S V, Ghosh B, et al. α-tocopherol succinate-anchored PEGylated Poly(amidoamine)dendrimer for the delivery of paclitaxel: assessment of in vitro and in vivo therapeutic efficacy[J]. Mol Pharm, 2019, 16(4): 1541-1554.

[40] Zhu J, Wang G, Alves C S, et al. Multifunctional dendrimer-entrapped gold nanoparticles conjugated with doxorubicin for pH-responsive drug delivery and targeted computed tomography imaging[J]. Langmuir, 2018, 34(41): 12428-12435.

[41] Pandey P K, Maheshwari R, Raval N, et al. Nanogold-core multifunctional dendrimer for pulsatile chemo-, photothermal- and photodynamic-therapy of rheumatoid arthritis[J]. J Colloid Interface Sci, 2019, 544: 61-77.

[42] Oliveira I M, Gonçalves C, Oliveira E P, et al. PAMAM dendrimers functionalised with an anti-TNF α antibody and chondroitin sulphate for treatment of rheumatoid arthritis[J]. Mater Sci Eng C, 2021, 121: 111845.

[43] Zhang D, Atochina-Vasserman E N, Maurya D S, et al. One-component multifunctional sequence-defined ionizable amphiphilic Janus dendrimer delivery systems for mRNA[J]. J Am Chem Soc, 2021, 143(31): 12315-12327.

[44] Selin M, Nummelin S, Deleu J, et al. High-generation amphiphilic Janus-dendrimers as stabilizing agents for drug suspensions[J]. Biomacromolecules, 2018, 19(10): 3983-3993.

[45] Xie Y, Yao Y. Octenylsuccinate hydroxypropyl phytoglycogen, a dendrimer-like biopolymer, solubilizes poorly water-soluble active pharmaceutical ingredients[J]. Carbohydr Polym, 2018, 180: 29-37.

[46] Xie Y, Yao Y. Octenylsuccinate hydroxypropyl phytoglycogen enhances the solubility and in-vitro antitumor efficacy of niclosamide[J]. Int J Pharm, 2018, 535(1-2): 157-163.

[47] Kesharwani P, Xie L, Banerjee S, et al. Hyaluronic acid-conjugated polyamidoamine dendrimers for targeted delivery of 3, 4-difluorobenzylidene curcumin to CD44 overexpressing pancreatic cancer cells[J]. Colloids Surf B Biointerfaces, 2015, 136: 413-423.

[48] López-Méndez L J, Cuéllar-Ramírez E E, Cabrera-Quiñones N C, et al. Convergent click synthesis of macromolecular dendritic β-cyclodextrin derivatives as non-conventional drug carriers: Albendazole as guest model[J]. Int J Biol Macromol, 2020, 164: 1704-1714.

[49] Mahmoudi A, Jaafari M R, Ramezanian N, et al. BR2 and CyLoP1 enhance in-vivo SN38 delivery using pegylated PAMAM dendrimers[J]. Int J Pharm, 2019, 564: 77-89.

[50] Chaudhary S, Gothwal A, Khan I, et al. Polypropyleneimine and polyamidoamine dendrimer mediated enhanced solubilization of bortezomib: Comparison and evaluation of mechanistic aspects by thermodynamics and molecular

simulations[J]. Mater Sci Eng C, 2017, 72: 611-619.

[51] Alfei S, Schito A M, Zuccari G. Considerable improvement of ursolic acid water solubility by its encapsulation in dendrimer nanoparticles: Design, synthesis and physicochemical characterization[J]. Nanomaterials, 2021, 11(9): 2196.

[52] Alfei S, Marengo B, Domenicotti C. Polyester-based dendrimer nanoparticles combined with etoposide have an improved cytotoxic and pro-oxidant effect on human neuroblastoma cells[J]. Antioxidants, 2020, 9(1): 50.

[53] Shi Y, Ye F, Chen Y, et al. Dendrimer-like glucan nanoparticulate system improves the solubility and cellular antioxidant activity of coenzyme Q10[J]. Food Chem, 2020, 333: 127510.

[54] Igartúa D E, Martinez C S, Temprana C F, et al. PAMAM dendrimers as a carbamazepine delivery system for neurodegenerative diseases: A biophysical and nanotoxicological characterization[J]. Int J Pharm, 2018, 544(1): 191-202.

[55] Hegde A R, Rewatkar P V, Manikkath J, et al. Peptide dendrimer-conjugates of ketoprofen: Synthesis and ex vivo and in vivo evaluations of passive diffusion, sonophoresis and iontophoresis for skin delivery[J]. Eur J Pharm Sci, 2017, 102: 237-249.

[56] Alfei S, Catena S, Ponassi M, et al. Hydrophilic and amphiphilic water-soluble dendrimer prodrugs suitable for parenteral administration of a non-soluble non-nucleoside HIV-1 reverse transcriptase inhibitor thiocarbamate derivative[J]. Eur J Pharm Sci, 2018, 124: 153-164.

[57] Mehrizi T Z, Ardestani M S, Khamesipour A, et al. Reduction toxicity of Amphotericin B through loading into a novel nanoformulation of anionic linear globular dendrimer for improve treatment of leishmania major[J]. J Mater Sci Mater Med, 2018, 29(8): 125.

[58] Zadeh Mehrizi T, Khamesipour A, Shafiee Ardestani M, et al. Comparative analysis between four model nanoformulations of amphotericin B-chitosan, amphotericin B-dendrimer, betulinic acid-chitosan and betulinic acid-dendrimer for treatment of Leishmania major: real-time PCR assay plus[J]. Int J Nanomedicine, 2019, 14: 7593-7607.

[59] Kaczorowska A, Malinga-Drozd M, Kałas W, et al. Biotin-containing third generation glucoheptoamidated polyamidoamine dendrimer for 5-aminolevulinic acid delivery system[J]. Int J Mol Sci, 2021, 22(4): 1982.

[60] Ooya T, Lee J. Hydrotropic hydrogels prepared from polyglycerol dendrimers: Enhanced solubilization and release of paclitaxel[J]. Gels, 2022, 8(10): 614.

[61] Liu J, Pang Y, Huang W, et al. Bioreducible micelles self-assembled from amphiphilic hyperbranched multiarm copolymer for glutathione-mediated intracellular drug delivery[J]. Biomacromolecules, 2011, 12(5): 1567-1577.

[62] Zeng Z, Qi D, Yang L, et al. Stimuli-responsive self-assembled dendrimers for oral protein delivery[J]. J Control Release. 2019, 315: 206-213.

[63] Zhao W, Yang S, Li C, et al. Amphiphilic dendritic nanomicelle-mediated delivery of gemcitabine for enhancing the specificity and effectiveness[J]. Int J Nanomedicine, 2022, 17: 3239-3249.

[64] Kirkby M, Sabri A B, Scurr D J, et al. Dendrimer-mediated permeation enhancement of chlorhexidine digluconate: Determination of in vitro skin permeability and visualisation of dermal distribution[J]. Eur J Pharm Biopharm, 2021, 159: 77-87.

[65] Venuganti V V K, Perumal O P. Effect of poly(amidoamine)(PAMAM)dendrimer on skin permeation of 5-fluorouracil[J]. Int J Pharm, 2008, 361(1-2): 230-238.

[66] Shah N, Steptoe R J, Parekh H S. Low-generation asymmetric dendrimers exhibit minimal toxicity and effectively complex DNA[J]. J Pept Sci, 2011, 17(6): 470-478.

[67] Mutalik S, Shetty P K, Kumar A, et al. Enhancement in deposition and permeation of 5-fluorouracil through human epidermis assisted by peptide dendrimers[J]. Drug Deliv, 2014, 21(1): 44-54.

[68] de Luca S, Seal P, Parekh H S, et al. Cell membrane penetration without pore formation: Chameleonic properties of dendrimers in response to hydrophobic and hydrophilic environments[J]. Adv Theory Simul, 2020, 3(7): 1900152.

[69] Chauhan A S, Sridevi S, Chalasani K B, et al. Dendrimer-mediated transdermal delivery: enhanced bioavailability of indomethacin[J]. J Control Release, 2003, 90(3): 335-343.

[70] Wang Z, Itoh Y, Hosaka Y, et al. Novel transdermal drug delivery system with polyhydroxyalkanoate and starburst polyamidoamine dendrimer[J]. J Biosci Bioeng, 2003, 95(5): 541-543.

[71] Borowska K, Wołowiec S, Rubaj A, et al. Effect of polyamidoamine dendrimer G3 and G4 on skin permeation of 8-methoxypsoralene—In vivo study[J]. Int J Pharm, 2012, 426(1-2): 280-283.

[72] Manikkath J, Hegde A R, Kalthur G, et al. Influence of peptide dendrimers and sonophoresis on the transdermal delivery of ketoprofen[J]. Int J Pharm, 2017, 521(1-2): 110-119.

[73] Cheng Y, Man N, Xu T, et al. Transdermal delivery of nonsteroidal anti-inflammatory drugs mediated by polyamidoamine(PAMAM)dendrimers[J]. J Pharm Sci, 2007, 96(3): 595-602.

[74] Shetty P K, Manikkath J, Tupally K, et al. Skin delivery of EGCG and silibinin: potential of peptide dendrimers for enhanced skin permeation and deposition[J]. AAPS PharmSciTech, 2017, 18: 2346-2357.

[75] Manikkath J, Parekh H S, Mutalik S. Surface-engineered nanoliposomes with lipidated and non-lipidated peptide-dendrimeric scaffold for efficient transdermal delivery of a therapeutic agent: Development, characterization, toxicological and preclinical performance analyses[J]. Eur J Pharm Biopharm, 2020, 156: 97-113.

[76] Chauhan S, Patel K, Jain P, et al. Matrix metalloproteinase enzyme responsive delivery of 5-fluorouracil using Collagen-I peptide functionalized Dendrimer-Gold nanocarrier[J]. Drug Dev Ind Pharm, 2022, 48(7): 333-342.

[77] Kosakowska K A, Casey B K, Kurtz S L, et al. Evaluation of amphiphilic star/linear-dendritic polymer reverse micelles for transdermal drug delivery: directing carrier properties by tailoring core versus peripheral branching[J]. Biomacromolecules, 2018, 19(8): 3163-3176.

[78] Pradhan D, Tambe V, Raval N, et al. Dendrimer grafted albumin nanoparticles for the treatment of post cerebral stroke damages: a proof of concept study[J]. Colloids Surf B Biointerfaces, 2019, 184: 110488.

[79] Zhong G, Long H, Zhou T, et al. Blood-brain barrier Permeable nanoparticles for Alzheimer's disease treatment by selective mitophagy of microglia[J]. Biomaterials, 2022, 288: 121690.

[80] Win-Shwe T T, Sone H, Kurokawa Y, et al. Effects of PAMAM dendrimers in the mouse brain after a single intranasal instillation[J]. Toxicol Lett. 2014. 228(3): 207-215.

[81] Dong Z, Katsumi H, Sakane T, et al. Effects of polyamidoamine(PAMAM)dendrimers on the nasal absorption of poorly absorbable drugs in rats[J]. Int J Pharm, 2010, 393(1-2): 245-253.

[82] El-Sayed M, Ginski M, Rhodes C, et al. Transepithelial transport of poly(amidoamine)dendrimers across Caco-2 cell monolayers[J]. J Control Release, 2002, 81(3): 355-365.

[83] Kitchens K M, Kolhatkar R B, Swaan P W, et al. Endocytosis inhibitors prevent poly(amidoamine)dendrimer internalization and permeability across Caco-2 cells[J]. Mol Pharm, 2008, 5(2): 364-369.

[84] Kolhatkar R B, Kitchens K M, Swaan P W, et al. Surface acetylation of polyamidoamine(PAMAM)dendrimers decreases cytotoxicity while maintaining membrane permeability[J]. Bioconjug Chem, 2007, 18(6): 2054-2060.

[85] Yang X, Wang L, Li L, et al. A novel dendrimer-based complex co-modified with cyclic RGD hexapeptide and penetratin for noninvasive targeting and penetration of the ocular posterior segment[J]. Drug Deliv, 2019, 26(1): 989-1001.

[86] Lancina M G, Wang J, Williamson G S, et al. DenTimol as a dendrimeric timolol analogue for glaucoma therapy: Synthesis and preliminary efficacy and safety assessment[J]. Mol Pharm, 2018, 15(7): 2883-2889.

[87] Sun D, Gao W, Hu H, Zhou S. Why 90% of clinical drug development fails and how to improve it[J]? Acta Pharm Sin B, 2022, 12(7): 3049-3062.

[88] Dowden H, Munro J. Trends in clinical success rates and therapeutic focus[J]. Nat Rev Drug Discov, 2019, 18(7): 495-496.

[89] Harrison R K. Phase II and phase III failures: 2013—2015[J]. Nat Rev Drug Discov, 2016, 15(12): 817-818.

[90] Liu K, Xiang J, Wang G, et al. Linear-dendritic polymer-platinum complexes forming well-defined nanocapsules for acid-responsive drug delivery[J]. ACS Appl Mater Interfaces, 2021, 13(37): 44028-44040.

[91] Zhu F, Xu L, Li X, et al. Co-delivery of gefitinib and hematoporphyrin by aptamer-modified fluorinated dendrimer for hypoxia alleviation and enhanced synergistic chemo-photodynamic therapy of NSCLC[J]. Eur J Pharm Sci, 2021, 167: 106004.

[92] Cho H, Kambhampati S P, Lai M J, et al. Dendrimer-triamcinolone acetonide reduces neuroinflammation, pathological angiogenesis, and neuroretinal dysfunction in ischemic retinopathy[J]. Adv Ther, 2021, 4(2): 2000181.

[93] Choi M, Thuy L T, Lee Y, et al. Dual-functional dendrimer micelles with glycyrrhizic acid for anti-inflammatory therapy of acute lung injury[J]. ACS Appl Mater Interfaces, 2021, 13(40): 47313-47326.

[94] Szota M, Reczyńska-Kolman K, Pamuła E, et al. Poly(Amidoamine)dendrimers as nanocarriers for 5-fluorouracil: Effectiveness of complex formation and cytotoxicity studies[J]. Int J Mol Sci, 2021, 22(20): 11167.

[95] Gallien J, Srinageshwar B, Gallo K, et al. Curcumin loaded dendrimers specifically reduce viability of glioblastoma cell lines[J]. Molecules, 2021, 26(19): 6050.

[96] Li L, Lei D, Zhang J, et al. Dual-responsive alginate hydrogel constructed by sulfhdryl dendrimer as an intelligent system for drug delivery[J]. Molecules, 2022, 27(1): 281.

[97] Sapra R, Verma R P, Maurya Govind P, et al. Designer peptide and protein dendrimers: a cross-sectional analysis[J]. Chem Rev, 2019, 119(21): 11391-11441.

[98] Medina S H, El-Sayed M E. Dendrimers as carriers for delivery of chemotherapeutic agents[J]. Chem Rev, 2009, 109(7): 3141-3157.

[99] Yang J, Zhang Q, Chang H, et al. Surface-engineered dendrimers in gene delivery[J]. Chem Rev, 2015, 115(11): 5274-5300.

[100] Akhtar N, Ashford M B, Beer L, et al. The global characterisation of a drug-dendrimer conjugate-PEGylated poly-lysine dendrimer[J]. J Pharm Sci, 2022, 112(3): 844-858.

[101] Huang S, Huang X, Yan H. Peptide dendrimers as potentiators of conventional chemotherapy in the treatment of pancreatic cancer in a mouse model[J]. Eur J Pharm Biopharm, 2022, 170: 121-132.

[102] Tallon C, Bell B J, Sharma A, et al. Dendrimer-Conjugated nSMase2 Inhibitor Reduces Tau Propagation in Mice[J]. Pharmaceutics, 2022, 14(10): 2066.

[103] Kong L, Fan D, Zhou L, et al. The influence of modified molecular(D/L-serine)chirality on the theragnostics of PAMAM-based nanomedicine for acute kidney injury[J]. J Mater Chem B, 2021, 9(43): 9023-9030.

[104] Fang X, Gao K, Huang J, et al. Molecular level precision and high molecular weight peptide dendrimers for drug-specific delivery[J]. J Mater Chem B, 2021, 9(41): 8594-8603.

[105] Foudah A I, Alqarni M H, Ross S A, et al. Site-specific evaluation of bioactive coumarin-loaded dendrimer G4 nanoparticles against methicillin resistant staphylococcus aureus[J]. ACS Omega, 2022, 7(39): 34990-34996.

[106] Garzon-Porras A M, Bertuzzi D L, Lucas K, et al. Nitric oxide releasing polyamide dendrimer with anti-inflammatory activity[J]. ACS Appl Polym Mater, 2020, 2(5): 2027-2034.

[107] Mai R, Deng B, Zhao H, et al. Design, synthesis, and bioevaluation of novel enzyme-triggerable cell penetrating peptide-based dendrimers for targeted delivery of camptothecin and cancer therapy[J]. J Med Chem, 2022, 65(7): 5850-5865.

[108] Russi M, Valeri R, Marson D, et al. Some things old, new and borrowed: Delivery of dabrafenib and vemurafenib to melanoma cells via self-assembled nanomicelles based on an amphiphilic dendrimer[J]. Eur J Pharm Sci, 2023, 180: 106311.

[109] Elsayyad N M E, Gomaa I, Salem M A, et al. Efficient lung-targeted delivery of risedronate sodium/vitamin D3 conjugated PAMAM-G5 dendrimers for managing osteoporosis: Pharmacodynamics, molecular pathways and metabolomics considerations[J]. Life Sci, 2022, 309: 121001.

[110] Yang X, Kuang Z, Yang X, et al. Facile synthesis of curcumin-containing poly(amidoamine)dendrimers as pH-responsive delivery system for osteoporosis treatment[J]. Colloids Surf B Biointerfaces, 2023, 222: 113029.

[111] England R M, Moss J I, Gunnarsson A, et al. Synthesis and characterization of dendrimer-based polysarcosine star polymers: Well-defined, versatile platforms designed for drug-delivery applications[J]. Biomacromolecules, 2020, 21(8): 3332-3341.

[112] Tripathi P K, Gupta S, Rai S, et al. Curcumin loaded poly(amidoamine)dendrimer-palmitic acid core-shell nanoparticles as anti-stress therapeutics[J]. Drug Dev Ind Pharm, 2020, 46(3): 412-426.

[113] Fruchon S, Caminade A M, Abadie C, et al. An azabisphosphonate-capped poly(phosphorhydrazone)dendrimer for the treatment of endotoxin-induced uveitis[J]. Molecules, 2013, 18(8): 9305-9316.

[114] Liaw K, Sharma R, Sharma A, et al. Systemic dendrimer delivery of triptolide to tumor-associated macrophages improves anti-tumor efficacy and reduces systemic toxicity in glioblastoma[J]. J Control Release, 2021, 329: 434-444.

[115] Lowell J A, Dikici E, Joshi P M, et al. Vaccination against cocaine using a modifiable dendrimer nanoparticle platform[J]. Vaccine, 2020, 38(50): 7989-7997.

[116] Sharma R, Kambhampati S P, Zhang Z, et al. Dendrimer mediated targeted delivery of sinomenine for the treatment of acute neuroinflammation in traumatic brain injury[J]. J Control Release, 2020, 323: 361-375.

[117] Liaw K, Reddy R, Sharma A, et al. Targeted systemic dendrimer delivery of CSF-1R inhibitor to tumor-associated macrophages improves outcomes in orthotopic glioblastoma[J]. Bioeng Transl Med, 2021, 6(2): e10205.

[118] Aleanizy F S, Alqahtani FY, Seto S, et al. Trastuzumab targeted neratinib loaded poly-amidoamine dendrimer nanocapsules for breast cancer therapy[J]. Int J Nanomedicine, 2020, 15: 5433-5443.

[119] Khoury E S, Sharma A, Ramireddy R R, et al. Dendrimer-conjugated glutaminase inhibitor selectively targets microglial glutaminase in a mouse model of Rett syndrome[J]. Theranostics, 2020, 10(13): 5736.

[120] Yamashita S, Katsumi H, Shimizu E, et al. Dendrimer-based micelles with highly potent targeting to sites of active bone turnover for the treatment of bone metastasis[J]. Eur J Pharm Biopharm, 2020, 157: 85-96.

[121] Falanga A, Del Genio V, Galdiero S. Peptides and dendrimers: How to combat viral and bacterial infections[J]. Pharmaceutics, 2021, 13(1): 101.

[122] Jebbawi R, Oukhrib A, Clement E, et al. An anti-inflammatory poly(phosphorhydrazone)dendrimer capped with azabisphosphonate groups to treat psoriasis[J]. Biomolecules, 2020, 10(6): 949.

[123] Ben-Zichri S, Meltzer M, Lacham-Hartman S, et al. Synergistic activity of anticancer polyphenols embedded in amphiphilic dendrimer nanoparticles[J]. ACS Appl Polym Mater, 2022, 4(12): 8913-8925.

[124] Pharma, S.; Available from: https://starpharma.com/company.

[125] Siriwardena T N, Capecchi A, Gan B H, et al. Optimizing antimicrobial peptide dendrimers in chemical space[J]. Angew Chem, 2018, 130(28): 8619-8623.

[126] Patrulea V, Gan B H, Perron K, et al. Synergistic effects of antimicrobial peptide dendrimer-chitosan polymer conjugates against Pseudomonas aeruginosa[J]. Carbohydr Polym, 2022, 280: 119025.

[127] Le M, Huang W, Ma Z, et al. Facially amphiphilic skeleton-derived antibacterial cationic dendrimers[J]. Biomacromolecules, 2023, 24(1): 269-282.

[128] Dhumal D, et al. Dynamic self-assembling supramolecular dendrimer nanosystems as potent antibacterial candidates against drug-resistant bacteria and biofilms[J]. Nanoscale, 2022, 14(26): 9286-9296.

[129] Mikagi A, Manita K, Tsuchido Y, et al. Boronic Acid-Based Dendrimers with Various Surface Properties for Bacterial Recognition with Adjustable Selectivity[J]. ACS Appl Bio Mater, 2022, 5(11): 5255-5263.

[130] Xie X, He J. Multivalent peptide dendrimers inhibit the fusion of viral-cellular membranes and the cellular NF-κB signaling pathway[J]. Eur J Med Chem, 2022, 230: 114140.

[131] Lopez P, Koh W H, Hnatiuk R, et al. HIV infection stabilizes macrophage-T cell interactions to promote cell-cell HIV spread[J]. J Virol. 2019. 93(18): e00805-19.

[132] Relaño-Rodríguez I, Espinar-Buitrago M S, Martín-Cañadilla V, et al. G2-S16 polyanionic carbosilane dendrimer can reduce HIV-1 reservoir formation by inhibiting macrophage cell to cell transmission[J]. Int J Mol Sci, 2021, 22(16): 8366.

[133] Jiang Y, Zhao W, Xu S, et al. Bioinspired design of mannose-decorated globular lysine dendrimers promotes diabetic wound healing by orchestrating appropriate macrophage polarization[J]. Biomaterials, 2022, 280: 121323.

[134] Erzina D, Capecchi A, Javor S, et al. An immunomodulatory peptide dendrimer inspired from glatiramer acetate[J]. Angew Chem Int Ed, 2021, 60(50): 26403-26408.

[135] Moslah W, Aissaoui-Zid D, Aboudou S, et al. Strengthening anti-glioblastoma effect by multi-branched dendrimers design of a scorpion venom tetrapeptide[J]. Molecules, 2022, 27(3): 806.

[136] Abd-El-Aziz A S, Benaaisha M R, Abdelghani A A, et al. Aspirin-based organoiron dendrimers as promising anti-inflammatory, anticancer, and antimicrobial drugs[J]. Biomolecules, 2021, 11(11): 1568.

[137] Liyanage W, Wu T, Kannan S, et al. Dendrimer-siRNA conjugates for targeted intracellular delivery in glioblastoma animal models[J]. ACS Appl Mater Interfaces, 2022, 14(41): 46290-46303.

[138] Almowalad J, Laskar P, Somani S, et al. Lactoferrin-and dendrimer-bearing gold nanocages for stimulus-free DNA delivery to prostate cancer cells[J]. Int J Nanomedicine, 2022, 17: 1409-1421.

[139] Tarach P, Janaszewska A. Recent advances in preclinical research using PAMAM dendrimers for cancer gene therapy[J]. Int J Mol Sci, 2021, 22(6): 2912.

[140] Ebrahimian M, Hashemi M, Farzadnia M, et al. Development of targeted gene delivery system based on liposome and PAMAM dendrimer functionalized with hyaluronic acid and TAT peptide: In vitro and in vivo studies[J]. Biotechnol Prog, 2022, 38(5): e3278.

[141] Dong Y, Chen Y, Zhu D, et al. Self-assembly of amphiphilic phospholipid peptide dendrimer-based nanovectors for effective delivery of siRNA therapeutics in prostate cancer therapy[J]. J Control Release, 2020, 322: 416-425.

[142] Rabiee N, Ahmadvand S, Ahmadi S, et al. Carbosilane dendrimers: Drug and gene delivery applications[J]. J Drug Deliv Sci Technol, 2020, 59: 101879.

[143] Thuy LT, Choi M, Lee M, et al. Preparation and characterization of polyamidoamine dendrimers conjugated with cholesteryl-dipeptide as gene carriers in HeLa cells[J]. J Biomater Sci Polym Ed, 2022, 33(8): 976-994.

[144] Mekuria S L, Li J, Song C, et al. Facile formation of PAMAM dendrimer nanoclusters for enhanced gene delivery and cancer gene therapy[J]. ACS Appl Bio Mater, 2021, 4(9): 7168-7175.

[145] Wang M, Liu H, Li L, et al. A fluorinated dendrimer achieves excellent gene transfection efficacy at extremely low nitrogen to phosphorus ratios[J]. Nat Commun, 2014, 5(1): 3053.

[146] Lv J, Wang H, Rong G, et al. Fluorination promotes the cytosolic delivery of genes, proteins, and peptides[J]. Acc Chem Res, 2022, 55(5): 722-733.

[147] Wang H, Wang Y, Wang Y, et al. Self-assembled fluorodendrimers combine the features of lipid and polymeric vectors in gene delivery[J]. Angew Chem, 2015, 127(40): 11813-11817.

[148] Tariq I, Ali M Y, Sohail M F, et al. Lipodendriplexes mediated enhanced gene delivery: A cellular to pre-clinical investigation[J]. Sci Rep, 2020, 10(1): 21446.

[149] Raval N, Jogi H, Gondaliya P, et al. Cyclo-RGD truncated polymeric nanoconstruct with dendrimeric templates for targeted HDAC4 gene silencing in a diabetic nephropathy mouse model[J]. Mol Pharm, 2020, 18(2): 641-666.

[150] Sharma R, Liaw K, Sharma A, et al. Glycosylation of PAMAM dendrimers significantly improves tumor macrophage

targeting and specificity in glioblastoma[J]. J Control Release, 2021, 337: 179-192.

[151] Azimifar M A, Salmasi Z, Doosti A, et al. Evaluation of the efficiency of modified PAMAM dendrimer with low molecular weight protamine peptide to deliver IL-12 plasmid into stem cells as cancer therapy vehicles[J]. Biotechnol Prog, 2021, 37(4): e3175.

[152] Lee J, Kwon Y E, Kim Y, et al. Enhanced transfection efficiency of low generation PAMAM dendrimer conjugated with the nuclear localization signal peptide derived from herpesviridae[J]. J Biomater Sci Polym Ed, 2021, 32(1): 22-41.

[153] Cooper R C, Yang H. Duplex of polyamidoamine dendrimer/custom-designed nuclear-localization sequence peptide for enhanced gene delivery[J]. Bioelectricity, 2020, 2(2): 150-157.

[154] Tan G, Li J, Liu D, et al. Amino acids functionalized dendrimers with nucleus accumulation for efficient gene delivery[J]. Int J Pharm, 2021, 602: 120641.

[155] Kim H, Nam K, Nam J P, et al. VEGF therapeutic gene delivery using dendrimer type bio-reducible polymer into human mesenchymal stem cells(hMSCs)[J]. J Control Release, 2015, 220(Pt A): 222-228.

[156] Nam J P, Nam K, Jung S, et al. Evaluation of dendrimer type bio-reducible polymer as a siRNA delivery carrier for cancer therapy[J]. J Control Release, 2015, 209: 179-185.

[157] Peng N, Yu H, Wang Z, et al. Dendrimer-grafted bioreducible polycation/DNA multilayered films with low cytotoxicity and high transfection ability[J]. Mater Sci Eng C, 2019, 98: 737-745.

[158] San Anselmo M, Postigo A, Lancelot A, et al. Dendron-functionalised hyperbranched bis-MPA polyesters as efficient non-viral vectors for gene therapy in different cell lines[J]. Biomater Sci, 2022, 10(10): 2706-2719.

[159] Laskar P, et al. Octadecyl chain-bearing PEGylated poly(propyleneimine)-based dendrimersomes: physicochemical studies, redox-responsiveness, DNA condensation, cytotoxicity and gene delivery to cancer cells[J]. Biomater Sci, 2021, 9(4): 1431-1448.

[160] Uchida H, Kabe Y, Yoshino K, et al. General strategy for the systematic synthesis of oligosiloxanes. Silicone dendrimers[J]. J Am Chem Soc, 1990, 112(19): 7077-7079.

[161] Gorzkiewicz M, Konopka M, Janaszewska A, et al. Application of new lysine-based peptide dendrimers D3K2 and D3G2 for gene delivery: Specific cytotoxicity to cancer cells and transfection in vitro[J]. Bioorg Chem, 2020, 95: 103504.

[162] Saviano F, Lovato T, Russo A, et al. Ornithine-derived oligomers and dendrimers for in vitro delivery of DNA and ex vivo transfection of skin cells via saRNA[J]. J Mater Chem B, 2020, 8(22): 4940-4949.

[163] Farbiak L, Cheng Q, Wei T, et al. All-in-one dendrimer-based lipid nanoparticles enable precise HDR-mediated gene editing in vivo[J]. Adv Mater, 2021, 33(30): 2006619.

[164] Abbasi J. Even mild COVID-19 may change the brain[J]. JAMA, 2022, 327(14): 1321-1322.

[165] Paull J R, Heery G P, Bobardt M D, et al. Virucidal and antiviral activity of astodrimer sodium against SARS-CoV-2 in vitro[J]. Antiviral Res, 2021, 191: 105089.

[166] Kandeel M, Al-Taher A, Park B K, et al. A pilot study of the antiviral activity of anionic and cationic polyamidoamine dendrimers against the Middle East respiratory syndrome coronavirus[J]. J Med Virol, 2020, 92(9): 1665-1670.

[167] Jeong W J, Bu J, Mickel P, et al. Dendrimer-peptide conjugates for effective blockade of the interactions between SARS-CoV-2 spike protein and human ACE2 receptor[J]. Biomacromolecules, 2022, 24(1): 141-149.

[168] Khaitov M, Nikonova A, Kofiadi I, et al. Treatment of COVID-19 patients with a SARS-CoV-2-specific siRNA-peptide dendrimer formulation[J]. Allergy, 2023, 78(6): 1639-1653.

[169] Eliezar J, Scarano W, Boase Nathan R B, et al. In vivo evaluation of folate decorated cross-linked micelles for the delivery of platinum anticancer drugs[J]. Biomacromolecules, 2015, 16(2): 515-523.

[170] Liu Y, Shah S, Tan J. Computational modeling of nanoparticle targeted drug delivery[J]. Rev Nanosci Nanotechnol, 2012, 1(1): 66-83.

[171] De Luca S, Seal P, Ouyang D, get al. Dynamical interactions of 5-fluorouracil drug with dendritic peptide vectors: the impact of dendrimer generation, charge, counterions, and structured water[J]. J Phys Chem B, 2016, 120(25): 5732-5743.

[172] Li Y, Hou T. Computational simulation of drug delivery at molecular level[J]. Curr Med Chem, 2010, 17(36): 4482-4491.

[173] Zloh M, Barata T S. An update on the use of molecular modeling in dendrimers design for biomedical applications: are we using its full potential[J]? Expert Opin Drug Discov, 2020, 15(9): 1015-1024.

[174] Ehsani E, Shojaie F. DFT computational investigation of the reaction behavior of polyamidoamine dendrimer as nanocarrier for delivery of melphalan anticancer drug[J]. J Mol Liq, 2021, 323: 114625.

[175] Phillips J C, Braun R, Wang W, et al. Scalable molecular dynamics with NAMD[J]. J Comput Chem, 2005, 26(16): 1781-1802.

[176] Vanommeslaeghe K, Raman E P, MacKerell A D Jr. Automation of the CHARMM General Force Field(CGenFF) II：

assignment of bonded parameters and partial atomic charges[J]. J Chem Inf Model, 2012, 52(12): 3155-3168.

[177] Best R B, Zhu X, Shim J, et al. Optimization of the additive CHARMM all-atom protein force field targeting improved sampling of the backbone ϕ, ψ and side-chain χ_1 and χ_2 dihedral angles[J]. J Chem Theory Comput, 2012, 8(9): 3257-3273.

[178] Vanommeslaeghe K, Hatcher E, Acharya C, et al. CHARMM general force field: A force field for drug-like molecules compatible with the CHARMM all-atom additive biological force fields[J]. J Comput Chem, 2010, 31(4): 671-690.

[179] Ouyang D, Zhang H, Herten D P, et al. Structure, dynamics, and energetics of siRNA-cationic vector complexation: A molecular dynamics study[J]. J Phys Chem B, 2010, 114(28): 9220-9230.

[180] Ouyang D, Zhang H, Parekh H S, et al. The effect of pH on PAMAM dendrimer-siRNA complexation: Endosomal considerations as determined by molecular dynamics simulation[J]. Biophys Chem, 2011, 158(2-3): 126-133.

[181] Bellini R G, Guimarães A P, Pacheco M A, et al. Association of the anti-tuberculosis drug rifampicin with a PAMAM dendrimer[J]. J Mol Graph Model, 2015, 60: 34-42.

[182] Barraza L F, Zuñiga M, Alderete J B, et al. Effect of pH on Eosin Y/PAMAM interactions studied from absorption spectroscopy and molecular dynamics simulations[J]. J Lumin, 2018, 199: 258-265.

[183] Caballero J, Poblete H, Navarro C, et al. Association of nicotinic acid with a poly(amidoamine)dendrimer studied by molecular dynamics simulations[J]. J Mol Graph Model, 2013, 39: 71-78.

[184] Otto D P, De Villiers M M. All-atomistic molecular dynamics(AA-MD)studies and pharmacokinetic performance of PAMAM-dendrimer-furosemide delivery systems[J]. Int J Pharm, 2018, 547(1-2): 545-555.

[185] Wang B, Sun Y, Davis T P, et al. Understanding effects of PAMAM dendrimer size and surface chemistry on serum protein binding with discrete molecular dynamics simulations[J]. ACS Sustain Chem Eng, 2018, 6(9): 11704-11715.

[186] Workineh Z G. Effect of surface functionalization on the structural properties of single dendrimers: Monte Carlo simulation study[J]. Comput Mater Sci, 2019, 168: 40-47.

[187] Kaminskas L M, Pires D E, Ascher D B. dendPoint: a web resource for dendrimer pharmacokinetics investigation and prediction[J]. Sci Rep, 2019, 9(1): 15465.

[188] Xu L, Wang H, Xu Y, et al. Machine learning-assisted sensor array based on poly(amidoamine)(PAMAM)dendrimers for diagnosing Alzheimer's disease[J]. ACS Sens, 2022, 7(5): 1315-1322.

[189] Jones D E, Ghandehari H, Facelli J C. Predicting cytotoxicity of PAMAM dendrimers using molecular descriptors[J]. Beilstein J Nanotechnol, 2015, 6(1): 1886-1896.

[190] Santos A, Veiga F, Figueiras A. Dendrimers as pharmaceutical excipients: synthesis, properties, toxicity and biomedical applications[J]. Materials, 2019, 13(1): 65.

[191] Chauhan A, et al. Dendrimer-based marketed formulations and miscellaneous applications in cosmetics, veterinary, and agriculture[M]. In: Pharmaceutical Applications of Dendrimers. Elsevier, 2020: 325-334.

[192] Viltres H, López Y C, Leyva C, et al. Polyamidoamine dendrimer-based materials for environmental applications: A review[J]. J Mol Liq, 2021, 334: 116017.

[193] Deng J, Ye Z, Zheng W, et al. Machine learning in accelerating microsphere formulation development[J]. Drug Deliv Transl Res, 2023, 13(4): 966-982.

[194] He M, Zheng W, Wang N, et al. Molecular dynamics simulation of drug solubilization behavior in surfactant and cosolvent injections[J]. Pharmaceutics, 2022, 14(11): 2366.

[195] Jiang J, Ma X, Ouyang D, et al. Emerging artificial intelligence(ai)technologies used in the development of solid dosage forms[J]. Pharmaceutics, 2022, 14(11): 2257.

第11章

人工智能与计算建模在经口吸入药物研发中的应用

李韧杰　莫纳什大学，澳大利亚
缪　浩　莫纳什大学，澳大利亚
周旭东　莫纳什大学，澳大利亚
邹瑞萍　莫纳什大学，澳大利亚
佟振博　东南大学，中国；东南大学－莫纳什大学联合研究院，中国

11.1 引言

慢性呼吸系统疾病是一种长期的肺部疾病,在全球范围内具有较高的发病及死亡率。不同于静脉注射或口服药剂,这些呼吸系统疾病[如哮喘和慢性阻塞性肺疾病(COPD)]的治疗通常需要将药物直接吸入人体肺部区域来控制与缓解。吸入装置是一种能够将药物以喷雾剂或气雾剂的形式直接递送至肺部的给药装置,对于吸入治疗起着至关重要的作用。传统的经口吸入药物研发过程较为冗长,大量的试错实验也极其依赖于研究人员的开发经验。近年来,计算建模和人工智能技术的高速发展为经口吸入药物的高效研发提供了很多实用的方法。本章将回顾这些模型是如何辅助/加速经口吸入药物的研发的,并探讨该类应用的未来前景和发展方向。

11.2 慢性呼吸系统疾病与吸入治疗

11.2.1 慢性呼吸系统疾病

慢性呼吸系统疾病会长期地影响肺部等呼吸系统器官。根据2017年发布的一项系统性研究,全球约有5.549亿人患有慢性呼吸系统疾病,相比1990年患者人数增加了39.8%[1]。由于其高发病率,慢性呼吸系统疾病被公认为是重要的全球公共卫生问题。

常见的呼吸系统疾病包括哮喘、慢性阻塞性肺疾病(COPD)、肺纤维化和肺炎等。在这些疾病中,COPD和哮喘具有最高的发病率[2]。哮喘的主要特征是反复发作的呼吸困难和喘息,患者可能在一天中会发作数次。COPD则是一种具有气流阻塞特征的慢性支气管炎或肺气肿的慢性疾病,随着疾病恶化,有可能会进一步发展为肺心病和呼吸衰竭。

11.2.2 吸入治疗

尽管许多慢性呼吸系统疾病无法完全治愈,但通过悉心护理和及时治疗,其恶化程度可以得到显著的控制[3,4]。预防和治疗慢性呼吸系统疾病的方法包括:减少或避免风险因素、接种疫苗和进行药物治疗等。其中风险因素包括吸烟(被动吸烟)、空气污染、过敏原等。而对于COPD患者,戒烟可以明显减缓疾病的进展。

吸入治疗被广泛应用于慢性呼吸系统疾病的药物治疗中,例如吸入皮质类固醇或吸入β受体激动剂,将药物直接输送到肺部。吸入治疗的目标是缓解和预防不良的肺部症状,如气道炎症和收缩。相较于全身给药,吸入给药可以实现更高的肺部药物浓度,避免肝脏的首过效应。因此在更低的剂量下,吸入给药仍可以与全身给药具有相近的治疗效果,进而降低了副作用的风险。对于吸入治疗,有经鼻和经口吸入两种常见手段,两者之间差异不大,本章将只讨论经口吸入药物开发中使用的计算模型方法。

11.2.3 吸入给药装置

不同于传统的给药模式，吸入治疗的药物是通过吸入装置直接递送至目标区域的。吸入装置可以根据不同的标准进行分类，如触发设备的方法（主动/被动）、单次/多次剂量、一次性/可重复补充使用等。本章根据药物制剂将吸入装置分类为四类（图11-1）：雾化器（nebulizer）、压力定量吸入器（pMDI）、干粉吸入器（DPI）和软雾吸入器（SMI）。

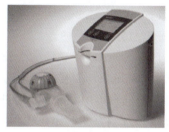 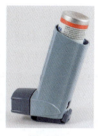 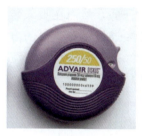 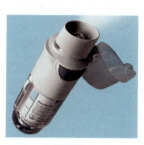

(A)雾化器　　　　　(B)pMDI　　　　　(C)DPI　　　　　(D)SMI

图11-1　四种吸入装置示例[5-7]

目前而言，每种吸入装置均不能广泛适用于所有患者。表11-1简要列出了不同吸入装置的优缺点[8]。为了达到满意的治疗效果，医生需要根据每个患者的情况选择适当的吸入装置。

表11-1　不同类型吸入装置的特点

类型	典型产品	优点	缺点
雾化器	Pari LC STAR（PARI，UK）	高递送量	耗时； 较低的递送效率
pMDI	pMDI（3M，USA）； Aerochamber（AbbVie，USA）	便携； 使用方法相对简单	需要使用者与器械具有良好的协调； 含有推进剂
DPI	Breezhaler（Novartis Pharma AG, Switzerland）； Diskus（GlaxoSmithKline，UK）； Handihaler（Boehringer Ingelheim GmbH, Germany）	便携； 不含推进剂； 对使用者与器械间的协调使用要求较低	递送效率相对较低； 对湿度较为敏感
SMI	Respimat（Boehringer Ingelheim GmbH, Germany）	便携； 不含推进剂； 不依赖于吸入流速	并非由呼吸触发； （目前）成本较高

11.3 计算建模简介

11.3.1 计算流体力学模型

在商业吸入装置的研发阶段,研究人员很难仅通过实验来了解装置内药物气溶胶的各项复杂性质。同样地,在患者通过吸入装置进行吸入后,药物气溶胶在人体呼吸道中的沉积与追踪也是一项极为棘手的任务。然而在吸入装置的开发以及优化过程中,上述参数均是非常重要的参考因素,因此需要通过计算建模的方法对上述参数进行定量研究。

计算流体力学(CFD)是一种用于模拟流体运动的数值模拟方法,并已被广泛应用于各个领域。通过解决描述流体运动的数学方程,CFD可以捕捉流场(flow field)的复杂物理特性[9]。具体而言,CFD将流场分成离散单元,然后为每个单元求解控制方程。而每个单元的解随后被组合在一起,从而获得整个流体域的解。由于在分析流体动力学方面的出色表现,CFD被认为是模拟药物气溶胶输送的有效工具[10]。

在吸入装置的相关研究中,CFD可用于模拟吸入装置中气体的流场("连续相")以及颗粒、液滴("离散相")的运动。对于层流流动的建模,CFD直接使用Navier-Stokes方程;对于湍流流动,则使用时间平均形式结合适当的模型来进行模拟[11]。通过CFD模拟,可以确定吸入装置的流场、压力损失和高湍流动能区域。

在模拟颗粒和液滴时,可以根据它们在装置中的浓度高低而采用不同的方法。当离散相的浓度较低(体积分数小于5%)时,离散颗粒模型(DPM)是理想的选择[12]。首先,确定流场,然后,通过该流场跟踪代表性颗粒,其运动路径由施加于颗粒上的力的平衡决定。DPM假设颗粒体积是可以忽略的,但这仅适用于低颗粒浓度的条件。对于更高的颗粒含量,其他模型例如密集离散颗粒模型(DDPM)[13]和欧拉-欧拉模型[14]则可以提供更可靠的结果。另一个经常使用的方法是离散元法(DEM)[15, 16],该模型则考虑了颗粒间和颗粒-壁面之间的相互作用。DEM常用于模拟像岩石和粉末这些颗粒介质的行为。在DEM模拟中,颗粒通常由简单的几何形状表示,如球体或多边形。每个颗粒的运动方程基于它与相邻颗粒的相互作用和任何施加于其上的外部力确定。在解决控制方程后,DEM可以相对精准地模拟颗粒随时间的运动轨迹。通过将CFD和DEM方法相结合,可以准确地跟踪颗粒在流场中的运动,并且还可以精确地模拟团聚体的分解。

11.3.2 生理药代动力学模型

经典的药代动力学(PK)建模是一种通过测试血浆或尿液中药物浓度来评估肺部药物吸收情况的体内方法,但它无法提供有关药物气溶胶在呼吸道内的区域沉积情况。基于生理的药代动力学(PBPK)建模是一种更先进的PK建模技术,用于计算体内药物吸收。PBPK模型是基于与药物物理化学性质以及吸收、分布、代谢和排泄(ADME)相关的属性构建的[17]。PBPK模型通常是个分区模型,即身体中的不同器官由单独的区域建模来表示。PBPK建模中使用的区域和参数具有生理意义,因此PBPK模型比经典PK模型更易解释。PBPK模型已被证明对于解释和预测口服药物的吸收非常有效[17]。最近,PBPK模型也被扩展应用到包括吸入药物在内的其他类型药物制剂。当给定吸入药物沉积数据时,肺部PBPK

模型可以预测肺组织浓度,并具有相当的准确度,这对于早期的药物开发非常有帮助。图11-2显示了吸入药物的肺部PK过程。

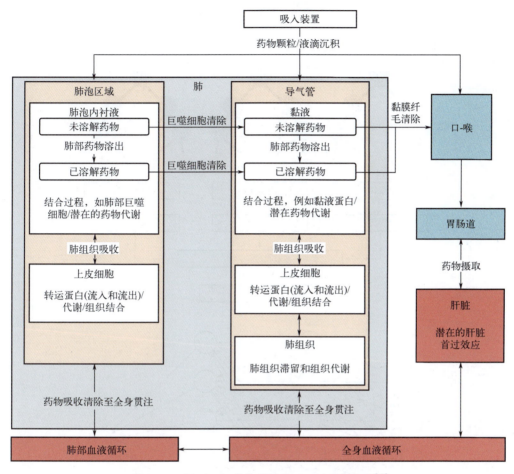

图11-2 针对吸入药物的肺部PK过程示意图[18]

11.3.3 人工智能模型

近十年来,人工智能(AI)在医学上的应用引起了广泛重视。机器学习是AI的一个重要分支,可以分析数据模式、拟合非线性方程,并基于大量数据进行预测。而深度学习则是机器学习的一个子集,当输入的数据量足够大的时候能够拥有更好的表现。在制药领域,流行使用的模型包括人工神经网络(ANN)、随机森林(RF)等。RF是一种流行的机器学习算法,可以用于处理分类和连续变量。RF首先创建大量决策树,其中每棵树都在数据集的随机特征子集上进行训练,并独立地学习基于给定特征进行决策。RF的最终预测是通过聚合所有树的预测来确定的。RF在分类和回归任务中均表现出不错的准确性。ANN受到人脑结构和功能的启发,模型中每个节点的行为类似于人类大脑中的神经元,并且它们通常在一个输入层、几个隐藏层和一个输出层中排列。数据首先从输入层传递到隐藏层,在传递到输出层之前进行复杂的计算。在训练过程中,神经元的权重将被调整以使预测输出与实际输出之间的误差最小化。图11-3展示了这两种AI模型的基本结构。值得注意的是,没有任何一种机器/深度学习算法可以适用于所有问题（也称为"无免费午餐定理"），研究人员应根据临床问题以及所拥有的数据格式来选择适当的算法。

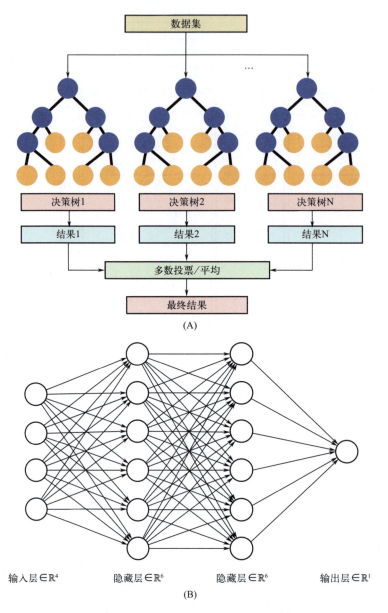

图11-3 （A）RF和（B）ANN的典型结构

过去在呼吸系统疾病和吸入药物研究领域，AI的应用主要与疾病诊断有关。如今，研究人员正在关注如何将实验结果、电子健康记录和电子医疗设备的数据结合到模型中，通过AI模型来改善吸入药物的研发和呼吸系统疾病的管理。

11.3.4 计算模型的验证与确认

对于基于机理的计算模型（如CFD和PBPK），在将其应用于实际场景之前，需要对模型的准确性进行验证与确认。对于CFD这类用于跟踪和预测药物颗粒运动的模型，通常通过将模拟得到的沉积分布与体内或体外实验数据进行比较来进行验证。体内数据是通过放射性标记颗粒的伽马闪烁法收集的，而体外数据通常是通过在真实人类呼吸道的模型上进行实验而得到的。例如：使用高效液相色谱法准确量化体外呼吸道模型各个区域的准确沉积值（体内体外实验方法将会在下一部分阐述）。对于PBPK模型，想要直接获得给药后肺部组织（经口吸入药物的目标区域）浓度数据非常困难，因此目前无法对模型进行直接验证。研究人员使用全身PK终点，如C_{max}（单剂量药物在血液中的最大浓度）和给药后时间-浓度曲线下面积（AUC）来验证PBPK模型[19]。

11.4 计算模型在吸入装置与制剂研发过程中的应用

在常见的计算方法中，CFD在吸入装置的研发过程中扮演着重要的角色，常见的应用包括：对现有商业吸入装置进行性能评估、吸入装置设计的优化以及对仿制吸入装置的生物等效性评估。AI模型则被应用于加速药物粉末处方的研发。相比之下，目前PBPK模型在吸入装置的几何设计和性能优化方面贡献有限[17]。

11.4.1 计算模型在雾化器研发过程中的应用

雾化器是一种通过压缩空气将液体药物分解成微小的气溶胶液滴的设备，通常用于治疗急性症状的患者。雾化器可以提供高剂量的药物，但传递效率较其他手持式吸入装置低，需要较长时间的给药和频繁的维护[20-22]。

CFD在研究雾化器开发方面的应用主要集中在分析设备性能和设计特征。研究人员利用CFD来研究雾化器的药物分散机理，证明了不同的雾化器罩[23]和波纹管[24]的设计都能够显著地影响雾化效果。CFD还被用于设计一种新型微型泵液滴发生器，以模拟气溶胶液滴的分散[25]。

11.4.2 计算模型在pMDI研发过程中的应用

相比起传统的雾化器，pMDI的设计更为紧凑且便携，通过计量装置能够准确地将特定剂量的药物以溶液或悬浮液的形式递送出去[26]。具体来说，当pMDI被激活时，药物和推进剂的混合物将会在压力的作用下从雾化罐中释放出固定的剂量[27]。

作为药物和辅料的溶解、分散介质，推进剂的选择在pMDI的研发过程中至关重要。研究人员通过CFD模拟比较了pMDI中不同推进剂的性能[28]。研究表明，氢氟烷（HFA）作为推进剂的pMDI相比于氯氟烃（CFC）作为推进剂的pMDI具有更好的性能，即有更多的药物被递送到了目标肺部区域。

然而，通过CFD来模拟pMDI中药物的流动具有很大的难度，因为从pMDI中释放的药物气溶胶是瞬态、不稳定的湍流状态[27]。在DPI研究中所采用的计算模型大多假设颗粒具有与气流相同的进入速度，然而pMDI产生的气溶胶速度高于气流速度，这大大增加了模拟运动的难度。在此等限制下，研究人员基于均质冻结模型（HFM）开发了一种内部流动模型

（IFM）[29, 30]来预测pMDI中的流动模式[31]。此外，最近的CFD研究发现，溶液的黏度和表面张力也影响pMDI产生的气溶胶尺寸[32]。

11.4.3　计算模型在SMI研发过程中的应用

SMI是最新型的雾化器，它以软雾的形式输送药物，且不含具有一定污染性的推进剂，并简化了使用方法。它可以以较低的剂量实现较高的肺部沉积效率，但目前相对较高的成本限制了其在许多国家的普及[33]。

在Respimat这个被广泛使用的SMI中，软雾通过两个液体射流在喷嘴处碰撞产生，药物溶液在此处分解成可吸入的、缓慢移动的软雾气溶胶[34]。为了优化设计，研究者通过CFD评估了Respimat的性能，发现大部分药物沉积发生在嘴部[35]。研究人员开发了VOF-to-DPM模型来模拟撞击雾化过程[36, 37]，揭示了撞击角度和速度分布如何影响雾化过程。基于这些CFD研究得到的改进策略，可以显著改善装置的递送效率。

11.4.4　计算模型在DPI研发过程中的应用

DPI常被用于替代含有推动剂的pMDI，以干粉颗粒的形式将药物递送至肺部。与pMDI相比，DPI的使用方法对患者更加友好[38]。根据其作用机制，DPI可以分为两种类型：①被动式DPI（患者提供能量将药物从装置中分散出来），适用于肺功能正常的患者；②主动式DPI（无须患者用力吸气），适合吸气能力较为低下的患者。

一个理想的DPI设计需要气流在装置的喷口附近具有高湍流水平，且在人体胸外区域的沉积损失较低[9]。DPI的性能受几何参数的影响极大，例如网格和喷口的几何形状[39]。CFD被广泛应用于指导装置设计和优化，例如优化商业吸入装置的性能[40]，以及优化装置的进气流动，从而减少患者吸入操作对于药物递送效率的影响[41]。同样，CFD被用于研究其他影响因素如网格结构[42]和空气旁路[43]等对装置性能的影响。

除了几何优化外，研究者也通过CFD对颗粒特性的机理进行了研究。对基于载体的DPI，其中细小的药物颗粒通常与较粗的载体（通常是α-乳糖一水合物）混合[44, 45]。通过CFD，研究者模拟了载体的物理特性对颗粒分散和输送的影响[46]。如图11-4所示，由CFD-DEM建模得到的结果表明，通过增加载体与药物的质量比，可以改善气溶胶性能。图11-5则展示了活性药物成分从载体上脱离的可视化过程[47]。

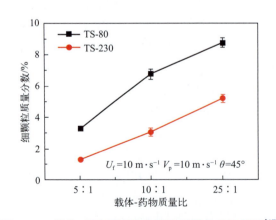

图11-4　载体-药物质量比与药物递送效率的关系[47]

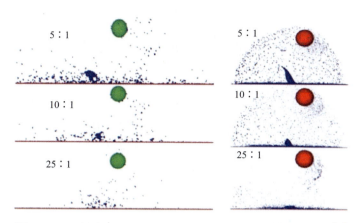

图11-5 颗粒在不同载体-药物质量比的处方下的脱离过程[47]

考虑到患者动作的差异性，吸入流速对颗粒分散的影响同样被广泛研究[48-50]。流速由装置的固有阻力以及患者吸入动作所导致的压降共同决定。研究发现，对于细小的药物颗粒，流速越低，聚集体的分散越困难[49]。然而，快速的流速却可能增加药物在口喉区的沉积，阻碍药物在肺部区域的输送效率（将在下一部分讨论）。因此，在设计或优化DPI时必须仔细考虑最佳吸入流速。

11.4.5 计算模型在吸入药物制剂研发过程中的应用

CFD不仅在优化吸入装置的设计方面表现出色[51]，在研究基于载体的药物制剂气溶胶机制方面也有所帮助。类似地，研究人员也通过AI模型来设计药物制剂并预测其气溶胶性能（主要是在DPI的开发中）[52]。

DPI的气溶胶性能可以通过质量中值气动直径（MMAD）、释放剂量（ED）、几何标准偏差（GSD）和细颗粒分数（FPF）等参数进行评估。ED表示从吸入装置中释放的药物量，而FPF表示质量小于5 μm的颗粒量，这个尺寸是最理想的送达至深肺的颗粒尺寸[53, 54]。ED可以通过剂量单位取样装置（DUSA）来测量[55]，而FPF和MMAD可以通过级联撞击器测试来表征，例如Andersen级联撞击器（ACI）和下一代撞击器（NGI）。

一组研究人员首先使用ANN模型来预测基于载体的干粉的ED和FPF[56]。他们使用扫描电子显微镜（SEM）图像中的关键物料属性（CMA）和衍生变量作为输入参数来预测ED和FPF。研究者从文献中收集了65个样本数据集作为训练样本。与其他经验建模方法相比，该模型显示出了更高的预测准确性。随后，进一步使用遗传算法（GA）开发了一个回归模型来更快地估算FPF和ED，也同样显示出良好的准确度。类似地，通过提取由薄膜冷冻（TFF）技术制备的134种干粉制剂和SEM图像的信息，研究者建立了一个气溶胶性能预测模型[57]。结果显示，RF模型在FPF预测方面表现最佳，而ANN和卷积神经网络（CNN）分别在对于MMAD数值的估计以及药物制剂的分类任务中表现最优。这些研究展示了AI模型在设计干粉制剂方面的潜力，未来可以极大地减少产品开发的工作量。

11.5 计算模型在吸入药物药效评价中的应用

与静脉或口服给药相比,吸入给药的疗效受多种外部因素影响,包括患者的依从性、患者吸入操作正确与否、药物颗粒的粒径分布等[58]。为了量化评估吸入给药的疗效,需要建立两种机理模型:一个是用于预测吸入药物沉积分布的药物气溶胶运动模型,另一个是可以预测给药后药物吸收浓度的PBPK模型。

11.5.1 药物沉积的预测模型

医学成像技术,例如二维伽马闪烁图像和三维单光子发射计算机断层扫描(SPETC),可以精确地捕捉到事先经过标记的颗粒在人体呼吸道中的位置[59],这也是追踪颗粒沉积最准确可靠的方法。然而,这些基于医学成像的方法受到多种客观因素的限制,例如相对高昂的实验成本,同时并非所有使用者都能够愿意承担辐射的风险。此外,这类方法仅仅能够捕获到吸入给药的最终沉积状态,而对于颗粒递送和沉积机理的研究无法提供帮助。

相较于上面的体内测量方法(*in vivo* method),体外方法(*in vitro* method)则是使用人体呼吸道的复制模型进行实验,进而研究颗粒的输送和沉积过程。这种方法相对廉价、易于实施,并且不受医学伦理的限制(除非使用患者真实呼吸道模型,需要通过伦理委员会的审批),同时,通过控制各种实验设备,也可以精准地控制颗粒属性和流速等参数。

除去上述的体内体外方法,计算方法(*in silico* method)对于药物颗粒的沉积分布预测也展示出了优势,相比实验方法,计算方法可以更高效、更准确地获取呼吸道每个部分的定量沉积分布数据。

(1)人体呼吸道结构

人类呼吸道可以分为三个区域:胸外(ET)、气管支气管(TB)和肺泡。ET区域,也称为上呼吸道,包括口腔和鼻腔、咽部和喉部。TB区域从气管延伸到末梢支气管,共有16级(第0~16级),其功能是将空气传导到肺泡区域。肺泡区域包括肺的第17~23级,是气体交换发生的地方。图11-6简要展示了人体呼吸道的结构。

(2)半经验&一维全肺模型

为了找到颗粒沉积分布规律与颗粒性质以及流速等参数的关系,研究人员首先尝试了去挖掘已有的体内体外实验数据中的规律。美国辐射防护与测量委员会(NCRP)[61]和国际辐射防护委员会(ICRP)[62]在20世纪90年代分别发布了关于呼吸道中吸入放射性气溶胶的剂量学模型。虽然这些模型最初是针对放射性气溶胶建立的,但经过验证这些半经验模型也适用于药物气溶胶[63]。在这些模型中,整个呼吸道被分成若干部分,每个部分的沉积量通过若干半经验方程(从已有的实验数据中推导得到)计算得出。类似地,研究者还提出了所谓的一维(1D)全肺沉积模型来计算药物沉积,如多径粒子剂量学模型(MPPD)[64]、随机模型[65]和Trumpet模型[66]。这些模型使用简单,计算量适中,但这些模型忽略了人体呼吸道的几何变化和流动的复杂性,因此当它们被应用在非标准情况时表现并不理想。基于这些模型,加拿大阿尔伯塔大学的气溶胶研究实验室(ARLA)开发了一个呼吸道沉积计算器,以便于对气溶胶沉积进行简便计算[67]。

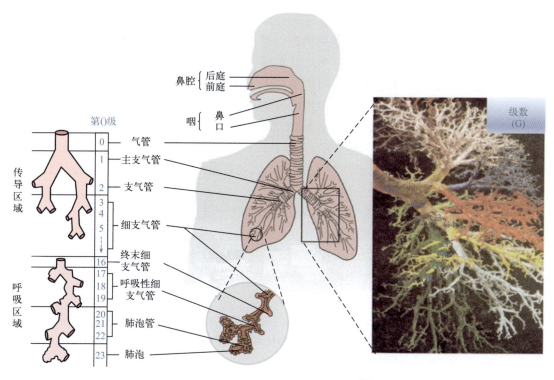

图 11-6 人体呼吸道结构示意图[60]

（3）基于 CFD 的预测模型

半经验和一维全肺模型的出现为吸入药物在呼吸道中的沉积分布预测提供了基础，但在实际应用过程中仍然存在改进空间：这两类模型只能预测 ET 或 TB 等区域的整体沉积情况，无法细化到肺部每一级的沉积分布。相比之下，CFD 建模可以提供关于气流和药物沉积的详细信息，从而实现进一步的参数研究。

研究 ET 区域的沉积模式至关重要，据估计 ET 区域的沉积分数为 20%~50%[68, 69]，该区域的沉积损失以及不同患者 ET 区域的几何形状差异使得在近似吸入条件下递送至不同患者肺部的药物剂量的差异性极大。许多研究人员在过去采用简化模型去研究沉积机制，但口咽部几何形状的关键细节却可能被忽略。基于此，一些研究人员使用从 CT 扫描中重建的患者特异性呼吸道模型进行研究，从而最大程度地保留所有几何参数。已有几位研究人员比较了真实口咽模型与简化模型的 CFD 预测结果，证实了真实口咽模型的预测结果更准确[70-72]，此外还发现沉积分布对呼吸道的几何尺寸变化非常敏感——真实模型中的沉积分数比简化模型高 25%~40%[73]。除此之外，研究者也研究了特定参数（如口腔容积[74]、声门开度[75] 和舌位[76]）对于药物沉积分布的影响。这些参数研究揭示了 ET 区域的几何尺寸变化对气溶胶动力学的显著影响。ET 区域几何尺寸的任何一点细微变化都会造成显著的沉积分布差异，因此，可以预见，建立一个定量评估几何尺寸影响的沉积模型是非常困难且复杂的。

在 ET 区域之后，TB 区域将空气传导到肺泡区域进行气体交换。同样，用于 CFD 建模的 TB 模型有各种各样的选择（从简化的 Weibel 模型到从 CT 扫描中重建的真实模型）。研究人员比较了在不同的吸气条件下各模型中的沉积分布，得到了和 ET 区域相似的结果，即 TB 区域的几何变化会显著影响沉积分布结果[77]。而在比简化 Weibel 模型更复杂的计算机生成模型中，研究员发现药物更多地沉积在分叉处。其他研究人员也得出了类似的结果[78]，表明TB区域的几何变化也可能导致更复杂的流动模式。

除了呼吸道几何变化外，沉积分布还受到吸气状态的影响。研究人员探讨了不同流速对气溶胶沉积的影响，发现喉部附近的狭窄收紧区域附近的气体流动为湍流状态[79]，而这种波动可以直接增加气溶胶沉积。类似地，研究者还比较了稳定和非稳定气流下的气溶胶运动，证明了非稳定气流可以增加ET区域的沉积，特别是在喉部区域[80]。对于某些吸入装置，如DPI，患者在使用后需要屏住呼吸几秒钟，研究者发现在屏住呼吸后，更多的气溶胶将沉积在支气管区域，而ET区域的沉积显著减少，这也从另一个角度证明了使用DPI时屏住呼吸的必要性[81]。

此外，颗粒本身的属性对其在人体呼吸道内的沉积也起着至关重要的作用。例如，大颗粒由于碰撞作用会停留在ET区域，而尺寸在0.01 mm到1 mm之间的颗粒将到达更深的肺部区域[82]。CFD模型验证了这一发现，揭示惯性碰撞是ET区域沉积的主要机制[83]。此外，其他性质如颗粒形状[84]、颗粒电荷[85]和湿化增长[86]等也在持续被研究着。

（4）基于AI的预测模型

与其他实验方法相比，CFD研究在吸入药物递送过程方面提供了更为详细的信息。然而，CFD同样存在一些弊端，例如需要大量的计算资源——一个算例可能需要数小时到数天的计算时间。鉴于计算资源的限制，研究人员开始尝试构建一个直接通过若干关键参数就能够预测药物沉积的人工智能模型。

研究者首先构建了三个独立的多层感知机（MLP）模型来分别预测ET、TB和肺泡区域的沉积，训练数据来自文献[87]中的实验数据。通过将呼吸模式、潮气量和颗粒尺寸作为输入参数，这些MLP模型实现了较高的预测精度，预测误差小于0.4%。该组研究者在后续研究中使用了单分散气溶胶沉积的实验数据作为训练数据，构建了一个ANN模型，该模型对肺部区域的多分散气溶胶沉积实现了更为准确的预测，误差小于0.025%[88]。

另一组研究也建立了一个ANN模型，试图通过DPI的体外实验结果来预测其在人体内的性能表现，即所谓的体内-体外相关性（IVIVC）[89]。这些模型对DPI的体内药物代谢动力学（PK）和药效动力学（PD）性能进行了良好的估计。最近，其他研究人员也建立了一个级联撞击器实验结果与基于放射显像数据的体内肺部沉积数据之间的相关模型，用于验证IVIVC[90]。他们也提出，ANN模型在建立处方属性和颗粒沉积之间的相关性模型方面具有巨大潜力，但前提是有足够多的训练样本。

上述研究通常侧重于从文献或体内实验中收集沉积数据，而有一个研究小组则直接试图使用CFD建模数据来预测人体呼吸道中的气溶胶输送[91]。通过使用其在前序研究中建立的数据库[92]，研究人员比较了K最近邻、高斯过程回归、RF和MLP四种机器学习算法的性能。MLP模型表现最佳，并能够准确地预测不同颗粒尺寸和流速下的颗粒沉积情况，这可以为药物研发实验中节省大量时间和成本。

11.5.2 吸入药物吸收与溶出的PBPK建模

在体外实验和计算模拟过程中，人们仅评估了吸入药物后呼吸道内药物的沉积分布情况，但并未考虑溶解和吸收等过程，这使得后续的药效评价难以被客观地描述[90]。为了量化评估吸入药物的药效，可以尝试将沉积分布数据与PK和PD结果相关联，因此研究者们开始尝试将PBPK模型与沉积预测模型相耦合,从而实现对于药效的定量评估。

一组研究人员通过PBPK模型将自制的体外溶解装置中经口吸入药物的溶解速率与体内实验结果进行比较[93],展示了体外实验与PBPK模型相结合的潜在应用。

另一组研究者使用商业PBPK软件Gastroplus中的肺部分区吸收和转运模型(PCAT),模拟了一种难溶化合物AZD5423在不同颗粒性质和吸入装置模型中的情况。沉积数据是通过体外级联撞击器的实验结果收集汇总得到的,但研究发现仅仅将沉积分布输入模型中并不能得到准确的PK数据,只有同时考虑沉积分布和药物(溶解)释放速率,该模型才可以准确得到准确可用的PK数据[94]。

在早期PBPK相关的研究中,人们对于沉积分布的处理更多的都是采用前述的经验模型或者体外实验数据。最近,研究人员开始将CFD模拟与PBPK模型结合使用。首先,使用CFD评估DPI设备的空气动力学性能,然后,使用级联撞击器产生的体外数据验证ED、MMAD和FPF等参数,确保CFD模拟的准确性。随后,这些参数被用作Gastroplus PCAT模块的输入,以计算药物的沉积分布,最终发现计算得到的C_{max}预测值与实际的PK数据非常相近[95]。

最新的另一系列研究中,研究人员利用准三维(Q3D)CFD建模来模拟人类呼吸道中的气溶胶输送和吸收,相比起全三维模型,Q3D模型拥有更高的效率[96-99]。传统的CFD建模可以提供高精度的沉积数据,但通常需要数天时间来模拟。Kannan等[97]通过将呼吸道表面网格简化为一组组互相连接的线段来优化呼吸道的几何模型,从而减少计算成本,但这种简化仍然保留了原始气道几何形状的所有基本特征(图11-7)。Q3D模型可以显著提高计算速度(比全三维CFD模拟快3000~25000倍),而最大的误差也仅小于15%。最初,Q3D模型仅限于人类气道的第7~9级(其余的气道和全身器官仍然使用传统的分区建模)[96, 97],后来通过创建"囊-喇叭"模型来代表肺泡,进而扩展到整个肺部[98]。在该研究中,肺部吸收模型和黏膜清除模型等PBPK模型直接采用了其他相关研究的模型。除了高计算效率之外,Q3D模型的优点是可以更准确地模拟黏液纤毛运输[19]。在未来,期待类似的模型能够更准确地模拟肺部和胃肠道的药物吸收过程。

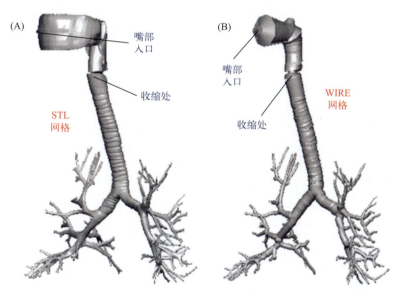

图11-7　人体呼吸道的(A)全三维模型与(B)准三维模型的比较[98]

11.6 计算模型在慢性呼吸系统疾病管理中的应用

正确的吸入治疗可以概括为三个阶段:患者学习如何用药、患者自行用药和后续居家定期坚持用药[100]。虽然通过各种研究和优化,吸入装置的性能已经得到了显著改善,但由于患者相对较低的依从性以及不正确的吸入技巧,吸入药物的实际疗效往往不令人满意。然而,这种低下的药物递送效率却存在着风险,如未来生活质量降低、恶化风险增加、住院甚至死亡[101]。万幸的是,与其他传统用药方法(患者只能自行记录每日是否准时地将药物服下)不同,吸入治疗中吸入装置的存在为研究人员提供了将用药追踪功能整合到装置中的机会,而装置所收集到的数据也可以在未来用作相关AI医疗数据大模型的训练样本。

11.6.1 基于吸入药物装置的电子检测设备

在传感技术和通信技术不断飞速进步的背景下,基于吸入装置的电子监测设备(IEMD)诞生了。这些设备通常是附加到吸入装置上或直接嵌入吸入装置中的一种外围(peripheral)设备。IEMD的主要作用有监测用药模式、提醒患者服药,并提供反馈以改进使用技巧。

第一个获得美国食品药品管理局(FDA)批准并上市的IEMD称为Nebulizer Chronolog[102]。该设备设计成可附加到MDI装置上的外壳,它是IEMD发展的一大飞跃。

在接下来的四十年中,各个公司、研发机构开发了许多具有不同功能的IEMD,不再仅限于记录用药的日期和时间,典型的新功能包括更紧凑的尺寸、计数功能、屏幕显示和移动手机端的APP支持。表11-2总结了一些典型IEMD所支持的功能。

表11-2 不同IEMD的功能比较

装置名称	发售时间	原吸入装置	记录使用次数	记录使用日期	屏幕显示	手机App
Nebulizer Chronolog[102]	1982	MDI		√		
MDILog[103]	1995	MDI		√	√	
Diskus Adherence Logger[104]	2004	DPI	√	√		
SmartDisk SmartTrack[105]	2009	DPI MDI		√	√	
INCA[106]	2014	DPI	√	√		√
Propeller Health[107]	2015	MDI	√	√		√
Proair DigiHaler[108]	2019	DPI	√	√		√

11.6.2 患者依从性的改善

近二十年来，研究者们采用了若干测量方法去监测慢性呼吸道疾病患者的用药依从性。结果表明，医生们的主观判断往往是不准确的[109]，而患者的自我报告同样不可靠，通常患者会高估或低估自己的依从性[110]。此外，用药补充记录等数据也容易受到数据完整性问题的影响，因为患者可能会选择不同的药房购买吸入药物，因此这样的用药补充数据在各国药物售卖系统均无法做到统一的情况下难以得到精准的监测[111]。

而一些研究则侧重于关注IEMD的使用能否真正干预/改善患者的依从性。这些所谓的干预行为包括临床医生的口头反馈/建议，或来自IEMD的直接反馈。表11-3总结了若干随机对照试验对患者依从性干预的结果。表11-3表明，IEMD的干预相较于传统的用药模式能更有效地改善患者的药物依从性。

表11-3 吸入治疗患者依存性的随机对照试验总结

入组人数	监测方法	依从性（干预）	依从性（正常使用）	改善	参考文献
50	IEMD 监测（DAL）	64.5%	49.1%	提高 32%	[112]
220	IEMD 监测（Smart Inhaler Tracker）	84%	30%	提高 180%	[113]
110	IEMD 监测	88%	66%	提高 33%	[114]
437	IEMD 监测（Propeller Health）	81%	69%	提高 17%	[115]
218	IEMD 监测（INCA）	73%	63%	提高 16%	[116]
1187	药房复购记录	44.5%	35.5%	提高 25%	[117]
2698	药房复购记录	21.3%	23.3%	无显著变化	[118]
103	患者自行报告	37.8%	62.2%	无显著变化	[119]

11.6.3 吸入参数的测量

虽然使用IEMD已被证明可以改善患者的药物依从性，但依从性和疾病进展之间的关系仍不明确。一项名为"关于使用电子监控设备来改善儿童依从性的临床试验"（E-Monitoring of Asthma Therapy to Improve Compliance in children trial，E-MATIC）的临床研究发现，虽然定期提醒患者可以改善依从性，但并没有降低疾病的急性加重率[120]。

在另一项名为"关于哮喘控制以及吸入装置错误使用的临床试验"（CRITical Inhaler mistaKes and Asthma controL，CRITIKAL）的研究中，研究者收集了来自5000多名患者的数据，研究了错误使用吸入装置与不良结果之间的关联[121]。除了装置使用错误，如"没有将嘴唇紧贴吸入装置导致漏气"，另一个关键发现是，约47%的COPD患者和35%的哮喘患者在使用吸入装置时未能产生足够的吸气力量，即峰值吸入流速低于要求以及吸气时间过短。

来自爱尔兰的INCA团队开发了一种名为吸入装置依从性评估设备（INCA）的装置，通过采集到的声音信号来跟踪从装置启动到患者进行吸入时的操作[106]。最初，这个基于声音的设备可以使用二次判别分析方法将采集到的声音分类为吸入和呼出等操作,并具有88.2%的准确度,接着通过将流量信号与吸入期间采集到的声音信号之间的对数关系相互关联,可以估算整个吸入过程的流量特征,得到的结果也相当准确,峰值吸入流速的估算正确率达到了88.2%,吸入量的估算准确率达到了83.94%[122-126]。

除了基于声音信号的INCA,Teva制药公司还设计制造了另一种基于压力传感器的吸入装置。该设备内置压力传感器,可以记录吸入流速和吸气时间的信息[108]。传感器的高灵敏度使其能够检测到极小的压力变化,从而增强了数据收集的可靠性。记录的吸入参数可以用于向患者提供建议或反馈,以改善他们的吸入技巧。

11.6.4　急性加重的预测模型

慢性呼吸道疾病患者如果未能按照药物治疗方案进行治疗,可能会出现急性加重。急性加重会导致肺功能下降、生活质量降低、更多的住院监测、增加的医疗支出和更高的死亡率[127]。如表11-4所示,许多研究人员成功建立了具有相当准确性的AI预测模型,通过使用自我用药监测数据预测患者健康状况的恶化。

表11-4　对于急性加重的AI预测模型

输入数据	模型	结果	参考文献
居家监测数据,如血氧浓度、心率等	循环神经网络	平均提前3天预警,88%准确度	[131]
居家监测数据,呼吸声	概率神经网络	平均提前4.43天预警,75.8%准确度	[132]
手机APP的电子问卷	模式识别	平均提前4.5天预警,84.7%准确度	[133]
自行记录的峰值吸入流速与哮喘症状	逻辑回归	平均提前3天预警,85%准确度	[134]
IEMD采集的吸入信息,临床数据,个人信息	XG-Boost	平均提前5天预警,83%准确度	[130]

另外,一些研究人员使用基于压力传感器的IEMD所收集的数据来将吸入参数与疾病加重程度进行关联[128-130]。在2022年的一项最新研究中[130],峰值吸入流速(PIF)、吸入量和吸入时间以及达到PIF的时间被用作输入参数,同时还收集了临床数据和人口统计信息,所建立的AI模型准确预测了接下来5天的急性加重情况,AUC值为0.83,其中每天布地奈德吸入次数是最强的预测参考因素。这项研究展示了基于IEMD数据的预测模型的潜力。

11.7　当前挑战与未来

表11-5总结了计算模型在经口吸入药物研发过程中的作用与贡献。这些模型一定程度上加快了药物研发过程,并提出了吸入治疗管理的新范式。然而,未来还仍有很多挑战等待解决,需要更多更深入的研究学习,以进一步提高吸入药物的疗效。

表11-5 计算模型在经口吸入药物研发过程中的应用

阶段		研发（药企）		市售（医院&居家）
目的		吸入装置设计药物制剂处方开发	给药效果评估	疾病管理与反馈
计算方法	CFD	优化吸入装置设计，提高装置给药效率	模拟药物沉积分布	N/A
	PBPK	N/A	估算药物溶出&吸收	N/A
	AI	设计干粉制剂处方	预测药物沉积分布	采集患者用药操作 预警急性发作

对于CFD建模，许多已发表的模型都使用简化的参数设置来加速计算。然而，如果想要更准确地捕捉人体呼吸道中颗粒的运动轨迹，则需要设置更为复杂、真实的参数，例如用移动的柔性表面替换静态的刚性边界，以及更精细的网格划分[60]。此外，受限于CT成像分辨率以及极高的计算资源需求，目前CFD模型无法精确预测呼吸道前几级以后的颗粒沉积，这使得患者个体差异性研究无法继续深入下去。

限制肺部PBPK模型进一步发展的因素是模型验证数据的欠缺。对于吸入治疗疗效最重要的评价数据——肺组织浓度的验证，目前主要是通过与全身PK数据进行比较，这无法保证肺浓度的准确性。

经口吸入药物中AI应用的主要问题和其他类似的数据驱动模型类似，主要受限于数据的缺乏以及不一致的数据格式。大型制药公司通常不会共享他们的实验数据，而对于个体研究人员来说，建立数据库的成本过高且时间耗费巨大。此外，许多研究选择从已发表论文中收集的实验结果作为训练数据，但应该选取/排除哪些参数，目前还没有共识。虽然现有的AI模型已经展示了出色的性能和未来应用的潜力，但构建一个具有解释性的吸入药物机制模型在未来仍然是一个巨大的挑战。

除了建模技术本身的限制，从模型整合的角度来看，同样有很多改进空间。现有的多数研究仅涉及一种或两种计算模型，从一种方法中得到的知识很难转移到另一种方法中。例如，急性加重的预测模型与颗粒沉积模型具有类似的输入参数，但是从颗粒沉积模型中总结出的沉积机制目前并没有被急性加重预测模型很好地利用。虽然研究者们已经在试图进行多方面的整合研究，例如已经有几项CFD研究将吸入装置和真实人类气道几何形状结合，以研究设备和处方的差异在人体的真实呼吸道中的表现[19]。类似地，将从CFD/AI预测模型中获得的沉积分布模型输入到PBPK模型中，也已成为经口吸入药物研发的趋势[17]。多种模型的整合不仅能够提高计算效率以及拓宽应用面，还可以让研究人员对经口吸入药物的潜在作用机制得到更为全面的理解。

随着建模技术的不断提高，我们也可以期待拥有更强功能的IEMD（按照如今时代的定义，可以被称为"智能吸入装置"）面世。通过传感器收集吸入参数，计算模型可以评估患者的吸入动作并向用户提供个性化使用反馈。吸入动作的量化评估也可以输入给急性加重的预测模型，使得患者能够在急性加重的若干天前就能够得到警告，并及时就医，改善患者的生活质量。

11.8 总结

本章回顾总结了计算建模方法在经口吸入药物研究和应用中的进展。计算建模方法提供了一种辅助/替代传统实验方法的思路，缩短了开发周期，并提供了对递送机制更深入的理解。为了实现更为精准的个性化治疗，如"智能吸入装置"，需要研究人员在后续的研究开发过程中不断优化和整合多种计算建模方法。整合多种模型无疑是极具挑战性的，因为研究人员需要精通每一个相关的研究领域，并且针对不同来源数据的处理也是一项极为繁琐的任务。然而，随着这个领域的人才不断涌现以及更多的用药数据被分享与公开，可以预见计算建模方法在经口吸入药物中的应用在不远的未来必将取得更大的突破，为更高效诊疗方案的制定以及以患者为中心的个性化医疗保健系统体系的建立提供更多帮助。

参考文献

[1] Soriano J B, Kendrick P J, Paulson K R, et al. Prevalence and attributable health burden of chronic respiratory diseases, 1990—2017: a systematic analysis for the Global Burden of Disease Study 2017[J]. Lancet Respir Med, 2020, 6(8): 585-596.

[2] Labaki W W, Han M K. Chronic respiratory diseases: a global view[J]. Lancet Respir Med, 20206(8): 531-533.

[3] Purdy S, Griffin T, Salisbury C, et al. Ambulatory care sensitive conditions: terminology and disease coding need to be more specific to aid policy makers and clinicians[J]. Public Health, 2008, 123(2): 169-173.

[4] Einarson T R, Bereza B G, Nielsen T A, et al. Utilities for asthma and COPD according to category of severity: a comprehensive literature review[J]. J Med Econ, 2015, 18(7): 550-563.

[5] Hertel S P, Winter G, Friess W.Protein stability in pulmonary drug delivery via nebulization[J]. Adv Drug Deliv Rev, 2014, 93: 79-94.

[6] Allan R, Newcomb C, Canham K, et al. Usability and Robustness of the Wixela Inhub Dry Powder Inhaler[J]. J Aerosol Med Pulm Drug Deliv, 2020, 34(2): 134-145.

[7] Dalby R, Spallek M, VoshaarT. A review of the development of Respimat® Soft Mist™ Inhaler[J]. Int J Pharm, 2004, 283(1): 1-9.

[8] P. Rogliani, Calzetta L, Coppola A, et al. Optimizing drug delivery in COPD: The role of inhaler devices[J]. Respir Med, 2017, 124: 6-14.

[9] Capecelatro J, Longest W, Boerman C, et al. Recent developments in the computational simulation of dry powder inhalers[J]. Adv Drug Deliv Rev, 2022, 188: 114461.

[10] Ruzycki C A, Javaheri E, Finlay W H. The use of computational fluid dynamics in inhaler design[J]. Expert Opin Drug Deliv, 2013, 10(3): 307-323.

[11] Wong W, Fletcher D F, Traini D, et al. The use of computational approaches in inhaler development[J]. Adv Drug Deliv Rev, 2011, 64(4): 312-322.

[12] Sommerfeld M. Modelling of particle-wall collisions in confined gas-particle flows[J]. Int J Multiph Flow, 1992, 18(6): 905-926.

[13] Popoff B, Braun M. A Lagrangian approach to dense particulate flows[C]. In: International Conference on Multiphase Flow, Leipzig, Germany, 2007.

[14] Ding J, Gidaspow D. A bubbling fluidization model using kinetic theory of granular flow[J]. AIChE J, 1990, 36(4): 523-538.

[15] Zhu H P, Zhou Z Y, Yang R Y, et al. Discrete particle simulation of particulate systems: A review of major applications and findings[J]. Chem Eng Sci, 2008, 63(23): 5728-5770.

[16] Tong Z B, Yang R Y, Yu A B, et al. Numerical study of effects of powder size and polydispersity on the dispersion of fine powders in a cyclonic flow[C]. In: AIP Conference Proceedings, 2009: 807-810.

[17] Wang W, Ouyang D. Opportunities and challenges of physiologically based pharmacokinetic modeling in drug delivery[J].

Drug Discov Today, 2022, 27(8): 2100-2120.

[18] Borghardt J M, Kloft C, Sharma A. Inhaled Therapy in Respiratory Disease: The Complex Interplay of Pulmonary Kinetic Processes[J]. Can Respir J, 2018, 2018: e2732017.

[19] Walenga R L, Babiskin A H, Zhao L. In silico methods for development of generic drug-device combination orally inhaled drug products[J]. CPT Pharmacomet Syst Pharmacol, 2019, 8(6): 359-370.

[20] Ibrahim M, Verma R, Garcia-Contreras L. Inhalation drug delivery devices: technology update[J]. Med Devices Auckl NZ, 2015, 8: 131-139.

[21] Geller D E. Comparing clinical features of the nebulizer, metered-dose inhaler, and dry powder inhaler[J]. Respir Care, 2005, 50(10): 1313-1321.

[22] Momin M A M, Tucker I G, Das S C. High dose dry powder inhalers to overcome the challenges of tuberculosis treatment[J]. Int J Pharm, 2018, 550(1-2): 398-417.

[23] Shakked T, Katoshevski D, Broday D M, et al. Numerical simulation of air flow and medical-aerosol distribution in an innovative nebulizer hood[J]. J Aerosol Med, 2005, 18(2): 207-217.

[24] Santati S, Thongsri J, Sarntima P. Modified small-volume jet nebulizer based on cfd simulation and its clinical outcomes in small asthmatic children[J]. J Healthc Eng, 2019, 2019: e2524583.

[25] Su G, Longest P W, Pidaparti R M. A novel micropump droplet generator for aerosol drug delivery: design simulations[J]. Biomicrofluidics, 2010, 4(4): 044108.

[26] H. S. Nelson, "Inhalation devices, delivery systems, and patient technique[J]. Ann Allergy Asthma Immunol Off Publ Am Coll Allergy Asthma Immunol, 2016, 117(6): 606-612.

[27] Crosland B M, Johnson M R, Matida E A. Characterization of the spray velocities from a pressurized metered-dose inhaler[J]. J Aerosol Med Pulm Drug Deliv, 2009, 22(2): 85-98.

[28] Kleinstreuer C, Shi H, Zhang Z. Computational analyses of a pressurized metered dose inhaler and a new drug-aerosol targeting methodology[J]. J Aerosol Med, 2007, 20(3): 294-309.

[29] Fletcher G. Factors affecting the atomization of saturated liquids[D]. Loughborough University, 1975.

[30] ClarkA R. Metered atomisation for respiratory drug delivery[D]. Loughborough University, 1991.

[31] Gavtash B, et al. CFD simulation of pMDI aerosols in confined geometry of USP-IP using predictive spray source[J]. J Aerosol Med Pulm Drug Deliv, 2015, 29.

[32] Gavtash B, Versteeg H K, Hargrave G, et al. A model of transient internal flow and atomization of propellant/ethanol mixtures in pressurized metered dose inhalers(pMDI)[J]. Aerosol Sci Technol, 2018, 52(5): 494-504.

[33] Lavorini F. The challenge of delivering therapeutic aerosols to asthma patients[J]. ISRN Allergy, 2013, 2013: 102418.

[34] Geller D E, Coates A L. Drug administration by inhalation in children[M]. In: Kendig & Chernick's Disorders of the Respiratory Tract in Children, Elsevier, 2012: 284-298.

[35] Longest P W, Hindle M. Evaluation of the Respimat Soft Mist inhaler using a concurrent CFD and in vitro approach[J]. J Aerosol Med Pulm Drug Deliv, 2009, 22(2): 99-112.

[36] Ge Y, Tong Z, Li R, et al. Numerical and experimental investigation on key parameters of the respimat® spray inhaler[J]. Processes, 2021, 9(1): 1-17.

[37] Jin W, Xiao J, Ren H, et al. Three-dimensional simulation of impinging jet atomization of soft mist inhalers using the hybrid VOF-DPM model[J]. Powder Technol, 2022, 407: 117622.

[38] Lavorini F, Pistolesi M, Usmani O S. Recent advances in capsule-based dry powder inhaler technology[J]. Multidiscip Respir Med, 2017, 12: 11.

[39] Tong Z, Yu A, Chand H K, et al. Discrete modelling of powder dispersion in dry powder inhalers-A brief review[J]. Curr Pharm Des, 2015, 21(27): 3966-3973.

[40] Suwandecha T, Wongpoowarak W, Srichana T. Computer-aided design of dry powder inhalers using computational fluid dynamics to assess performance[J]. Pharm Dev Technol, 2016, 21(1): 54-60.

[41] Kopsch T, Murnane D, Symons D. Optimizing the entrainment geometry of a dry powder inhaler: methodology and preliminary results[J]. Pharm Res, 2016, 33(11): 2668-2679.

[42] Leung C M S, , Tong Z, Zhou Q, et al. Understanding the different effects of inhaler design on the aerosol performance of drug-only and carrier-based DPI formulations. Part 1: Grid structure[J]. AAPS J, 2016, 18(5): 1159-1167.

[43] Kopsch T, Murnane D, Symons D. A personalized medicine approach to the design of dry powder inhalers: Selecting the optimal amount of bypass[J]. Int J Pharm, 2017, 529(1-2): 589-596.

[44] Malcolmson R J, Embleton J K. Dry powder formulations for pulmonary delivery[J]. Pharm Sci Technol Today, 1998, 1(9): 394-398.

[45] Telko M J, Hickey A J. Dry powder inhaler formulation[J]. Respir Care, 2005, 50(9): 1209-1227.
[46] Donovan M J, Kim S H, Raman V, et al. Dry powder inhaler device influence on carrier particle performance[J]. J Pharm Sci, 2012, 101(3): 1097-1107.
[47] Tong Z B, Yang R Y, Yu A B. CFD-DEM study of the aerosolisation mechanism of carrier-based formulations with high drug loadings[J]. Powder Technol, 2016, 314: 620-626.
[48] Yang J, Wu C Y, Adams M. Numerical modelling of agglomeration and deagglomeration in dry powder inhalers: a review[J]. Curr Pharm Des, 2015, 21(40): 5915-5922.
[49] Tong Z, Zhong W, Yu A, et al. CFD-DEM investigation of the effect of agglomerate-agglomerate collision on dry powder aerosolisation[J]. J Aerosol Sci, 2016, 92: 109-121.
[50] Wong W, Fletcher D F, Traini D, et al. Particle aerosolisation and break-up in dry powder inhalers 1: evaluation and modelling of venturi effects for agglomerated systems[J]. Pharm Res, 2010, 27(7): 1367-1376.
[51] de Boer A H, Hagedoorn P, Woolhouse R. Computational fluid dynamics(CFD)assisted performance evaluation of the Twincer^{TM} disposable high-dose dry powder inhaler[J]. J Pharm Pharmacol, 2012, 64(9): 1316-1325.
[52] Jiang J, Ma X, Ouyang D, et al. Emerging artificial intelligence(ai)technologies used in the development of solid dosage forms[J]. Pharmaceutics, 2022, 14(11): 2257.
[53] Zeng X M, Martin G P, Tee S K, et al. Effects of particle size and adding sequence of fine lactose on the deposition of salbutamol sulphate from a dry powder formulation[J]. Int J Pharm, 1999, 182(2): 133-144.
[54] Shekunov B Y, Chattopadhyay P, Tong H H Y, et al. Particle size analysis in pharmaceutics: principles, methods and applications[J]. Pharm Res, 2007, 24(2): 203-227.
[55] Abadelah M, Chrystyn H, Bagherisadeghi G, et al. Study of the emitted dose after two separate inhalations at different inhalation flow rates and volumes and an assessment of aerodynamic characteristics of Indacaterol Onbrez Breezhaler® 150 and 300 μg[J]. AAPS PharmSciTech, 2018, 19(1): 251-261.
[56] Farizhandi A A K, Alishiri M, Lau R. Machine learning approach for carrier surface design in carrier-based dry powder inhalation[J]. Comput Chem Eng, 2021, 151: 107367.
[57] Jiang J, Peng H H, Yang Z, et al. The applications of Machine learning(ML)in designing dry powder for inhalation by using thin-film-freezing technology[J]. Int J Pharm, 2022, 626: 12217.
[58] Hajian B, De Backer J, Vos W, et al. Efficacy of inhaled medications in asthma and COPD related to disease severity[J]. Expert Opin Drug Deliv, 2016, 13(12): 1719-1727.
[59] Jaafar-Maalej C, Andrieu V, Elaissari A, et al. Assessment methods of inhaled aerosols: technical aspects and applications[J]. Expert Opin Drug Deliv, 2009, 6(9): 941-959.
[60] Huang F, Zhu Q, Zhou X, et al. Role of CFD based in silico modelling in establishing an in vitro-in vivo correlation of aerosol deposition in the respiratory tract[J]. Adv Drug Deliv Rev, 2021, 170: 369-385.
[61] Bailey M, Birchall A. Deposition, retention and dosimetry of inhaled radioactive substances[J].J Radiol Prot, 1998, 18(1): 022.
[62] Bair W J. The ICRP human respiratory tract model for radiological protection[J]. Radiat Prot Dosimetry, 1995, 60(4): 307-310.
[63] Cheng Y S. Mechanisms of pharmaceutical aerosol deposition in the respiratory tract[J]. AAPS PharmSciTech, 2014, 15(3): 630-640.
[64] Anjilvel S, Asgharian B. A multiple-path model of particle deposition in the rat lung[J]. Fundam Appl Toxicol, 1995, 28(1): 41-50.
[65] Koullapis P, Ollson B, Kassinos S C, et al. Multiscale in silico lung modeling strategies for aerosol inhalation therapy and drug delivery[J]. Curr Opin Biomed Eng, 2019, 11: 130-136.
[66] Yu C. Exact analysis of aerosol deposition during steady breathing[J]. Powder Technol, 1978, 21(1): 55-62.
[67] Finlay W H, Martin A R. Recent advances in predictive understanding of respiratory tract deposition[J]. J Aerosol Med Pulm Drug Deliv, 2008, 21(2): 189-206.
[68] Fleming J, Conway J, Majoral C, et al. Controlled, parametric, individualized, 2-D and 3-D imaging measurements of aerosol deposition in the respiratory tract of asthmatic human subjects for model validation[J]. J Aerosol Med Pulm Drug Deliv, 2015 28(6): 432-451.
[69] Carrigy N B, Martin A R, Finlay W H.Use of extrathoracic deposition models for patient-specific dose estimation during inhaler design[J]. Curr Pharm Des, 2015, 21(27): 3984-3992.
[70] Longest P W, Xi J. Effectiveness of direct Lagrangian tracking models for simulating nanoparticle deposition in the upper airways[J]. Aerosol Sci Technol, 2007, 41(4): 380-397.

[71] Xi J, Longest P. Transport and deposition of micro-aerosols in realistic and simplified models of the oral airway[J]. Ann Biomed Eng, 2007, 35(4): 560-581.

[72] Huang F, Zhang Y, Tong Z B, et al. Numerical investigation of deposition mechanism in three mouth-throat models[J]. Powder Technol, 2021, 378: 724-735.

[73] Longest P W, Hindle M, Choudhuri S D, et al. Comparison of ambient and spray aerosol deposition in a standard induction port and more realistic mouth-throat geometry[J]. J Aerosol Sci, 2008, 39(7): 572-591.

[74] Xi J, Yuan J E, Yang M, et al. Parametric study on mouth-throat geometrical factors on deposition of orally inhaled aerosols[J]. J Aerosol Sci, 2016, 99: 94-106.

[75] Brouns M, Verbanck S, Lacor C. Influence of glottic aperture on the tracheal flow[J]. J Biomech, 2007, 40(1): 165-172.

[76] Xi J, Yang T. Variability in oropharyngeal airflow and aerosol deposition due to changing tongue positions[J]. J Drug Deliv Sci Technol, 2019, 49: 674-682.

[77] Kim Y H, Tong Z B, Chan H K, et al. CFD modelling of air and particle flows in different airway models[J]. J Aerosol Sci, 2019, 134: 14-28.

[78] Poorbahrami K, Oakes J M. Regional flow and deposition variability in adult female lungs: A numerical simulation pilot study[J].Clin Biomech, 2019, 66: 40-49.

[79] Kleinstreuer C, Zhang Z. Laminar-to-turbulent fluid-particle flows in a human airway model[J]. Int J Multiph Flow, 2003, 29(2): 271-289.

[80] Grgic B, Martin A R, Finlay W H. The effect of unsteady flow rate increase on in vitro mouth-throat deposition of inhaled boluses[J]. J Aerosol Sci, 2006, 37(10): 1222-1233.

[81] K. Kadota, Imanaka A, Shimazaki M, et al. Effects of inhalation procedure on particle behavior and deposition in the airways analyzed by numerical simulation[J]. J Taiwan Inst Chem Eng, 2018, 90: 44-50.

[82] Phalen R F, Hinds W C, John W, et al. Rationale and recommendations for particle size-selective sampling in the workplace[J]. Appl Ind Hyg, 1986, 1(1): 3-14.

[83] Jayaraju S T, Brouns M, Verbanck S, et al. Fluid flow and particle deposition analysis in a realistic extrathoracic airway model using unstructured grids[J]. J Aerosol Sci, 2007, 38(5): 494-508.

[84] Feng Y, Kleinstreuer C. Analysis of non-spherical particle transport in complex internal shear flows[J]. Phys Fluids, 2013, 25(9): 091904.

[85] Piemjaiswang R, Shiratori S, Chaiwatanarat T, et al. Computational fluid dynamics simulation of full breathing cycle for aerosol deposition in trachea: Effect of breathing frequency[J]. J Taiwan Inst Chem Eng, 2019, 97: 66-79.

[86] Chen X, Feng Y, Zhong W, et al. Numerical investigation of the interaction, transport and deposition of multicomponent droplets in a simple mouth-throat model[J]. J Aerosol Sci, 2017, 105: 108-127.

[87] Nazir J, Barlow D J, Lawrence M J, et al. Artificial neural network prediction of aerosol deposition in human lungs[J]. Pharm Res, 2002, 19(8): 1130-1136.

[88] Nazir J, Barlow D J, Lawrence M J, et al. Artificial neural network prediction of the patterns of deposition of polydisperse aerosols within human lungs[J]. J Pharm Sci, 2005, 94(9): 1986-1997.

[89] de Matas M, Shao Q, Richardson C H, et al. Evaluation of in vitro in vivo correlations for dry powder inhaler delivery using artificial neural networks[J]. Eur J Pharm Sci, 2008, 33(1): 80-90.

[90] Chow M Y T, Tai W, Chang R Y K, et al. In vitro-in vivo correlation of cascade impactor data for orally inhaled pharmaceutical aerosols[J]. Adv Drug Deliv Rev, 2021, 177: 113952.

[91] Islam M S, Husain S, Mustafa J, et al. A novel machine learning prediction model for aerosol transport in upper 17-generations of the human respiratory tract[J]. Future Internet, 2022, 14(9): 247.

[92] Islam M S, Saha S C, Sauret E, et al. Ultrafine particle transport and deposition in a large scale 17-generation lung model[J]. J Biomech, 2017, 64: 16-25.

[93] Hassoun M, Malmlöf M, Scheibelhofer O, et al. Use of PBPK modeling to evaluate the performance of dissolv it, a biorelevant dissolution assay for orally inhaled drug products[J]. Mol Pharm, 2019, 16(3): 1245-1254.

[94] Bäckman P, Tehler U, Olsson B. Predicting exposure after oral inhalation of the selective glucocorticoid receptor modulator, azd5423, based on dose, deposition pattern, and mechanistic modeling of pulmonary disposition[J]. J Aerosol Med Pulm Drug Deliv, 2017, 30(2): 108-117.

[95] Vulović A, Šušteršič T, Cvijić S, et al. Coupled in silico platform: Computational fluid dynamics(CFD)and physiologically-based pharmacokinetic(PBPK)modelling[J]. Eur J Pharm Sci, 2018, 113: 171-184.

[96] Kannan R, Chen Z J, Singh N, et al. A quasi-3D wire approach to model pulmonary airflow in human airways[J]. Int J Numer Methods Biomed Eng, 2017, 33(7): e2838.

[97] Kannan R, Singh N, Przekwas A. A compartment-quasi-3D multiscale approach for drug absorption, transport, and retention in the human lungs[J]. Int J Numer Methods Biomed Eng, 2018, 34(5): e2955.

[98] Kannan R, Singh N, Przekwas A, et al. A quasi-3D model of the whole lung: airway extension to the tracheobronchial limit using the constrained constructive optimization and alveolar modeling, using a sac-trumpet model[J]. J Comput Des Eng, 2021, 8(2): 691-704.

[99] Kannan R, Arey R, Przekwas A, Berlinski A, Singh N. Evaluating drug deposition patterns from Turbuhaler® in healthy and diseased lung models of preschool children[J]. J Pulm Med Respir Care, 2022, 4(1): 1008.

[100] Vrijens B, Dima A L, Van Ganse E, et al. What we mean when we talk about adherence in respiratory medicine[J]. J Allergy Clin Immunol Pract, 2016, 4(5): 802-812.

[101] Vestbo J, Anderson J A, Calverley P M, et al. Adherence to inhaled therapy, mortality and hospital admission in COPD[J]. Thorax, 2009, 64(11): 939-943.

[102] Tashkin D P, Rand C, Nides M, et al. A nebulizer chronolog to monitor compliance with inhaler use[J]. Am J Med, 1991, 91(4A): 33S-36S.

[103] Julius S M, Sherman J M, Hendeles L. Accuracy of three electronic monitors for metered-dose inhalers[J]. Chest, 2002, 121(3): 871-876.

[104] Bogen D, Apter A J. Adherence logger for a dry powder inhaler: A new device for medical adherence research[J]. J Allergy Clin Immunol, 2004, 114(4): 863-868.

[105] Foster J M, Smith L, Usherwood T, et al. The reliability and patient acceptability of the smarttrack device: a new electronic monitor and reminder device for metered dose inhalers[J]. J Asthma, 2012, 49(6): 657-662.

[106] D'Arcy S, MacHale E, Seheult J, et al. A method to assess adherence in inhaler use through analysis of acoustic recordings of inhaler events[J]. PLoS One, 2014, 9(6): e98701.

[107] Merchant R K, Inamdar R, Quade R C. Effectiveness of Population health management using the propeller health asthma platform: A randomized clinical trial[J]. J Allergy Clin Immunol Pract, 2016, 4(3): 455-463.

[108] Chrystyn H, Safioti G, Buck D, et al. Real-life inhaler technique in asthma patients using the electronic ProAir Digihaler[J]. Eur Respir J, 2019, 54(suppl 63): PA4258.

[109] Zeller A, Taegtmeyer A, Martina B, et al. Physicians' ability to predict patients' adherence to antihypertensive medication in primary care[J]. Hypertens Res Off J Jpn Soc Hypertens, 2008, 31(9): 1765-1771.

[110] Bender B, Wamboldt F S, O'Connor S L, et al. Measurement of children's asthma medication adherence by self report, mother report, canister weight, and Doser CT[J]. Ann Allergy Asthma Immunol, 2000, 85(5): 416-421.

[111] Jentzsch N S, Camargos P A M. Methods of assessing adherence to inhaled corticosteroid therapy in children and adolescents: adherence rates and their implications for clinical practice[J]. J Bras Pneumol Publicacao of Soc Bras Pneumol E Tisilogia, 2008, 34(8): 614-621.

[112] Bender B G, Apter A, Bogen D K, et al. Test of an interactive voice response intervention to improve adherence to controller medications in adults with asthma[J]. J Am Board Fam Med, 2010, 23(2): 159-165.

[113] Chan A H Y, Stewart A W, Harrison J, et al. The effect of an electronic monitoring device with audiovisual reminder function on adherence to inhaled corticosteroids and school attendance in children with asthma: a randomised controlled trial[J]. Lancet Respir Med, 2015, 3(3): 210-219.

[114] Charles T, Quinn D, Weatherall M, et al. An audiovisual reminder function improves adherence with inhaled corticosteroid therapy in asthma[J]. J Allergy Clin Immunol, 2007, 119(4): 811-816.

[115] Moore A, Preece A, Sharma R, et al. A randomised controlled trial of the effect of a connected inhaler system on medication adherence in uncontrolled asthmatic patients[J]. Eur Respir J, 2021, 57(6): 2003103.

[116] Sulaiman I, Greene G, MacHale E, et al. A randomised clinical trial of feedback on inhaler adherence and technique in patients with severe uncontrolled asthma[J]. Eur Respir J, 2018, 51(1): 1701126.

[117] Bender B G, Cvietusa P J, Goodrich G K, et al. Pragmatic trial of health care technologies to improve adherence to pediatric asthma treatment: a randomized clinical trial[J]. JAMA Pediatr, 2015, 169(4): 317-323.

[118] Williams L K, Peterson E L, Wells K, et al. A cluster-randomized trial to provide clinicians inhaled corticosteroid adherence information for their patients with asthma[J]. J Allergy Clin Immunol, 2010, 126(2): 225-231.

[119] Koufopoulos J T, Conner M T, Gardner P H, et al. A web-based and mobile health social support intervention to promote adherence to inhaled asthma medications: randomized controlled trial[J]. J Med Internet Res, 2016, 18(6): e4963.

[120] Vasbinder E C, Goossens L M, Rutten-van Mölken M P, et al. e-Monitoring of Asthma Therapy to Improve Compliance in children(e-MATIC): a randomised controlled trial[J]. Eur Respir J, 2016, 48(3): 758-767.

[121] Price D B, Román-Rodríguez M, McQueen R B, et al. Inhaler errors in the CRITIKAL study: type, frequency, and

association with asthma outcomes[J]. J Allergy Clin Immunol Pract, 2017, 5(4): 1071-1081.

[122] Taylor T E, Zigel Y, Looze C D, et al. Advances in audio-based systems to monitor patient adherence and inhaler drug delivery[J]. Chest, 2018, 153(3): 710-722.

[123] Sulaiman I, Cushen B, Greene G, et al. Objective assessment of adherence to inhalers by patients with chronic obstructive pulmonary disease[J]. Am J Respir Crit Care Med, 2017, 195(10): 1333-1343.

[124] Taylor T E, Zigel Y, Egan C, et al. Objective assessment of patient inhaler user technique using an audio-based classification approach[J]. Sci Rep, 2018, 8(1): 2164.

[125] O'Dwyer S M, Mary S, Machale E, et al. The effect of providing feedback on inhaler technique and adherence from an electronic audio recording device, INCA®, in a community pharmacy setting: study protocol for a randomised controlled trial[J]. Trials, 2016, 17(1): 226.

[126] Sulaiman I, Seheult J, Sadasivuni N, et al. The impact of common inhaler errors on drug delivery: investigating critical errors with a dry powder inhaler[J]. J Aerosol Med Pulm Drug Deliv, 2017, 30(4): 247-255.

[127] Shah S A, Velardo C, Farmer A, et al. Exacerbations in chronic obstructive pulmonary disease: Identification and prediction using a digital health system[J]. J Med Internet Res, 2017, 19(3): e69.

[128] Merchant R, et al. An updated model for prediction of asthma exacerbations using albuterol electronic multi-dose dry powder inhaler[J]. CHEST, 2020, 158(4): A48-A49.

[129] Snyder L D, et al. A predictive model for copd exacerbations using proair digihaler: a 12-week, open-label study, in: C15. Predicting outcomes in copd[M]. In: American Thoracic Society International Conference Abstracts. American Thoracic Society, 2020: A4485-A4485.

[130] Lugogo N L, DePietro M, Reich M, et al. A predictive machine learning tool for asthma exacerbations: Results from a 12-week, open-label study using an electronic multi-dose dry powder inhaler with integrated sensors[J]. J Asthma Allergy, 2022, 15: 1623-1637.

[131] Nunavath V, Goodwin M, Fidje J T, et al. Deep neural networks for prediction of exacerbations of patients with chronic obstructive pulmonary disease, in Engineering Applications of Neural Networks, Pimenidis E, Jayne C, Eds[M]. In: Communications in Computer and Information Science. Cham: Springer International Publishing, 2018: 217-228.

[132] Fernandez-Granero M A, Sanchez-Morillo D, Leon-Jimenez A. An artificial intelligence approach to early predict symptom-based exacerbations of COPD[J]. Biotechnol Biotechnol Equip, 2018, 32(3): 778-784.

[133] Sanchez-Morillo D, Fernandez-Granero M A, Jiménez A L. Detecting COPD exacerbations early using daily telemonitoring of symptoms and k-means clustering: a pilot study[J]. Med Biol Eng Comput, 2015, 53(5): 441-451.

[134] Zhang O, Minku L L, Gonem S. Detecting asthma exacerbations using daily home monitoring and machine learning[J]. J Asthma, 2021, 58(11): 1518-1527.

第12章

使用3D打印技术的数字处方开发：人工智能与建模

蒂莫西·特雷西（Timothy Tracy） 南京三迭纪医药科技有限公司，中国；
Tracy Consultants，美国

吴　磊　南京三迭纪医药科技有限公司，中国

成森平　南京三迭纪医药科技有限公司，中国

李霄凌　南京三迭纪医药科技有限公司，中国；太平洋大学，美国

12.1 引言

将药物配制成患者可以安全和便利使用的产品的实践可以追溯到公元前，涵盖了中国、印度、埃及和西方国家等多个文化。西方国家的药剂师实践是最早以试验结果为基础标准化制剂实践的例子。在20世纪50年代末到60年代初，物理药学奠基人Takeru Higuchi引入了现代科学应用于药物研究和产品开发中[1, 2]。将科学原理应用于药物处方和产品开发，彻底改变了以往基于经验的处方工作，构建了现代制药处方的框架。尽管制药产品的处方现在在很大程度上是由科学原理驱动的，但当前的处方开发过程仍然依赖于科学家的经验，而且在一定程度上仍然涉及由于材料和生物系统中固有变量的不确定性而导致的试错。因此，即使在今天，制剂过程可能需要多次迭代才能实现所期望的处方。尽管取得一定成功，但这种经验法存在一些局限性。首先，这种策略高度依赖于制剂工作者的知识和经验。例如，制剂工作者可能会专门研究某种类型的处方，如缓释制剂，但对延迟释放、控制释放或增溶技术可能研究经验较少。因此，尽管制剂工作者在某个领域非常有经验，但他们可能没有针对具体研究挑战所需的全部专业知识。其次，这种方法可能需要多次迭代，直到选择了正确的参数组合。例如，为了避免药物在胃部分解和实现所期望的肠道吸收，人们可能需要尝试多种肠溶包衣。由于需要多次迭代，因此这种经验法的第三个局限性随之产生，即需要生产一致性的多批次药片。即使小规模的制片设备也需要一定数量的活性物质成分和赋形剂才能进行一次"生产"，通常需要生产数十个或更多的药片。尽管可以手动一次制作一片药片，但这种方法也有其局限性，比如不同参数的预测/猜测性、劳动密集和低再现性，使其可能不能产生一个真正具有代表性的产品。因此，当前的制剂开发过程并不理想，也可能需要大量时间和资源。

为了解决这些局限性，研究人员已经开始探索各种方法和技术，以实现更快速、更准确的理想处方预测和更高效的试验处方生产。其中许多研究工作集中在利用迅速发展的人工智能（AI）和数学建模技术，以先验方式预测理想处方。大量关于产品性能的信息，如赋形剂和活性药物成分，以及存储和处理这些大量数据的能力，为制剂工作者提供了以前无法获得的工具。通过挖掘文献，结合大型合作机构或在线共享数据，已大大扩展了供制剂者使用的信息，并将知识基础扩展到个体、制剂部门甚至公司。这些成果，再加上前面提到的计算方法和计算/存储方法，大大丰富了所有研究者可以使用的工具，不仅能够解决复杂的处方问题，还能够创造全新的药物递送技术，这在以前是难以想象的。有关AI和数学建模在传统片剂生产方法中剂型设计和开发方面的应用示例，读者可以参考已发表的文献[3, 4]。

尽管使用人工智能和数学建模大大增加了供制剂工作者使用的信息量，但仍然不能解决当前处方开发方法的某些局限，如灵活和快速的原型制作。采用3D打印的数字药物开发和生产过程可以补充人工智能和数学建模在药物处方方面的工作。使用3D打印的优势包括明确定义和可重复的工艺参数、快速原型制作、连续加工、构建复杂内部结构的能力、增材制造以及在扩大规模时使用相同的参数。通过实现快速原型制作，3D打印有助于生产小批量，甚至只有几片药片，最大限度减少了辅料/活性药物成分（API）的使用，并允许在一个工作日内进行多次生产和溶解测试。此外，一些3D打印技术可通过不同的物料供给机制将常见的赋形剂混合物甚至多个混合物输入同一台机器，从而可以快速制备含不同成分的制剂。

本章将探讨制剂科学家如何利用3D打印药品的优势，结合人工智能和数学建模，快速、经济并更高效地开发和生产药物产品。这些研究成果可以通过缩短开发时间、降低成本和加速审批过程来使公司受益，最终使患者受益。

12.2 药物制剂处方中的3D打印方法

将3D打印技术应用于药物生产的首次报告可以追溯到1996年，出自麻省理工学院的Michael Sima博士的实验室[5]。这项工作促成了Aprecia制药公司的成立，并推动了首个3D打印药物Spritam在2015年获得FDA批准。自这项早期研究工作以来，科学家们已经应用了多种3D打印技术来制备药物。美国材料试验协会（American Society for Testing and Materials，ASTM）将3D打印方法分为七种[6]。根据这些方法在制药处方中的应用，相关方法可以分为四类：挤出法、粉末法、液体法和板材层压法。这些方法的优势和局限性总结见表12-1[7]。

表12-1 制药应用中代表性3D打印技术的比较（已授权转载[7]）

分类		技术	基本原理	优势	局限
挤出法	材料挤出	熔融沉积建模（FBD）	载药的丝材被加热至临界状态，使其变为半流体状态，然后根据模型参数从打印喷嘴中挤出	● 设备多样性（多个喷嘴） ● 设备价格低廉 ● 机械性能良好	● 难以扩大规模 ● 载药量低
		半固体挤出（SSE）	半固体挤出通过一个基于注射器的打印头，在压力或螺旋齿轮旋转的作用下均匀挤出糊状物，并逐层沉积在打印平台上	● 载药量高 ● 打印工艺温和 ● 辅料范围广泛	● 需要后处理 ● 分辨率低 ● 效率低
		熔融挤出沉积（MED）	熔融挤出沉积是将粉末供料转化为软化/熔融状态，然后通过精确的逐层沉积来制造具有所需结构的物体	● 无后处理 ● 易于放大 ● 设备多样性（多个喷嘴）	● 载药量低
粉末法	黏结剂喷射	喷墨3D打印	首先制备一个二维基于粉末的层，然后喷射黏合剂溶液图案化和固化粉末床中的特定区域，从而组装三维物体	● 易于放大 ● 产量高 ● 载药量高	● 需要后处理 ● 粉末使用效率低
	粉末床熔合	选择性激光烧结（SLS）	使用聚焦的能源（例如激光或电子束）有选择地将粉末颗粒固化成实体物体	● 分别率高 ● 无须支撑材料	● 药物降解风险 ● 需后处理

续表

分类	技术	基本原理	优势	局限
液体法	槽光聚合	立体光刻术，数字光处理（DLP）	基于使用紫外线激光源对液体光敏树脂进行选择性光聚合的原理	● 分辨率与准确度高 ● 具有印刷微型结构的能力	● 需后处理 ● 潜在材料毒性 ● 有限的光敏树脂
	材料喷射	连续或按需喷射	通过打印头进行沉积，然后通过溶剂蒸发或在紫外光下固化来干燥，从而逐层构建对象	● 分辨率高 ● 印刷片的表面质量高	● 需后处理 ● 有限的辅料
板材层压法	板材层积	丝网印刷创新药物技术	将印刷浆料通过印刷屏幕的不同开口传送到给定的基材上进行打印	● 易于放大 ● 打印速度高	● 需后处理

12.2.1 挤出法

挤出法是目前应用于制备药物制剂最广泛的3D打印技术之一。正如其名称所示，该方法通过从喷嘴挤出材料，逐层形成物体或药片，从而实现具有各种内部和外部几何形状的自由形式片剂的生产。可以利用多个喷头来形成片剂的不同部分，以控制药物释放特性，或将多种API合并到单个片剂中。片剂的内部几何形状可以配置为具有独特性能的多层，具有各自释放特性的多个隔室，或者可以提供胃内滞留的浮力等。在同一片剂的不同部分内具有独立的药物递送表现的能力，尤其对于具有同一种API的多种处方或具有多个API且需要每个API具有独立释放特性的情况具有明显优势，因此可以在单个片剂内实现独立优化。

挤出式3D打印的两种最常见的应用是熔融沉积建模（FDM）和半固态挤出（SSE）[8]。近年来，该方法的更多应用已经得到了开发，其中包括熔融挤出沉积（MED）[9]、直接粉末挤压[10]、直接粉末打印[11]以及Arburg塑料自由成型[12]。在FDM和SSE方法中，使用在X、Y和Z方向移动的喷嘴（打印头）来挤出含药物的材料到板上，逐层形成药片。可以使用多个喷嘴将不同组成的辅料或不同的药物注入到同一个药片中。在熔融沉积建模中，药物被浸渍到聚合物丝中，由滚筒移动，加热，然后挤出到板上。在半固态挤出中，药物被并入半固态基质中，然后通过喷嘴挤出到板上。熔融挤出沉积（MED）允许药物和辅料的干粉在线混合，熔化成可挤出的形式，然后通过喷嘴连续挤出到在X、Y和Z方向上连续移动的板上。

12.2.2 粉末法

粉末法通常在高载药量和/或需要易分散的多孔结构时使用。尽管相对于挤出法，粉末法应用可能性较小，灵活性较差，但此法可以生产多个层次来改变药物的释放。粉末法有粉末喷墨（也称为喷墨粉末）和粉末床熔合两种方法。喷墨粉末类似于熟知的喷墨打印过程，液体黏合剂被喷射到包含药物和辅料的粉末表面上[13]。喷射过黏合液的粉末在干燥后会粘合在一起，留下未被打印的粉末。此法需要后期处理和加工，多余的含药粉末也需要重点考虑。在粉末床熔合技术中，选择性激光烧结（SLS）是最广泛使用的方法[14]。激光束的高能量被用来固化载药粉末。SLS的高分辨能力使其能够构建复杂和精确的结构。SLS还需要进行后期处理过程来去除未黏合的粉末。最后,必须考虑由高能量输入可能导致的药物降解。

12.2.3 液体法

液体法适用于制造具有精细细节的复杂结构,从而具备生产非常复杂的内部和外部结构的能力。在液体法中,药物通常包含在液体中,一般是一些单体或聚合物,然后采用添加或去除的工艺。立体光刻法是用于制药业的最常用的液体法,它涉及将药物溶解在聚合物树脂溶液中,然后使用激光束进行光聚合以产生物体[15]。树脂的单体可以被改变以改善释放动力学。数字光处理、液晶显示和体积三维打印方法也已被用于制备药物制剂。液体法的第二常见应用是按需滴加[16],在液体中含有药物,类似于前面所描述的按需滴加方法,药物是通过喷墨喷头以薄层的形式沉积的。立体光刻法则适用于制药应用受到制药反应中产生的中间体与药物可能发生的相互作用的限制,同时还需要考虑激光产生的热量对药物稳定性的影响。

12.2.4 板材层压法

板材层压法具有一个优点,即能够大规模生产药片[17, 18]。在这个过程中,药物被并入一个糊状物质中,然后将这个糊状物质涂抹在一个筛网上(类似于将墨水印在纸上的丝网印刷过程),药物会以薄层的形式沉积到筛网的离散开口中。然后重复这个过程,直到形成所需数量的层,并完成药片的制作。制成的药片在包装之前需要进行干燥。

12.3 使用3D打印技术实现新颖的片剂结构

3D打印技术具有制造复杂的外部形状和复杂的几何内部结构的能力,这使得研究者可以采用新的方法来控制药物释放速率以及药物在胃肠道中的释放位置、释放的起始时间、释放方式,甚至在一个单元中结合多种释放特性。这种水平的控制通常是通过使用多种材料和精确控制材料沉积来实现的。

12.3.1 使用3D打印技术构建独特的片剂外部几何结构

3D打印药物技术可以制造片剂的复杂的外部形状,开辟了许多传统片剂制造设备无法实现的可能性。对于传统药片压制而言,只能通过冲头和模具来创造有限的外形,从而产生平滑的表面。而3D打印是一种无须传统模具的增材自由形式制造方法,因此可以节省大量时间和成本。在传统的制剂工艺中,除了通过减小或增大片剂的表面积来进行表面微调或添加涂层(如肠溶包衣或缓释包衣)之外,几乎没有其他可以从几何角度改变药物释放的方法[19, 20]。使用3D打印技术,能够逐层创建药片而无须压制,可以设计具有可以穿过部分或整个药片的通道的片剂,并且可以设计成蜂窝或编织的形状(见图12-1)。这些开放式结构设计允许在相同的整体药片尺寸内增加表面积,甚至可以通过不同通道或编织部分的药片溶解特性的差异来精确控制药物的释放速率或释放动力学类型。此外,3D打印技术还允许以咀嚼片、软糖形式打印独特的形状,尤其适合儿童给药。

12.3.2 使用3D打印技术构建独特的片剂内部几何结构

3D打印片剂也可以通过控制以产生非常复杂的内部结构,从而实现前所未有的药物控制释放。这些内部结构可以非常简单,例如均一高度多孔的结构,也可以非常复杂,例如多层或多隔室结构(见图12-1)。多孔设计可以用于制备口崩片,这些口崩片在口腔中迅速分解,只需要少量水即可帮助轻松吞咽[21]。多层片剂可以通过多种方式进行设计,以实现多种不同的释放特性。例如,可以通过调整时间控制层的厚度来延迟活性药物成分的释放,以将其传送到胃肠道的特定部位,如结肠,从而实现更局部地治疗疾病,如溃疡性结肠炎[22]。药物的快速释放,或者更为缓慢和持续的释放,可以通过具有不同载药隔室表面积的多层结构来实现[20]。单一活性成分的释放可以通过具有不同释放动力学特性的多个隔室进行微调[23]或者每个隔室可以包含不同的活性成分,每种活性成分都具有自己独特的释放特性[24, 25]。多个隔室还可以通过灵活调整每个单独隔室中延迟层的组成或厚度,从而实现两次或三次脉冲释放模式[26, 27]。另外,其中一个隔室可以制成空心,以提供浮力,使药片能够在胃中漂浮并实现胃滞留[28, 29]。上述只是一些如何调节药物释放以产生所需的药代动力学特性的示例。3D打印片剂的结构控制为剂型设计的数字化提供了潜力,并为药物释放特性的控制增加了新的维度。

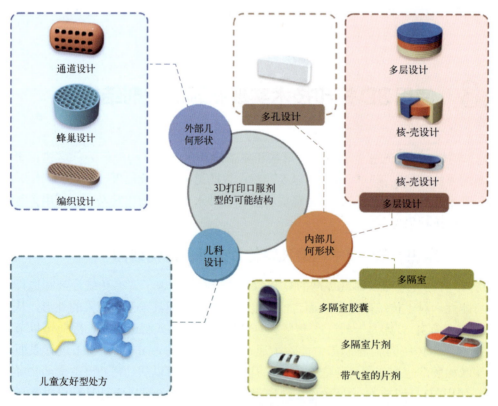

图12-1　3D打印片剂的可能结构[7]

12.4 使用3D打印进行处方开发的人工智能

12.4.1 辅料选择

辅料及其性能一直是处方开发中对试错过程产生影响的变量。选择合适的辅料，可以使制剂制备更容易，选择与活性药物成分兼容的辅料并达到期望的药物释放特性，这是一直以来制剂开发的挑战。即使对经验丰富的制剂科学家来说，每种API都是不同的，选择最佳的辅料组合是一个更为经验主义的过程，可能需要大量时间和多次迭代才能找到正确的组合。幸运的是，基于大量辅料、API和释放特性数据库的算法正在不断发展，以改善这个过程。例如，巴斯夫（BASF）的Zoomlab[30]就是这样一个对于制剂科学家可获得的资源库。通过先进的算法，Virtual Pharma Assistant Zoomlab™根据API的特性提供了最佳辅料组合的建议。制剂科学家输入API的性质和目标释放特性。根据这些信息，算法会建议使用哪些辅料，并提供结果，指导该组合在实现目标释放特性方面的表现。除了已经包含在数据库中的信息外，用户还可以输入其他辅料的化学信息或已记录的辅料的其他信息，以帮助算法指导辅料选择。这种定制化还可以用于改变辅料的比例/百分比，或者增加或减少辅料，以观察这些变化会如何改变预测的释放结果。通过采用这种快速且可定制的过程，制剂科学家可以在很短的时间内测试许多"虚拟"的辅料组合和组成百分比，从而减少了实验室测试的数量，并减少了购买大量辅料进行测试的需求。尽管最初是为传统的药物制剂开发的，但Zoomlab现在也被用于药物的3D打印。M3DISEEN是一种基于网络的制药软件，旨在利用人工智能机器学习技术加速FDM 3D打印[31]。通过输入制剂成分，这款软件可以预测机械特性、挤出温度、可打印性和打印温度，从而加速了选择适用于FDM 3D打印辅料的过程。

最近，多个机器学习（ML）模型被成功构建，用于预测结晶药物制剂的无定形和随后通过热熔挤出（HME）制备的无定形固体分散体（ASD）的化学稳定性，并已证明具有高度的预测准确性[32]。与化合物无定形和化学稳定性相关的API的亚结构已经可以准确的确定，并确定了HME过程的关键属性。这些结果也可能适用于使用挤出法3D打印技术的制剂开发。

12.4.2 使用3D打印的制剂开发

材料和生理系统引起的变量通常导致在制剂开发过程中进行不断试错。3D打印可以创建结构，减少某些变量对药物释放的影响。推进制药3D打印材料评估方法可以进一步减少这些变量的影响。将人工智能方法应用于3D打印药物制剂的开发是一个相对较新的发展，但是同时也是该方法的逻辑延伸。由于构成3D打印过程的参数数量以及通过调整这些参数改变控制程度和定制程度，人工智能方法是将其能力应用于3D打印药物开发的合乎逻辑的选择。除了选择适当的辅料外，还必须选择许多其他参数，如打印参数，包括打印温度、打印速度、打印路径、喷嘴直径等。鉴于外部和内部药片几何形状的几乎无限的可能性，使用大型数据集的人工智能方法可以帮助选择最佳的药片配置。而且，用于选择所有这些因素（辅料、打印参数和药片几何形状）的最佳组合以产生所需的溶解特性（或所选参数将产生的特性）的方法对于制定3D打印药物的科学家来说是一个巨大的可用资源。以下是将人工智能应用于3D打印药物开发的几个示例。这些研究的关键信息总结在表12-2中。

表12-2 AI和ML在3D打印药物领域的应用

3D打印技术	剂型（API）	AI/ML方法	输出	参考文献
DLP	速释片与缓释片（阿托莫西汀）	ANN	● 溶出行为	[33]
DLP	缓释片（布洛芬）	ANN	● 溶出行为	[34]
FDM	缓释片（地西泮）	ANN	● 溶出行为（五个时间点的药物释放百分比）	[35]
	速释，延时和逐步释放片	进化算法	● 溶出行为	[36]
DLP	缓释片（对乙酰氨基酚、茶碱或卡马西平）	多元线性回归，SVM	● 溶出行为 ● 释放动力学模型	[37]
FDM	ns	SVM，RF，ANN，KNN，LR	● 可打印性 ● 丝材机械特性 ● HME和FDM工艺温度 ● 溶出行为	[38]
FDM	ns	SVM，RF，KNN，MLR，神经网络，DL	● 可打印性 ● 丝材机械特性 ● HME和FDM工艺温度	[39]
FDM	ns	SVM，RF，ANN	● 可打印性 ● 丝材机械特性 ● HME和FDM工艺温度 ● 溶出行为	[40]

注：DL：深度学习（deep learning）；SVM：支持向量机（support vector machines）；RF：随机森林（random forests）；ANN：人工神经网络（artificial neural networks）；KNN：K最近邻（K-nearest neighbor）；MLR：多元线性回归（multivariate linear regression）；LR：逻辑回归（logistic regression）；ns：无（not supplied）。

Muniz Castro及其同事[38]已经应用机器学习方法来预测FDM打印方法中的丝材性能、丝材可打印性、各种打印条件/参数以及预期的溶出曲线。这些研究人员从114篇使用FDM 3D打印技术的出版物中收集了数据，涵盖了968种不同的处方。关于用于制造丝材的热熔挤出工艺的信息包括挤出机型号、挤出速度、挤出温度、挤出扭矩和丝材机械特性。关于FDM打印工艺，收集的信息包括打印机品牌和型号、喷嘴直径、打印速度、打印温度、平台温度以及给定处方可打印性。与处方的关键组成有关的信息也涵盖在数据库中，包括处方中每个组分的百分比组成，以及片剂的形状、尺寸、重量、层厚度，是否包含外壳（如果包含外壳，则包括其厚度和填充百分比）。如果药物在水中的溶解度在文章中不可用，那么将使用文献值。如果文章中包括溶出测试的信息，那么这些信息将被输入模型。通过研究考察五种不同的机器学习技术：支持向量机（SVM）、随机森林（RF）、人工神经网络（ANN）、K最近邻（KNN）和逻辑回归（LR）。从中发现，ANN是最准确的，可以用于预测处方的打印参数和溶出特性。例如，使用ANN，可以以94%的准确度预测丝材的机械特性和可打印性。挤出温度预测误差为±5℃，打印温度预测误差为±6.9℃。除了在预测打印参数方面的准确性外，ANN方法还能够在±24.3 min内预测T20、T50和T80的溶解时间。这些结果表明，应用ANN技术的机器学习方法可能在制药3D打印中具有重要应用，此方法很有潜力通过减少处方所需性能特性的迭代次数来加速处方开发过程。

与这项研究工作相辅相成，该研究团队开发了一个基于网络的软件程序M3DISEEN，制剂科学家可以使用它来预测FDM打印成片的API和辅料组合的性能特性[39]。使用AI和ML技术，该软件可分析大量的API特性、赋形剂特性和打印参数信息。为了最初填充数据集，研究人员开发了614种含药丝材处方，使用了145种不同的赋形剂，将这些处方打印成片，并评估了它们的性能特性。使用这个软件，用户可以选择数据库中已经包含的分子，或者输入自己的分子和其多种理化特性。然后，用户可以选择一组辅料，并使用这个组合来预测生成的丝材的可打印性、丝材的热熔挤出的最佳温度以及最佳的打印温度等特性。这个软件使用AI和ML技术来分析和监测与API、辅料和打印参数相关的大量数据。为了评估模型的性能，从开发的处方中使用了75%的信息作为训练集，其余的作为测试集。该模型能够以可接受的准确度预测多个参数。例如，可打印性的预测准确度为76%，丝材特性的准确度为67%。热熔挤出温度的预测均方根误差为8.9℃，而模型能够在8.3℃的绝对误差内预测FDM加工温度。通过这个软件，用户还可以快速而容易地改变组分的组成，并预测这些改变对溶解特性的影响。这种方法可以减少处方测试的迭代次数，以实现所需的制剂产品。

Ong及其同事[40]的一份有趣的报告应用了机器学习方法来预测FDM打印的片剂性能。通过整合阳性和阴性的实验结果，创建了一个更加异质化的数据集。数据集包括了在实验室内打印和测试的片剂信息，以及文献中的片剂性能数据。数据集包括通过HME和FDM创建的1594种独特处方，十分广泛。同时，对SVM、RF和ANN三种不同的机器学习模型进行了评估。针对每个建模参数，RF模型显示出了最佳的预测性能。处方的可打印性和丝材的机械特性可以以84%或更高的准确度进行预测，具体取决于参数。HME加工温度的预测均方根误差为5.5℃，FDM加工温度的预测均方根误差为8.4℃。这些结果比以前的工作更准确，显示了使用更大、更异质的数据集的价值。

AI方法还被应用于预测片剂内部结构，以实现所需的API释放曲线。Grof和Štěpáne[36]应用AI和进化算法来预测3D打印片剂的结构。尽管可能适用于其他片剂的外部结构，但这项工作将其应用关注于圆柱形片剂结构上，并对患者可能喜欢或可以接受的形状和尺寸设置了边界。这个计算模拟使用了二维和三维片剂形状，但在这两种情况下，药物只被认为是从片剂的侧面释放，而不是从顶部或底部释放。随后，研究人员创建了理论上快速溶解和慢溶解部分的片剂，有的带有API，有的没有。这些仅从片剂的侧面释放的片剂结构被设计用来控制溶剂的进入，从而控制各种片剂释放特性。然后，对这些结构和API的释放进行建模，以预测理论释放特性。例如，API可以以"阶跃函数"的方式释放、延迟释放、缓慢释放以及各种组合释放形式。尽管这些结果仅仅是计算模拟的，还没有经过实验验证，但这个过程在片剂结构设计中实现所需的释放特性和片剂性能特性方面可能会有用。这些预测建模工作的数据已经包含在M3DISEEN在线软件程序中[39]。

利用机器学习方法来预测和调整药物释放速率，也已应用于采用数字光处理（DLP）方法制备的速释和缓释3D打印片剂[33]。研究人员使用了人工神经网络（ANN）的机器学习方法来预测达到所需释放特性的最佳载药量和片剂厚度。以亲脂性弱碱阿莫西林作为模型药物，制备了直径恒定但厚度和载药量不同的圆柱形片剂，以实现阿莫西林的速释或缓释。片剂厚度从0.75 mm到3 mm不等，载药量从5%到20%不等。使用广义回归神经网络（GRNN）方法对包含23个实验的数据集进行了处理，其中17个实验数据被包括在训练集中，4个实验数据被包括在验证集中，2个实验数据被包括在测试集中。在完成数据集训练后，训练集的RMS为0.126，验证集为0.040，测试集为0.035。GRNN模型能够合理地预测基于片剂厚度和载药量的药物释放特性。对于两个测试曲线，通过比较预测的释放曲线与实际释放曲线，得到f_2分别为51.05和70.13，表明两者具有相似性。这些结果证明了本方法预测基于DLP 3D打印所制备的速释和缓释片剂的整体释放特性的能力。

同一研究小组还使用了人工神经网络和DLP 3D打印来优化和预测弱酸性药物布洛芬的释放[34]。在布洛芬的恒定载药量（5%）下，在11种不同的训练处方和3种测试处方中变化聚合物浓度、水浓度和核黄素浓度。使用线性和对数S型激活函数，采用反向传播算法开发了两种不同的人工神经网络（ANN）。然后，将预测的释放曲线与给定的辅料和布洛芬的实际释放曲线进行比较。对于神经网络1，预测与实验值的R^2值为0.9811；对于神经网络2，预测与实验值的R^2值为0.9960。神经网络1采用了多层感知机网络、反向传播算法和线性激活函数，根据f_1差异值（14.30）和f_2相似度值（52.15）判断能够产生最具预测性的结果。以上阿莫西林的结果表明，可以使用ANN来预测包含酸性或碱性药物的DLP 3D打印片剂的药物释放。

深度学习神经网络是机器学习的一个子领域，与传统的人工神经网络相比，它使用更多的隐藏层和更多的神经元来传递数据。深度学习神经网络也被用于预测FDM打印片剂的药物释放[35]，这是为了改进和克服实验设计（DoE）模型的局限性而采取的措施。在这项研究中，研究人员使用FDM打印含地西泮的片剂，旨在研究深度学习模型描述片剂的表面积体积比和打印参数（填充密度和填充模式）的影响的能力。研究者使用了自组织映射（SOM）神经网络来可视化各种参数之间的关系，并使用多层感知机网络来预测药物释放性质。含地西泮的片剂以圆柱形打印而成，内含0~4个孔（图12-2），填充密度在20%~100%变化，填充模式为锯齿或线条。当片剂含有一个孔时，孔直径为4 mm，而当片剂含有2个或更多孔时，孔直径为1.5 mm。总的来说，填充密度较低且采用锯齿填充模式的片剂释放速率较快。然而，对于采用线条填充模式的片剂，较高的填充密度观察到了更快的释放速率。具有较高表面积体积比（例如，带有孔的片剂）的片剂产生了更快的药物释放。这些数据随后被输入到深度学习模型中。使用SOM绘制数据可视化了各种参数对药物释放的影响。通过测试几个深度学习ANN模型，以描述表面积体积比和填充密度对药物释放的影响。然后，选择在训练集、验证集和测试集的RMS值最低的网络模型。该模型的训练集、验证集和测试集的RMS值分别为0.143、0.140和0.093。将两种测试处方的实验溶解曲线与这些配置的模型预测的溶解曲线进行比较，得到相似性因子f_2分别为70.24和77.44。

Tagami及其同事[37]还评估了用机器学习方法预测DLP 3D打印制造的片剂性能特征的应

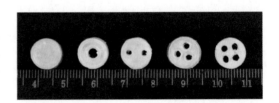

图12-2　3D打印片剂的图像（从左到右：圆柱形片剂，带有一个孔的片剂，带有两个孔的片剂，带有三个孔的片剂和带有四个孔的片剂）[35]

用。研究人员在片剂特性方面采用了不同的方法，通过制造所谓的"幽灵片剂"，旨在释放药物但不会崩解。ML 模型使用多元线性回归模型来预测指定时间的药物释放情况，并使用 SVM 模型来预测药物释放动力学。使用的三种模型药物分别是对乙酰氨基酚、茶碱和卡马西平。ML 模型中共输入了六个变量：药物浓度、聚乙二醇二丙烯酸酯[poly（ethylene glycol）diacrylate，PEGDA]浓度、水的用量、打印期间的光照时间以及对乙酰氨基酚和茶碱的用量。最佳拟合是通过包含除光照时间以外的所有变量获得的。该 108 个样本的数据集被随机分为已知数据的训练集和未知数据的测试集，据此评估了不同比例的训练数据和测试数据。线性回归模型平均 R^2 值在多个测试条件中都大于 0.900，并且在其中一个排列中高达 0.944。在药物释放动力学的预测中，两种非线性核（高斯径向偏差函数和多项式函数）的得分为 0.926。为了评估 ML 模型的先验应用，随机选择了含有三种药物之一的打印墨水的新组成。含对乙酰氨基酚或卡马西平的片剂表现出与预测相似的药物释放，其 f_2 值分别为 82.8 和 69.9。然而，含茶碱的片剂与预测的药物释放相似性较低，f_2 值为 25.2。这项工作表明，ML 可以至少有效地预测 DLP 3D 打印的含对乙酰氨基酚和卡马西平的片剂的药物释放。

有关应用 AI 和机器学习于制剂 3D 打印药物的优质综述，请参考已发表的参考文献[41, 42]。

12.5 使用 3D 打印进行处方开发中的数学建模

除了 AI 和 ML 数据驱动方法在 3D 打印药物处方开发中应用之外，基于机制的数学建模也可用来预测最佳打印参数和溶出曲线。本节描述了数学建模在这两种情况下的示例应用。

12.5.1 预测可打印性

与片剂处方一样，若能够预测最佳的打印条件也可以加速开发过程。由于 3D 打印涉及多个可修改的参数，增加了其灵活性，这也意味着人们必须深刻理解改变每个参数会如何影响最终产品。了解打印速度、喷嘴直径、挤出温度等变量对特定 API 和辅料组合以产生所需的外部和内部几何形状的影响至关重要。幸运的是，数学建模已应用于这些过程，且提供了一些初步框架，可以事先预测打印参数，从而减少了过程的经验性，并为制剂研究者提供了加快开发最终处方开发的更多工具。

例如，Zidan 和同事们[43]对用于 3D 打印缓释片的载药糊状物料的挤出性能进行了广泛的分析。用于 3D 打印的糊状物料可能不具备标准流变测试中易于通过的流变特性，微挤出过程可能导致糊状物料在喷嘴孔口被迫剪切和变形，而在糊状物料流动和墨盒壁之间没有薄的滑移层。研究人员研究了 19 种不同的辅料（Avicel PH101、Avicel PH105、乳糖和卡波姆 794 等）和双氯芬酸钠（模型药物）组合，并开发了一个适用于微挤出方法（喷嘴直径为 0.4 mm 或 0.6 mm）的本构流变模型。然后，基于挤出性数据，使用包括流量、喷嘴和墨盒直径、打印压力和滑移角参数的本构方程计算了材料参数。该模型随后用于预测糊状物料的屈服应力、黏稠度和流动指数。所有三个参数都具有较低的相对均方根误差（RMSE）；屈服应力值为 0.0691 bar，黏稠度指数值为 0.034，流动指数为 6.3 bar/sn。可溶性和可膨胀辅料的百分比都对屈服应力、流动性和黏稠度参数有显著影响。喷嘴直径只影响流动指数，而不影响黏稠度指数。由此得出结论，可以开发一个能够充分表征使用微挤出工艺进行药物3D打印的糊状物流变行为的数学模型。

用于3D打印参数以及FDM 3D打印片剂的后打印特性的预测模型也已构建[44]。研究人员首先创建了一个数据库，其中包括通过所采用的不同打印框架创建的产品特性。然后，通过设计实验的方式比较了不同比例的丙烯腈丁二烯苯乙烯（ABS）、聚乳酸（PLA）和高冲击聚苯乙烯（HIPS）聚合物对于片重、片重差异、打印时间和孔隙度等参数的影响，以确定对片剂参数最关键的打印因素。然后，筛选了以下因素，以初步评估其对片剂参数的影响：每个板上的打印片剂数量、形状、填充图案、打印机品牌、层高、尺寸、填充密度、温度和速度。接着，通过进行更多的更为密集的实验来优化模型，只考虑了其中三个变量：每个板上的打印片剂数量、打印片剂的尺寸比例和打印片剂的填充密度，同时控制其他变量保持不变，并监测相同的参数（片重、片重差异、打印时间和孔隙度）。最后，通过将模型应用于两种不同处方[包括不同数量的片剂、不同量的活性药物成分（美沙酮）以及不同范围的孔隙度]来验证模型。每个板上的打印片剂数量对片重产生了显著影响，增加打印片剂的数量会使平均片重减小。同样，增加打印速度会导致片重的降低。片剂的样式对片重产生了显著影响，因为内部空间的差异对于填充所用空间的影响很大。最后，打印机品牌对片重产生了显著影响，但层高和填充图案对片重没有影响。

再如，Tabriz等[45]评估了用于FDM 3D打印载药丝材的一系列聚合物。研究人员评估了超过二十种不同的聚合物，并通过热熔挤出制备了丝材。他们对所得丝材进行了一系列打印参数、物理化学性质和力学性能的评估，包括玻璃化转变温度、降解温度、最高挤出温度、3D打印温度、热稳定性、差示扫描量热谱、抗拉强度、流变学行为等。随后，使用主成分分析来评估可打印的聚合物与不可打印的聚合物之间的差异。此外，研究还发现，韧性是与可打印性最相关的力学性能，而脆性和韧性无法明确区分不可打印的聚合物。因此，得出结论，只需要抗拉强度这一个力学性能参数，即可评估聚合物的可打印性。这一研究有助于更好地理解不同聚合物在3D打印中的适用性，从而优化制药产品的制备过程。

12.5.2 溶出曲线预测

与预测打印参数类似，数学建模也被应用于预测药物溶出曲线。例如，Zheng等[20]进行了一项广泛的研究，分析了通过MED 3D打印制备的不同药物释放和溶出曲线的各种情况。这些制成的片剂包含一个支撑的、不溶解的外壳结构，药物只能从片剂的底部或顶部释放，而不能从侧面释放。在支撑的外壳结构内，包含了一系列具有不同表面积的药物核心层，药物可以从这些层中释放出来，也就是说，表面积是决定药物释放的因素（图12-3）。使用美托洛尔作为活性药物成分，并测量了每种制剂的释放情况。由此建立了一个数学模型，使用层厚和表面积设计这两个变量，以预测随时间变化的理论释放百分比 $Q_{(t)}$。随时间的 $Q_{(t)}$ 用一个通用方程表示：

$$Q_{(t)} = \frac{D_{(t)}}{D_{\text{total}}} = \frac{R_{\text{D}}\int_0^t S_{(t)}\mathrm{d}t}{V} \times 100\% \tag{12-1}$$

式中，$D_{(t)}$ 是时间 t 时从药物隔室释放的药物量；D_{total} 是药物隔室中所含的总剂量；R_D 是单位时间内深度上的矩阵溶解速率；t 是溶解时间，$S_{(t)}$ 是时间 t 时药物隔室的暴露表面积；V 是药物隔室的总体积。

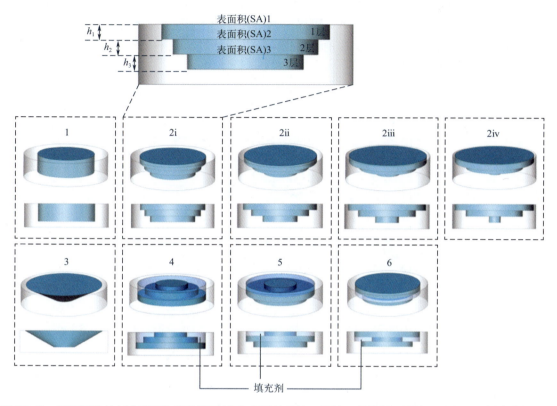

图12-3 用于评估片剂表面积与药物释放速率之间关系的不同核-壳片剂配置的图形表示。其中药物隔室为青绿色，外壳为浅白色，填充剂为蓝色[20]

此项研究测试了八种不同的模型，其中表面积或呈阶梯状增加，或呈阶梯状减少，或先增加后减少，或不断减少，或在整个片剂中表面积保持不变。在整个片剂中表面积保持不变的情况下，美托洛尔以零阶方式释放，与预测一致。图12-4中为以图形表示的每种片剂配置的释放速率。对于其他每种模型，药物释放速率与预测一致，绘制出线性关系（R^2 = 0.9832），这进一步证明了预测释放速率与观察释放速率之间的强相关性。

Tagami 等[46]还研究了FDM 3D打印片剂中表面积对药物释放的影响。使用FDM 3D打印并以钙黄绿素作为模型药物，研究人员评估了暴露的药物组分的表面积（片剂的顶部和底部，药物不会从侧面释放）对药物释放的影响。如图12-5所示，片剂中含药物的部分由片剂的红色部分表示，并且作为表面层的一部分而变化。活性药物成分与辅料/填充剂的比例保持2∶3（V/V）不变，以便直接比较药物的溶出。另外，使用两种类型的聚合物，即聚乙烯醇（PVA）或聚乳酸（PLA），来进行研究聚合物组成对药物释放的影响。研究发现，PVA可溶于水，而随着聚合物的溶解，阻止药物释放的能力会随时间而减弱。相反，PLA不溶于水，降解非常缓慢。因此，通过改变这两种聚合物的比例，可以改变药物释放。然后，对片剂进行溶出测试，测量了随时间释放的药物量。当层中含药物的组分在整个层中保持不变时，片剂表现出零级释放特性。通过改变含药物的表面积所占暴露表面积的比例，研究人员能够控制药物释放曲线。钙黄绿素/PVA的表面积与溶解速率高度相关（$R^2 = 0.9162$），而暴露的药物组分的表面积与溶解速率也高度相关（$R^2 = 0.9985$）。这些研究人员还证明，通过在暴露的药物表面上加入一层PVA，可以引入药物开始溶解之前的滞后时间。这项研究工作与上述工作相辅相成，因为改变片剂表面积，以及在这种情况下，药物暴露的表面积，可以用来可预测地控制药物释放。

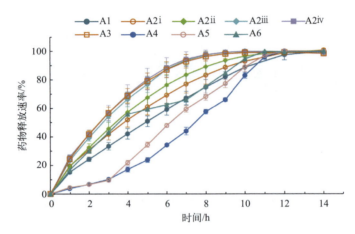

图12-4 图12-3中每种片剂配置的释放速率。数据以均值 ± 标准差表示（$n = 6$）[20]

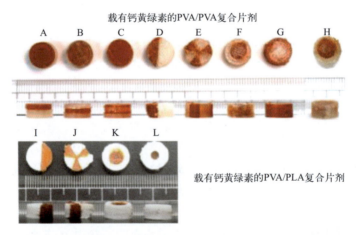

图12-5 直径为10 mm、厚度为5 mm的3D打印复合片剂的照片。这些复合片剂的红色组分含有钙黄绿素–PVA，而淡蓝色的部分仅含有PVA填充物（实际打印颜色为半透明白色）和PLA填充物（实际打印颜色为白色）[46]

试图根据片剂几何形状的表面积与体积比来预测生物药剂学分类系统（BCS）Ⅰ类（高溶解性，高渗透性）和BCS Ⅱ类（低溶解性，高渗透性）药物的释放曲线的工作也在进行中[47]。在评估各种药物的溶解度时，重要的是要考虑溶解性差异可能对释放特性产生重要影响。在这项工作中,研究人员选择普拉克索(pramipexole)和左旋多巴(levodopa)代表BCS Ⅰ类药物,吡喹酮(praziquantel)代表BCS Ⅱ类药物。通过热熔挤压制备了每种药物的含药丝材,并使用FDM技术打印制备了多种形状/配置的药片,如立方体形状、中空圆柱体、圆柱体和金字塔形,以涵盖广泛的表面积/体积比范围。然后对每种处方进行了溶出测试。有趣的是,剂量和药片大小并没有显著影响药物释放,只有表面积/体积比对药物释放速率产生了影响。平均溶出时间与表面积/体积比密切相关,R^2为0.998。研究人员尝试开发了几种数学模型以拟合数据并建立药物释放的预测模型。模型包括Korsmeyer-Peppas方程、Peppas Sahlin方程、Higuchi方程、修改的Higuchi方程、Hixson Crowell方程、Hopfenberg方程和Weibull方程。适用于可膨胀羟丙甲基纤维素片剂的改良Higuchi方程如下:

$$\frac{M_t}{M_0} = 2 \times \left(\frac{SA}{V}\right) \times \left(\frac{D \times t}{\pi}\right)^{0.5} \qquad (12\text{-}2)$$

在这个方程中,M_t代表时间t时已释放的API量;M_0表示片剂中初始API的量;D表示API在基质中的扩散系数;SA和V分别表示片剂的表面积和体积。BCS Ⅰ类药物最适合使用Peppas Sahlin方程进行拟合[48],然而,对于BCS Ⅱ类药物,Weibull函数更适合[48]。这些模型随后用于预测以前未经测试的其他片剂组成的药物释放曲线。相对均方根误差百分比(RMSEP)通常小于2%,尽管在具有较高SA/V比率的处方中稍高(约3% RMSEP)。研究者假设较高SA/V比率的较大误差可能是药物释放更快导致在完整的释放百分比范围内更难拟合。这些结果表明,由于它们在溶解度上的差异,不同的BCS类药物可能适用于不同模型。

此外,研究人员还评估了预测控释药物递送系统的释放动力学的能力[49]。他们再次使用热熔挤出和FDM打印生产的丝材,以茶碱作为模型药物,但这次通过控制密度来改变片剂内的网络结构,同时保持表面积/质量比恒定。片剂为壳厚400 μm的椭圆形设计,内部网络为直角。偶数层的丝材以90度的角度打印,与奇数层的丝材重叠,形成重叠的填充网络。片剂的重量(263 mg至668 mg)和剂量与填充密度成正比,而网络的比表面积随填充密度变化不大。使用自定义的溶出装置进行溶出实验,该装置允许将片剂侧向放置,以适应片剂的编织设计,结果显示随着网络密度的增加,药物释放速率较慢。研究人员试图应用Higuchi模型[48]来预测药物释放,但由于不同填充密度产生不同的释放动力学,该模型不足以适用。通过使用线性插值法来预测填充密度从15%到25%变化的样品片剂的药物释放发现,两者具有非常强的相关性,预测均方根误差(RMSEP)较低,在1.4%到3.7%之间,表明本法具有良好的预测能力。

其他研究组也开发了预测3D打印片剂药物释放的方法。Sun等[50, 51]制作了构造为"胶囊中的片剂"或"片剂中的圆盘"的3D打印剂型,也就是制备一个完全可定制的含药插入物,然后将其放入胶囊形状或片剂形状的外壳中,旨在创建一种个性化药物制备方法(图12-6)。通过修改插入物的配置,可以定制药物释放速率,以实现目标释放曲线。这些片剂由三个部分组成,即含药的表面侵蚀聚合物,不含药的表面侵蚀聚合物以及作为片剂涂层的不透水但可生物降解的聚合物。与上述3D打印示例相反,3D打印机用于制作所需的药物释放配置的模具,然后将药物溶液倒入模具中并使其硬化,而不是直接用3D打印机打印配置。3D打印机还用于制作外壳,其开口大小与形成的含药/不含药侵蚀部分的尺寸相匹配,然后将插入物手动插入外壳中。利用这项技术，通过改变插入物的配置，能够产生各种各样的药物释放模式，例如零阶释放，多脉冲释放，不断增加或不断减少的释放速率，甚至是步进函数释放，每个步骤的幅度不同（图12-7）。由此研究人员开发出了一个根据片剂的厚度、体积以及含药基质的尺寸来预测药物释放百分比的数学模型。药物释放百分比（PR）可以通过以下方程式从含药基质的几何形状中计算出来。

$$\mathrm{PR} = \frac{R_\mathrm{d} T \int_0^t (W_\mathrm{D} - W_n)\mathrm{d}t}{V_\mathrm{T}} \times 100\% \qquad (12\text{-}3)$$

在这个方程中，W_D 和 W_n 分别代表片剂的不同部分的宽度；T 代表片剂的厚度；V_T 代表含药基质的总体积；t 代表时间。使用模型药物对乙酰氨基酚和苯肾上腺素，成功地预测了各种释放曲线，如恒定释放、增大和减小释放速率的释放以及脉冲释放，预测准确度较高。然后，紧接着扩展了这项工作，包括由同一片剂释放两种药物，这些药物具有相似或不同的释放曲线，例如两种不同的恒定释放速率的药物，一种恒定释放速率、另一种减小释放速率的药物，一种增大释放速率和一种减小释放速率的两种药物，甚至一种恒定释放速率、另一种分段释放速率的两种药物，均能准确预测药物释放。

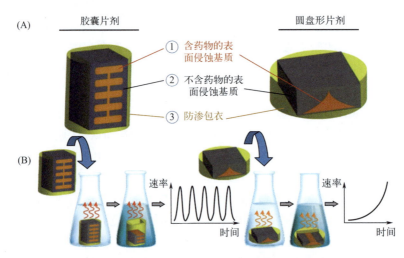

图12-6 可完全定制的药物片剂设计。（A）药物片剂的内部组分可以呈胶囊或圆盘形。专门设计的含药物的表面侵蚀基质的形状以按所需的释放曲线释放药物。除了顶部的开口，该片剂的所有侧面都由不透水的涂层保护。（B）示意图用于说明按照含药物基质的形状在溶解介质中释放具有可定制释放曲线的胶囊和圆盘形药物片剂[51]

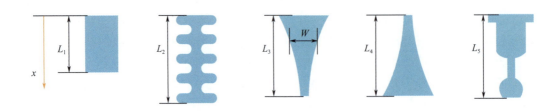

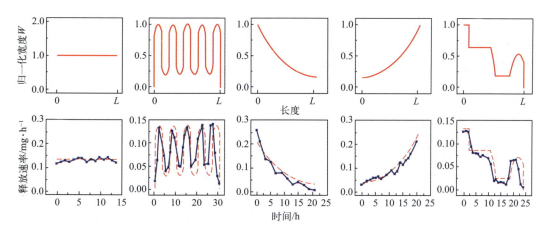

图12-7 药物片剂中染料的预期释放速率和实验测定的速率。顶部一行：使用五种不同形状的片剂。W 表示 x 轴上任意点处含染料聚合物的宽度（即片剂降解方向）。片剂的长度分别为 L_1 = 5.5 mm，L_2 = 9.0 mm，$L_3 = L_4$ = 8 mm 和 L_5 = 8.2 mm。中间行：以 W 对长度作图，其中通过将 W 除以每种形状的最大 W 来对 W 进行了归一化。如底部一行图中的红色虚线所示，可以将 W 转换为预期的释放速率[50]。

用于预测打印性能和释放曲线的模型为减少在处方开发中导致不确定性的变量提供了基础，从而实现了高效和可预测的产品开发。

12.6　3D打印处方源于设计

12.6.1　3D打印处方源于设计（3DFbD®）的方法

基于应用人工智能于处方开发的概念，并利用全面的辅料性能特性、打印参数和其他关键属性数据库，3D打印处方源于设计（3DFbD®）的概念已经发展起来，以减少工作量并通过使用3D打印来加速药物的处方开发和打印。这一方法包括八步流程，从目标药代动力学曲线开始，迅速高效地预测最佳处方，以实现预测的药物释放曲线，从而实现所需的目标药代动力学曲线。图12-8中呈现了这一过程的示意图，下面将提供更详细的描述，并附带一个示例说明。

只有溶解的药物才能被吸收，这个过程起始于定义目标药代动力学曲线和相应的药物释放曲线，该曲线预计将支持实现体内药代动力学曲线。接下来，定义外部和内部的药片结构，以实现所需的药物释放曲线。例如，是否需要延迟释放曲线、缓慢释放曲线或多次脉冲释放曲线？相应地，释放曲线是否需要实现特定的体内 C_{max}、最小化 C_{max} 和 C_{min} 之间的差异，或在整个给药间隔期间保持高于 C_{min}？回答这些关键问题可以为设计满足这些要求的片剂结构提供必要的信息。正如在 Zheng 等[20]的文章中所描述的开发药片结构和相应的释放性能的数学模型对于设计最佳的药片结构至关重要。一旦几何结构确定，人工智能可以根据其性能特性数据库，单独或组合使用辅料，以及在可能的情况下与指定API结合使用，来评估所需的辅料及其比例。

在定义了药片结构和辅料组成之后，将这些信息输入到3D打印软件中，以生成所需的药片制备打印指令。从这些指令中，生产原型药片，并将其进行溶解测试，并与期望的体外药物释放曲线进行比较。假设达到了期望的体外药物释放曲线，那么该处方将在动物或人类中进行测试，以评估达到目标药代动力学曲线的程度。这个过程利用了大量关于材料和药片结构的信息数据库，因此可以在很少的迭代甚至只有一次迭代中实现目标曲线，从而大大加快了处方开发过程。

作为这个流程的最后说明，3D药片设计的额外好处是，可以考虑将药片的构建类比"乐高"积木以实现设计（见图12-8第3步）。通过这个概念框架，可以"连接"或"组合"具有不同性能特征的组件，通过微调药物释放以实现期望的剖面。例如，如果需要迅速达到药物水平但需要维持这个浓度一段时间，可以将药片的一部分制备成含有足够API以快速达到期望的C_{max}的快速释放部分，然后再设计第二个含有不同API量并具有延迟释放特性以维持这个浓度的部分。同样，可以设想模拟每天三次服药而伴随着药物浓度的高峰和低谷，但用此方法只需每天服药一次。为了实现这一点，可以设想创建三个部分，每个部分都含有相同量的API，但释放的API具有不同的延迟，以使来自每个部分的API的释放在几小时内依次发生。Zheng等应用了这些方法，使用了"乐高"模型，将具有不同特性的部分组合在一起，以实现期望的体外溶出曲线和目标体内药代动力学曲线[20]。

设计驱动的制剂使得数字化的制剂开发流程成为可能，它利用了计算机辅助设计（CAD）、物质数据库、药代动力学建模和模拟。将这些数学/数字化方法纳入传统的基于经验的制剂开发流程中，实现了制剂开发的可预测性、成本效益和时间效率的飞跃。

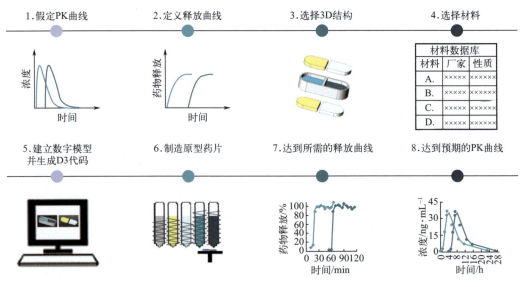

图12-8 3D打印设计制剂方法的示意图[20]

12.6.2 3DFbD®对质量源于设计的贡献

质量源于设计（QbD）的概念最早由Juran于1992年提出[52]，这种以质量和创新为目标的设计过程已经被美国食品药品管理局（FDA）采纳，并作为药物的发现、开发和生产的一部分。特别值得注意的是，FDA在其《行业指南Q8（R2）药物开发》文件中明确支持了

QbD原则的使用[53]。QbD方法评估多个变量，并允许分析这些变量是否有相互作用而对整个过程产生影响，从而更全面地理解关键质量属性（CQA）。这种更全面的方法允许建立一个"设计空间"，在这个空间中，可以了解各种变量组合的完整范围，以获得符合目标产品概况的产品，使制药者和制造商能够比"可接受范围"更灵活的方式进行操作。QbD概念还被提议作为药物处方开发这一更具体任务的框架[54]。

QbD方法已经应用于3D打印片剂的开发中。例如，Than和Titapiwatanakun采用了QbD方法来开发FDM 3D打印速释片剂[55]。最初，研究人员采用了一种实验设计（DoE）方法，独立确定了不同载药量和辅料组成的关键物料属性（CMA）。D-最佳混合设计解释了不同组成对药物释放的影响，并为从少量计算中开发高度预测性模型以及速释片剂的最佳处方奠定了基础。此外，研究人员还将QbD方法应用于控释3D打印处方的设计[56]。同样地，采用FDM 3D打印和类似的设计，涉及九种处方的混合设计表明，药物释放受不同聚合物的协同作用影响，并成功地预测出最佳处方。这些研究为使用QbD进行速释和控释制剂开发提供了实际场景。

3DFbD®方法可以帮助确定产品几何设计、关键物料属性和关键工艺参数对产品CQA（如溶解度）的影响过程。建立数学模型，可以根据外部和内部3D几何结构对溶解曲线进行先验预测，并利用AI/ML加速辅料选择。3DFbD®是QbD的补充，重要的是，3DFbD®充当QbD框架下制剂开发的重要补充，提供数字溶出判断、片剂结构设计和辅料选择。使用3DFbD®方法，基于对相关因素的系统和全面了解，实现了制剂开发的可预测，且具有成本效益。3DFbD®方法还可以利用实验设计方法来提供尽可能稳健的信息集，以实现最准确的预测。因此，3DFbD®方法是一种有前景的工具，可减轻工作量并加速口服固体剂型的开发。

12.7 总结

药物3D打印技术的蓬勃发展以及该工艺的灵活性和可定制性，使得药物释放曲线和由此产生的体内药代动力学以及制剂开发结果的可预测性成为可能，而这在传统的制片和制剂方法中是不可能实现的。结合数字制造、人工智能、机器学习和数学建模，制剂开发出现了一个新方向，并提供了一种方法，减少当前的试错式制剂开发方法的使用，将制药产品开发过程推进了一步。3D打印技术刚刚起步，因此不仅需要确定辅料的性能特点和可打印性、打印参数，还需要确定所使用的片剂结构及其对药物释放曲线的影响。通过使用AI和ML方法，以及利用与产品性能相关的不断增长的信息数据库的数学模型，以提供有关片剂药物释放性能的准确、高效的先验预测，加速了这项工作的进展。进一步的研究不仅可以更好地了解辅料的性能、打印参数的作用，还能建立更广泛的生产剂型及其性能特征数据库，这将为进一步开发人工智能方法提供必要的信息，从而优化3D打印方法和所生产的剂型。随着这些信息和相关数据库的不断增长，不仅预测结果将不断改进，药物制剂研发过程也将不断加快，从而缩短将药物推向市场造福患者的时间并降低成本。

参考文献

[1] Higuchi T.Rate of release of medicaments from ointment bases containing drugs in suspension[J].J Pharm Sci, 1961, 50(10): 874-875.

[2] Stella V J.My mentors[J].J Pharm Sci, 2001, 90(8): 969-978.

[3] Bannigan P, Aldeghi M, Bao Z, et al.Machine learning directed drug formulation development[J].Adv Drug Deliv Rev, 2021, 175: 113806.

[4] Gao H, Wang W, Dong J, et al.An integrated computational methodology with data-driven machine learning, molecular modeling and PBPK modeling to accelerate solid dispersion formulation design[J].Eur J Pharm Biopharm Off J Arbeitsgemeinschaft Pharm Verfahrenstechnik EV, 2021, 158: 336-346.

[5] Wu B M, Borland S W, Giordano R A, et al.Solid free-form fabrication of drug delivery devices[J].J Controlled Release, 1996, 40(1): 77-87.

[6] ISO/ASTM, 2021. Additive manufacturing — General principles — Fundamentals and vocabulary [WWW Document]. ISO. URL https://www.iso.org/standard/74514.html(accessed 3.6.23)

[7] Tracy T, Wu L, Liu X, et al.3D printing: Innovative solutions for patients and pharmaceutical industry[J].Int J Pharm, 2023, 631: 122480.

[8] Azad M A, Olawuni D, Kimbell G, et al.Polymers for extrusion-based 3D printing of pharmaceuticals: A holistic materials process perspective[J].Pharmaceutics, 2020, 12(2): 124.

[9] Cheng S, Li X, DENG F, et al.3D printing device and method[P].US11364674B2, 2018.

[10] Goyanes A, Allahham N, Trenfield S J, et al.Direct powder extrusion 3D printing: Fabrication of drug products using a novel single-step process[J].Int J Pharm, 2019, 567: 118471.

[11] Fanous M, Gold S, Muller S, et al.Simplification of fused deposition modeling 3D-printing paradigm: Feasibility of 1-step direct powder printing for immediate release dosage form production[J].Int J Pharm, 2020, 578: 119124.

[12] Zhang B, Nasereddin J, McDonagh T, et al.Effects of porosity on drug release kinetics of swellable and erodible porous pharmaceutical solid dosage forms fabricated by hot melt droplet deposition 3D printing[J].Int J Pharm, 2021, 604: 120626.

[13] Sen K, Mehta T, Sansare S, et al.Pharmaceutical applications of powder-based binder jet 3D printing process: A review[J]. Adv Drug Deliv Rev, 2021, 177: 113943.

[14] Awad A, Fina F, Goyanes A, et al.Advances in powder bed fusion 3D printing in drug delivery and healthcare[J].Adv Drug Deliv Rev, 2021, 174: 406-424.

[15] Deshmane S, Kendre P, Mahajan H, et al.Stereolithography 3D printing technology in pharmaceuticals: a review[J].Drug Dev Ind Pharm, 2021, 47(9): 1362-1372.

[16] Tam C H, Alexander M, Belton P, et al.Drop-on-demand printing of personalised orodispersible films fabricated by precision micro-dispensing[J].Int J Pharm, 2021, 610: 121279.

[17] Awad A, Trenfield S J, Goyanes A, et al.Reshaping drug development using 3D printing[J].Drug Discov Today, 2018, 23(8): 1547-1555.

[18] Schneeberger A, Kühne K, Kerschbaumer H, et al. Method for producing a drug delivery system[P].US20220387331A1, 2022.

[19] Patel S K, Khoder M, Peak M, et al.Controlling drug release with additive manufacturing-based solutions[J].Adv Drug Deliv Rev, 2021, 174: 369-386.

[20] Zheng Y, Deng F, Wang B, et al.Melt extrusion deposition(MED^{TM})3D printing technology: A paradigm shift in design and development of modified release drug products[J].Int J Pharm, 2021, 602: 120639.

[21] Pyteraf J, Jamróz W, Kurek M, et al.Preparation and advanced characterization of highly drug-loaded, 3D printed orodispersible tablets containing fluconazole[J].Int J Pharm, 2023, 630: 122444.

[22] Melocchi A, Uboldi M, Briatico-Vangosa F, et al.The Chronotopic^{TM} system for pulsatile and colonic delivery of active molecules in the era of precision medicine: Feasibility by 3D printing via fused deposition modeling(FDM)[J]. Pharmaceutics, 2021, 13(5): 759.

[23] Khaled S A, Burley J C, Alexander M R, et al.3D printing of five-in-one dose combination polypill with defined immediate and sustained release profiles[J].J Control Release Off J Control Release Soc, 2015, 217: 308-314.

[24] Awad A, Fina F, Trenfield S J, et al.3D Printed pellets(miniprintlets): A novel, multi-drug, controlled release platform technology[J].Pharmaceutics, 2019, 11(4): E148.

[25] Goh W J, Tan S X, Pastorin G, et al.3D printing of four-in-one oral polypill with multiple release profiles for personalized

delivery of caffeine and vitamin B analogues[J].Int J Pharm, 2021, 598: 120360.

[26] Maroni A, Melocchi A, Parietti F, et al.3D printed multi-compartment capsular devices for two-pulse oral drug delivery[J].J Controlled Release, 2017, 268: 10-18.

[27] Melocchi A, Uboldi M, Parietti F, et al.Lego-Inspired capsular devices for the development of personalized dietary supplements: Proof of concept with multimodal release of caffeine[J].J Pharm Sci, 2020, 109(6): 1990-1999.

[28] Charoenying T, Patrojanasophon P, Ngawhirunpat T, et al. Fabrication of floating capsule-in-3D-printed devices as gastro-retentive delivery systems of amoxicillin[J].J Drug Deliv Sci Technol, 2020, 55: 101393.

[29] Jeong H M, Weon K Y, Shin B S, et al.3D-printed gastroretentive sustained release drug delivery system by applying design of experiment approach[J].Mol Basel Switz, 2020, 25(10): E2330.

[30] ZoomLab [WWW Document], 2023. URL https: //virtualpharmaassistants.basf.com/s/(accessed 3.6.23).

[31] M3DISEEN [WWW Document], 2020. URL https: //m3 diseen.com/predictions/(accessed 3.6.23).

[32] Jiang J, Lu A, Ma X, et al.The applications of machine learning to predict the forming of chemically stable amorphous solid dispersions prepared by hot-melt extrusion[J].Int J Pharm X, 2023, 5: 100164.

[33] Stanojević G, Medarević D, Adamov I, et al.Tailoring atomoxetine release rate from dlp 3D-printed tablets using artificial neural networks: Influence of tablet thickness and drug loading[J].Mol Basel Switz, 2020, 26(1): 111.

[34] Madzarevic M, Medarevic D, Vulovic A, et al.Optimization and prediction of ibuprofen release from 3 d dlp printlets using artificial neural networks[J].Pharmaceutics, 2019, 11(10): 544.

[35] Obeid S, Madžarević M, Krkobabić M, et al.Predicting drug release from diazepam FDM printed tablets using deep learning approach: Influence of process parameters and tablet surface/volume ratio[J].Int J Pharm, 2021, 601: 120507.

[36] Grof Z, Štěpánek F.Artificial intelligence based design of 3D-printed tablets for personalised medicine[J].Comput Chem Eng, 2021, 154: 107492.

[37] Tagami T, Morimura C, Ozeki T.Effective and simple prediction model of drug release from "ghost tablets" fabricated using a digital light projection-type 3D printer[J].Int J Pharm, 2021, 604: 120721.

[38] Muñiz Castro B, Elbadawi M, Ong J J, et al.Machine learning predicts 3D printing performance of over 900 drug delivery systems[J].J Control Release Off J Control Release Soc, 2021, 337: 530-545.

[39] Elbadawi M, Muñiz Castro B, Gavins F K H, et al.M3DISEEN: A novel machine learning approach for predicting the 3D printability of medicines[J].Int J Pharm, 2020, 590: 119837.

[40] Ong J J, Castro B M, Gaisford S, et al.Accelerating 3D printing of pharmaceutical products using machine learning[J].Int J Pharm X, 2022, 4: 100120.

[41] Elbadawi M, McCoubrey L E, Gavins F K H, et al.Harnessing artificial intelligence for the next generation of 3D printed medicines[J].Adv Drug Deliv Rev, 2021, 175: 113805.

[42] Elbadawi M, McCoubrey L E, Gavins F K H, et al.Disrupting 3D printing of medicines with machine learning[J].Trends Pharmacol Sci, 2021, 42(9): 745-757.

[43] Zidan A, Alayoubi A, Coburn J, et al.Extrudability analysis of drug loaded pastes for 3D printing of modified release tablets[J].Int J Pharm, 2019, 554: 292-301.

[44] Pires F Q, Alves-Silva I, Pinho L A G, et al.Predictive models of FDM 3D printing using experimental design based on pharmaceutical requirements for tablet production[J].Int J Pharm, 2020, 588: 119728.

[45] Tabriz A G, Scoutaris N, Gong Y, et al.Investigation on hot melt extrusion and prediction on 3D printability of pharmaceutical grade polymers[J].Int J Pharm, 2021, 604: 120755.

[46] Tagami T, Nagata N, Hayashi N, et al.Defined drug release from 3D-printed composite tablets consisting of drug-loaded polyvinylalcohol and a water-soluble or water-insoluble polymer filler[J].Int J Pharm, 2018, 543(1-2): 361-367.

[47] Windolf H, Chamberlain R, Quodbach J. Predicting drug release from 3D printed oral medicines based on the surface area to volume ratio of tablet geometry[J].Pharmaceutics, 2021.13(9): 1453.

[48] Bruschi M L eds.5-Mathematical models of drug release.In: Strategies to modify the drug release from pharmaceutical systems[M].Woodhead Publishing, 2015: 63-86.

[49] Korte C, Quodbach J.3D-printed network structures as controlled-release drug delivery systems: Dose adjustment, api release analysis and prediction[J].AAPS PharmSciTech, 2018, 19(8): 3333-3342.

[50] Sun Y, Soh S.Printing tablets with fully customizable release profiles for personalized medicine[J].Adv Mater, 2015, 27(47): 7847-7853.

[51] Tan Y J N, Yong W P, Kochhar J S, et al.On-demand fully customizable drug tablets via 3D printing technology for personalized medicine[J].J Controlled Release, 2020, 322: 42-52.

[52] Juran J M.Juran on Quality by Design: The new steps for planning quality into goods and services[M].Free Press, Maxwell

Maxmillan Canada, 1992.

[53] Guidance for Industry: Q8(R2)Pharmaceutical Development.U.S. Food and Drug Administration, 2009.

[54] Singh B, Kapil R, Nandi M, et al. Developing oral drug delivery systems using formulation by design: vital precepts, retrospect and prospects[J].Expert Opin Drug Deliv, 2011, 8(10): 1341-1360.

[55] Than Y M, Titapiwatanakun V.Tailoring immediate release FDM 3D printed tablets using a quality by design(QbD) approach[J].Int J Pharm, 2021, 599: 120402.

[56] Than Y M, Titapiwatanakun V.Statistical design of experiment-based formulation development and optimization of 3D printed oral controlled release drug delivery with multi target product profile[J].J Pharm Investig, 2021, 51: 715-734.

第13章

专家系统在药物处方工艺设计中的研究与应用

杜若飞　上海中医药大学，中国；中药现代制剂技术教育部工程研究中心，中国
张　裕　上海中医药大学，中国；中药现代制剂技术教育部工程研究中心，中国

13.1 引言

专家系统（expert system，ES）是一种以专业知识和专家经验为基础和依据，模拟专家思维模式的智能计算机系统。作为人工智能（AI）的重要分支之一，专家系统能够利用现有的知识和经验进行推理、判断和决策，具有良好的启发性。并且专家系统的各功能模块都可以在不影响其他部件运行的同时进行修改，使得用户可以灵活地更新每个部分。此外，它还可以为用户提供更清晰的推理和判断过程，帮助用户更好地理解工作流程，并提高他们对给定结果的信任度。因此可以认为专家系统具有启发性、灵活性、透明度、可解释性等特点[1]。不同于决策支持系统仅能辅助用户进行决策，专家系统可通过自主推理功能给出决策结果，发挥人类专家的作用，并具备人类专家无法做到的收集与分析处理大数据的优势[2]。随着人工智能技术的越发成熟，专家系统、决策支持系统等智能技术在各领域的研究与应用日渐广泛，为解决特定领域内复杂问题提供了新的选择。如以指导药物处方设计为目的的专家系统可有效减少实验次数，降低传统试错实验的时间、耗材成本，提高处方设计的合理性与高效性，同时降低研究对人类经验的依赖程度，提高结果的真实性与准确性[3]。

按照发展阶段，专家系统一般可以分为4类：基于规则的专家系统、基于框架的专家系统、基于案例的专家系统和基于语义网络的专家系统[4]。20世纪60年代，费根鲍姆等成功研发了世界上首个可根据化合物分子式和质谱数据推断分子结构的专家系统DENDRAL[5]，也是最早的基于规则的专家系统。在此基础上，基于规则的专家系统MYCIN[6]与EMYCIN[7]也相继诞生，MYCIN是早期最具代表性的医学诊断专家系统，专家系统的研究热潮由此展开。随着各领域对机器学习研究的不断深入，将两者相结合正成为当下热门趋势，基于模型的专家系统与基于网络的专家系统就是采用了机器学习、深度网络、决策树等算法构建而成。专家系统发展至今，已广泛应用于各个领域。在医药领域，专家系统已逐渐渗透药物研发、制剂生产、临床用药等各个环节。

质量源于设计（QbD）理念最早由FDA提出，并已经成为全球制药领域的行动指南。该原则是一种以预定目标为始，强调对产品、原料、工艺的深刻理解和控制的系统开发方法，有助于提高研发和生产效率并降低时间物料成本。其关键要素包括目标产品质量概况（quality target product profile，QTPP）、关键质量属性（critical quality attributes，CQA）、关键物料属性（critical material attributes，CMA）、关键工艺参数（critical process parameter，CPP）、设计空间（design space）、风险评估（risk assessment）和控制策略（control strategy）等[8]。随着其在药物开发、制剂生产、循环、临床应用等领域的渗透和应用[9]，基于原辅料药性能的药物处方设计逐渐成为高效、优质、低成本生产的关键。专家系统等智能技术的引入可以极大促进QbD理念在研究和生产中的应用，为制药领域，尤其是中药产业的现代化转型提供有力支持[10-12]。因此，用于药物发现、开发和处方设计的专家系统的开发与优化拥有巨大潜力。

本文将简要汇总国内外药学领域专家系统的研究成果，并针对中药制剂专家系统的各组成部分进行介绍，同时结合具体案例详细说明中药制剂专家系统的运作流程，以期为新的制药专家系统的研究与开发提供启发和借鉴。

13.2 专家系统的结构

专家系统通常由数据库、规则库、推理引擎和人机互动界面四个部分构成。数据库和规则库又可统称为知识库。知识库主要用于收集、储存和管理用于解决该领域问题可能需要的相关专家知识、专家经验和根据知识经验总结归纳的规则。知识库与推理引擎分属于独立模块，这使得专家系统具有较高的灵活性与可解释性[13]。其工作流程一般如下：首先由用户在用户界面输入某一专业领域的相关信息，然后通过推理引擎以数据库和规则库为依据，对用户输入的信息进行反复匹配和分析，从而模拟专家的思维方式进行逻辑推理，并通过解释器输出至用户界面（图13-1），为用户提供推荐方案或建议。因此，专家系统的各部分中又以知识库和推理引擎最为核心。下文将对各模块的构建方法和药学相关研究成果进行详尽的归纳总结。

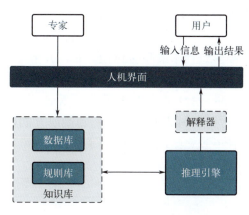

图13-1 专家系统的结构简图

13.2.1 数据库

13.2.1.1 概念与作用

数据库是传统专家系统运行的基础，主要用于储存该专业领域相关信息数据，如药学领域专家系统的数据库往往收集了大量药物的基本性质、作用功能、不良反应等信息。数据库的规模和准确性决定了专家系统运行结果的可信度、准确度、可行性等系统质量[14]。对于化学药物相关的专家系统，数据库具有非必要性，一般通过收集化学反应规则或反应机理作为规则库，即可支持专家系统的推理运作。而对于中药制剂专家系统，数据库仍然发挥了重要作用。尽管原辅料的基本性质和相关信息通常可从国家法定标准或法规、现行版《中国药典》等权威文件中获得，但此类途径信息往往分布零散，无法快速获得并分类归纳。并且由于国内相关研究起步较晚，药物本身又存在成分复杂、理化性质不稳定、质量差异大、质量标准不统一等问题，数据难以收集全面，通用性、系统性的规则和规律总结仍然相对欠缺，无法借鉴化学药品的专家系统模式辅助指导制剂研发过程。因此需要大量实验数据积累，不断扩大具有参考性的数据库容量，并通过数学建模等方式寻找可以指导中药制剂研究的一般性规律，从而建立性能良好的中药制剂专家系统，为提高制剂研发效率提供有效助力。

13.2.1.2 数据库内容

中药制剂中，以颗粒剂、片剂、胶囊剂为代表的口服固体制剂是目前已上市的中成药的主要剂型[15]，同时基于QbD理念[16]和相关文献报道[17,18]，原料药与辅料的流动性等粉体性质对口服固体制剂的制备工艺和成品质量有较大影响，属于CMA。因此，相对完整的数据库内容应囊括中药原料药和药用辅料的理化性质、药辅相容性等信息。曹君杰[19]等建立的iTCM数据库就是由此开发而来，该数据库中除了载有SeDeM专家系统的12个粉体物性参数外，还包括粉体粒径分布、真密度、固相分数、质构参数、近红外光谱[20]和形貌等参数，是目前为止相对全面的中药原辅料数据库。

此外，制剂制备过程中的工艺参数也很大程度上影响着产品质量。因此，制剂关键工艺过程参数的确定和数值量化或将成为未来中药专家系统数据库进一步优化与拓展的研究方向之一。如为了更好地理解流化床制粒过程并控制颗粒的质量，曾佳等[21]展开了中药流化床制粒工艺粒子聚集过程的数值模拟研究，分别测定了黏合剂溶液的密度、比热容、黏度、沸点和表面张力和其在流化床喷雾过程中的喷雾粒径分布，并依此构建了黏合剂溶液特性数据库。同时，制剂的关键质量属性等内容也应纳入数据库，作为判断制剂质量的参考之一。如片剂的硬度、崩解度；颗粒剂的粒径粒形、颗粒得率，等等。

表13-1简要列举了部分常用辅料数据库和中药制剂研究的药辅数据库及其特点，这些数据库都为中药制剂处方设计专家系统的构建提供了养料。

表13-1 药物和药用辅料的常用数据库

类别	数据库	特点
药用辅料	获批药品非活性成分库	提供各种检索方式，包括辅料名称（中英文）、CAS编号、UNII、给药途径、剂型等
	常用辅料数据库[22]	包含常用辅料的基本辅料信息、理化信息和结构信息
	ACDINA[23]	建立了处方药物辅料与药物活性成分之间的连接网络 可以促进发现未知的药用赋形剂-蛋白质的相互作用
	国际药物制剂网	包含几乎所有可用的药物辅料、中间体、药物物质相关信息和处方
中药+辅料	iTCM[19]	包括SeDeM系统的12个参数和粉末粒径分布、真密度、质构参数、近红外光谱等参数
	中药口服固体制剂原辅料近红外光谱（NIR）数据库[20]	扩展了iTCM数据库物性参数类型

13.2.1.3 数据来源

中药数据库的数据来源主要有以下几种方式：①对已公开的药物、辅料理化性质等信息及已有的小型数据库中的信息整合筛选；②对实验数据和经验进行总结分类分析等。上述数据经统计分析处理、数学建模、机器学习模型建立与训练后，可进一步形成规则库中的规则和推理机制。

第一种途径是较为传统的数据库构建方法，往往需要人工收集与数据挖掘、网络爬虫等技术相结合。在2013年，冯怡等[24]就提出可以将原料药理化特性、已上市药物的处方、常用辅料信息以及制剂相关文献数据收集归类后，借助计算机编程将其转化为原料药数据库、处方数据库、辅料数据库和文献数据库，共同构成专家系统数据库。但该方法存在效率较低、容量有限等不足，逐渐被研究者淘汰。

第二种途径是总结分析实验数据以得到数据库，是一种更符合中药制剂研究的一般过程的方式。与化学药品相比，中药原料药的物理化学性质具有更大的不确定性和不稳定性，无法像化学药品一样仅仅通过文献总结或反应规则、特征官能团等得到普遍规律，相关数据主要来源于基于经验的实验积累，而缺乏更加科学、系统的数据整合与规律总结。因此通过收集大量基于科学可靠的表征方法的实验数据来构建中药原辅料数据库，是目前更主流的方式之一。数据收集流程包括选择适宜表征方法和指标参数、验证方法科学性与可行性、建立各类指标参数间的相关性模型，总结普遍性规律，使用编程语言进行转换，作为数据库的一部分。准确的表征结果决定了数据的准确性和专家系统的可靠性，因此应该结合物料种类和剂型特点选择合适的参数和表征方法以获得数据。

中药多以浸膏粉作为中间体制成不同剂型，具有易吸湿、成分复杂等特性，容易导致制剂过程控制困难和产品质量不稳定，因此在中药制剂中，粉体的物性表征尤为重要，表征内容一般包括粒径粒型、流动性、吸湿性等。以粉体流动性为例，常用的表征方法包括：通过霍尔流量计测量、质量流率测量等方法获得颗粒的质量流量；通过静力学休止角、剪切流变力学等方法测量颗粒摩擦等[25]。通常用于评价粉体流动性的指标包括休止角、压缩度、平板角、均齐度、黏聚力等。

由于中药粉体普遍存在较强的吸湿性且极大影响制剂过程与制剂质量，准确地表征吸湿性是优化制剂处方与工艺的前提。常见的表征方法主要基于吸湿量、临界相对湿度、吸湿曲线等评价指标，但大都操作繁琐、测定周期长。基于此，付小菊等[26]采用平衡吸湿量、吸湿初速度、吸湿加速度为特征参数，量化表征物料吸湿性，通过聚类分析等方法筛选出与中药粉体吸湿性相关性大且测定简便的物性，建立了一种基于粉体含水量、粒径、黏性、水溶特性的吸湿性表征方法。宁汝曦等[27]通过拟合吸湿率-时间动态曲线，以平衡吸湿率（F^∞）、半吸湿时间（$t_{1/2}$）描述动态吸湿过程，并将粉体按吸湿行为划分为4类（图13-2），构建了一种更为直观的吸湿性表征方法。赵樱霞等[28]同样采用F^∞和$t_{1/2}$对不同中药提取物干燥粉体的吸湿行为进行表征。

传统专家系统数据库往往需要人工定期整理更新，随着机器学习的兴起，与之相结合的专家系统的数据更新可以实现数据挖掘、自主学习等功能。如使用模糊聚类分析、人工神经网络等技术获取数据等，或利用Python等计算机编程工具以网络爬虫、数据挖掘等方式获取知识数

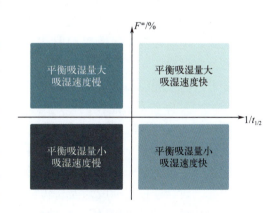

图13-2 物料吸湿性二维表征示意图

据[29]。此外，数据库的构建也离不开管理开发工具的支持，常用的工具有SQL SERVER系列等[30]。

13.2.2 规则库

13.2.2.1 概念与作用

在讨论规则库的概念与作用之前，首先应了解何谓知识表示。在信息学中，所谓知识，就是把有关信息关联在一起所形成的信息结构，客观世界中事物之间的不同关系形成了不同的知识，并具有可表示性和可利用性。知识表示是指将知识以计算机能识别的方式进行表示和储存，可用于解决复杂问题，常用于专家系统的构建，也是专家系统知识库的构建基础。常用的知识表达方法有产生式规则、谓词逻辑、语义网络、框架表示等[31]。

规则库主要用于存放基于专业知识和经验总结归纳而成的相关规则，用于指导专家系统的逻辑推理过程，可与数据库共同构成知识库，也是推理机制和推理引擎运行的基础。

13.2.2.2 类型

每个专家系统的规则库内容取决于该系统应用的专业领域，与数据库相比，更加重视各因素间的逻辑关系，且不同专家系统的规则库专一性的特点更显著。规则库根据规则内容的来源和类型主要可以大致分为三类：产生式规则、数学建模和AI建模。

（1）产生式规则

产生式规则是常见的知识表示形式之一，也是产生式系统的主体，产生式系统又是专家系统的运行基础之一。产生式系统由多个产生式规则组成，一个产生式生成的结论可作为已知事实供另一个产生式使用。其产生主要是将已有知识库或数据库中的信息进行整合后得到普遍规律，或人工归纳实验数据与经验后总结得到特定领域内的规律与规则，通常使用二叉树数据结构，即"IF-THEN"形式进行表示。

应用于制剂处方开发或药物发现的专家系统，其规则库内容一般包括药物相互作用规则、药物配伍规则、原辅料相容性等规则。以PharmDE等专家系统为例，其规则库总结收集了以往研究报道中一般储存条件下的药物-赋形剂不相容机制、药物间相互作用和药物研发经验，包括60条药物相互作用规则、17种相互作用类型和22种化学反应特征结构。

但此类规则库主要依赖于人工输入，无法自主学习并更新知识，规则库规模也相对较小，且运行效率较低，虽然在临床诊断方面表现良好[32]，但在制剂研发等领域的应用中无显著优势，逐渐被数学建模和AI技术代替。

（2）数学建模

随着医药产业现代化进程的加快，数学建模等技术在药物开发与制造等研究中得到了广泛应用，并发挥着不可忽视的作用[33]，根据需要解决的问题构建数学模型，并通过模型的相关数据归纳总结相应的规则，也是常见的规则库构建方法之一。尤其在尚未形成规模性数据库、规则库的中药制剂领域，数学建模可基于物料属性和工艺参数预测产品的质量属性，形成更符合中药制剂开发的规则库，对于完善专家系统的推理基础具有重要意义。

因此，数学建模逐渐成为提高药物研发效率、指导制剂生产和控制产品质量的主要工具之一。如曾佳等[21]针对流化床制粒过程的雾化压力、进风温度等工艺参数，建立了相应的数学预测模型。这些模型可与决策树等方法相结合，对黏合剂浓度等物料属性分别进行分类，并得到相应的雾化压力、进风温度等制粒工艺参数的选择或计算规则，当用户输入物料参数时，系统可利用建立的数学模型计算得到其他关键参数的预测值，并根据规则推理分析，给出最佳制粒处方和工艺参数。

（3）AI建模

随着机器学习、深度学习、ANN等技术的研究与发展，与之相结合的数据库、规则库构建方法的应用日渐广泛，AI也逐渐成为构建规则库的重要工具之一。在药物发现或计算机辅助药物设计过程中，机器学习等AI技术的应用大大提高了药物开发效率，在药物研发中具有广阔应用前景[34]。Yang等[35]提到的AI算法过程包括定义问题、数据收集、AI建模、模型训练与评估等，其中模型构建是最为重要的部分，由于其所用的方法与专家系统规则库的构建方法有较多重叠，对规则库的构建具有一定借鉴和参考意义。构建模型后还需要收集与目标问题相关的专业知识与数据，并对其进行模型训练和评估以减小系统运行误差，规则库中的规则可通过对数据集训练归纳获得[36]，数据集可沿用已构建的数据库，也可重新收集获得。

设计并建立一个合适的模型体系首先需要选择合适的算法，如SVM、RF、ANN等，此类算法在已报道的规则库中也有所应用。深度学习技术是基于神经网络发展而来的新体系结构，常见架构有循环神经网络（RNN）、卷积神经网络（CNN）、生成深度神经网络（DNN）等[37]，由于其具有可分析处理大量数据并能实现自主学习的优势，在专家系统的构建中受到越来越多研究者的青睐。2019年，Han等[38]运用深度学习、随机森林等机器学习算法建立了固体分散体物理稳定性的预测模型。

13.2.3 推理引擎

13.2.3.1 概念与作用

推理引擎又称推理机，是模拟专家思维给出方案的核心部分，可根据用户输入的信息进行推理，从而给出解决问题的方案或预测结果，推理机指挥并控制着整个推理的过程和方向，也直接影响着专家系统进行辅助决策的能力。推理机的关键在于基于数据库与规则库的推理机制。在经过推理机处理得到结论后，建立解释机可以为用户提供该结论的简单易懂的解释说明，让用户更清晰直观地理解专家系统的推理过程。

13.2.3.2 推理机制

推理机制是利用已获取的知识获得新的知识、得到新的结论并解决提出问题所使用的推理方法和控制策略，即专家系统得到最终结论所依据的规则与逻辑。专家系统中的推理机制通常是基于演绎推理的正向推理[39]，其结论具有一定不确定性和不准确性。专家系统的推理流程大致如下：将用户输入的内容与数据库和规则库进行匹配，选择适宜规则进行推理，并得到最终结论。常见的推理方法包括逻辑推理、定性推理、本体推理、概率推理、机器推理。

综上所述，推理机制可以分为基于规则的推理机制、基于案例的推理机制、基于模糊逻辑的推理机制和基于机器学习的推理机制，下文将分别进行介绍。

（1）基于规则的推理机制

基于规则的推理机制是指以产生式规则或大量具体规则为主体进行演绎推理的过程，此过程通常运用产生式结构[40]的逻辑推理，因此也称产生式系统的专家系统。产生式系统推理机由匹配、选择（冲突解决）、执行3个阶段组成。根据需求的不同，专家系统应用的推理方式也不同，可分为正向推理、反向推理和双向推理3种形式[41]。该过程通常需要使用决策树等分类分析方法对数据库和规则库中的知识进行处理分析，得到逻辑规则，如"IF……THEN……"等规则。基于规则的推理具有简单迅速的特点，但当几条依靠同一事实的规则同时被触发时，无法进行有效地筛选，因此往往会与其他几种推理机制联合运用。基于规则的推理机制通常用于以产生式规则或数学建模等内容为规则库的专家系统，在药学和临床诊断用的医学专家系统中均有所应用。脂质体专家系统[42]中建立的推理机就采用了基于规则的推理机制，可根据不同条件选择性地调用某个数据库中的内容，得到更为准确的推荐结果。

（2）基于案例的推理机制

基于案例的推理机制是一种以具体案例组成的案例库作为核心主体，对案例进行分析和关联后得到相应的一系列规则，并以此为依据进行类比推理，为用户提供解决方案的方法[43]。其核心思想是通过重用或修改以前解决相似问题的方法来解决新的问题[44-46]。

以此机制构建的专家系统应具有分析现有案例与先前案例的相似性或差异性的能力，该机制的推理准确性取决于案例库的规模以及专家的经验知识，因此对案例数量和质量要求较高。该机制适用于明确的理论模型难以建立、领域规则难以形式化等较为复杂的情况[47]，较多应用于医学临床诊断、法学、环境等领域，在药学领域中应用较少[48]。其中以薛启隆等[49]的研究较为典型。该研究结合深度学习、案例推理、仿真建模等技术，以中药带式干燥工艺为研究对象初步构建了中药制药工艺知识库，并基于案例推理构建了较为完整的工艺优选过程。

在案例收集的基础上，结合深度学习、ANN等机器学习方法，可进一步对大量具体案例分析处理，得到更加庞大、可靠的案例库与规则库。或通过案例检索、案例重用、案例修改、案例调整过程，为难以得到完备规则的问题提供解决方案[50]，为药物发现与开发提供便利。

（3）基于模糊逻辑的推理机制

基于模糊逻辑的推理机制是指使用模糊理论或模糊逻辑将语言变量转换为数学变量后进行分析推理的方法[51, 52]。模糊理论将事物的属性以集合的形式构成各个模糊集，对集合内的元素赋予隶属度，通过模糊集和隶属度函数之间的集合运算得出目标集合中各个元素的模糊值，该值在一定程度上反映了各元素出现的概率。这种机制适用于信息不确定或不完整的情况，以及难以确定数据间相关性的情况[53]，因此在临床诊断方面的应用较为常见，而在药学领域较为少见。

（4）基于机器学习的推理机制

基于机器学习的推理机制是指利用ANN、深度学习等技术自主学习、获得知识，然后通过分析处理和训练数据集，得到一个预测结果或可能的解决方法的机制。此类推理机制的核心在于数据准备和模型的建立与训练。知识学习的结果，即模型的准确性，取决于知识库中知识或数据的数量和质量。其在药物开发与制剂研究专家系统中的应用也日渐广泛，涉及的技术与算法同规则库的构建相似，也可与规则库中的规则或模型相结合，共同完成推理机的运行。曹韩韩[54]在干法制粒处方工艺专家系统推理机的构建中主要运用了人工神经网络中的BP神经网络算法（图13-3），以五倍子浸膏粉和金钱草浸膏粉为原料，将中药浸膏粉与常用的微晶纤维素按照不同比例混合，通过测量混合粉体的松密度，建立了混合粉体松密度的预测模型。该技术可以任意精度逼近任意的连续函数，广泛应用于非线性建模。

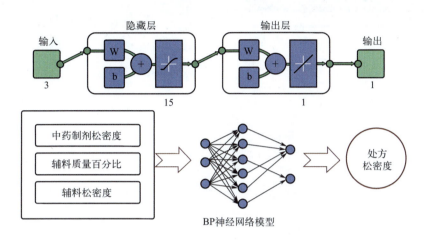

图13-3　松密度BP神经网络预测模型的网络结构[54]

上述推理机制各有优劣，仅使用单一机制可能无法得到准确结果，选择多种推理机制联合运用可有效提高推理机的运行准确性，因此在设计开发专家系统时应根据需要解决的问题选择适宜机制。对于药物发现、开发和制剂研究而言，基于规则的推理机制和基于机器学习的推理机制是更高效、更具可行性的选择之一。

13.2.4　用户界面

用户界面是用户与计算机进行信息传递、交换的媒介和接口，也称"人机界面"。简洁而便于操作的用户界面可以更高效地帮助用户解决问题，对专家系统运行过程的可视化、可操作和可控制有着重要意义。专家系统的人机界面通常包括Windows软件界面、线上网页界面和移动应用程序等形式，其设计与实现主要取决于不同编程语言等开发工具。按照构建载体的不同，用户界面主要可以分为两类：利用编程软件构建以用户为中心、以Windows窗口为载体的操作界面；利用Web开发工具构建以浏览器或应用程序为载体的用户界面。

随着互联网的发展与普及，基于Web的人机界面也成为主要形式之一。中药指纹图谱方法推荐系统中，在浏览器/服务器架构的帮助下，建立了一个基于Web的用户界面[55]。此类界面依托于浏览器或移动端，不受计算机限制，具有更高的操作灵活性和便捷性，对用户更加友好。

明良山等[56]构建的专家系统的人机界面（图13-4）主要依托于应用程序，不依赖于网络即可运行，用户登录后可根据需要选择不同模式，系统界面包括流化床模式选择、制粒方式确定、系统推荐处方与工艺、系统推荐干燥时间等模块，各模块又分别包括输入界面和输出界面。根据用户输入的物料信息，各模块将分别调用系统数据库与规则库中相应内容，为用户提供合理的推荐方案，并给予清晰的推理过程及解释。

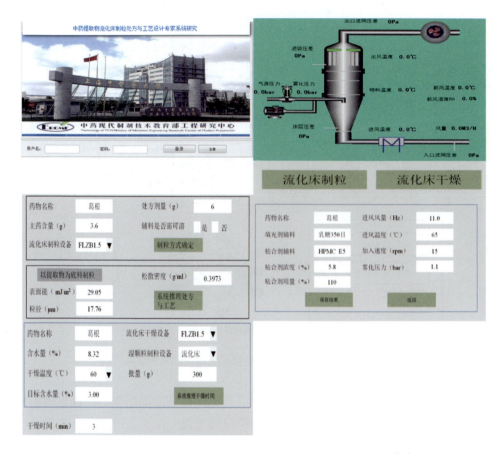

图13-4　流化床制粒处方与工艺设计专家系统的用户界面[56]

近年来,数字孪生技术的相关研究势头正盛,该技术是一种通过计算机进行高精度、多维度、全方面的动态仿真,将处于物理世界的实体按照一定映射规则在虚拟世界中建立模型,并实现物理世界和虚拟世界之间的实时交互通信、虚实互控、自我迭代优化更新[57-59]。其结构包括物理实体、虚拟实体和连接两者的数据接口。与以预测为主要目的的数值模拟、仿真建模等技术相比,数字孪生所建立的模型具有动态实时性的特点,可以跟随实体实时演化,适用于解决传统静态模型难以解决的问题。基于以上特点,该技术在工业生产等领域的应用日益广泛,将其与专家系统结合应用在制剂生产中,从而实现生产过程的可视化和实时可控制,或将为中药制剂生产过程的控制与优化提供新的思路。

13.3　应用

PubMed是世界上最权威的文摘类医学文献数据库之一,MEDLINE数据库提供生物医学和健康科学领域的文献搜索服务工具,以"Expert system/Pharmaceutics expert system/Medical expert system"为关键词进行检索,PubMed中近10年所报道的专家系统的相关研究文献数量见图13-5。相关文献数量在2021年前后到达峰值,而在2022年后略有下降。在中国知网数据库中,以"Expert system"为关键词的检索结果中,学科分布占比最多的主要为自动化、计算机、电力工业等领域(图13-6),与医药领域相关的前10类学科分布如图13-7所示,主要集中于医学、生物学、计算机等领域,药学领域的专家系统研究仅占所有研究的很小一部分,仍然有较大的发展空间。

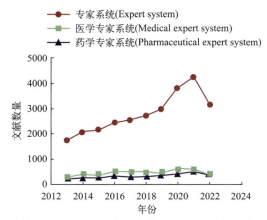

图13-5　以不同关键词检索PubMed中专家系统相关文献数量的近10年走势

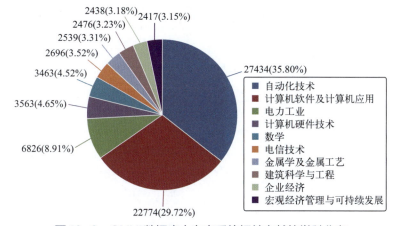

图13-6　CNKI数据库中专家系统相关文献的学科分布

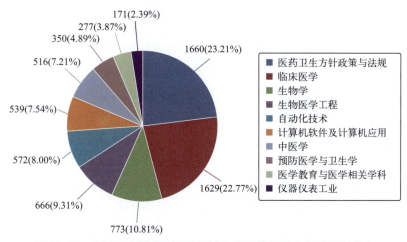

图13-7　CNKI数据库中医学领域专家系统相关文献的学科分布

表13-2展示了较为典型的国内外药学领域专家系统的研究与应用。专家系统在制剂研究中的应用相对较少，且专属性明显，不同剂型间不具有通用性。Pilar Pérez等[60]开发的图谱专家系统SeDeM是一个特例，尽管不具有专家系统的基本构成，但具有良好的实用性和更广的应用范围，在化学药物和中药领域都有所应用，尤其适用于片剂、胶囊剂等粉末相关固体制剂研发[61]。

表13-2 国内外制剂领域专家系统研究的部分汇总

研究机构	剂型	解决问题	知识表达方法	开发工具	时间	文献
德国海德堡大学	气雾剂、片剂、胶囊剂	生产方法、包装、产品的预测性能	策略、公式和规则	C/Small talk	1990	[62] [63]
印度Cadila实验室	片剂	辅料与药物的最佳相容性配比	物理、化学和生物学相关描述	Prolog	1992	—
伦敦大学	胶囊剂	预测新药和辅料混合物的性质，推荐粉末加工方式	问卷、决策树和生产规则	C	1996	—
巴塞罗那大学	片剂	直压片剂预处方开发	线性组合	无	2005	—
波兰雅盖隆大学	微乳，固体分散体	模型在计算机中实现的问题	分子描述符	Java	2006	[64]
巴塞罗那大学	片剂等与粉末相关制剂	研究物料粉体性质	SeDeM图	—	2006	[60]
苏州大学	脂质体	辅料选择与制备技术	归纳、产生式规则	C+	2007	[42]
沈阳药科大学	渗透泵片	双层渗透泵片处方设计	归纳前期经验	VB	2009	—
泰国清迈大学	片剂	片剂处方和生产设计的框架	描述性语言	无	2011	—
上海中医药大学	中药硬胶囊	处方与工艺设计	规则和数学模型	Matlab	2014	—
上海中医药大学	颗粒剂（干法制粒）	处方与工艺设计	规则和数学模型	Matlab	2015	—
上海中医药大学	粉末为原料的制剂	粉体可压性评价和缺陷校正	经验/统计函数关系	Matlab/C++	2017	—
上海中医药大学	颗粒剂（流化床制粒）	处方与工艺筛选优化	规则和数学模型	Matlab	2018	—
上海中医药大学	固体分散剂	处方设计	分子描述符	Python	2019	—
上海中医药大学	颗粒剂（流化床制粒）	微观层面预测或判断处方工艺的适宜性	计算机数值模拟技术	ANSYS等	2020	[21]
上海中医药大学	中药粉末直压片剂	处方设计	规则和数学模型	Java	2021	—
上海中医药大学	颗粒剂（湿法制粒）	处方与工艺设计	规则和数学模型	Java	2022	—

13.3.1 SeDeM 专家系统

SeDeM 是一种基于 QbD 理念的简便高效的处方预筛选工具，主要用于评估药物与辅料的直接压片性能。研究表明，原辅料的粒径、流动性等粉体性质很大程度上影响了直接压片过程[65, 66]。该系统通过对药物及辅料的粉体性质进行评估和赋值[61]，将原辅料 CMA 与制剂的 CQA 建立联系，进而辅助片剂、胶囊剂等制剂的开发和优化处方设计，为固体制剂的处方研究提供了较为系统化标准化的物料数据收集方法[67]。基于过往研究，SeDeM 选取了多个代表性物性参数作为评价指标，包括振实密度（D_c）、堆密度（D_a）、卡尔指数（CI）、豪斯纳比（IH）、休止角（α）、粒径与粒度分布（%Pf）等 12 个参数，从粉体密度、流动性、可压性等多个维度进行评价，并以雷达图的形式呈现（图 13-8）。根据剂型的不同，研究者还可以在上述参数的基础上添加和优化，以得到更加准确的结果[68]。表 13-3 汇总了近年来 SeDeM 用于药物处方设计研究的相关应用。

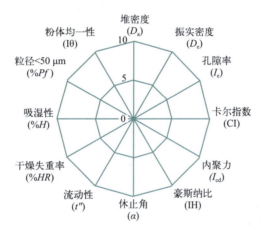

图 13-8　SeDeM 专家系统的参数图谱

表 13-3　近年来 SeDeM 在药物处方设计中的应用

时间	药物	辅料	研究目的	文献
2017	无水茶碱	新型聚合物 PU（二硫代二乙醇 DTDI）（PU4）、PU[(^{i}Pr) Man-DTDI]（由分子质量分别为 40000 Da（PU5）和 90000Da（PU5′）的分子合成	开发两种新型生物可降解聚氨酯作为制备稳定基质的辅料，并研究其在直接压片中的适用性	[69]
2017	瑞舒伐他汀钙	乳糖-预胶化玉米淀粉喷雾干燥混合物 预胶化玉米淀粉 交联聚维酮	应用 SeDeM 表征辅料物性特征，并基于此开发优化瑞舒伐他汀钙口服分散片的处方	[70]
2018	葡糖盐胺 F0357	微晶纤维素（Avicel®PH101） β-环糊精（Kleptose®，ROQUETTE） 共聚维酮（Kollidon®VA64）等	利用 SeDeM 研究 6 种稀释剂用于直接压片的适用性； 获得计算直接压片所需填充剂用量的数学方程	[3]
2018	氯沙坦	微晶纤维素（Avicel PH 101） 乳糖 玉米淀粉等	利用 SeDeM 辅助药物研发，考察原料药和辅料用于直接压片的适用性，并制备适宜直接压片的混合物	[71]

续表

时间	药物	辅料	研究目的	文献
2018	二盐酸西替利嗪	硬脂酸镁 二氧化硅 甘露醇等	研究 SeDeM 在表征活性物质物理特性中的作用，并基于此进行二盐酸西替利嗪的口服冻干剂的处方开发	[72]
2019	双氯芬酸钾	埃洛石纳米管 淀粉 1500 微粉硅胶 200 等	利用 SeDeM 研究埃洛石纳米管作为直接压片的多功能赋形剂的适用性	[73]
2019	溶菌酶冻干	高分散性二氧化硅 硬脂酸镁	研究 SeDeM 在直接压片的药用口香糖片处方开发中的应用与优化	[74]
2019	三七皂苷提取物	HPMC K4M HPMC K15M 乳糖等	采用 SeDeM 方法对原辅料的物理性能进行表征，阐明原辅料的理化性质变化对三七皂苷基质片的体外溶出图谱的影响，由此建立一种可以优选能够达到目标体外溶出曲线的最佳赋形剂及用量的指导模型	[75]
2019	利巴韦林	微晶纤维素 硬脂酸镁 结晶乳糖（Tablettose-80）等	应用 SeDeM-ODT 专家系统优化压片过程的工艺参数，并制备具有更好流动性、可压缩性和崩解行为的颗粒	[76]
2019	齐多夫定	乳糖 甘露醇 微粉硅胶等	利用 SeDeM 表征齐夫多定与辅料的理化性质，基于此开发优化其直接压片的适宜处方	[77]
2019	红景天提取物	微晶纤维素 乳糖 淀粉等	利用 SeDeM 表征红景天提取物及其与辅料的混合物的物性特征，并预测原料药与药辅混合物的直接压片性能	[78]
2020	托卡朋	微晶纤维素（Vivapur® 102/Avicel® PH 101） 麦芽糊精（Kleptose®） 聚维酮（Kollidon® VA 64）等	利用 SeDeM 筛选直接压缩制备的托卡酮缓释片的最优处方，并研究托卡朋粒径对缓释片缓释作用的影响	[79]
2021	—	玉米淀粉（CDH Chemicals） 微晶纤维素（Avicel® PH101）	研究 SeDeM 专家系统在以玉米淀粉（致密性差）和微晶纤维素（高可压缩性）粉末为模型辅料开发一种新型共加工辅料方面的适用性	[80]
2021	—	HPMC （K4M/K15M/K100M）	利用 SeDeM 表征来自不同制造商、不同黏度等级 HPMC 的不同材料属性	[81]
2021	偏硅酸铝镁 Neusilin® US2（50NEU）	聚乙二醇 400 微晶纤维素（Avicel® PH102） 单水乳糖	通过增加两个重要的压缩特性：平均屈服压力 P_y 和可压性参数 σt_{max} 以改进 SeDeM 专家系统，并优选最适宜的偏硅酸铝镁直接压片的稀释剂处方	[82]
2021	香茅油	二氧化硅 200/300/30 高吸油性二氧化硅 Sipernat 22S 微粉硅胶 244 FP 等	以挥发油释放率代替 SeDeM 中的干燥失重指数，以吸附率代替内聚力指数，优化 SeDeM 利用 SeDeM-SLA 优选适宜的香茅油载体，探究香茅油的吸附机制，提供一种新的液体成分固体化的评价手段	[83]
2021	姜黄提取物粉末	微晶纤维素 PH101 微粉硅胶 N20 交联聚维酮	使用纳米二氧化硅对姜黄提取物粉末的粉体质地和表面性能进行改性，利用 SeDeM 辅助评价改性后的提取物粉末的直接压片的性能	[84]

续表

时间	药物	辅料	研究目的	文献
2021	阿替洛尔	微晶纤维素 硬脂酸镁 羧甲基淀粉钠	根据 SeDeM-ODT 专家系统表征颗粒特性，优化高剪切湿法造粒工艺，并对片剂特性进行预测	[85]
2021	大麻二酚	乳糖 微晶纤维素 山梨醇等	利用 SeDeM 优选合适的直接压片辅料制备含大麻二酚的口腔分散片	[86]
2021	盐酸二甲双胍（结晶，90.0% 直接压缩）	滑石粉 微粉硅胶 硬脂酸镁	利用粉末 X 射线衍射法、SeDeM、Heckel 方程、Ryshkewitch-Duckworth 方程评价和比较盐酸二甲双胍结晶和直接压片用盐酸二甲双胍粉末的压片性能	[87]
2021	布洛芬	微晶纤维素（Avicel PH101） 交联聚维酮（Kollidon CL-SF） 微粉硅胶等	考察 SeDeM 专家系统在湿法挤出制粒过程中的适用性，并对软材和制得颗粒进行表征评价	[88]
2021	对乙酰氨基酚	水稻淀粉	利用 SeDeM 专家系统获得辅料和原料药的粉末特性，确定对乙酰氨基酚直接压片所需的赋形剂用量的计算规则	[89]
2021	千屈菜干燥提取物	—	利用 SeDeM 专家系统探究原料药物理性质与药材有效成分的相关性，并基于 SeDeM 及其他表征结果促进植物药的标准化	[90]
2022	瑞舒伐他汀钙	单水乳糖 微晶纤维素 磷酸氢钙等	利用 SeDeM 优化更合适的无定形型瑞舒伐他汀钙片的辅料和处方，以达到理想的生物利用度	[91]
2022	布洛芬/咖啡因	聚合物氧化物 乙基纤维素 甲基丙烯酸-丙烯酸乙酯共聚物	采用选择性激光烧结法制备不同尺寸的多颗粒单元，并应用 SeDeM 专家系统对制得的多颗粒单元进行表征评价	[92]
2022	格列美脲	交联羧甲基纤维素钠 微晶纤维素 聚乙二醇等	利用 SeDeM-ODT 专家系统优化稀释剂特性（流动性、可压缩性和崩解行为），改善药物的直接压片性能	[93]
2022	盐酸曲马朵	微晶纤维素（Avicel ™ PH-101） 硬脂酸镁 二氧化硅（Aerosil ™ 200）	利用 SeDeM 专家系统开发控释盐酸曲马朵渗透片的直接压片处方并优化； 建立一种基于计算机的 PBPK 模型用以评价体内药动学	[94]
2022	奈韦拉平	交联聚维酮 交联羧甲基纤维素钠 羧甲基淀粉钠	利用固体分散体增强 BCS Ⅱ类药物奈韦拉平的溶解度； 利用 SeDeM 表征辅料和固体分散体的物性特征，优选直接压片的最佳处方并制备口服分散片	[95]

尽管 SeDeM 在片剂等口服固体制剂的研究中有较多应用，但由于其不具有专家系统的基本结构，与一般意义上的专家系统存在较大差异，对于制剂专家系统的研究与设计的参考意义有限，因此下文将选择具有代表性的典型专家系统，就其在中药研究各阶段中的应用及其构建与组成进行详细介绍。

13.3.2 中药质量控制专家系统

13.3.2.1 中药原料药质量控制

中药最终产品的质量很大程度上取决于中药原料药以及辅料的质量，而中药材与前处理中间体的质量又是保证中药原料药质量的前提。利用基于红外光谱、X射线衍射技术的专家系统等技术可极大地提高中药材的分析鉴定效率，促进原料药的质量一致性和标准化，加速中药现代化进程。由于不同中药的成分各不相同，其实验方法与条件也有所区别，相应的指纹图谱也具有一定特异性，因此可通过指纹图谱对中药材进行鉴定。

基于此，孙国祥等[30, 96]先后构建了用于鉴别中药真伪优劣的X射线衍射指纹图谱专家系统（TCM-XFP-ESG）和中药红外光谱指纹图谱专家系统（TCM-IRFP-ESG），为用户提供推荐的实验方法与评价结果。以TCM-XFP-ESG为例，研究者利用VB. NET 2.0和SQL Server 2003软件开发专家系统，包括查询系统、推荐系统、优化系统等模块。数据库中包括甘草等40味临床常用中药的X射线衍射法信息，然后基于产生式规则构建规则库，包括了X射线衍射法的原理、中药指纹图谱技术和中药提取方法等内容。此外，王海慧等[97]采用了典型的产生式规则来构建中药指纹图谱专家系统。上述研究都一定程度上促进了专家系统在中药原药材质量控制中的应用，为提高中药产品质量提供了前期保障。

13.3.2.2 处方设计

基于QbD理念的中药药物设计、中药剂型设计等中药产品设计，以及药辅合一理论指导下的中药制剂处方设计、中药制药工艺路线设计等中药工艺设计，在保障中药产品的有效性、安全性和质量可控性等方面有着重要意义。下文将分别选择针对不同剂型的处方设计专家系统，对其构建与运行流程简要说明。

（1）片剂

中药粉体由于特有的易吸湿、黏度大等特点，大多无法用于直接压片，但直接压片在制剂生产中可有效提高生产效率、提高制剂质量一致性，因此关于中药粉体直接压片的相关研究的需求较为迫切。但已有研究大多独立进行，尚无汇总性的研究成果，尤其是专家系统方面的研究相对缺乏，无法为中药直接压片提供较为系统、全面的参考和指导。

基于此，中药现代制剂技术教育部工程研究中心的研究人员基于原辅料物理性质和压片功能属性设计开发了中药粉末直接压片的处方工艺设计和片剂质量调控的专家系统，并在研究考察粉体流动性、压缩性、成型性等压片功能属性的同时，探究了中药粉末直接压片的压缩成型机制，并利用聚类分析将其分类为Ⅰ～Ⅴ类。其中，辅料筛选规则主要包括填充剂、崩解剂、润滑剂、助流剂对中药粉体及片剂质量的调控规律。以填充剂为例，研究者[98]考察了Ⅱ～Ⅳ类粉体不同处方比例进行压片的压缩过程参数和抗张强度、崩解时限等片剂质量属性，然后采用线性模型、二次多项式模型等进行拟合，得到适合不同粉体类型的预测模型和实验设计空间，并针对不同粉体类型推荐基础处方，进而构建了适用于粉末直接压片工艺的中药片剂品质调控专家系统。

不同类型粉体的拟合模型差异显著，具体模型如下所示：Ⅱ类粉体中，$DT = 133.09A + 62.06B + 110.27C + 85.60D - 335.36AB - 257.39AC - 190.54AD - 131.77BD - 108.67CD$；$TS =$

13.12A + 6.14B + 4.26C + 6.58D − 36.29AB − 43.85AC。而在Ⅳ类粉体中，TS = 8.66A + 6.96B + 6.37C + 6.94D − 39.46AC − 37.18AD − 47.29BCE − 44.58BD − 44.63CD；DT = 69.26A + 38.62B + 62.78C + 45.54D − 104.43AC；TW = 2.41A + 4.87B + 11.43C + 24.67D-127.09BD-176.45CD；Sqrt（Fri）= 2.04A + 4.51B + 6.89C + 7.46D。其中，TS 为抗张强度，DT 为崩解时限，A、B、C、D 分别为不同填充剂。

（2）颗粒剂

① 高剪切湿法制粒专家系统　颗粒是颗粒剂、片剂、胶囊剂等常见中药固体剂型的中间体，制得颗粒的质量很大程度上决定着最终制剂的质量，而高剪切制粒是常见的湿法制粒方法之一，具有高载药量、高效率、低能耗等优点，且在连续化生产上也有较大潜力，是中药制剂生产的重要工序，但在制粒过程中，往往存在粘壁、重复性差等问题，且由于中药成分复杂、种类多样，影响颗粒成型和颗粒质量的因素众多，尚未形成较为系统、高效的质量调控策略。因此，为了更深刻地了解中药提取物高剪切湿法制粒过程，并优化制粒处方、控制颗粒质量，刘斌斌等[99]探究了原辅料的CQA与高剪切制粒中的CPP间的相关性，并基于此建立了中药提取物高剪切湿法制粒处方工艺设计专家系统。

首先，对具有一定代表性的35种中药提取物粉体和13类辅料的含水量、真密度等基础物性参数进行表征，构建中药原辅料物性数据库。此外，由于软材对于颗粒质量也发挥了重要作用，适宜的软材评价指标也有必要纳入数据库，基于文献报道，选择物料黏性与浸润性作为评价指标。利用混合扭矩流变仪（mixer torque rheometer，MTR）模拟高剪切湿法制粒过程，以最大扭矩力（TRQ_{max}）和相应液固比（L/S）作为CMA，分别表征物料黏性和浸润性，在此基础上建立了中药提取物粉体物理药剂学分类系统（physicalpharmaceutics classification system，PCS），将数据库中的物料分为4类（图13-9），构建了一个相对系统的中药原辅料数据库。

基于TRQ_{max}与L/S数据和PCS，建立相应的辅料筛选原则：Ⅰ类中药提取物应选择Ⅲ类辅料；Ⅱ类中药选择Ⅳ类辅料；Ⅲ类中药选择Ⅳ类辅料；Ⅳ类中药选择Ⅲ类辅料。基于中药原辅料的显著色差，采用数字图像处理技术中的灰度值法表征物料的混合状态，并以原辅料的真密度、卡尔指数等11个参数为自变量，以混合均匀度的相对理论值偏差为因变量，采用偏最小二乘法、随机森林算法建立相关性预测模型，探究了影响物料混合均匀度的主要因素。

然后，分别考察PCS分类中Ⅱ～Ⅳ类中药的载药量、L/S、黏合剂添加速度、搅拌速度、剪切速度等处方工艺参数对颗粒得率、团块率、粒径、真密度等CQA的影响，进而建立了针对中黏性和高黏性中药提取物的高剪切制粒关键质量属性的处方设计与优化模型，包括颗粒得率模型、颗粒粒径大小模型、颗粒堆密度模型、颗粒卡尔指数模型等处方设计模型（表13-4）。上述模型与原辅料筛选原则共同构成了该专家系统的规则库。

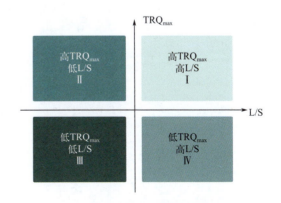

图13-9　中药提取物粉体物理药剂学分类系统（PCS）（高TRR_{max}：TRQ_{max} > 0.930 N·m；高L/S：L/S > 0.060 mL·g^{-1}）[99]

表13-4 PCS Ⅱ~Ⅳ类中药的颗粒关键质量属性模型（a：主药含量；b：乙醇浓度；c：L/S）[99]

药物类型	颗粒得率模型	颗粒粒径大小模型	颗粒堆密度模型	颗粒卡尔指数模型	颗粒真密度模型	颗粒硬度模型
PCS Ⅱ	$GY=-591.05+43.67a-16.50b+1934.50c+0.32ab-108.81ac+26.27bc-0.26a^2$	$D_{50}=2269.47-208.11a+116.42b-9716.51c-1.98ab+842.33ac-241.33bc$	$\rho_b=0.0365-4.8197\times10^{-3}b+1.7702c$	$CI=+51.30-0.41a+0.25b-82.27c$	$\rho_{真实}=1.2991+4.4425\times10^{-3}a-2.0774\times10^{-4}b+1.0831c+4.2537\times10^{-3}bc-1.0100\times10^{-4}a^2-3.1750\times10^{-5}b^2-1.6039c^2$	$Hd=-20892.42+357.76a+42.80b+81940.03c-6.10a^2-1.60b^2-96930.25c^2$
PCS Ⅲ	$GY=159.54+8.18a+1.18b+269.76c-0.09ab$	$D_{50}=5278.44+96.21a-174.68b+2506.20c-1.85ab+1.19a^2+1.39b^2$	$\rho_b=3.2295+0.0198a-0.0245b-13.0435c-2.4750\times10^{-4}ab-0.0777bc+3.0623\times10^{-4}b^2+31.7935c^2$	$CI=-48.79-1.22a-0.89b+782.55c+0.01ab+3.63bc-1823.71c^2$	$\rho_{真实}=-0.7953-1.3025\times10^{-3}a+8.9671\times10^{-3}b+2.3659c-0.0298bc$	$Hd=2198.36+28.01a-28.64b$
PCS Ⅳ	$GY=-119.12+10.12b-1993.13c+24.16bc-0.09b^2$	$D_{50}=141.98+126.73a-1.04b+3285.37c-1.54ab$	$\rho_b=2.6660+0.0130a-0.0547b-1.1224c-0.0003ab+0.0561ac+0.0004b^2$	$CI=-13.54+0.78a+0.30b+63.88c-4.66ac$	$\rho_{真实}=2.8935-0.0160a-0.0341b+0.0001ab+0.0001a^2+0.0002b^2$	$Hd=-4536.81+162.42a-18867.46c+228.70bc-1.25b^2$

推理机作为数据库与规则库的串联主体，是主导专家系统运行的关键构成。与上述片剂专家系统类似，研究者采用决策树算法构建了运行框架，并且考虑到规则的交互与重复匹配等问题，设定了推理顺序的优先级。系统推理逻辑主要包括原辅料分类与筛选、物料混合均匀度预测和最佳处方工艺设计三部分。系统可根据用户输入信息和储存的预测模型得到推荐的辅料用量、乙醇浓度、L/S等处方工艺参数。同时，针对制粒过程中可能出现的意外情况，采用正向演绎推理法建立了原因分析模块与解决方案模块。

综上，一个具有一定可行性的基于规则的中药高剪切制粒处方与工艺设计专家系统被成功开发，为中药制粒提供了较为实用的辅助工具。

② 流化床制粒专家系统　流化床制粒是目前常见的制粒方法之一，广泛应用于中药固体制剂生产，集混合、润湿、制粒和干燥于一体，传热性能好、混合能力强，但同时也存在所制颗粒粒度不均、粒径控制困难等局限，探究流化床制粒过程中影响颗粒质量的关键因素，进而优化制粒过程、控制颗粒质量，是提高流化床制粒生产效率与质量的重要途径之一。基于此，明良山等[56]以原辅料物性表征结果建立数据库，对流化床制粒过程中关键因素建立数学模型构成规则库，开发了中药流化床制粒处方与工艺设计专家系统，为该过程的控制和优化提供了新方法，促进了中药流化床制粒的进一步发展与应用。数据库中主要收集了中药提取物粉末与辅料的接触角、表面能，混合粉体的含水量、流动性等物理性质，以及黏合剂的溶液黏性、表面张力等溶液性质（表13-5）。

表13-5　流化床制粒专家系统数据库内容与表征方法

数据库内容	属性参数	表征方法
原料药与辅料表面能	接触角	探测液体：水／二碘甲烷 测定方法：静滴法（视频接触角测量仪）
	表面能	基于接触角结合 Owens、Wendt、Rebel 和 Kalbel 法（OWRK）计算表面自由能
混合粉体的物理性质	含水量	干燥失重测定法（红外水分测定仪）
	密度	松密度、振实密度、真密度
	流动性	流动性指数：休止角、压缩性、平板角、黏附度或均齐度，每项综合加权
	引湿性	《中国药典》（2025版）四部　药物引湿性试验指导原则
	粒形粒径	扫描粒形粒径测定仪、马尔文激光粒度仪
黏合剂	流变类型	旋转流变仪
	溶液黏度	旋转流变仪
	表面张力	铂金板法（表面张力仪）
	溶液密度	常规法：质量／体积

规则库的整体构成如图13-10所示，包括基于表面能的原料药与辅料分类筛选规则和处方工艺筛选规则。处方工艺筛选部分主要基于进风风量、进风温度等工艺参数建立了各类相关性模型，简化了专家系统的推理与计算过程。规则库中的相关性模型主要采用曲线拟合等方法进行构建。

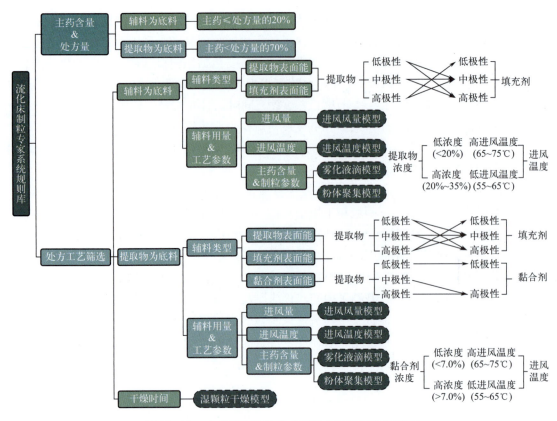

图13-10 中药提取物流化床制粒专家系统的规则库

此外,还可利用数值模拟技术构建相关性模型。以曾佳等[100]建立的雾化液滴粒径模型为例,该模型可以预测并控制制粒过程中黏合剂的雾化液滴粒径和雾化角,对于颗粒成型有重要意义。根据文献报道和前期研究,采用高分辨率的扫描粒形粒径测定仪表征雾化液滴的粒径和雾化角,为建模提供可靠数据支持。随后,采用响应面中心复合试验设计(central composite design,CCD),研究了黏合剂浓度(X_1)、雾化压力(X_2)和喷雾速率(X_3)对雾化液滴的影响,进而采用二次回归的方法计算工艺参数对液滴尺寸和喷雾角的影响,如式(13-1)所示

$$d_p = \beta_0 + \sum_{i=1}^{n} \beta_i X_i + \sum_{\substack{i=1 \\ i<j}}^{n-1} \sum_{j=2}^{n} \beta_{ij} X_i X_j + \sum_{i=1}^{n} \beta_{ii} X_i^2 + \varepsilon \tag{13-1}$$

式中,X为自变量;d_p为平均液滴直径;β_0、β_i、β_{ii}和β_{ij}分别表示回归方程的截距、线性、二次项和相互作用项的系数。N和ε表示自变量的个数和实验误差。根据过程参数对雾化液滴的影响程度结果显示,黏合剂黏度、雾化压力和喷雾速率均对雾化液滴粒径具有显著性影响(图13-11),因此以上述3个参数为自变量,采用逐步回归分析法建立黏合剂溶液的雾化液滴模型,得到拟合回归方程:

标准化方程:

$$d_p = -1.76 \times e^{-10} + 0.44 \times \eta - 0.81 \times p + 0.28 \times n \tag{13-2}$$

数据还原：

$$d_p = 158.10 + 0.09 \times \eta - 72.73 \times p + 0.83 \times n \tag{13-3}$$

式中，η 为黏度（mPa•s）；p 为雾化压力（bar）；n 为黏合剂加入的喷雾速率（r•min^{-1}）。相关系数为 0.93（$R^2=0.93$，$P < 0.0001$），表明模型拟合精度良好。

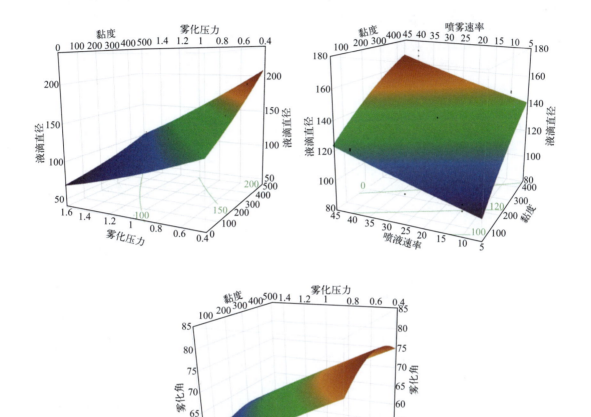

图13-11 黏合剂黏度、雾化压力、喷雾速率对雾化液滴粒径的影响[100]

以上数学模型能够准确预测流化床制粒过程中雾化喷嘴在不同工艺参数范围内的雾化性能。通过对雾化性能的控制进而控制物料在制粒过程中聚集成核，最终达到对制粒过程粒径的控制。通过上述数学建模、数值模拟等技术，可有效提取流化床制粒过程中各 CMA、CQA、CPP 间的关联性与一般规律，基于此构建的专家系统对于流化床制粒的过程控制和质量保障有着重要意义。

（3）胶囊剂

胶囊剂是中药制剂的常见剂型之一，但相比于化药胶囊剂，中药胶囊剂存在装量差异大的问题。因此，杜若飞等[101]开发了基于神经网络理论的中药硬胶囊剂处方设计专家系统，以期改善中药胶囊剂装量差异大及吸湿吸潮等问题，并为推动中药胶囊剂的智能化研发与生产提供新思路。该研究采用激光粒径测试仪、质构仪等设备表征中药原料药的物理性质，这些数据与大量辅料的理化性质一起构成专家系统的数据库，并以人工神经网络为核心算法，建立了5个"制剂原料-辅料-硬胶囊剂质量"相关性数学模型，以此构建规则库。该系统以硬胶囊剂的质量和稳定性为评价指标，借助规则库中的模型进行模拟专家决策的推理过程，为用户提供筛选最优处方条件。

以上研究一定程度上加快了中药现代化、智能化的步伐，但大多仍停留在实验阶段，如何将专家系统应用于实际仍然是巨大的挑战，有待进一步完善与拓展。

13.4 总结

随着研究的深入以及与机器学习的结合，各种类型的ES层出不穷，逐渐渗透到越来越多的领域中，为人们的生活、生产提供了极大便利。但目前大部分专家系统研究主要针对医学临床诊断、工业生产等方面，制药领域的专家系统研究尚有较大的研究空间和提升可能；且除少量网站可对用户开放外，大多数研究仍然处于实验室阶段，暂未投入实际应用。因此，如何将研究成果更好地应用于实际也成为当前必须突破的主要瓶颈问题之一。

近年来，越来越多的研究者已经开展了相关研究并取得了一定成果，但专家系统仍然存在知识数据量小、可解决的问题相对单一、运营成本高等局限性。以基于人工神经网络的专家系统为例，虽然它可以实现自适应推理和联想推理，但由于其需要大量知识数据进行模型训练，其运算准确性在一定程度上取决于数据库的容量。此外，作为工作基础之一的知识库的知识获取主要依赖于人工输入和更新，数据量小且无法做到自主学习，有一定滞后性，随着知识库的扩大，其工作效率也会受到影响，对于数据量巨大的领域，专家系统的可应用性和优势较小。

得益于机器学习的发展，专家系统与机器学习结合的研究开始激起研究者们的兴趣，但能否实现知识库的自主更新、推理机制的进一步完善等，有待进一步深入探索验证。对于中药制剂而言，由于其生产过程复杂、环节多样，系统全面的物性数据库的开发有利于促进中药生产的信息化与智能化，因此，数据库的拓展和优化是亟待发展的研究方向之一，需完善的内容包括：①扩展物料库中样本的多样性，如纳入中药材、中药复方制剂中间体、新型药用辅料等更多粉体类型，以及各种原辅料、中间体和剂型的质量评价标准与指标；②物性参数的表征与分析的标准化，有助于扩大数据库在该领域的权威性与适用性；③深化与机器学习等AI工具的结合，通过自主迭代实现数据库信息的更新优化，实现灵活动态的处方工艺研究。

由于专家系统的上述限制，其发展进程渐缓，同时随着各行业的智能化改造不断深入，知识图谱逐渐受到越来越多研究者的青睐。知识图谱是一种结构化的语义知识库，与基于语义网络的专家系统类似，其核心为"实体"-"关系"-"实体"的三元组（图13-12），图中"原辅料属性参数"与"表征方法"等即为实体，连接两者的线即为关系，可用于迅速描述物理世界中的概念及其相互关系，将复杂数据清晰化可视化，并实现知识的快速响应和推理。与以推理为核心的传统专家系统相比，具有储存数据类型多样、数据获取迅速智能、数据可视化等优势。

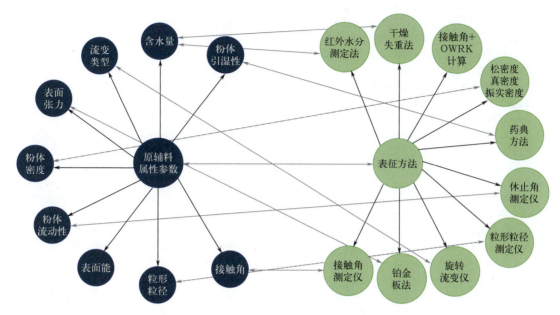

图13-12　模拟具有不同类型实体和概念的知识图谱

近年来，知识图谱在药学领域的应用也在逐渐拓展，其中以基于数据挖掘和文献分析的研究现状分析最为常见[102, 103]。此外，知识图谱在药物相互作用、药物重定位的研究发现中也有所应用[104, 105]。将知识图谱应用于数据库、规则库的构建，同时结合深度学习等机器学习技术或将有利于专家系统知识库的自主学习和更新，成为未来专家系统的发展方向之一。

参考文献

[1] Yang X, Zhu D Q, Sang Q B. Research and prospect of expert system[J]. Jisuanji Yingyong Yanjiu 2007, 24(5): 4-9.

[2] Tang H J. Similarities and differences between expert systems and decision support systems and their applications[J]. Zhongguo Nongye Ziyuan yu Quhua 1995, (3): 56-60.

[3] Suñé-Negre J M, Pérez-Lozano P, Miñarro M, et al. Application of the SeDeM Diagram and a new mathematical equation in the design of direct compression tablet formulation[J]. Eur J Pharm Biopharm, 2008, 69(3): 1029-1039.

[4] Zhang Y D, Wu L N, Wang S H. Survey on development of expert system[J]. Jisuanji Gongcheng yu Yingyong(Computer Engineering and Applications), 2010, 46(19): 43-47.

[5] Lindsay R K, Buchanan B G, Feigenbaum E A, et al. DENDRAL: a case study of the first expert system for scientific hypothesis formation[J]. Artificial intelligence, 1993, 61(2): 209-261.

[6] Shortliffe E H, Davis R, Axline S G, et al. Computer-based consultations in clinical therapeutics: explanation and rule acquisition capabilities of the MYCIN system[J]. Computers and biomedical research, 1975, 8(4): 303-320.

[7] Van Melle W, Shortliffe E H, Buchanan B G. EMYCIN: A knowledge engineer's tool for constructing rule-based expert systems[M]. In: Rule-based expert systems: The MYCIN experiments of the Stanford Heuristic Programming Project, 1984: 302-313.

[8] Li S W, Yang Y. Application of quality by design in the supervision of complex generic drugs in the united states[J]. Chin J Pharm, 2021, 52(6)846-854.

[9]   Liu Y J, Wang Y J, Deng L L, et al. Research on chinese medicine preparation process based on quality by design concept: A review[J]. Mod Chin Med, 2022, 24(03): 523-528.

[10] Yu J Q, Xu B, Yao L, et al. Chinese medicine quality derived from design methods and applications for-(Ⅶ): intelligent manufacturing[J]. World Chin Med, 2018, 13(3): 574-579.

[11] Shi G L, Xu B, Lin Z Z, et al. Chinese medicine quality derived from design methods and applications for-(Ⅲ): Process Modeling[J]. World Chin Med, 2018, 13(3): 543.

[12] Jiang J L, Xuan J B, Zhang K X, et al. The application and genaralization of mathematical models in QbDs[J]. Chin New Drugs J, 2018, 27(4): 429-436.

[13] Buchanan B G. Expert systems: working systems and the research literature[J]. Expert systems, 1986, 3(1): 32-50.

[14] Wang N N, Sun H M, Dong J, et al. PharmDE: A new expert system for drug-excipient compatibility evaluation[J]. Int J Pharm, 2021, 607: 120962.

[15] Qi F Y, Li W J, Zhao X Q, et al. Manufacturing classification system for oral solid dosage forms of traditional Chinese medicines(Ⅰ): classification of processing routes[J]. China J Chin Mater Med, 2023, 48(12): 3169-3179.

[16] Pi T H, Dai Y H, Wang D K. Quality by design in the application research progress of formulation design[J]. Chin J Pharm, 2022, 20: 129-138.

[17] Wang L, Chen F X, Zeng H X, et al. Application of powder characterisation to implementation of quality by design(QbD)[J]. Chin J Pharm, 2014, 45(11): 1086-1089.

[18] Gao D. Research on the Correlation among Powder Properties of Component Traditional Chinese Medicine, Process Parameters and Quality of Dry Granules and Construction of Prediction Models based on QbD Concept. 2021.

[19] Cao J J, Xu B, Dai S Y, et al. Construction and application of iTCM material database for pharmaceutical excipients of chinese medicine oral solid dosage forms[J]. Chin Herb Med, 2021, 52(17): 5166-5175.

[20] Zhang K F, Wang Z, Cao J J, et al. Establishment and application of a near infrared spectral database for pharmaceutical excipients of chinese medicine pral solid dosage forms[J]. Journal of Instrumental Analysis, 2021, 40(1): 1-9.

[21] Zeng J. Numerical simulation technology traditional chinese medicine based on computer investigation on fluidized bed granulation process for traditional chinese medicine based on computer numerical simulation technology[D]. Shanghai: Shanghai University of Traditional Chinese Medicine, 2020.

[22] Ding Z, Dai X, Shi X, et al. Design and development of pharmaceutical excipients database[J]. World Science and Technology, 2011, 13(4): 611-615.

[23] Zhang C Y. Construction and Application of Pharmaceutical Excipients Bioactivity Database[D].Hangzhou: Zhejiang University, 2023.

[24] Feng Y, Du R F, Hong Y L, et al. Thoughts on construction of expert system for the preparation process design of traditional chinese medicine[J]. World Science and Technology-Modernization of Traditional Chinese Medicine, 2013, 15(01): 25-28.

[25] Du Y, Zhao L J, Feng Y, et al. Characterization methods of flowability of traditional chinese medicine powders[J]. China J Chin Mater Med, 2012, 37(05): 589-593.

[26] Fu X J, Feng Y, Xu D S, et al., Further study of the characterization method of hygroscopic characteristics of traditional chinese medicine extracts[J]. Chin Tradit Pat Med, 2010, 32(12): 2075-2079.

[27] Ning R X, Xiong Z W, Zhao Y X, et al. Dynamic two-dimensional characterization technique and influencing factors analysis of the hygroscopicity of Chinese medicine extracts[J]. Acta Pharmaceutica Sinica, 2022, 57(6): 1887-1894.

[28] Zhao Y X, Xiong Z W, Hu X X, et al. Study on anti-hygroscopic technology based on correlations between particle spatial properties and hygroscopicity of Chinese medicinal extracts[J]. China J Chin Mater Med, 2021, 46(23): 6020-6027.

[29] Feng G. In implementation of Web data mining technology based on Python[M]. IOP Publishing, 2021: 012033.

[30] Sun G X, Hu Y S, Jin J, et al. Construction and application of TCM X-ray diffraction fingerprint expert sytem Grid[J]. Cent South Pharm, 2009, 7(10): 766-769.

[31] Wang R T. Design and implementation of the expert system based on the framework knowledge structure[D]. Nanjing University of Posts and Telecommunications, 2017.

[32] Pal D, Mandana K M, Pal S, et al. Fuzzy expert system approach for coronary artery disease screening using clinical parameters[J]. Knowledge-Based Systems 2012, 36: 162-174.

[33] Destro F, Barolo M. A review on the modernization of pharmaceutical development and manufacturing: trends, perspectives, and the role of mathematical modeling[J]. Int J Pharm, 2022, 620: 121715.

[34] Schuhmacher A, Gassmann O, Hinder M, et al. The present and future of project management in pharmaceutical R&D[J]. Drug discovery today 2021, 26(1): 1-4.

[35] Yang X, Wang Y, Byrne R, et al. Concepts of artificial intelligence for computer-assisted drug discovery[J]. Chemical

reviews, 2019, 119(18): 10520-10594.

[36] Worth A P. ECVAM's activities on computer modelling and integrated testing[J]. Alternatives to Laboratory Animals, 2002, 30(2_suppl): 133-137.

[37] Jing Y, Bian Y, Hu Z, et al. Deep learning for drug design: an artificial intelligence paradigm for drug discovery in the big data era[J]. The AAPS journal 2018, 20: 1-10.

[38] Han R, Xiong H, Ye Z, et al. Predicting physical stability of solid dispersions by machine learning techniques[J]. Journal of Controlled Release, 2019, 311；16-25.

[39] Stephens R G, Dunn J C, Hayes B K. Are there two processes in reasoning？ The dimensionality of inductive and deductive inferences[J]. Psychological Review, 2018, 125(2): 218.

[40] Jiang N, Dong H Y. Construction of an expert system inference machine for liquid chromatography selection optimization[J]. Guide of China Medicine, 2012, 10(01): 265-267.

[41] Zhao X, Wang Y D, Guo L J. Prospects and general methods of designing medical expert system inference machine[J]. Yiliao Weisheng Zhuangbei, 2013, 34(12): 100-102+114.

[42] Shen Z. Preliminary study of the construction of expert system and its application for liposome preparation[D].Zhenjiang: Jiangsu University, 2007.

[43] Sarabi S, Han Q, de Vries B, et al.The nature-based solutions case-based system: a hybrid expert system[J]. J Environ Manage, 2022, 324: 116413.

[44] Miao H Z. Overview of case-based reasoning[J]. Journal of Qufu Normal University (Natural Science) 2014, 40(03): 59-62.

[45] Ji S H, Ahn J, Lee E B, et al. Learning method for knowledge retention in CBR cost models[J]. Automation in Construction, 2018, 96: 65-74.

[46] Chergui O, Begdouri A, Groux-Leclet D. Integrating a Bayesian semantic similarity approach into CBR for knowledge reuse in community question answering[J]. Knowledge-Based Systems, 2019, 185: 104919.

[47] Liu D. Logical reasoning and argumentation of the new generation of legal intelligence systems[J]. China Legal Science, 2022, (03): 145-164.

[48] Zhou S, Chen C, Meng Q. Exploration on applications of case-based reasoning in field of chinese medicine[J]. Chin Arch Tradit Chin Med, 2018, 36(09): 2223-2226.

[49] Xue Q, Wang B, Miao K, et al. Construction of knowledge base of chinese medicine manufacturing[J]. China J Chin Mater Med, 2022, 47(12): 3402-3408.

[50] Feng C. Research on emergency decision methods based on case-based reasoning[D]. Xi'an: Northwestern Polytechnical University, 2020.

[51] Ozsahin D U, Ozsahin I. A fuzzy PROMETHEE approach for breast cancer treatment techniques[J]. Int J Med Res Health Sci, 2018, 7(5): 29-32.

[52] Boadh R, Grover R, Dahiya M, et al. Study of fuzzy expert system for the diagnosis of various types of cancer[J]. Mater Today Proc, 2022, 56: 298-307.

[53] Murugesan G, Ahmed T I, Bhola J, et al. Fuzzy logic-based systems for the diagnosis of chronic kidney disease[J]. BioMed Res Int, 2022, 2022(1): 1-15.

[54] Cao H. Research on the expert system of dry granulation prescription and process design of traditional Chinese medicine[D]. Shanghai: Shanghai University of Traditional Chinese Medicine, 2015.

[55] Wang H, Liang J, Dong H, et al. Design and application of recommended system of traditional chinese medicine fingerprints based on web platform[J]. Cent South Pharm, 2010, 8(07): 538-541.

[56] Ming L. Study on an expert system for the design of formulation and operational parameters in fluidized bed granulation of traditional chinese medicine(TCM)extract[D]. Shanghai: Shanghai University of Traditional Chinese Medicine, 2018.

[57] Rosen R, Von Wichert G, Lo G, et al. About the importance of autonomy and digital twins for the future of manufacturing[J]. IFAC-Papers Online, 2015, 48(3): 567-572.

[58] Grieves M, Vickers J. Digital twin: Mitigating unpredictable, undesirable emergent behavior in complex systems[M]. In: Transdisciplinary perspectives on complex systems. Springer Nature, 2017, 85-113.

[59] Liu D, Guo K, Wang B, et al. Summary and perspective survey on digital twin technology[J]. Chin J Sci Instrum, 2018, 39(11): 1-10.

[60] Pérez P, Suñé-Negre J M, Miñarro M, et al. A new expert systems(SeDeM Diagram)for control batch powder formulation and preformulation drug products[J]. Eur J Pharm Biopharm, 2006, 64(3): 351-359.

[61] Singh I, Thakur A K, Bala R, et al. SeDeM expert system, an innovative tool for developing directly compressible tablets: a review[J]. Current Drug Research Reviews Formerly: Current Drug Abuse Reviews, 2021, 13(1): 16-24.

[62] Haux R, Wetter T, Stricker H, et al. Knowledge-based galenical development of drug products: An overview on the design of the galenical development system Heidelberg[J]. Medical Informatics Europe, 1991: 204-208.

[63] Stricker H, Haux R, Wetter T, et al. Das《Galenische Entwicklungs-System Heidelberg》[J]. Pharm Ind, 1991, 53(6): 571-578.

[64] Mendyk A, Jachowicz R. Unified methodology of neural analysis in decision support systems built for pharmaceutical technology[J]. Expert Systems with Applications, 2007, 32(4): 1124-1131.

[65] Li Z, Zhang M, Zhou M, et al. Application of hydroxypropyl methylcellulose in the direct pressing process of surface modification of traditional Chinese medicine powder[J]. Chin Tradit Pat Med, 2021, 43(10): 2755-2759.

[66] Dhondt J, Bertels J, Kumar A, et al. A multivariate formulation and process development platform for direct compression[J]. Int J Pharmaceut, 2022, 623: 121962.

[67] Gaikwad S S, Kothule A M, Morade Y Y, et al. An overview of the implementation of SeDeM and SSCD in various formulation developments[J]. Int J Pharmaceut 2023: 122699.

[68] Nofrerias I, Nardi A, Suñé-Pou M, et al. Optimization of the Cohesion Index in the SeDeM Diagram expert system and application of SeDeM Diagram: An improved methodology to determine the Cohesion Index[J]. PLoS One, 2018, 13(9): e0203846.

[69] Campiñez M D, Benito E, Romero-Azogil L, et al. Development and characterization of new functionalized polyurethanes for sustained and site-specific drug release in the gastrointestinal tract[J]. Eur J Pharm Sci, 2017, 100: 285-295.

[70] Dasankoppa F S, Sajjanar V M, Sholapur H, et al. Application of SeDeM ODT expert system in formulation development of orodispersible tablets of antihyperlipidemic agent[J]. J Young Pharm, 2017, 9(2): 203.

[71] Tadwee I, Shahi S. Formulation development of losartan potassium immediate release tablets and process optimization using SeDeM expert system[J]. J Appl Pharm. Sci, 2018, 8(2): 033-043.

[72] Flórez Borges P, García-Montoya E, Pérez-Lozano P, et al. The role of SeDeM for characterizing the active substance and polyvinyilpyrrolidone eliminating metastable forms in an oral lyophilizate—A preformulation study[J]. PLoS One, 2018, 13(4): e0196049.

[73] Ahmed F R, Shoaib M H, Yousuf R I, et al. Clay nanotubes as a novel multifunctional excipient for the development of directly compressible diclofenac potassium tablets in a SeDeM driven QbD environment[J]. Eur J Pharm Sci, 2019, 133: 214-227.

[74] Zieschang L, Klein M, Jung N, et al. Formulation development of medicated chewing gum tablets by direct compression using the SeDeM-Diagram-Expert-System[J]. Eur J Pharm Biopharm, 2019, 144: 68-78.

[75] Zhang Y, Xu B, Wang X, et al. Optimal selection of incoming materials from the inventory for achieving the target drug release profile of high drug load sustained-release matrix tablet[J]. AAPS PharmSciTech, 2019, 20: 1-13.

[76] Khan A. Optimization of the process variables of roller compaction, on the basis of granules characteristics(flow, mechanical strength, and disintegration behavior): an application of SeDeM-ODT expert system[J]. Drug Dev Ind Pharm, 2019, 45(9): 1537-1546.

[77] Nofrerias I, Nardi A, Suñé-Pou M, et al. Formulation of direct compression Zidovudine tablets to correlate the SeDeM diagram expert system and the rotary press simulator Styl'ONE results[J]. AAPS PharmSciTech, 2020, 21: 1-9.

[78] Wan S, Yang R, Zhang H, et al. Application of the SeDeM expert system in studies for direct compression suitability on mixture of rhodiola extract and an excipient[J]. AAPS PharmSciTech, 2019, 20: 1-10.

[79] Nardi-Ricart A, Nofrerias-Roig I, Suñé-Pou M, et al. Formulation of sustained release hydrophilic matrix tablets of tolcapone with the application of sedem diagram: influence of tolcapone's particle size on sustained release[J]. Pharmaceutics, 2020, 12(7): 674.

[80] Salim I, Olowosulu A K, Abdulsamad A, et al. Application of SeDeM Expert System in the development of novel directly compressible co-processed excipients via co-processing[J]. Futur J Pharm Sci, 2021, 7: 1-12.

[81] Wan S, Dai C, Bai Y, et al. Application of multivariate methods to evaluate differential material attributes of HPMC from different sources[J]. ACS omega 2021, 6(43): 28598-28610.

[82] Mamidi H K, Mishra S M, Rohera B D. Application of modified SeDeM expert diagram system for selection of direct compression excipient for liquisolid formulation of Neusilin® US2[J]. J Drug Deliv Sci Tec, 2021, 64: 102506.

[83] Shah D S, Jha D K, Gurram S, et al. A new SeDeM-SLA expert system for screening of solid carriers for the preparation of solidified liquids: A case of citronella oil[J]. Powder Technology, 2021, 382: 605-618.

[84] Zhang Y, Li Y, Wu F, et al. Texture and surface feature-mediated striking improvements on multiple direct compaction properties of *Zingiberis rhizoma* extracted powder by coprocessing with nano-silica[J]. Int J Pharmaceut, 2021, 603: 120703.

[85] Khan A. Prediction of quality attributes(mechanical strength, disintegration behavior and drug release)of tablets on the basis of characteristics of granules prepared by high shear wet granulation[J]. Plos one, 2021, 16(12): e0261051.

[86] Vlad R A, Antonoaea P, Todoran N, et al. Pharmacotechnical and analytical preformulation studies for cannabidiol orodispersible tablets[J]. Saudi Pharm J, 2021, 29(9): 1029-1042.

[87] Castaneda Hernandez O, Caraballo Rodriguez I, Bernad Bernad M J, et al. Comparison of the performance of two grades of metformin hydrochloride elaboration by means of the SeDeM system, compressibility, compactability, and process capability indices[J]. Drug Dev Ind Pharm, 2021, 47(3): 484-497.

[88] Vasiljević I, Turković E, Nenadović S, et al. Investigation into liquisolid system processability based on the SeDeM Expert System approach[J]. Int J Pharmaceut, 2021, 605: 120847.

[89] Trisopon K, Kittipongpatana N, Wattanaarsakit P, et al. Formulation study of a co-processed, rice starch-based, all-in-one excipient for direct compression using the sedem-odt expert system[J]. Pharmaceuticals 2021, 14(10): 1047.

[90] Iancu V, Iancu I M, Roncea F N, et al. In Pharmaco-technical profile of Lythri herba freeze-dried extract based on SeDeM methodology[J]. IEEE, 2021: 1-4.

[91] González R, Peña M Á, Torres N S, et al. Design, development, and characterization of amorphous rosuvastatin calcium tablets[J]. Plos one, 2022, 17(3): e0265263.

[92] Vasiljević I, Turković E, Piller M, et al. Processability evaluation of multiparticulate units prepared by selective laser sintering using the SeDeM Expert System approach[J]. Int J Pharmaceut, 2022, 629: 122337.

[93] Khan A, Qayum M, Ahmad L, et al. Optimization of diluents on the basis of SeDeM-ODT expert system for formulation development of ODTs of glimepiride[J]. Adv Powder Technol, 2022, 33(2): 103389.

[94] Saleem M T, Shoaib M H, Yousuf R I, et al. SeDeM tool-driven full factorial design for osmotic drug delivery of tramadol HCl: Formulation development, physicochemical evaluation, and in-silico PBPK modeling for predictive pharmacokinetic evaluation using GastroPlus™[J]. Frontiers in Pharmacology, 2022, 13: 974715.

[95] Rao M R P, Sapate S, Sonawane A. Pharmacotechnical evaluation by SeDeM expert system to develop orodispersible tablets[J]. AAPS PharmSciTech, 2022, 23(5): 133.

[96] Sun G X, Wang Z, Jin J, et al. Study on IR fingerprint expert system Grid[J]. Cent South Pharm, 2009, 7(08): 622-625.

[97] Wang H, Dong H Y, Jin J, et al. Knowledge base structure research of traditional chinese medicine fingerprint expert system[J]. Heilongjiang Medicine Journal, 2010, 23(01): 13-16.

[98] Yu Y, Zhao H, Shi C, et al. Study on the effect of different fillers on tablet properties of natural plant products: Quality regulation and formulation recommendation[J]. J Drug Deliv Sci Technol, 2023, 84: 104444.

[99] Liu B. Research on expert system for the design of formulation and process in high shear wet granulation of traditional chinese medicine extract[D]. Shanghai : Shanghai University of Traditional Chinese Medicine, 2022.

[100] Zeng J, Ming L, Wang J, et al. Empirical prediction model based process optimization for droplet size and spraying angle during pharmaceutical fluidized bed granulation[J]. Pharm Dev Technol, 2020, 25(6): 720-728.

[101] Du R F. A dissertation presented to shanghai university of traditional chinese medicine[D]. Shanghai: Shanghai University of Traditional Chinese Medicine, 2014.

[102] Han S, Dai Y, Ding Y, et al. CiteSpace knowledge map analysis of research progress on *Tripterygium wilfordii* Toxicity[J]. China J Chin Mater Med, 2022, 47(04): 1085-1094.

[103] Tang R, Wei X, Ma J, et al. Research status and hotspot of *Granati Pericarpium* based on CiteSpace scientific knowledge graph analysis[J]. Chin Herb Med, 2023, 54(12): 3949-3961.

[104] Zhang J, Chen M, Liu J, et al. A Knowledge-graph-based multimodal deep learning framework for identifying drug-drug interactions[J]. Molecules, 2023, 28(3): 1490.

[105] Ghorbanali Z, Zare-Mirakabad F, Akbari M, et al. DrugRep-KG: Toward learning a unified latent space for drug repurposing using knowledge graphs[J]. J Chem Inf Model, 2023, 63(8): 2532-2545.

第14章

固体片剂药物生产工艺研发及其多尺度模型

陈锡忠　上海交通大学，中国；谢菲尔德大学，英国
刘　锴　谢菲尔德大学，英国
王利戈　山东大学，中国
李　亮　上海交通大学，中国
罗正鸿　上海交通大学，中国

14.1 引言

片剂通常由活性药物成分和固体辅料组成，目前被广泛用于口服给药。药片一般可以通过压缩一定体积的粉末、颗粒或其他适当的方法（例如3D打印）来制备[1]。根据制造步骤或制药的特性，片剂可以分为不同类型，包括压制片、包衣片、多层片、舌下片、泡腾片、舌下崩解片、溶解口服片和可咀嚼片。片剂的优点包括剂量精度高、易于制造、良好的物理及化学稳定性和便携性。此外，片剂可以根据需要进行设计，以控制药物释放速率，增加生物利用度或针对特定区域进行药物递送[2, 3]。另一方面，尽管片剂作为一种剂型具有多种优点，但也存在一些缺点，例如处方选择有限和起效慢[4]。表14-1列出了片剂的主要优点和缺点。

表14-1 片剂的主要优点和缺点

优点	缺点
● 方便：片剂易于吞咽，可用水或不用水服用。包衣技术可以掩盖难闻气味和苦味。	● 某些患者吞咽困难：一些患者，特别是儿童和老年人，可能吞咽片剂会有困难。
● 精准性：片剂的设计包含精确的药物量，这使得患者更容易服用正确的剂量。	● 有限的处方选择：对于溶解度差或在胃中易降解的药物，片剂可能难以配制。
● 稳定性：片剂相对稳定，可以保存很长一段时间而不会降解，使其成为需要长期服用的药物的一个很好的选择。	● 起效缓慢：一些片剂可能比其他剂型（如液体制剂或注射剂）需要更长的时间才开始起效。
● 灵活性：片剂的处方可以使药物以特定的速率或在体内的特定位置释放，有助于提高治疗效果。	● 与食物或饮料的相互作用：有些片剂可能与特定的食物或饮料相互作用，从而影响其吸收和有效性。
● 成本效益：片剂的制造成本通常低于其他剂型。包装和剥离最简单也最便宜，这可以帮助降低患者的用药成本	● 无法调整剂量：一旦片剂生产出来，如果不重新生产新的批次，就很难调整剂量

片剂有很多特性方面的差异，包括大小、形状、重量、硬度、厚度、脆性、孔隙度、崩解时间、溶解速率等，这些特性取决于其用途和所采用的制造工艺。从大小的角度来看，片剂可以分为标准尺寸片和小型片。片剂的大小影响其在咽喉和食管内的通过情况，也影响患者吞咽片剂的能力。较大的片剂可能导致药片在食管内通过延迟，从而导致药片在食管中破裂，并可能引起不适、局部食管炎症和其他不良反应。另一方面，片剂过小可能难以操作和包装，并可能导致剂量错误。此外，片剂的大小还会影响溶解速率和崩解速率，进而影响活性药物成分的生物利用度。片剂的大小可以通过长度、宽度、高度、直径等多个指标来衡量，这些指标取决于片剂的形状。Vallet等[5]得出结论，直径大于6.5 mm的片剂对于年长的人来说难以服用。Kenji等[6]建议片剂的阈值大小是长度、宽度和高度的总和，应该小于21 mm。

片剂的形状是另一个重要特性，不仅因为它对吞咽能力的影响，还因为它与片剂的拉伸强度有直接关系。片剂的形状还被证明会影响药物释放的特性。在给定的大小和重量下，某些形状的片剂更容易被吞咽。片剂有几种形状，包括平面圆形、凸圆形、椭圆形、长方形和胶囊形状[7]。Jørgensen等[8]通过研究得出结论，椭圆形片剂通过食管的时间较短，可能更容易被吞咽。除了通过时间，片剂的拉伸强度也可以根据片剂的形状进行数学计算（例如，参考Pitt和Heasley关于凸面药片的研究[9]）。同时，对于包衣片，片剂的形状和大小也会对包衣性能产生影响。Kandela等[10]研究发现，没有锐利边缘或球度接近1的片剂应该具有最好的包衣均匀性。片剂的力学性质不仅受材料属性影响，还受片剂的形状和大小影响。Lura 等[11]提出了一种用于测试片剂强度的变形行为测试。结果表明，在大多数情况下，小型片剂的屈服压力显著高于常规尺寸的药片。

片剂孔隙率是指在片剂结构中含有孔隙或空隙的程度。片剂孔隙率会影响片剂的溶出和崩解速率，进而影响活性药物成分的生物利用度。孔隙率较高的片剂可以更快地溶解和崩解，起效更快，而孔隙率较低的片剂会更慢地溶解和崩解，起效较慢。此外，片剂孔隙率会影响片剂的物理稳定性，如抗机理应力和吸湿性。孔隙率过高或过低的药片在制造、储存或运输过程中更容易损坏或变质[12]。

14.2 片剂的药物制造过程

传统的药品生产过程由图14-1所示的批量模式下的一系列独立单元操作组成（例如，配药、混合、高剪切造粒、干燥、压片）。相比之下，连续制造（CM）流程将所有单元操作集成到单个生产流程中，单元操作之间无须启动或停止过程（图14-1）。由于原材料通过集成工艺流程直接转化为片剂，因此CM无须处理工艺中间体，从而加快了制造过程。目前，有三种典型的制片方法，即湿法制粒压片法、干法制粒压片法和直接压片法。这些方法中的每一种在压片过程中使用的具体程序和物理机制方面都有所不同（见图14-1）。在这些过程之后，片剂可能会经历各种整理步骤，如包衣、抛光或压印。

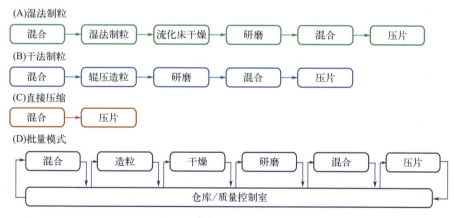

图14-1　片剂连续制造流程示意：（A）湿法制粒压片；
（B）干法制粒压片；（C）直接压片；（D）批量模式

湿法制粒压片涉及将活性药物成分与润湿剂混合形成颗粒，然后将颗粒干燥并压缩成片剂。湿法制粒主要有两种类型，即高剪切和低剪切。在高剪切制粒过程中，将聚乙烯吡咯烷酮（polyvinylpyrrolidone）或羟丙甲基纤维素（HPMC）等黏合剂溶解在液体中（通常是水），然后喷洒到已在容器中混合的粉末床上。容器内设有由电机驱动的刀片或叶轮系统，可产生高剪切力作用。这确保了粉末床均匀地被黏合剂溶液湿润，在混合物颗粒之间产生液体连接，形成湿颗粒。然后，湿颗粒通常使用流化床干燥器进行干燥，得到用于压片的干颗粒。通过对干燥后的颗粒进行研磨，可以使颗粒的大小均匀，便于压片。另一种湿法制粒的方法是流化床制粒，这是一种低剪切过程。它涉及使粉末混合物流态化，并以雾化黏合剂溶液使湿粉末形成颗粒。这个过程的优点在于将制粒和干燥结合在一个设备中[13]。在连续生产过程中，通常使用双螺杆制粒机进行湿法制粒。表14-2列出了湿法制粒压片工艺的优缺点。

表14-2 湿法制粒压片工艺的优缺点

优点	缺点
● 提高粉末混合物的流动性和可压缩性 ● 增强活性和非活性成分的均匀性 ● 减少对工人有害的粉尘产生 ● 增加片剂强度，降低易碎性 ● 允许添加湿敏感或疏水化合物 ● 适用于热敏性药物 ● 可与多种辅料和原料药配合使用	● 过程较长，比其他方法需要更多的时间和设备 ● 难以控制颗粒的大小和形状 ● 需要小心处理湿颗粒，以避免损坏或粘住。在润湿和干燥过程中，原料药可能发生化学或物理降解 ● 溶剂和黏合剂的需求会增加生产成本，并影响最终产品的稳定性 ● 所产生的颗粒可能是吸湿的，需要仔细包装以防止吸湿

作为湿法制粒的替代方法，干法制粒是一种在不使用液体黏合剂的情况下形成颗粒的过程。在干法制粒中，最常用的设备是辊压制粒机。它通过使用一对相互旋转的辊轮将粉末混合物压缩成一张致密的片状颗粒。然后，通过研磨或筛分的过程将致密的片状颗粒分解成所需大小的颗粒。干法制粒通常用于对湿度、热量或压力敏感的材料，并相比湿法制粒具有以下几个优点：首先，它省去了干燥步骤，从而节省时间和降低成本；其次，由于没有使用液体黏合剂，不存在微生物污染的风险，这使得最终产品更加稳定。然而，与湿法制粒压片法相比，该过程可能导致较低的产量，并且颗粒的密度可能会因材料性质和工艺中施加的压缩力而有所不同。表14-3列出了干法制粒压片工艺的优缺点。

表14-3 干法制粒压片工艺的优缺点

优点	缺点
● 避免使用液体黏合剂，液体黏合剂在某些处方中可能不稳定或发生反应 ● 能生产出密度和压缩性可控的颗粒 ● 避免了干燥步骤，可以减少加工时间和成本 ● 适用于湿敏或热敏化合物 ● 对于溶解度差或低剂量制剂的药物，这可能是一个很好的选择	● 可能会产生颗粒大小和形状不均匀，影响含量均匀性和溶出度 ● 需要更大的压缩力才能形成片剂，这会导致设备的磨损 ● 在产量和生产率方面，通常比湿法造粒效率低 ● 可能不适合某些处方或成分

与湿法和干法制粒压片法相比，直接压片法是一种相对简单而直接的过程，是制造片剂的最优选途径。直接压片包括将原料药和其他赋形剂直接压缩成片剂，而不需要造粒或其他加工步骤。将活性药物成分（API）、赋形剂和任何必要添加剂的均匀混合物混合在一起，然后使用压片机压缩成片剂。直接压缩有几个好处，比如更短的处理时间、更低的成本和更少的处理步骤。然而，这种方法需要适当的材料性能，并不适用于所有类型的处方，因为某

些材料可能具有较差的流动性能或不易压缩。此外，到达所需的片剂硬度和崩解时间对某些制剂可能具有挑战性。表14-4列出了直接压片过程的优缺点。

表14-4 直接压片过程的优缺点

优点	缺点
● 过程简单直接，不需要任何中间步骤，如制粒或碾磨，减少了处理时间和成本 ● 需要更少的辅料，这可以节省成本 ● 可用于热敏性或湿性等不能经受湿法制粒工艺的药物	● 需要高质量和特性良好的原料，以确保片剂性能的一致性和可重复性 ● 可能不适用于流动性较差的材料 ● 可能导致片剂机理强度差，封盖或粘连问题，特别是高剂量或强效药物

片剂的生产工艺最终需要确保每次剂量的一致性，即每次剂量应包含一致的成分分布。此外，应该有统一的溶出度和生物利用度，以确保药品的安全性和有效性。制造工艺的选择取决于原料药的物理和化学性质、目标产品概况和成本效益等因素。在选择合适的片剂生产路线时，需要考虑以下因素[4]。

① 药物的物理和化学性质：药物的性质，如溶解度、稳定性和粒度，会影响不同制造路线的适用性。

② 期望的片剂特性：通过特定的制造工艺可以更好地实现片剂的期望特性，如硬度、崩解时间和溶出度。

③ 成本效益：应考虑制造过程的成本，包括设备、人工和材料。

④ 法规要求：片剂的重量和药物含量必须一致。在选择生产路线时，应考虑药品生产工艺的法规要求，如GMP指南。

⑤ 环境影响：还应考虑制造过程对环境的影响，例如能源消耗和废物产生。

在片剂生产过程中，过程分析技术（PAT）是生产合格最终产品过程监控的重要和有效的工具。PAT可以定义为通过及时测量原材料或过程中的关键物料属性、关键工艺参数、关键质量属性来设计、分析和控制制造过程的系统，目的是确保最终产品质量[14]。PAT由测量硬件和分析与存储结果的软件组成。PAT包括直接测量的工具，如在线pH计，或使用红外或拉曼光谱进行在线分析。根据测量方法，PAT可分为近线（at line）、随线（on line）、在线（in line）和离线（off line）四种类型。在PAT工具中，近红外或拉曼光谱可用于制药行业的大部分单元操作，如测量水分含量[15]、密度和孔隙率[16]、混合均匀性[17]、片剂含量和均匀性[18]、片剂包衣厚度[19]等。这两种方法之间的选择通常取决于辅料和原料药的光谱范围，依赖于吸收特性以及所需的分析速度。

14.3 计算模型

片剂生产是一个复杂的过程，涉及各种单元操作，每个单元都需要适当的监控和控制，以确保最终产品符合所需的规格。该过程需要大量的专业知识、设备和资源来获得高质量的最终产品，并且必须满足严格的监管标准。由于制造过程的复杂性，不同类型的模型，从经验到第一性原理的方法，已经发展到包括预测和优化过程、减少实验次数、提高过程效率等方面。一个好的模型应该捕捉原料药、辅料等关键物料属性和关键工艺参数之间复杂的相互作用，提供对关键质量属性的洞察。通过建模，制造商可以减少昂贵和耗时的实验数量，并优化生产高质量片剂的过程，同时最大限度地减少浪费和成本。数值建模可以帮助优化工艺设计流程，加深对工艺的理解，并在投入生产前发现潜在问题、降低未知风险。这样可以有效避免代价高昂的失误和生产事故。然而，在过程和产品开发中使用的模型类型可能会因公司而异，甚至在同一组织内的不同项目团队之间也会有很大差异[20]。有些群体可能严重依赖经验研究和先验知识，虽然这可以解决遇到的生产问题，但往往效率低下。其他人可能根据过去的经验或"直觉"工作，由于缺乏广泛性，可能失效或不适用。有些团队采用更合理的方法，系统地将科学和工程原理应用于开发过程。一般来说，建模方法可分为机理建模、数据驱动建模和混合建模[21]。

机理模型是利用物理和化学原理来描述和预测系统行为的数学方程，可用于模拟不同片剂生产加工步骤中的颗粒行为。有限元法（FEM）、离散元法（DEM）和种群平衡模型（PBM）是片剂生产过程中典型的机理模型。有限元法是一种利用Galerkin法求解复杂数学问题的数值方法，适用于涉及应力、变形和流体流动等现象的问题。有限元模型可以考虑材料性能、设备几何形状和工艺条件（如压缩力、速度和温度）的影响。因此，它已被广泛应用于模拟和分析颗粒在片剂压缩和干法制粒过程中的行为[22, 23]。它还有助于优化设备设计，降低生产过程中片剂或胶囊破损的风险，最大限度地减少封盖、层压等缺陷的发生[24]。Abaqus和Ansys是两种商用有限元软件，已广泛用于片剂压缩模拟。图14-2是基于Abaqus的有限元法在辊压制粒机卷压过程中的应用实例，模拟可以跟踪并显示卷压过程中的应力分布。对应力演化的研究有助于预测压缩过程中潜在的失效机制，也有助于深入了解卷压材料密度变化的潜在原因。

离散元法（DEM）是一种数值模拟技术，用于模拟单个颗粒的行为及其相互作用。在DEM中，系统被分成大量的单个颗粒，每个颗粒都有自己的属性，如大小、形状和表面属性。然后根据物理定律，如牛顿运动定律和库仑摩擦定律，对每个颗粒的行为进行建模。颗粒之间通过接触力（如法向力和切向力）相互作用，这些力可由颗粒的物理性质计算得出。DEM的主要优点是它可以提供对单个颗粒行为及其相互作用的详细理解，这是实验难以实现的。DEM模拟可用于研究口服固体制剂的各种工艺，如粉末混合、颗粒形成、片剂压缩和包衣[25]。它可以帮助优化工艺参数或筛选材料属性，如粒度、形状和表面性能，以提高最终产品的质量。常用的商业和开源的DEM软件包，包括Altair EDEM、Ansys Rocky、LIGGGHTS、MUSEN和MercuryDPM。对于模具填充模拟，可以研究多分散颗粒的流动和偏析行为，并预测填充率。对于片剂包衣，DEM可用于研究片剂间和片剂内的变化。在销磨过程中，通过数值模拟可以直接或间接地预测破碎后的粒度分布。在螺旋进给过程中，采用合适的DEM接触模型可以预测黏性粉末的进给速度。对于制粒过程，DEM可用于研究混合和团聚机制。对于压片机，DEM可以跟踪单个颗粒运动、颗粒-颗粒和颗粒-壁面相互作用，因此可以定量研究原料药和辅料的压缩特性[26]。图14-3是一个应用DEM模拟针式研磨过程中颗粒破碎的例子。

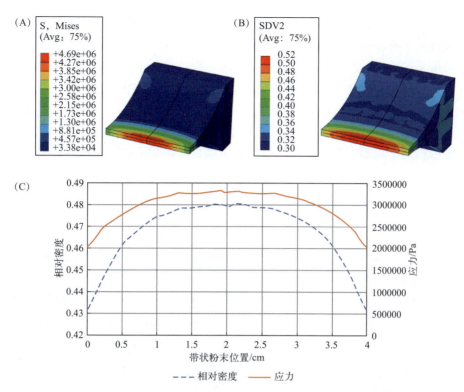

图14-2 有限元法在压实过程中的应用：（A）带状粉末应力等值线图；（B）带状粉末相对密度等高线图；（C）带状材料中部的应力和相对密度分布

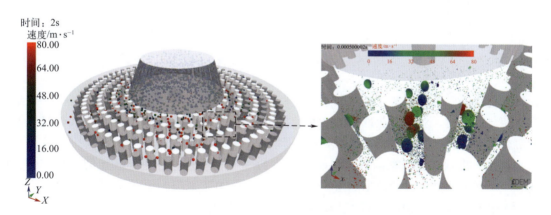

图14-3 利用DEM模拟针式研磨过程中颗粒破碎过程

种群平衡模型（PBM）通过计算在每个粒度区间中形成的颗粒数量的变化和离开该粒度区间的颗粒数量的变化来描述每个粒度段中颗粒数量的数学方程。这些模型假设每个粒径分数中的颗粒有相互作用并与周围环境相互作用，从而导致该粒径分数中的颗粒数量随时间变化[27]。PBM通过模拟颗粒的破碎、团聚和磨损来描述粉末在加工过程中粒度分布的演变。例如，PBM可用于优化制粒过程，通过预测最佳操作条件，如叶轮速度、喷雾速率和黏合剂浓度，以达到所需的粒度分布和流动性。此外，在Aspen Plus、gPROMS

FormulatedProducts、Dyssol等流程模拟软件中通常采用PBM模型[28]。流程模拟是一种集成完整生产过程的工具，可用于预测受物料特性和各单元操作条件影响的动态过程。此外，该流程模型可用于综合工艺分析，包括灵敏度分析、设计空间识别和优化。这有助于通过识别过程特征和瓶颈来制定控制策略[29]。图14-4为一个使用基于PBM的流程模拟对连续湿法制粒压片生产过程进行敏感性分析的例子[30]。流程图模型可以帮助更深入地理解各种跨工艺操作的关键工艺参数和关键质量属性之间复杂的相互作用。本章14.4节将介绍一个研究案例，说明如何应用全局敏感度分析方法系统地识别显著影响所需过程响应的关键工艺参数。

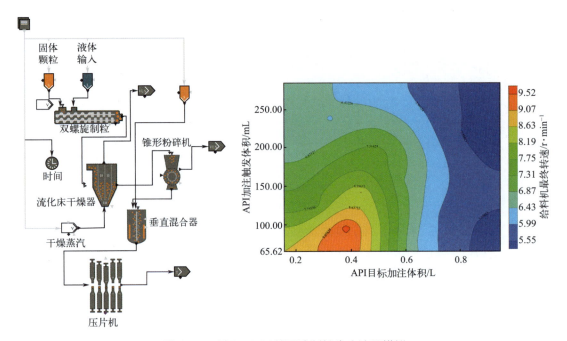

图14-4　基于PBM的湿法制粒生产流程模拟

机理建模的一个主要缺点是，如果对过程机制不完全了解，模型预测的误差和不确定性将会很明显。同时，对于商业规模的全面模拟机理建模方法的计算成本通常很高，这就需要使用高性能计算来生成预测[31]。数据驱动模型具有较低的计算复杂度，但其可靠性和有效性很大程度上取决于源数据的数量和质量。在21世纪，制药行业已经开始经历数字化、自动化和生产过程中产生大量数据的重大转变。在工业4.0和制药4.0时代，数据驱动、人工智能（AI）和机器学习（ML）方法已被用于分析大数据或开发数字孪生等多项任务。人工神经网络是一种有效的过程预测数据驱动模型，通常用于描述采用机理模型计算成本高或无法准确预测过程的复杂过程。人工神经网络的创建受到了人脑信息处理行为的启发，其中的基本计算单元被称为人工神经元或人工节点。神经元可以将接收到的输入转换为期望的输出，为此，首先使用激活函数对输入进行加权和求和，然后使用输出传递函数进一步计算输出。通常，人工神经网络的结构由三个不同的层组成：输入层、隐藏层和输出层，每一层由一系列节点组成。

人工神经网络已被用于预测各种药物制造过程，包括粉末混合、制粒、研磨、压片和涂层。例如，已报道的人工神经网络模型在预测制粒方面的两种应用研究。Shirazian等[32]最近创建了一个人工神经网络模型来预测双螺杆制粒机操作中的粒度分布。他们设计了一系列的测试,来测量表示颗粒粒径分布的 d 值。将液固比(L/S)、螺杆转速、进料流量、螺杆构型作为4个输入,d10、d50、d90作为3个输出。人工神经网络结构每层最多使用四个节点和两个隐藏层。添加更多的节点和层是可能的,但这会增加求解时间。Millen 等[33]应用梯度增强回归树(GBRT)来表征颗粒粒径分布,如片剂抗拉强度、片剂直径和干法制粒过程中的厚度。与其他机器学习算法相比,GBRT在湿法制粒CQA的预测中最为成功。同时,人工神经网络模型也可以与机理模型相结合,即所谓的混合模型。例如,对于人工神经网络的混合应用,Hamza[34]开发了PBM-ANN混合模型,用于模拟双螺杆制粒机进行连续湿法造粒。利用种群平衡模型(PBM)预测颗粒粒径分布,并利用人工神经网络估计平均停留时间,平均停留时间是求种群平衡模型数值解的必要条件。模型以液体进料流量、固体进料流量和螺杆转速为输入,以粒度分布为主要输出。通过模型标定和验证表明,混合模型能较准确地预测颗粒粒度分布,而L/S是双螺杆制粒中最重要的工艺参数。在下游工艺中,压片通常是制造的最后一个工艺单元,这确保了患者收到的片剂能够满足严格的质量要求。当构建压片工艺时,首要考虑的是压缩粉末混合物如何在压片机内反应。Zawbaa 等[35]提出了一种基于进化算法的人工神经网络计算智能模型,通过轧辊压实来预测片剂孔隙率和抗拉强度。以不同的药用辅料(MCC、甘露醇、乳糖和二元混合物)、粒径上限和不同的压缩压力为输入,采用灰狼优化(GWO)、蝙蝠优化(bat)、遗传算法(GA)和粒子群优化算法(PSO)等多种生物优化算法选择最佳输入组合,并利用人工神经网络模型对片剂孔隙度和抗拉强度进行预测。

Roggo 等[36]将深度神经网络(deep neural network,DNN)用于连续湿法制粒生产线生产固体剂型,选择PAT实时监测的7个关键工艺参数和8个关键质量属性。基于这些关键工艺参数,采用深度学习技术预测关键质量属性。优化后,选择了具有3个隐藏层和6个隐藏神经元的神经网络。API含量、PSD值和LOD值的预测校准误差小于10%。一般来说,数据驱动模型,如人工神经网络,已经成为处理大数据和实施工业/制药4.0原则的数据分析工具。从上面的应用中可以发现,人工神经网络和混合模型几乎应用于所有的制药步骤。表14-5总结了数据驱动模型在片剂生产过程中的应用。

表14-5　数据驱动模型在片剂制造过程中的使用

单元操作	模型	关键工艺参数	关键质量属性	参考文献
API 合成	BP-FNN	反应时间、反应温度、酶量和底物摩尔比	酯的分离收率	[37]
API 合成	CFD-GA-FNN	温度、流速和进料组成	反应器性能指标(转化率、产率和选择性)	[38]
结晶	GA-FNN	温度、含水量、体积、溶剂浓度和加入时间、pH 和搅拌速率	晶体密度	[39]
结晶	ResNet CNN	PVM 探针和原位成像	污染物分类	[40]
双螺杆造粒	BP-FNN	液固比、螺杆、速度、进料速率和螺杆配置	粒径分布	[32]
干法制粒	GBRT	粒径分布	抗张强度、直径、厚度	[33]

续表

单元操作	模型	关键工艺参数	关键质量属性	参考文献
双螺杆造粒	PBM-FNN	进料流速、液体流速和螺杆速率	TSG 中颗粒的停留时间	[34]
辊压	EA-FNN	药用辅料、颗粒尺寸的上限和压缩压力	片剂孔隙率和抗张强度	[35]
湿法制粒	BP-FNN	API 和辅料的进料器流速，液体进料速率和挤出机转速以及干燥器的转速、温度、气流流速	混合后、干燥后、压片进料和片剂中的 API 含量，干燥失重（LOD）和粒径分布	[36]
高速混合制粒	多项式回归	搅拌桨转速、给料速率、切割器速度和湿法混合时间、制粒时间、处方	粒径分布、堆积系数和颗粒强度	[41]
高速混合制粒	PCA 和 MLR	搅拌桨转速、液体添加速率和湿法混合时间	颗粒硬度、片剂抗张强度、颗粒平均粒径	[42]
辊压	多项式回归和 MLR	液压压力、辊速和螺杆速率	带状物应力及密度	[43]
直接压片	PCA 和 PLS	材料材质、冲头速度、润滑剂比例	片剂抗张强度	[44]

目前，还没有一个通用的模型可以用于所有的药品生产过程。以上描述的每个模型都有其优点和缺点。每种方法的适用性取决于所建模的具体过程、可用数据、研究目标和要解决的潜在问题陈述。在选择适当的流程建模方法时，考虑这些限制是很重要的，因为它们会影响模型在制药制造和相关领域的准确性、可靠性和适用性。表14-6 概述了制造过程中不同模型的优缺点。此外，通常这些方法的组合可以获得对制造过程更全面的理解。

表14-6 制造过程的不同模型概述

模型	优点	缺点
有限元模型	● 提供系统的力、应变和应力的详细时空信息 ● 提供灵活地处理复杂的几何形状和边界条件 ● 适用于粉末压实、流动和失效问题	● 假设粉末是连续介质，可能无法捕捉到单个颗粒或离散现象的详细行为 ● 需要准确的材料特性和边界条件的知识来获得可靠的结果
离散元模型	● 允许对单个颗粒及其相互作用进行建模，捕获详细的颗粒流动行为 ● 可以洞察颗粒材料微观尺度的现象和行为	● 计算需求随着系统中粒子数量的增加而增加，因此模拟的规模受到限制 ● 需要关于粒子特性和相互作用的详细信息
种群平衡模型	● 可以提供粒子属性分布的详细信息，如大小和形状 ● 允许预测复杂的现象，如聚集和断裂 ● 对整个系统的全局优化非常有用	● 要求核函数来封闭粒子尺度现象 ● 没有明确考虑设备的结构信息 ● 需要大量的实验数据进行参数估计
数据驱动模型	● 利用可用的过程数据来创建模型，减少对底层机制详细知识的需求 ● 能捕捉非线性和复杂关系 ● 在无法很好地理解底层机制时非常有用	● 在很大程度上依赖于现有数据的质量和代表性 ● 数据范围外的外推能力有限 ● 可能无法提供对潜在物理过程的详细见解

14.4 研究案例

14.4.1 谢菲尔德大学的中型试验工厂

2018年，谢菲尔德大学建立了一个中型试验工厂（DiPP）用于开发粉末制药流程，其中包括主要用于制药行业的大量操作单元。DiPP是一个独特的工业4.0的示范，用于谢菲尔德大学的本科教学和研究任务。DiPP由一个连续结晶装置、一个过滤干燥器和一个大型GEA Consigma 25粉末到片剂生产线组成，这是制药行业连续制造过程的一个例子。连续过滤干燥器和连续振荡挡板结晶器都用于制造高纯度晶体和药用化合物，这些材料可作为药物制造中的活性成分。试验工厂的Consigma 25连续粉末到片剂生产线具有一系列同时运行的单元操作，其中包括双螺杆制粒机、流化床干燥机、锥磨机、垂直搅拌机和旋转压片机。在单元过程之间，物料以气动和重力方式移动。DiPP从料斗和减重给料器开始，将预混合的粉末输送到双螺杆制粒机（TSG）。在双螺杆制粒机中，使用具有不同混合元件（输送元件和捏合元件）的共流螺杆将粉末与添加的液体混合。随着处方内组分的不断润湿，通过搅拌使初级粉末颗粒聚结或固结，以产生湿颗粒。湿颗粒在制粒后要经过干燥阶段以便蒸发水分，形成干燥的颗粒。在干燥过程中，使用带有六个分段干燥器的流化床干燥器，以降低颗粒和粉末的水分含量。然后，将干燥的颗粒从流化床干燥器气动输送到锥磨机以将颗粒磨碎。在干燥装置和锥磨机之间，利用近红外光谱（NIR）来检测干燥后颗粒的水分含量。近红外光谱用作PAT工具，用于监测产品质量，特别是湿度水平，并向系统提供反馈，指示产品是否应保留或作为废物丢弃。碾磨后，颗粒移动到下一步的混合单元，在到达旋转压片机之前，可以添加其他材料和润滑剂。该设施的示意图和详细的过程视频介绍可在谢菲尔德大学化学工程系的网站上获得。

旋转压片机对确定片剂的性质至关重要，图14-5说明了旋转压片机的工作原理。压片机包括一个主料斗、12 mm模具和20个凹模。该工艺开始时，混合粉末从主料斗流向给料架，在给料架上，两个共流旋转桨将粉末送入模具。第一个桨片最初在过填充凸轮位置时提供过量的粉末，而第二个桨片在填充凸轮位置填充和刮取所需的粉末量。在移动到最终压实阶段之前，模具经过预压缩，其中两个辊施加压力以去除多余的空气。然后，在最后的压实阶段，通过压实力冲孔模具，从而确定压片强度。最后，顶出阶段的下冲头将压缩片剂推出生产线[7]。

除了Consigma 25连续粉末到片剂生产线外，DiPP的工业控制室还专门设计了先进的控

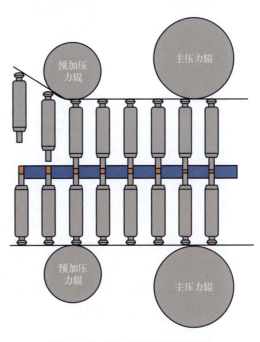

图14-5　压片压实过程示意图

制系统和整个试验工厂的数字孪生系统。谢菲尔德大学（University of Sheffield）、Perceptive Engineering 和西门子（Siemens）合作开发了一种创新的解决方案，将从结晶到压片的整个连续药物生产过程数字化，是当前世界领先的工业4.0示范产品。该项目的主要目标是采用以数据为中心的方法和人工智能技术，为现实场景中潜在的物联网应用提供测试和验证设施[45]。

14.4.2 连续直接压片过程的模拟

图14-6显示了连续直接压片过程的流程图模拟。该过程包括通过各自的给料器进料和混合各种粉末，然后使用压片机将混合物压缩成片剂的过程。所得片剂具有关键质量属性（CQA），如片剂孔隙率和抗拉强度。在每个工作流程的单元中，有几个可操纵的输入可能对CQA产生影响，例如螺杆速度、填充量、停留时间和压片压力。连续直接压片过程的流程仿真在西门子过程系统企业（SPSE）开发的过程建模仿真软件平台 gPROMS FormulaProducts 中进行[46]。该软件可用于化学、制药和能源行业，对化工过程进行建模和模拟，以及设计和优化工艺设备和操作。通过流程模拟，可以系统地研究关键物料属性（CMA）和关键工艺参数（CPP）对最终片剂关键质量属性（CQA）的影响。

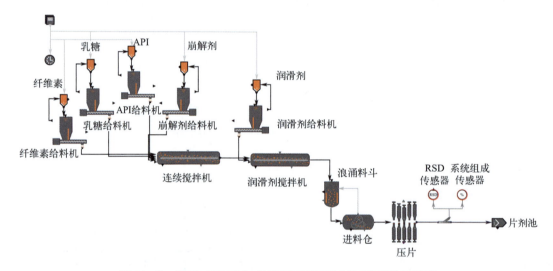

图14-6　使用gPROMs的连续直接压片过程模拟的流程图

模拟使用的材料如表14-7所示，采用的模型分别列示下：
① 给料器所用模型：

$$ff = ff_{\max} - (ff_{\max} - ff_{\min})e^{-\beta m_{给料器}} \tag{14-1}$$

式中，$ff_{\max}$表示在给料器中观察到的最大给料因子；$ff_{\min}$表示在机组重量接近零时推断出的最小给料因子；β是基于料斗质量的给料因子衰减率；$m_{给料器}$表示给料器中的物料质量。在仿真中，$ff_{\max}$、$ff_{\min}$和β的值分别为 1 g·rev^{-1}、0.2 g·rev^{-1}、3.3 kg^{-1}。

② 搅拌机所使用的模型：

$$E_\theta(\theta) = f(Pe, \theta)$$

$$Pe = \frac{uL}{D_p} \quad \theta = \frac{t}{\tau}$$

式中，E_θ 为无因次停留时间分布；Pe 为小颗粒数；θ 为无因次停留时间；D_p 为主流物料弥散系数；u 为主流流速；L 为机组混合长度；τ 为平均停留时间。D_p 和 τ 分别为 $0.4\ \text{cm}^2 \cdot \text{s}^{-1}$ 和 $100\ \text{s}$。

③ 片剂压实模型为：

$$T_p = T_{0\_p} e^{-k_{b-p} \varepsilon_p}$$

式中，T_p 为初生相的抗拉强度；T_{0_p} 为在初生相为零孔隙度时的抗拉强度；k_{b-p} 为初生相的结合能力；ε_p 为初生相的孔隙率。T_{0_p} 为 20 MPa，k_{b-p} 为 8。

表14-7　模拟中使用的材料特性总结

	MCC	乳糖	API	崩解剂	润滑剂
堆密度 /kg·m^{-3}	280	660	600	500	500
粒径分布 25% 分位数 / μm	2.12	2.27	2.74	13.38	10.75
粒径分布 50% 分位数 / μm	10.31	10.66	11.71	33.87	26.93
粒径分布 75% 分位数 / μm	44.52	45.50	48.52	72.22	57.96
质量分数 /（kg/kg）	1.00	1.00	1.00	1.00	1.00
颗粒内部孔隙率（m^3/m^3）	0.01	0.01	0.01	0.01	0.01
体积形状因子	0.52	0.52	0.52	0.52	0.52
表面形状因子	3.14	3.14	3.14	3.14	3.14

在使用流程模拟软件预测实际制造过程前，采用的机理模型参数需要通过实验数据进行校准和验证，以确保准确可靠地捕获制造过程重要的单元，并评估无法直接测量的模型参数。在给料单元中，选取机理模型中的最大给料因子、最小给料因子和给料因子衰减率作为标定参数。在连续混合装置中，用实验数据标定了 Peclet 数和平均停留时间。图14-7 和图 14-8 显示了在给料器和搅拌器单元中校准模型与实验结果的比较。从图中可以看出，校正后的模型能够很好地捕捉实验数据的趋势。

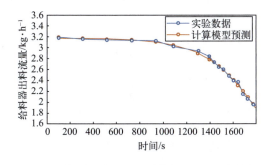

图14-7　给料器流量实验数据与模型预测对比

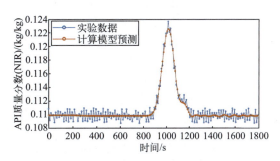

图14-8　搅拌器实验数据与模型预测对比

在对给料器和搅拌器模型进行标定后,可以通过全局敏感度分析(GSA)来探索该工艺的设计空间。GSA 提供了一种方法来检查系统的整体行为,并通过考虑输入变量(CPP)和输出变量(CQA)的选定子集来调查系统行为,并以清晰简洁的方式分析结果。由此产生的结果可以用于多个目的,如确定满足所需出口规格的操作制度,以及支持执行额外实验的决策。在 gPROMS 中,使用蒙特卡洛方法对不同输入的多个模型进行评估,样本生成方法可以选择 Sobol 采样和 Pseudo-Random 采样。图 14-9 和图 14-10 显示了原料药加注设置的 GSA 结果,包括原料药加注触发量和 API 目标加注量对原料药给药机螺杆转速和给料器出药流量的影响。图 14-11 显示了 API 给料机的螺杆转速随补料设置的等高线图。从图 14-9 可以看出,随着原料药加注触发量的增加,原料药给料机的螺杆转速也随之升高,这一点从图 14-11 也可以观察到。相比之下,图 14-10 中的散点表明,原料药流量与加注设置参数之间没有很强的相关性。图 14-12 显示了压实压力对最终片剂抗拉强度和 API 分数的全局敏感度分析。可以看出,压实压力的提高使压片的抗拉强度不断提高。通过 GSA 计算得到压片操作设计空间,可以确定最佳工艺条件。

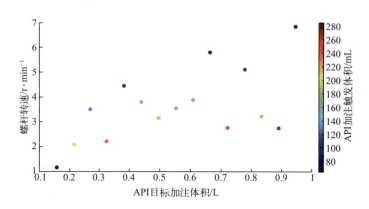

图 14-9　原料药填充设置对原料药给料器螺杆转速的全局敏感度分析

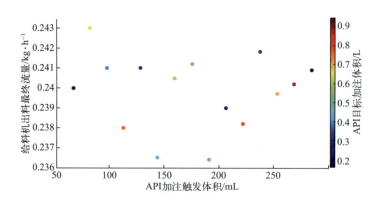

图 14-10　API 加注设置对 API 流量的全局敏感度分析

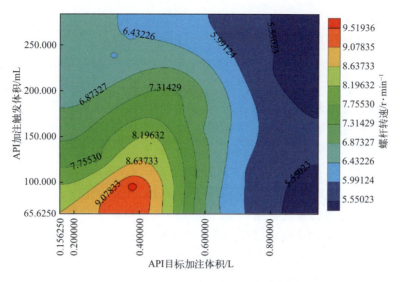

图14-11　GSA中原料药螺杆转速对填充量影响的等高线图

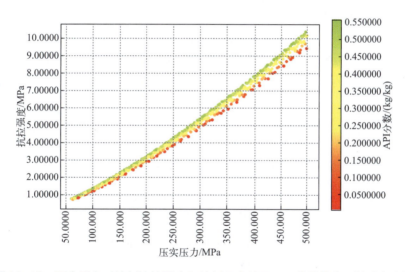

图14-12　压实压力对片剂抗拉强度和片剂压实单元API分数的全局敏感度分析

14.5　总结

片剂是药物最广泛使用的剂型之一，因为它们易于管理，稳定性好，便于患者接受。片剂可以使用多种技术进行制造，包括直接压片、湿法制粒和干法制粒。采用最先进的片剂制造工艺，如连续制造工艺和过程分析技术（PAT），可以提高质量、效率和成本效益。然而，尽管片剂在制造方面取得了较大进展，但片剂在处方和工艺设计的建模方法方面仍存在不足。首先，片剂制造过程非常复杂，涉及多种物理现象，如颗粒-颗粒相互作用、颗粒-黏合剂相互作用、流体流动、传热传质等。准确地对这些过程建模需要对底层物理有深刻的理解。其次，片剂生产中使用的原材料的性质，如粒度、形状和密度，通常会有很大的变化，导致最终产品的变化。这种可变性需要在模型中加以考虑，以确保其准确性。再次，针对片剂生产过程建立的模型通常只反映具体的处方和操作条件，因此需要更严格地研究其通用性和预测的不确定性。总的来说，这些挑战需要多学科合作，结合实验数据，理论模型和数值模拟，以准确地模拟片剂制造过程。

近年来，口服固体片剂的数字化制造工艺和分析技术的重大发展提高了对工艺和产品的理解，基于这些发展提供了一个良好的实时释放测试平台，可以消除全部或部分线下终端产品测试，确保片剂产品达到预期质量。随着物联网（Internet of Things，IoT）的出现，我们可以获取大量片剂制造商的工艺数据，实现实时在线模型评估和更新[47]。此外，虚拟现实（VR）和增强现实（AR）的使用可以提供多样化和清晰的过程可视化。随着人工智能（AI）的最新进展，数据驱动模型和混合模型在帮助实现智能、自主的制药生产线方面越来越受关注。此外，实时释放测试（RTRT）已成为一种先进的质量控制方法，用于片剂制造商快速检测和解决偏离目标CQA的问题，降低产品不合格的风险[48]。通过使用RTRT，制造商可以更全面地了解工艺参数对片剂性能的影响，从而更准确地预测溶出度和其他CQA，这将有助于提高片剂产品的质量和一致性，减少生产完成后测试和调整的需要。RTRT还可以促进连续制造工艺的实施，从而进一步提高片剂生产的效率和质量。通过过程分析技术和数字模型的输入，RTRT可以通过对连续制造过程的性能提供实时反馈，显著提高片剂制造的质量和效率，在未来这将为患者带来更安全、更有效的药物。

参考文献

[1] Ubhe T S, Gedam P. A brief overview on tablet and it's types[J]. Journal of Advancement in Pharmacology, 2020, 1(1): 21-31.

[2] Al-Achi A. Tablets: a brief overview[J]. Journal of Pharmacy Practice and Pharmaceutical Sciences, 2019, (1): 49-21.

[3] Lachman L, Lieberman H A, Kanig J L. The theory and practice of industrial pharmacy[M]. third eds. Lea & Febiger Philadelphia, 1976.

[4] Harbir K. Processing technologies for pharmaceutical tablets: a review[J]. Int Res J Pharm, 2012, 3: 20-23.

[5] Vallet T, Michelon H, Orlu M, et al. Acceptability in the older population: the importance of an appropriate tablet size[J]. Pharmaceutics, 2020, 12(8): E746.

[6] Kabeya K, Satoh H, Hori S, et al. Threshold size of medical tablets and capsules: based on information collected by Japanese medical wholesaler[J]. Patient preference and adherence, 2020, 14: 1251-1258.

[7] Wang L G, Omar C, Litster J D, et al. Tableting model assessment of porosity and tensile strength using a continuous wet granulation route[J]. International Journal of Pharmaceutics, 2021, 607: 120934.

[8] Hey H, Jørgensen F, Sørensen K, et al. Oesophageal transit of six commonly used tablets and capsules[J]. Br Med J(Clin Res Ed), 1982, 285: 1717-1719.

[9] Pitt K G, Heasley M G. Determination of the tensile strength of elongated tablets[J]. Powder technology, 2013, 238: 169-175.

[10] Kandela B, Sheorey U, Banerjee A, Bellare J. Study of tablet-coating parameters for a pan coater through video imaging and Monte Carlo simulation[J]. Powder technology, 2010, 204: 103-112.

[11] Lura A, Tardy G, Kleinebudde P, Breitkreutz J. Tableting of mini-tablets in comparison with conventionally sized tablets: A comparison of tableting properties and tablet dimensions[J]. International Journal of Pharmaceutics: X, 2020, 2: 100061.

[12] Adolfsson Å, Nyström C. Tablet strength, porosity, elasticity and solid state structure of tablets compressed at high loads[J]. International journal of pharmaceutics, 1996, 132: 95-106.

[13] Burcham C L, Florence A J, Johnson M D. Continuous manufacturing in pharmaceutical process development and manufacturing[J]. Annual review of chemical and biomolecular engineering, 2018, 9: 253-281.

[14] Watts C. PAT–A framework for innovative pharmaceutical development manufacturing and quality assurance. FDA/RPSGB Guidance Workshop, 2004.

[15] Peters J, Teske A, Taute W, et al. Real-time process monitoring in a semi-continuous fluid-bed dryer–microwave resonance technology versus near-infrared spectroscopy[J]. International Journal of Pharmaceutics, 2018, 537: 193-201.

[16] Singh R, Román-Ospino A D, Romañach R J, et al. Real time monitoring of powder blend bulk density for coupled feed-forward/feed-back control of a continuous direct compaction tablet manufacturing process[J]. International journal of pharmaceutics, 2015, 495 : 612-625.

[17] Simonaho S P, Ketolainen T, Ervasti M, et al. Continuous manufacturing of tablets with PROMIS-line: Introduction and case studies from continuous feeding, blending and tableting[J]. European Journal of Pharmaceutical Sciences, 2016, 90 : 38-46.

[18] Roggo Y, Pauli V, Jelsch M, et al. Continuous manufacturing process monitoring of pharmaceutical solid dosage form: A case study[J]. Journal of Pharmaceutical and Biomedical Analysis, 2020, 179 : 112971.

[19] Hattori Y, Sugata M, Kamata H, et al. Real-time monitoring of the tablet-coating process by near-infrared spectroscopy-Effects of coating polymer concentrations on pharmaceutical properties of tablets[J]. Journal of Drug Delivery Science and Technology, 2018, 46 : 111-121.

[20] Qiu Y, He X, Zhu L, et al. Product and process development of solid oral dosage forms[M]. Developing solid oral dosage forms. Elsevier, 2017: 555-591.

[21] Simon L L , Kiss A A, Cornevin J, et al. Process engineering advances in pharmaceutical and chemical industries: digital process design, advanced rectification, and continuous filtration[J]. Current opinion in chemical engineering, 2019, 25: 114-121.

[22] Mazor A, Perez-Gandarillas L, De Ryck A, et al. Effect of roll compactor sealing system designs: A finite element analysis[J]. Powder Technology, 2016, 289: 21-30.

[23] Wu C Y, Ruddy O, Bentham A, et al. Modelling the mechanical behaviour of pharmaceutical powders during compaction[J]. Powder technology, 2005, 152: 107-117.

[24] Han L, Elliott J, Bentham A, et al. A modified Drucker-Prager Cap model for die compaction simulation of pharmaceutical powders[J]. International Journal of Solids and Structures, 2008, 45: 3088-3106.

[25] Yeom S B, Ha E S, Kim M S, et al. Application of the discrete element method for manufacturing process simulation in the pharmaceutical industry[J]. Pharmaceutics, 2019, 11: 414.

[26] Ponginan R. Optimizing pharmaceutical manufacturing processes using EDEM simulation, 2019.

[27] Wang Z, Escotet-Espinoza M S, Ierapetritou M. Process analysis and optimization of continuous pharmaceutical manufacturing using flowsheet models[J]. Computers & Chemical Engineering, 2017, 107: 77-91.

[28] Dosta M, Litster J D, Heinrich S. Flowsheet simulation of solids processes: Current status and future trends[J]. Advanced Powder Technology, 2020, 31: 947-953.

[29] Nishii T, Matsuzaki K, Morita S. Real-time determination and visualization of two independent quantities during a manufacturing process of pharmaceutical tablets by near-infrared hyperspectral imaging combined with multivariate analysis[J]. International Journal of Pharmaceutics, 2020, 590: 119871.

[30] Metta N, Ghijs M, Schäfer E, et al. Dynamic flowsheet model development and sensitivity analysis of a continuous pharmaceutical tablet manufacturing process using the wet granulation route[J]. Processes, 2019, 7: 234.

[31] Pandey P, Bharadwaj R, ChenX. Modeling of drug product manufacturing processes in the pharmaceutical industry[M]. Predictive Modeling of Pharmaceutical Unit Operations, Elsevier, 2017: 1-13.

[32] S. Shirazian, M. Kuhs, S. Darwish, D. Croker, G.M. Walker, Artificial neural network modelling of continuous wet granulation using a twin-screw extruder[J]. International journal of pharmaceutics, 2017, 521 : 102-109.

[33] Millen N, Kovačević A, Djuriš J, et al. Machine learning modeling of wet granulation scale-up using particle size distribution characterization parameters[J]. Journal of Pharmaceutical Innovation, 2020, 15: 535-546.

[34] Ismail H Y, Singh M, Shirazian S, et al. Development of high-performance hybrid ann-finite volume scheme(ann-fvs)for simulation of pharmaceutical continuous granulation[J]. Chemical Engineering Research and Design, 2020, 163: 320-326.

[35] Zawbaa H M, Schiano S, Perez-Gandarillas L, et al. Computational intelligence modelling of pharmaceutical tabletting processes using bio-inspired optimization algorithms[J]. Advanced Powder Technology, 2018, 29 : 2966-2977.

[36] Roggo Y, Jelsch M, Heger P, et al. Deep learning for continuous manufacturing of pharmaceutical solid dosage form[J]. European journal of pharmaceutics and biopharmaceutics, 2020, 153: 95-105.

[37] Moghaddam M G, Ahmad F B H, Basri M, et al. Artificial neural network modeling studies to predict the yield of enzymatic synthesis of betulinic acid ester[J]. Electronic Journal of Biotechnology, 13(2010)3-4.

[38] Gbadago D Q, Moon J, Kim M, et al. A unified framework for the mathematical modelling, predictive analysis, and optimization of reaction systems using computational fluid dynamics, deep neural network and genetic algorithm: A case of butadiene synthesis[J]. Chemical Engineering Journal, 2021, 409 : 128163.

[39] Velásco-Mejía A, Vallejo-Becerra V, Chávez-Ramírez A, et al. Modeling and optimization of a pharmaceutical crystallization process by using neural networks and genetic algorithms[J]. Powder Technology, 2016, 292 : 122-128.

[40] Salami H, McDonald M A, Bommarius A S, et al. In situ imaging combined with deep learning for crystallization process monitoring: application to cephalexin production[J]. Organic Process Research & Development, 2021, 25: 1670-1679.

[41] Bajdik J, Baki G, Szent-Királlyi Z, et al. Evaluation of the composition of the binder bridges in matrix granules prepared with a small-scale high-shear granulator[J]. Journal of Pharmaceutical and Biomedical Analysis, 2008, 48 : 694-701.

[42] Thapa P, Choi D H, Kim M S, et al. Effects of granulation process variables on the physical properties of dosage forms by combination of experimental design and principal component analysis[J]. Asian journal of pharmaceutical sciences, 2019, 14: 287-304.

[43] Reddy J P, Phanse R, Nesarikar V. Parameter estimation for roller compaction process using an instrumented vector TF mini roller compactor[J]. Pharmaceutical Development and Technology, 2019, 24 : 1250-1257.

[44] Haware RV, Tho I, Bauer-Brandl A. Multivariate analysis of relationships between material properties, process parameters and tablet tensile strength for α-lactose monohydrates[J]. European Journal of Pharmaceutics and Biopharmaceutics, 2009, 73 : 424-431.

[45] Ntamo D, Lopez-Montero E, Mack J, et al. Industry 4.0 in Action: Digitalisation of a continuous process manufacturing for formulated products[J]. Digital Chemical Engineering, 2022, 3 : 100025.

[46] S.P.S.E. Ltd., gPROMS Formulated Products.

[47] Boukouvala F, Niotis V, Ramachandran R, et al. An integrated approach for dynamic flowsheet modeling and sensitivity analysis of a continuous tablet manufacturing process[J]. Computers & Chemical Engineering, 2012, 42: 30-47.

[48] I.H.T. Guideline, Pharmaceutical development, Q8(2R). As revised in August, 2009.

第15章

药物开发中的机器学习

约翰·伯特克（Johan Bøtker）　　哥本哈根大学，丹麦
尤卡·兰塔宁（Jukka Rantanen）　　哥本哈根大学，丹麦
安德斯·马德森（Anders Madsen）　　哥本哈根大学，丹麦

15.1 引言

机器学习（ML）为制药界利用不断增加的医疗保健服务和制药开发相关数据开辟了新的可能。设计一种新的医药产品往往涉及基于知识的决策，而要将决策过程记录下来是具有挑战性的，并且这一过程往往带有试错的成分。数据驱动的产品（制剂）设计可以作为一种替代方法来记录这种基于知识的过程，并摆脱以基于试错的实验工作。

本章将重点概述ML在药物产品设计中的不同应用，涵盖了与材料科学（处方前研究）、产品（制剂）设计以及药物产品的制造和质量控制方面有关的实例。本章并不详细介绍具体的方法和算法，而是侧重于制药科学家可以使用ML方法的领域。相关药典章节（如《欧洲药典》5.21应用于分析数据的化学计量学方法）已经介绍了这些方法和最佳实践过程。需要注意的是，本章中部分示例与现有产品开发直接相关，而有些示例则更具探索性，作为药物开发的一部分，其全面商业化应用的道路更为漫长。在这里，首先提醒读者要了解一般的ML工作流程（图15-1）[1]。下面将介绍一个基于所选物质的理化特性对活性物质（溶胶）溶解度进行监督预测的示例。该示例重点介绍了监督式ML工作中的典型步骤：

第一步，收集、整理和清洗数据集（图15-1，步骤Ⅰ）。在这一步骤中，重要的是要严格把关，只选取具有相关性的特征。分子建模软件可用于生成大量可能有用的特征（分子描述符）。与药品设计相关的数据也可以是源于实验的（例如，体外药物释放实验），但这会耗费大量时间来构建数据集。另一个复杂的因素是，药物数据并不总是数字化为简单的格式。药典中的数据结构就是一个例子，其中的数据挖掘并不简单。值得注意的是，在药品开发过程中应用机器学习的一个关键因素是缺乏结构化的制剂和产品成分数据库。下文将对此进行讨论。

第二步，模型的评估和选择（图15-1，Ⅱ）。这一步首先要将收集和清洗后的数据集分为训练集和测试集。重要的是要选定测试集，使其能够涵盖所有潜在的未来可应用场景以及模型的最终用途。之后使用训练集建立模型，并使用测试集测试模型性能，从而达到对不同建模方法和算法进行比较的目的。

最后，对最优模型进行模型解释（图15-1，Ⅲ）。当模型在测试集上的预测性能达到可接受的水平后，统计的相关性和每个特征的重要性就可以通过一些相对简单的指标可视化。

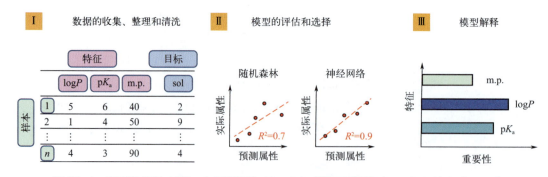

图15-1 根据物质的辛醇-水分配系数（log$P$）、酸解离常数（pK_a）和熔点（m.p.）监督预测活性物质溶解度（sol）的ML工作流程[1]

以上是机器学习的典型工作流程，以下各节将介绍机器学习应用于药物开发和商业化生产中的实例。

15.2 制药材料科学

处方前研究阶段需要大量材料信息，如水溶性、pK_a、盐型、溶解特性、粉末流动性、片剂的压缩性以及与辅料的相容性。这些可用于机器学习的信息并不总是容易获得的，因为手中必须有大量的数据集，而如何获得这些合适的数据是目前机器学习在制药材料科学研究领域中应用的最大挑战。其中主要的障碍在于数据需要经过仔细清洗和标记才可以用于机器学习模型的训练。

数据的整理（图15-1第Ⅰ步给出了一个数据示例）通常是机器学习流程的主要部分。在很多情况下数据有许多不同的来源，例如不同的仪器、数据库或研究小组。数据也可能是在不同温度下收集的，或使用了来自不同供应商的化学品。所有数据都应根据这些相关信息进行标注以解释数据的变化，否则将会被视为垃圾信息，或在解释机器学习结果时导致错误的结论。

精确的模型需要大量的样本，并且样本应涵盖所有可能的实验结果，即在示例中，样本应涵盖整个$\log P$、pK_a和m.p.范围，从而得到高溶解度和低溶解度的目标值。

接下来的章节将概述一些获取此类标注数据的重要方法，即使用数据库和模拟数据。在更之后的章节中，再对高通量分析的情况进行介绍。以下所述的研究范例重点关注固态药品，但必须强调的是，这些方法适用于所有类型的药品。

15.2.1 与制药相关的数据库实例

如表15-1所示，已有一系列的数据库能够提供固态剂型的相关数据。然而，在许多情况下，这些数据结构不完善，标注不充分，无法立即用于更高级的数据分析。将制剂数据库中的信息与化学数据库连接起来是一项具有挑战性的工作。典型的药典数据通常包含数千个条目，而化学数据库通常有数百万个条目。

表15-1 一些常用的包含固体制剂信息的数据库[2]

	一些常用的固体制剂数据库		
	名称	规模	出版商
原料药（API）/化学物质	美国药典（USP）	>5000	美国药典公约
	PubChem 数据库	>1.11亿	美国国家生物技术信息中心（NCBI）
	剑桥结构数据库（CSD）	>900000	剑桥大学
	SciFinder 数据库	1.42亿	化学文摘（CAS）
	默克索引	>10000	英国皇家化学学会（RSC）
辅料	非活性成分数据库	9438	美国食品药品管理局（FDA）

一些常用的固体制剂数据库			
	名称	规模	出版商
处方	Drugs@FDA（FDA 批准药物）	>20000	美国食品药品管理局（FDA）
	橙皮书	N/A	美国食品药品管理局（FDA）
	DrugBank 数据库	>500000	阿尔伯塔大学
	Dissolution Methods 数据库	1388	美国食品药品管理局（FDA）
	MedlinePlus® 数据库	~1500	美国国立卫生研究院
	Drug Information Portal 数据库	>49000	美国国立卫生研究院

要将制药材料研究作为合理设计的指导，就必须从原子级结构入手，建立构效关系。原子结构决定了大量重要的制药材料特性，如溶解性、力学稳定性和热稳定性。基本的结构知识并不涉及分子结构，而是对固态分子三维堆积的全面描述。固态材料可分为晶体和无定形物质。大多数制药材料都以晶体为主，也就是说，虽然颗粒表面和界面可能是高度无序的，但主体材料可以被定性为晶体。

晶体中分子间的作用力决定了晶体的堆积能以及晶体的晶格振动。基于对这些力的计算（例如，使用周期性密度泛函理论计算），可以确定晶体的自由能。晶体的自由能与其熔点、固态相变温度（例如与多晶型转变或脱水有关的温度）以及溶解度直接相关。分子堆积模式还决定了晶体材料的力学性能，如体积模量和剪切强度。

目前已发现的晶体结构大约有一百万个，包括14000多种通过衍射实验确定的药物结构，都存放在一系列数据库中，如剑桥结构数据库（CSD）、无机结构数据库（ICSD）和晶体学开放数据库（COD）。对于基于蛋白质的处方，蛋白质数据库（PDB）提供了蛋白质分子结构和可能的堆积模式，即四级结构，这在非晶体制剂中是可以实现的。Ayres等[3]介绍了其他来源的可用的化学信息。与产品（制剂）设计相关的药物数据所面临的一个挑战是关键材料的结构信息过时，例如赋形剂分类法[4]。

这些数据库中蕴含的结构化的信息非常适合机器学习方法，其中的数据高度结构化，并且数据库努力遵循FAIR原则：可查找（findable）、可访问（accessible）、可交互（interoperable）和可重复使用（resuable）。这些重要原则使科学家能够轻松地访问数据。从研究人员的角度来看，可视性增加了合作机会，促进了跨学科研究。可交互使研究人员能够将不同来源的数据集结合起来，促进新见解和创新方法的产生。晶体学信息文件（CIF）是一种由国际晶体学联合会定义的非常灵活并且明确的晶体结构数据交换格式，它是晶体学数据交换的标准格式。在化学和生物结构领域有众多的软件支持该格式。用于导入、操作和导出CIF文件的计算机程序库非常丰富（例如PyCifRW，一个开放式的Python库），从而为机器学习提供了一个方便的起点。在许多方面，CIF格式可以作为在制药数据科学领域建立数据存储和交换格式的灵感来源和指南。

当纯药物晶体表现出溶解性差或片剂性差等问题时，形成共晶是提高药物晶体性能的一种有前景的方法。Devogelaer和其合作者[5]对CSD数据库进行了数据挖掘，共研究了9222种共晶，发现了69种经常出现的共形物。根据这些共形物与同其形成共晶体的药物，对这些共形物进行了网络和聚类分析。由此得出的聚类图（见图15-2）可作为共晶药物设计的基础。

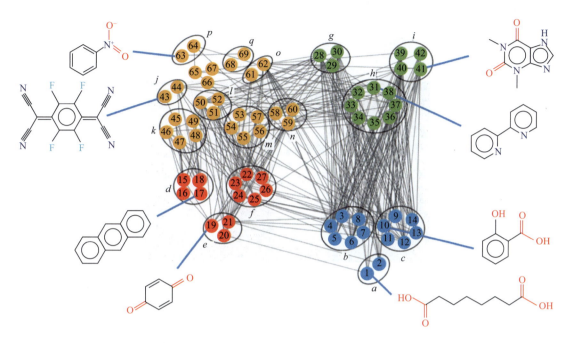

图15-2　CSD数据分析示例：根据与特定药物形成共晶体的倾向性的网络分析，对最常见的共形物进行聚类[5]

15.2.2　模拟

将机器学习与原子级模拟相结合是在自然科学领域中使用ML的一种新兴方法。因为数据可以由计算机生成，而且可以探索更大范围的参数，这种基于模拟的机器学习可以用于快速开发模型，并可能使ML模型具有更好的外推特性。这种方法在制药领域的发展中并不常用，因为计算机信息必须从催化剂、热电、二维材料等其他材料设计领域转化[6,7]。

许多应用于制药科学的分析方法都可以通过计算机模拟来解释。例如，如果已知晶体结构，就可以模拟X射线衍射数据以及紫外光谱、拉曼光谱、红外光谱和固态核磁共振光谱。当分析信号中出现新特征时，模拟就可用于指导解释。也可以通过在模拟数据上训练过的ML模型来指导解释。最近的一个例子就是粉末X射线衍射数据分析。Suzuki等[8]模拟了约200000个粉末的XRD图谱作为训练数据集。为了按照晶体对称性对XRD图谱进行分类，研究人员对几种ML算法进行了测试，后续在实际系统中的应用非常成功。核磁共振数据的处理也可以用ML方法来辅助，最近一种名为DU8ML的方法就应用在了复杂生物碱上[9]。

利用定量构效关系和构性关系（QSAR/QSPR）模型对晶体性质[如溶解度[10]、熔点、油水分配系数（$\log P$）[11]和屏障渗透性（$\log BB$）[12]]进行分类和预测是一个活跃且重要的领域。这种方法使用了化学描述符，如分子式、几何构造和官能团。尽管许多此类模型都取得了一定的成功，但哪些描述符对溶解度和熔点预测最重要仍存在疑问。事实上，这些ML方法可能需要更加全面地描述分子的性质以及其在固态和液态下的相互作用[13]。以晶体结构预测[14]和密度泛函理论形式的高级计算和模拟是有希望产生这种输入的方法，但计算的成本相当高。基于力场的方法计算成本较低，例如蒙特卡洛模拟和MD模拟，已被证明可用于计算晶癖[15]（图15-3）、溶解度[16]和力学性质[17]。当前正是将此类计算与机器学习技术相结合，实现高质量制药材料开发的好时机。

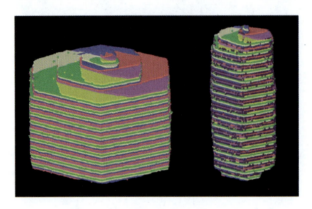

图15-3 加入（右）和未加入（左）影响晶体长宽比的生长调节剂（暗色球体）的L-胱氨酸晶体生长模拟[15]

15.3 产品设计

在产品设计或制剂设计中，传统的工作方式一直依赖于试错实验。此外，在药物制剂领域，人们还经常使用不同的分类方法，如生物药剂学分类（BCS）系统和Lipinski五规则，这些方法主要是经验性分类。这些分类系统旨在评估一种化合物是否有可能作为口服给药发挥作用。然而，据观察，美国食品药品管理局批准的许多药物并不符合Lipinski五规则[18]，并且关于改进BCS分类方法的建议也在反复提出[19-21]。因此，这些传统的分类系统可能还有改进的余地。人工智能可能会对这些传统方法提出挑战，在过去的几十年中，人们已经注意到研究工作正在转向一种比预测和试错试验更系统的方法。

利用实验设计（design of experiments，DoE）方法进行制剂设计的可能性在多年前就有所介绍，然而，这些方法要求在进行分析之前必须进行特定的实验。因此，DoE并不是筛选大量变量以设计新制剂的最佳途径，因为在此过程中所需的实验数量会突然急剧增加。ML提供了无须实验设计数据就能对药物制剂的特性进行 in silico 预测的可能性，这一特性有效地缩短了药物开发的时间，同时还传递了优化信息，克服了药物产品开发中高失败率的困境，提高了产品的一致性，所有这些都将使整个社会受益匪浅。

ML已被证明在设计无定形固体分散体时具有一定优势，因为ML可以用来预测无定形固体分散体的稳定性。研究表明，使用随机森林模型预测无定形固体分散体的稳定性可以达到82%的准确率。随机森林模型还进一步提供了每个处方特征的重要性，这种重要性评估可直接用于设计新的无定形固体分散体。这是因为目前对无定形固体分散体稳定性的实验评估需要3到6个月的时间。如果实验不成功，还需要再进行3到6个月的实验[22]。由此可见，利用ML可以大大缩短药物开发的时间。此外，随机森林模型所提供的每个制剂特征的重要性可以用于确定特定优化需求中最重要的特征，所以也提供了直接途径来优化制剂。通过识别最重要的特征，还可以提高产品的一致性，因为最重要的特征对关键质量属性的影响最大。因此，为了获得产品的一致性，了解并能够控制这些特征是非常重要的。

ML还被用于研究脂质纳米颗粒的药物输送策略。神经网络在阐明数据变量中蕴含的关系方面优于传统的响应面方法，能够更高效地优化脂质纳米颗粒药物处方[23]。

然而，在制剂科学中应用ML还存在一些障碍。这些挑战主要来自必须具有应用于ML知识和处方知识的多学科专业知识。因此，进行分析的个人或研究团队必须同时具备数据科学和制剂科学领域的知识。多年来，物理学、生物学和化学等领域都存在这种对双重领域知识的要求，这些领域和期刊包括计算物理学、计算生物学和计算化学。因此，可以鼓励在药学教育中开设相关课程来应对对ML知识和经验的需求。此外，已经在个人或公共部门工作的专业人员也需要终身学习，以提高他们在ML方面的知识和经验，从而可以从这些数据处理方法中获益。

在药物制剂领域实施ML的另一个障碍是，目前可用的数据集规模较小，并且生成起来既费时又费力。在整个制药领域，数据集从本地实验室创建的单个产品的小型实验数据集到从数据库中提取的患者群体的基因组序列不等（图15-3）。

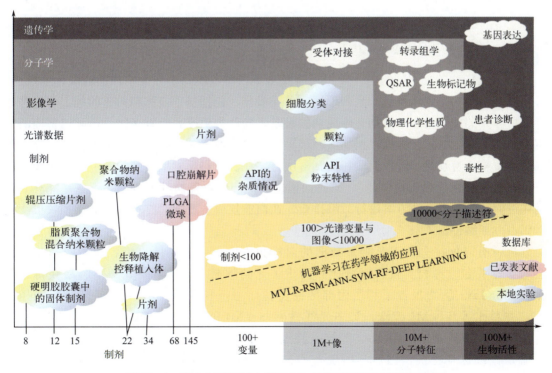

图15-4 整个制药领域中用于ML的数据规模和来源示意图

从图15-4中可以明显看出，ML的应用是随着数据量和数据可用性的增长而增加的，因此ML更适用于患者诊断等领域，而相对并不适用于药物制剂。由于ML可以直接洞察数据中的关系，因此它与分析化学（见第15.5节）密切相关，从图15-4中可以看出，分析化学涵盖了从分子到处方的所有领域。还应该指出的是，几十年来，在分析化学领域，ML一直是以"化学计量学"和"多元数据分析"等术语来描述的，以便读者在文献中进行更深入的搜索。与分析化学的直接联系还强调了ML与制药材料科学（见第15.2节）和药品制造（见第15.4节）都有密切联系，在这两个领域中，分析化学的应用非常广泛，有助于了解材料特性和工艺参数对特定药品关键质量属性的影响。

此外，除了对可用数据的要求外，还要求这些数据应结构化、经过清理和标注，以便于机器阅读。目前，专利和学术出版物中的处方数据没有经过结构化、清理和标注，因此无法进行机器读取。为了利用专利和学术出版物等来源的数据，必须投入大量的工作，因为定量数据通常以数字的形式呈现，只有通过图像分析等方法才能提取出数值。当然，学术出版物和专利从来都不是数据源，而是用来阐明观点、进行讨论和得出结论的。与出版物相关的数据存储库等新举措可能会缓解其中的一些障碍，但如果要从众多论文中合并数据，则可能需要对数据进行大量的结构化处理、清理和标注，例如，必须预见并妥善处理不同论文之间单位变更等障碍。

15.4 药品制造

15.4.1 过程数据和预测模型

药品制造包括各种不同的单元操作，涉及从蛋白质发酵到小分子实体的合成化学反应。活性物质的下游加工也涉及另一系列不同的单元操作，包括基于液体和粉末的加工。这些单元操作所涉及的加工设备通常都是由成熟的设备供应商提供，并配有高级仪器和过程监测与控制选项。所有这些工艺数据，例如实时药品释放测试数据，在制药行业都没有得到充分利用来提高质量。特别是，过程监测和控制解决方案在制药科学领域受到的关注相对较少，这部分开发通常被视为"工程实践"。还应该指出的是，所收集的过程数据并不总是能够充分利用先进的数据分析解决方案进行故障排查。在商业规模生产中，终产品分析和相关批次的放行仍占主导地位。

分析带有时间序列的工艺测量数据的内部数据库可用于支持决策。大型制药公司通常会收集这类包含原材料批次间变化和历史工艺的数据，但学术研究却不容易获得这些数据。Elbadavi等[24]报告了利用内部数据支持熔融沉积建模（FDM）工艺参数选择的情况，并对比了几种ML方法，如多元线性回归（MLR）、K最近邻（KNN）、支持向量机（SVM）、随机森林（RF）、（传统）神经网络（NN）和深度学习（DL）。这项工作的基础是仔细选择特征，然后利用现有的ML Python库预测FDM流程中的打印温度等（图15-5）。

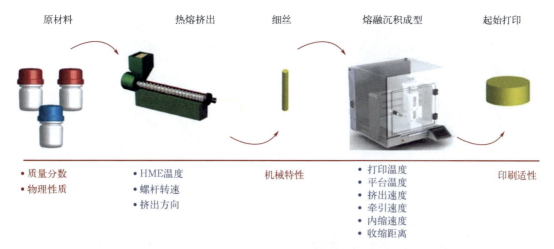

图 15-5 用于收集建立熔融沉积建模（FDM）过程的机器学习模型的变量（蓝色文本）和产品/中间特征（红色字体）的工作流程[24]

15.4.2 作为数据源的过程分析

在制药科学领域，有一些过程工程的先驱范例。Watano 等[25]在 20 世纪 90 年代提出了使用模糊逻辑来控制制粒工艺，其中创新的过程分析技术（PAT）工具和直接过程接口的使用发挥了关键作用。这种基于 PAT 和数据驱动过程控制的理念基本上可用于控制所有与制药相关的单元操作。如《欧洲药典》（*European Pharmacopoeia*）中所规定的那样，有一个明确的监管框架来执行。多变量统计过程控制（MSPC）专著 5.28 提供了这样的一个框架。该专著还强调了 PAT 在实现连续生产和实时释放测试（RTRT）时的重要性。目前已有多种成熟的 PAT 工具，如文献中记载的用于固体制剂下游加工的工具[26, 27]。最常见的 PAT 解决方案之一是近红外光谱（NIR）法，通常涉及光谱数据的多元分析。

PAT 工具可用于收集工艺流中移动物料的细粒度细节。De Beer 研究小组记录了连续运行的双螺杆制粒机中物料特性的可视化（图 15-6）。研究者基于近红外光谱（NIR）成像技术实现了这一过程中活性物质停留时间分布（RTD）的可视化，并描绘了移动颗粒流中的水含量（湿度图）。化学图谱不仅可以观察加工过程中材料化学成分空间位置的变化，还可以监控加工过程中材料的细微变化。近红外光谱和拉曼光谱可用于观察材料固态成分的变化。这种详细程度可将药品生产和新型 RTRT 解决方案的质量提高到一个新的水平。

熟练的工艺操作员通常使用视觉信息来控制制药工艺。例如，在制粒过程中，颗粒的外观可与制粒状态联系起来[29]，同样的，在包衣工艺中，包衣的视觉外观可用于检测工艺终点[30]。要模仿人类流程操作员的视觉观察，需要使用专用的数据科学工具，如支持向量机（SVM）技术。从移动材料中收集时间序列图像数据存在一些挑战。这将增加收集的数据量，并导致对稳健数据存储解决方案的需求增加。处理这类时间序列数据需要高效的数据缩减方法。

然而，对历史过程数据进行更详细的分析可以为特定产品的故障排除提供完全独特的机会。例如，使用 Kohonen 自组织图（SOM）来探索湿法制粒过程的历史过程数据，就证明了这一点[31]。

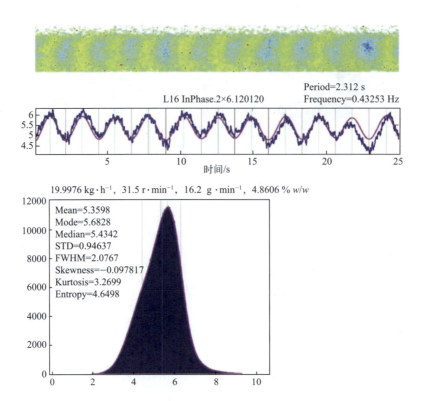

图15-6 基于近红外光谱的双螺杆制粒机颗粒湿度图、平均时间水分曲线和直方图（底部）[28]

15.4.3 与个性化药品生产系统有关的方面

未来的药品将越来越具有个性化，在目前的大规模生产模式下，这是一个挑战。因此，应开发未来的生产系统，使该领域向个性化产品发展。即时诊断和可穿戴传感器可提供患者更精细的健康数据[32]，这些数据可用于开发医药产品的大规模定制模型（图15-7）。人工智能/ML方法对于分析健康数据和指导包含所有这些数字元素的新供应链解决方案至关重要。

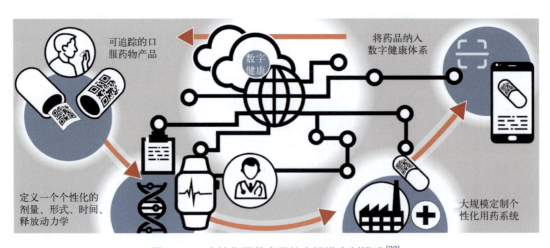

图15-7 个性化医药产品的大规模定制模式[32]

15.5 制药环境中的分析化学

人工智能/ML技术为分析化学领域提供了许多机遇。这与机器学习从多方面推动药物开发过程有关：人们可以利用高端分析工具对剂型进行更精细的分析，从而开发出越来越复杂的给药系统。此外，还可以分析更多的剂量单位，甚至可以在单一剂量单位层面分析个性化产品，并将其与大规模定制方案连接起来。相关的分析实例包括图像分析、振动光谱和质谱分析[3, 33]，以及许多其他分析化学领域。此外，AI/ML方法也长期受到分析化学学会的关注，其期刊包括Journal of Chemometrics、Journal of Chemical Information and Modeling、Chemometrics and Intelligent Laboratory Systems[34]。生物、医学和环境领域的样品基质复杂，需要越来越复杂的仪器和分析方法才能从这些样品中提取相关信息。高通量样品处理和机器人技术也在不断增加可分析的样品数量，这就凸显了高效算法在这一领域的重要性。人工智能/成像技术解决的常见难题包括信噪比低、分析信号重叠、峰值选取以及难以从复杂的分析反应中提取信息。将成像技术与化学图谱相结合，为了解现实生活中的样品开辟了一条全新的途径。然而，基于软件的经典方法可能比较复杂，二维成像（逐像素光谱）和三维成像通常需要特殊的编程经验。

制药科学界熟知的技术，如红外/紫外光谱、粉末衍射、单晶衍射、小角散射和层析成像等，都可以在大型设施如同步加速器和中子散射设施中进行。然而，同步加速器的高通量所提供的空间和时间分辨率要比内部技术高出几个数量级。同步辐射的这些优点提供了非凡的可能性：可以在运行状态下研究药物材料的生产；也可以作为复杂药物递送系统原位研究的一部分，例如作为时间、压力、湿度、温度和pH的函数；并且可以在平衡和非平衡的情况下进行研究。中子可对X射线实验进行补充研究。中子具有非破坏性和批量分析的优势，结合独特的光谱分析和同位素信息，可产生与X射线不同的元素灵敏度。

高时间分辨率和/或超大型探测器意味着同步加速器和中子设施的实验会产生大量数据。基于ML的数据处理和分析可以在实验过程中即时做出决策。事实上，高斯回归已被证明对开发大型设施的自主数据采集算法非常有效[35]。这些方法有利于高通量实验设置，并能更深入地了解相关系统的时间分辨数据。

15.6 总结

人工智能和ML为制药领域的发展提供了巨大的潜力，并将影响我们未来设计制药产品的方式。基于数据科学的方法可以解决这些产品日益个性化的需求。在制药科学领域应用人工智能/移动式人工智能（AI/ML）也存在一定阻碍，这主要与训练此类模型所需的大量数据有关。此外，数据需要结构化和标签化，这本身就可能成为在特定环境中实施人工智能/ML的巨大障碍。建立实验和模拟数据的公共数据库需要被更加重视。有必要在该领域开展更多教育，并从更广泛的意义上将数据科学纳入教学课程。这不仅应在本科教育中进行，还应在博士培训和终身学习计划中进行。为确保人工智能/ML 能够在制药领域中成功应用，将数据科学融入制药科学是学术界、工业界和监管机构的共同任务。

参考文献

[1] Bannigan P, Aldeghi M, Bao Z, et al. Machine learning directed drug formulation development[J]. Advanced Drug Delivery Reviews, 2021, 175: 113806.

[2] Jiang J, Ma X, Ouyang D, et al. Emerging artificial intelligence(AI) technologies used in the development of solid dosage forms[J]. Pharmaceutics, 2022, 14(11): 2257.

[3] Ayres L B, Gomez Federico J V, Linton J R, et al. Taking the leap between analytical chemistry and artificial intelligence: A tutorial review[J]. Analytica Chimica Acta, 2021, 1161: 338403.

[4] Hancock B C, Goldfarb D J. Excipient taxonomy for the 21 st century[J]. Journal of Pharmaceutical Sciences, 2023, 112(3): 626-633.

[5] Devogelaer J J, Meekes H, Vlieg E, et al. Cocrystals in the Cambridge Structural Database: a network approach[J]. Acta Crystallographica Section B, 2019, 75(3): 371-383.

[6] Toyao T, Maeno Z, Takakusagi S, et al. Machine learning for catalysis informatics: Recent applications and prospects[J]. ACS Catalysis, 2020, 10(3): 2260-2297.

[7] Schleder G R, Padilha A C M, Acosta C M, et al. From DFT to machine learning: Recent approaches to materials science–a review[J]. Journal of Physics: Materials, 2019, 2(3): 032001.

[8] Suzuki Y, Hino H, Hawai T, et al. Symmetry prediction and knowledge discovery from X-ray diffraction patterns using an interpretable machine learning approach[J]. Scientific Reports, 2020, 10(1): 21790.

[9] Novitskiy I M, Kutateladze A G. DU8ML: machine learning-augmented density functional theory nuclear magnetic resonance computations for high-throughput in silico solution structure validation and revision of complex alkaloids[J]. The Journal of Organic Chemistry, 2022, 87(7): 4818-4828.

[10] Schroeter T S, et al. Estimating the domain of applicability for machine learning QSAR models: a study on aqueous solubility of drug discovery molecules[J]. Journal of Computer-Aided Molecular Design, 2007, 21(9): 485-498.

[11] Hughes L D, Schwaighofer A, Mika S, et al. Why are some properties more difficult to predict than others？A study of qspr models of solubility, melting point, and log$P$[J]. Journal of Chemical Information and Modeling, 2008, 48(1): 220-232.

[12] Muehlbacher M, Spitzer G M, Liedl K R, et al. Qualitative prediction of blood–brain barrier permeability on a large and refined dataset[J]. Journal of Computer-Aided Molecular Design, 2011, 25(12): 1095-1106.

[13] Xiouras C, Cameli F, Quilló G L, et al. Applications of artificial intelligence and machine learning algorithms to crystallization[J]. Chemical Reviews, 2022, 122(15): 13006-13042.

[14] Reilly, A.M., et al., Report on the sixth blind test of organic crystal structure prediction methods[J]. Acta Crystallographica Section B, 2016. 72(4): 439-459.

[15] Hill A R, Cubillas P, Gebbie-Rayet J T, et al. CrystalGrower: a generic computer program for Monte Carlo modelling of crystal growth[J]. Chemical Science, 2021, 12(3): 1126-1146.

[16] Schnieders M J, Baltrusaitis J, Shi Y, et al. The Structure, thermodynamics and solubility of organic crystals from simulation with a polarizable force field[J]. J Chem Theory Comput, 2012, 8(5): 1721-1736.

[17] Brunsteiner M, Nilsson-Lil S, Morgan L M, et al. Finite-temperature mechanical properties of organic molecular crystals from classical molecular simulation[J]. Crystal Growth & Design, 2023, 23(4): 2155-2168.

[18] Zhang M Q, Wilkinson B. Drug discovery beyond the 'rule-of-five'[J]. Current Opinion in Biotechnology, 2007, 18(6): 478-488.

[19] Fagerholm U. Evaluation and suggested improvements of the biopharmaceutics classification system(BCS)[J]. Journal of Pharmacy and Pharmacology, 2007, 59(6): 751-757.

[20] Larregieu C A, Benet L Z. Distinguishing between the permeability relationships with absorption and metabolism to improve BCS and BDDCS predictions in early drug discovery[J]. Mol Pharm, 2014, 11(4): 1335-1344.

[21] DeGoey D A, Chen H J, Cox P B, et al. Beyond the Rule of 5: Lessons learned from AbbVie's drugs and compound collection[J]. Journal of Medicinal Chemistry, 2018, 61(7): 2636-2651.

[22] Han R, Xiong H, Ye Z, et al. Predicting physical stability of solid dispersions by machine learning techniques[J]. Journal of

Controlled Release, 2019, 311-312: 16-25.

[23] Li Y, Abbaspour M R, Grootendorst P V, et al. Optimization of controlled release nanoparticle formulation of verapamil hydrochloride using artificial neural networks with genetic algorithm and response surface methodology[J]. European Journal of Pharmaceutics and Biopharmaceutics, 2015, 94: 170-179.

[24] Elbadawi M, Castro B M, Gavins F K H, et al. M3DISEEN: A novel machine learning approach for predicting the 3D printability of medicines[J]. International Journal of Pharmaceutics, 2020, 590: 119837.

[25] Watano S, Fukushima T, Miyanami K. Application of fuzzy logic to bed height control in agitation-fluidized bed granulation[J]. Powder Technology, 1994, 81(2): 161-168.

[26] Laske S, Paudel A, Scheibelhofer O, et al. A review of PAT strategies in secondary solid oral dosage manufacturing of small molecules[J]. Journal of Pharmaceutical Sciences, 2017, 106(3): 667-712.

[27] Markl D, Warman M, Dumarey M, et al. Review of real-time release testing of pharmaceutical tablets: State-of-the art, challenges and future perspective[J]. International Journal of Pharmaceutics, 2020, 582: 119353.

[28] Vercruysse J, Toiviainen M, Fonteyne M, et al. Visualization and understanding of the granulation liquid mixing and distribution during continuous twin screw granulation using NIR chemical imaging[J]. European Journal of Pharmaceutics and Biopharmaceutics, 2014, 86(3): 383-392.

[29] Laitinen N, Antikainen O, Rantanen J, et al. New perspectives for visual characterization of pharmaceutical solids[J]. Journal of Pharmaceutical Sciences, 2004, 93(1): 165-176.

[30] Hirschberg C, Edinger M, Holmfred E, et al. Image-based artificial intelligence methods for product control of tablet coating quality[J]. Pharmaceutics, 2020, 12(9): 877.

[31] Rantanen J T, Laine S J, Antikainen O K, et al. Visualization of fluid-bed granulation with self-organizing maps[J]. Journal of Pharmaceutical and Biomedical Analysis, 2001, 24(3): 343-352.

[32] Raijada D, Katarzyna W, Greisen E, et al. Integration of personalized drug delivery systems into digital health[J]. Advanced Drug Delivery Reviews, 2021, 176: 113857.

[33] Debus B, Parastar H, Harrington P, et al. Deep learning in analytical chemistry[J]. TrAC Trends in Analytical Chemistry, 2021, 145: 116459.

[34] Baum Z J, Yu X, Ayala P Y, et al. Artificial intelligence in chemistry: Current trends and future directions[J]. Journal of Chemical Information and Modeling, 2021, 61(7): 3197-3212.

[35] Noack M M, Zwart P H, Ushizima D M, et al. Gaussian processes for autonomous data acquisition at large-scale synchrotron and neutron facilities[J]. Nature Reviews Physics, 2021, 3(10): 685-697.

第16章

生物医药专利大数据分析及应用

徐佳琪　澳门大学，澳门，中国
袁嘉璐　澳门大学，澳门，中国
蔡　鸿　澳门大学，澳门，中国
胡元佳　澳门大学，澳门，中国

16.1 引言

知识产权包括专利权、商标权、著作权。知识产权能够反映一个国家和地区的经济和科学技术的发展水平。新兴技术专利在一定程度上反映了国家生产力和创新技术研发环境和行业现状。适当的知识产权保护有利于科学研究的可持续性，也有助于提高商业投资的驱动力。因此，全世界对知识产权日益关注与重视。

专利文件作为一个巨大的数据源，整合了技术、商业、法律和经济信息，包含结构化数据和非结构化数据各种数据格式。在某一领域的专利数据中，除了可以观察科学研究进展之外，还可以评估及预测其创新前沿趋势。近十年来，全球生物医药行业的专利申请量和申请人量稳步增长。根据《2021年世界知识产权报告》[1]，2020年全球专利申请数量超过320万，这意味着平均每天产生近万份专利申请。因此，专利数据具有海量增长、高速发展的特点。值得注意的是，专利申请流程一般较为完整、规范，保证了数据的真实性。此外，专利信息是一种易于获取的公共资源，保证了数据的可获得性。因此，专利数据具有大数据"5V"（Volume、Value、Velocity、Veracity、Variety）特征。

专利大数据蕴藏着大量的前沿知识，无论从学术角度，还是商业价值都十分值得研究。首先，专利数据有助于了解先进的研究趋势。根据前沿趋势评估产业前景，辅助学术研究及科研成果转化。其次，通过专利数据可以了解目标领域行业内参与者的协作模式和竞争格局，有利于决策调整、风险管理和竞争力提升。第三，目标领域的自由实施（free to operate，FTO）是初步药物发现后进一步可行性研究的关键前提之一，有助于避免重复投资，防范专利侵权风险。因此，蓬勃发展的专利数据具有巨大的潜力，非常值得关注。

16.1.1 专利数据的应用现状

如前所述，专利数据蕴含海量信息，具有大数据特征。然而，专利数据的应用十分有限。首先，主观与客观的数据噪音以及大量未标记数据，导致专利数据处理困难。其次，专利文件通常以非常复杂的形式呈现，涉及跨学科知识，时间跨度一般较长，成文形式又与通用语言有很大不同，造成数据提取困难。此外，光学字符识别（optical character recognition，OCR）和机器翻译使得专利文献中经常出现印刷错误和检索错误。因此，专利文献的实际使用并不常见，很少有专利被学术论文引用。由此产生了专利数据应用现状的矛盾：一方面，专利是学术研究和产品商业化之间不可或缺的桥梁，是先进技术和创新的丰富数据源。另一方面，如上所述，由于数据结构的复杂性和数据处理的困难度，专利数据并未得到充分利用。但显而易见，学术界和工业界均可获益于专利数据的挖掘与研究。因此，建立专利数据挖掘的分析标准和开发相关计算工具是十分必要的。

16.1.2 专利数据在生物医药研究中的应用

由于生物医药研发通常具有高投入、高风险、长周期的特点，知识产权对于创新药物至关重要。美国专利法要求专利说明中必须要包含"最佳实施例"（best mode），即发明人在申请专利时，认为可以实施发明最好的方式。在"最佳实施例"要求下，临床前候选药物

（preclinical candidate，PCC）的关键信息必须包含在相关专利申请文件中，也就是说，PCC将在最初申请专利时即被涵盖在专利内。相比之下，出于商业保护目的的研究论文一般并不会公开PCC的全部信息。因此，有效、合理的生物医药专利数据挖掘，可以揭示不包含在研究论文中的PCC信息，具有启发药物研究和支持决策的潜在价值。此外，还可以利用专利挖掘来避免研究重叠和知识产权侵权。一般来说，在一项技术或候选药物商业化之前，需要进行专利FTO分析。FTO分析可以通过侵权风险和障碍评估来识别专利申请的可操作性。在美国，FTO报告具有法律效力，在一定程度上有助于避免在诉讼中被法院认定为故意侵权而导致赔偿金额的增加。

生物医药专利数据挖掘具有探索技术前沿的潜在价值，可用于行业研究、技术挖掘、FTO分析、PCC预测等方面。然而，生物医药专利内容通常比其他领域的专利更冗长、更复杂。生物医药专利的分析高度依赖于目标领域的专家知识和经验。单个分支领域通常包含成百上千个同族专利。为了保护关键信息，专利申请人会有意识地对专利施加大量人为噪音。根据以往研究经验，数据噪音率可达50%~80%。因此，数据筛选、降噪和技术标引对于数据处理至关重要。越来越多的计算工具和相关算法被开发用于专利的数据挖掘，包括但不限于图论、机器学习、深度学习和自然语言处理（NLP）等。

16.1.3 概念框架

生物医药专利数据挖掘的概念框架包含三个部分：宏观数据分析处理、微观技术挖掘和方法选择。具体内容见图16-1。

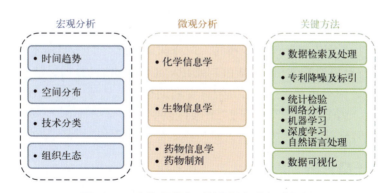

图16-1 生物医药专利数据挖掘的概念框架

左侧蓝色方框为生物医药专利宏观格局分析。中间红框为生物医药专利微观分析，包括化学信息学、生物信息学、药物制剂。右侧绿色框包含生物医药专利分析的关键方法

16.2 专利格局分析

专利格局分析是一种针对专利的综合性分析方法。可大致分为时间、空间、技术、组织生态四个维度。专利分析的标准和指南《专利情况报告准备指南》（Guidelines for Preparing

Patent Landscape Reports）由世界知识产权组织（World Intellectual Property Organization，WIPO）制定[2]。相关论文研究已指出详细标准和专利分析检查清单，如系统评价和荟萃分析的首选报告项目（Systematic Reviews and Meta-Analyses，PRISMA）和专利格局分析的报告项目（Reporting Items for Patent Landscapes，RIPL）[3,4]。例如，标准中提到，专利分析应考虑专利格局的完整性和可靠性，以确保研究的可比性。PRISMA 和 RIPL 中包含 20 多个项目，涵盖了标准研究论文从标题到结论的整个框架结构。通过减少重复性和研究偏差，提供了对专利格局分析进行系统审查的具体方法。这些方法得到了大多数研究人员和学术组织的认可。此外，PRISMA 还提供了流程图，方便研究设计每一步的逻辑判断。2020 年，我国国家知识产权局发布了《专利导航指南》（GB/T 39551—2020），明确了我国专利分析的国家标准。生物医药专利分析的流程见第 6 部分"实务操作及相关问题"（图 16-17）。

16.2.1　数据收集和标准化处理

专利收集应遵循 RIPL 和 PRISMA 标准。该流程图由 PRISMA 提供，用于数据检索。在专利数据库中检索标题、摘要和权利要求时，应包含特定技术或检索目标的正式名称、缩写、派生词和同义词。在研究报告或学术论文中应披露完整的检索词。数据筛选过程中需要有详细的流程图，并披露剔除重复、无关记录的标准，并在专利家族或专利文件中明确指明用于进一步研究的专利。专利文献中经常出现错误、前后不一致和公司名称混乱等现象，因此必须进行数据标准化。在数据分析前对专利权人和发明人姓名进行标准化、专利标引原则标准化，以准确评估某个组织或单个发明人在某一领域的影响力。

RIPL 中详细确定了在标准专利格局分析中应呈现的研究结果。合格的专利格局分析应检查 20 多个列出的项目，包括但不限于清晰且内容丰富的标题、简明扼要表达研究目的和发现的摘要、使用的数据库和涵盖的专利局、选择和排除标准的详细描述、专利家族生成方法的说明[如德温特世界专利索引（DWPI）或 IPADOC 索引]、数据标准化的详细流程、分析说明（如空间或时间分析等）、研究中所有专利的列表（专利号、公开年、摘要等信息）以及研究的局限性。PRISMA 也列出了 27 个项目以供分析结果检查，这些检查项目也应在一个标准的专利格局分析中纳入考量。

16.2.2　文献计量分析

文献计量分析是一种研究大量文献数据的定量方法，涉及数学、统计学、语言学等多个学科。专利格局分析包含基于专利文献的计量分析。通过统计分析以及各种信息的比较和排序，能够揭示目标行业发展的动态特征，展示具有时间趋势的技术演变等。

16.2.3　专利格局分析标准

基于 RIPL 定义的专利格局分析，专利格局应从时间、空间、组织、技术等多个维度建立，旨在提供全方位的专利景观，消除信息不对称，支持相关决策。时间分析包括区位优势、智能定位、分工、溢出效应等。空间分析则涉及特定领域的里程碑、高峰、平台、趋势等。组织生态系统指目标领域内的参与者模式，包括竞争者、合作者、先驱者、领导者、追随者等。技术分类则应通过技术集群、核心技术、边缘技术、交叉技术等方面进行分析。通过专利导航，揭示目标领域的整体发展情况，包括行业模式、利益相关者、潜在的机遇和挑战等。

16.2.3.1 时间-空间分析

专利格局研究的时间分析通常以年份为基础进行。生物医药专利中,产品生命周期及里程碑收集通常能够持续数十年。专利数据时间分析的年份有申请年、公开年和优先权年三种选择。一旦做出选择,年份格式应在研究中保持一致。申请年是指公司或组织向专利局提交申请和投入的年份。然而,由于申请年份存在18个月的延迟公布,使用申请年进行时间分析时,近年的专利数量经常出现下降趋势。这种下降趋势很容易被误认为是近年来某个行业的萧条。专利公开年是指专利公开或被授权的年份。使用公开年进行时间分析时,近年的专利数量不会出现下降趋势。然而,世界各地专利局的专利申请和专利授权之间的时间差距明显不同。此外,无论是已授权的申请还是待审的申请,专利数据中的公布年份都很难解释。优先权年是专利时间分析的第三个选择。优先权年是指最初向某个专利局提交某项专利申请的年份。优先权年对于澄清某项专利作为现有技术与其后申请专利的关系至关重要,特别是当该专利在国内申请之前已通过国际或国外专利局申请时。优先权年的缺点是相关同族专利造成的时间偏差。由于较大的专利家族通常处于长期发展中,优先权年无法反映单项专利的增长情况。如果选择优先年作为时间分析的输入变量,则应在同族专利合并后再使用。在时间分析中,如何选择年份作为输入变量并没有非常严格的限制,在保证输入变量的准确性和一致性的情况下,可根据具体的研究背景和研究目的做出选择。

16.2.3.2 组织生态分析

专利数据组织生态分析包含组织协作和技术引用等相关分析。网络分析是展示组织生态系统的复杂关系和高维度的有效方法。通常有两种应用:发明人或受让人合作网络和专利文件引用网络。发明人或受让人网络揭示了目标领域的主导者、合作者和竞争模式。在大多数情况下,网络节点代表该领域的参与者,而网络中的边代表两个参与者之间的协作。对于引用网络,最简单的引用网络结构由代表专利文献的节点和代表定向引用关系的边构成。基于最简单的专利文件引用网络,可进一步扩展为专利家族或专利权人合作网络。专利合作网络揭示了行业内部组织之间的潜在合作和共同发展关系,而引用网络则显示了特定领域的技术演变。这几类网络都可以作为专利组织生态的展示。

16.2.3.3 技术分类

在大多数生物医药专利研究中,应提供广泛、全面的技术分类,以洞察特定领域的发展趋势和研究热点。技术类别可以通过不同的方法来识别。第一种方法,可使用专利分类代码进行技术分类。专利分类代码一般直接包含在专利文件中,表示特定专利的主要分类,非常容易获取,可以作为技术分类的依据。然而,使用分类代码来比较不同的专利文献是有一定难度的。由于这些分类码是由不同的专利局生成的,通常应用于不同的系统,分类级别多样化,统一起来十分困难。因此,在大多数情况下,通常采用第二种方法,即人工手动进行专利的技术分类。根据专家意见以及对主题行业的理解,从主观角度对专利技术进行分类。基于这种方法,技术分类依赖于人工识别,所有入选的专利文件都需要人工单独逐个阅读,然后人工识别和总结出关键信息。手动方法将大大提高类别分组的完整性和准确性,但这项工作非常耗时且费力,特别是进行大型专利数据集的分析。

第三种方法是近年来日益发展起来的半自动或全自动分类方法。这种方法是随着人工智能的发展而逐渐可行并被具体化、任务化。专利类别分组任务中涉及机器学习、深度学习和文本挖掘等方法。该方法更省时、省力，但可能不如手动方法精确、灵活。此外，这些计算模型需要进行修正和迭代，以满足各种个性化的分析应用场景。

技术分类的另一个需要考虑的问题是单个专利应归属于唯一的类别还是可以归属于多个不同类别。事实上只要技术映射完全清晰，这两种情况都是可以接受的。如果一项专利只能归入单一类别，则应明确专利的研究重点。如果一项专利可归属于多个类别，则应清楚地说明类别之间的关系，清晰地描述和可视化类别间的交互作用。例如，一项关于siRNA递送系统的专利格局分析采用了弦图进行类别间相互作用的可视化，完整地呈现了类别间的关系和交互作用[5]。

16.2.4 专利检索数据库

16.2.4.1 PATENTSCOPE数据库

PATENTSCOPE数据库是WIPO开发的免费专利数据库，拥有来自73个国家和地区专利局的约1.25亿条记录。PATENTSCOPE数据库将专利文件分为不同的部分，包括专利标题、描述、权利要求、专利家族和附图（通常包含示例中的实验结果）等。PATENTSCOPE数据库的界面非常简洁，使用起来十分便利。全文及补充材料汇总为PDF格式，可实现一键下载。PATENTSCOPE数据库还可用于搜索化学结构[6]，数据库中已包含从专利文本中识别出的化合物名称和文本附图中嵌入的化学结构。用户可以上传、绘制结构，或将输入的结构转换为化合物名称、商业名称或通用名称。可以针对确切的结构进行检索，也可通过使用"Search Scaffold"选项搜索分子的基本骨架来进行结构检索。检索范围包括专利的标题、摘要、权利要求和描述字段，数据库涵盖国际专利申请（patent cooperation treaty，PCT）（自1978年起）以及美国、英国、德国等多个国家的专利（自1979年起）。结果以列表形式呈现，并且可以显示检索结果中的化学结构。分析功能还能够对结果进行排序，例如按发明人或申请人排序，提供一些基本的专利信息等。结构检索可与其他检索功能相结合，例如结构检索结合分类代码或关键字检索。还可以搜索特定专利中的全部结构。一旦找到专利，可以分别查看说明书和权利要求中的化学结构，并提供定位功能，查找该结构在专利中的具体位置。更重要的是，PATENTSCOPE数据库中提供了所有可能的马库什结构，所有结构都会自动集成并枚举到数据库中。PATENTSCOPE数据库中化学结构检索使用起来简单直观，为研究人员提供了有用的开源数据来识别潜在的相关专利。

16.2.4.2 FreePatentsOnline数据库

FreePatentsOnline数据库由Patents Online LLC开发。该数据的特点是首页的专利按照行业进行分类，每个行业又分为若干子行业。还支持按专利号快速搜索。专利内容显示在单个页面上。适用于对目标行业有一定了解后精准查找相关专利的需求。

16.2.4.3 Lens数据库

Lens数据库由独立非营利机构Cambia开发，包含来自106个国家和地区的超过1.38亿条专利记录,可免费访问并进行研究。除了重点介绍专利的基本信息,如标题、摘要、权利要求和描述之外,Lens数据库还额外提供专利中生物信息检索,包括专利中的生物序列,如核苷和蛋白质序列等。序列被格式化为FASTA文件。数据库操作界面简洁友好,通过在快速检索中输入专利号,专利信息会被分类到不同的信息标签中,非常便于查找。

16.2.4.4 德温特世界专利索引(Derwent Innovation Index,DI)数据库

DI数据库涵盖来自59个国家和地区的超过1400万项专利。作为商业数据库,DI以英语为基本语言提供独有的专利改写功能,对专利的标题、摘要等进行自动和手动改写,以提高用户专利阅读、数据筛选和标引的效率。专利信息可以Excel文件形式下载,并按文档的组成进行个性化分隔,实现分批下载。

16.2.4.5 IncoPat数据库

IncoPat数据库是由北京INCOPAT有限公司开发的商业数据库。该数据库涵盖来自157个机构的超过1.2亿件专利文件。IncoPat数据库以中国用户为中心,引入中文DWPI数据,提供DWPI信息的机器翻译,并支持全数据库范围的全球专利中文检索,以提高中国用户的专利阅读速度和使用体验。

16.3 从专利数据中挖掘化学信息

科技的进步使研究人员能够更方便、更快捷、更高效地获取世界各地的科学数据、方法和成果。对于化学家来说,获取化合物的最新信息非常重要。专利的特点是信息更及时、更可靠、更全面,具有可合成特性和靶向特异性的关键活性候选分子只有在专利中才会公开。平均而言,一个新化合物出现在专利中的时间要比出现在科学文献中的时间早2~3年[7]。只有6%的专利生物活性化合物能在文献中找到[8]。因此,化学专利是化学家非常重要的信息来源。

16.3.1 专利中的化学信息

化学专利通常包含两类化学信息。第一类是用于描述化学物质、化学反应、化合物性质、实验数据等的文字。由于缺乏标准化的命名规定,化合物的文字表述千差万别,容易引起歧义和法律纠纷。因此,专利中还加入了第二类信息,即化学结构的图像,以准确表示化学物质的具体结构。

16.3.1.1 化学命名实体

化学专利中基于文本信息的学术表达是化学命名实体。命名实体是指用名称标识的实体,在化学专利中则指化学物质等化学实体。具体来说,包括化学物质(化合物、化学元素、试剂或反应、溶剂)、化学反应、化合物性质和实验数据、化学形容词及其他(如化学族名称等)[9]。

16.3.1.2　化学结构图像

专利中的化学结构图像通常包括两类。第一类是受专利保护的化学结构，包括以下内容：

① 具体实施方式，也称为"最佳模式"：要求申请人必须在说明书中公开发明人在提交化学专利申请时已知的实施发明的最佳模式或最佳方法。化合物专利中的"最佳模式"是指一种或多种特定的化学结构。

② 马库什结构：这是一种化学结构表示法，用于表示一组相关的化合物。马库什结构描述了多个独立的可变基团，如R基团，其中一个侧链可以有不同的结构[10]。

第二类是非专利保护结构，通常是反应物、试剂、中间体、取代基团等。它们用于描述受保护分子的制备过程或受保护非专利结构中的可变取代基，是对受专利保护的实体的说明和描述。

16.3.2　化学信息数据挖掘方法

专利中两种不同类型的化学信息（化学命名实体、化学结构图像）有不同的挖掘方法和工具。挖掘化学命名实体的方法是文本挖掘中命名实体识别（named entity recognition，NER）中的分支化学命名实体识别（chemical named entity recognition，CNER）。挖掘化学结构图像的方法是基于光学字符识别（OCR）的光学化学结构识别（optical chemical structure recognition，OCSR）。

16.3.2.1　化学命名实体识别（CNER）

目前已开发出多种CNER方法，可分为四种类型：基于词典的系统、基于规则的系统、基于统计的系统和同时使用多种方法的组合系统。

① 基于词典的系统：词典是特定领域的词汇集合。基于词典的系统使用词典中的术语列表来识别文本中出现的实体。识别分为精确匹配和近似匹配。精确匹配是从给定的术语列表中根据文本对同义词进行精确的文本搜索。而近似匹配则不要求给定术语与文本完全匹配，而是执行模糊匹配，允许插入、删除或替换某些字符。大多数基于词典的CNER方法都使用近似匹配。Hettne等[11]结合了来自UMLS、MeSH、ChEBI、DrugBank、KEGG、HMDB和ChemIDplus的信息，编制了一本词典，用于识别文本中的小分子和药物。

② 基于规则的系统：使用人类开发的规则来提取实体名称。该模型由一组使用句法和语法规则的规则组成，通常与词典相结合。规则分为基于上下文的规则和基于模式的规则（单词拼写或形态模式）。基于上下文的规则的一个例子是"如果一个专有名词跟在一个人的头衔后面，那么专有名词就是一个人的名字"[12]。例如，Narayanaswamy等[13]不仅成功地根据一套人工制定的规则识别了化学物质，还提高了蛋白质名称检测的准确性。

③ 基于统计的系统：使用统计模型来识别特定的实体名称。通过使用注释过的高质量文档，基于数据的特征表示可以创建一个可通用的统计模型。最流行的统计方法是机器学习监督学习模型，如条件随机场（conditional random field，CRF），以及隐式标记模型和最大熵马尔可夫模型。Leaman等[14]利用BioCreative V的化合物和药物名称识别（CHEMDNER）任务提供的语料库，结合集合学习和CRF算法，描述了一个针对专利的CNER系统，其精

确度为0.8752，召回率为0.9129，F值为0.8937，取得了BioCreative Ⅴ任务中的最高性能。

④ 组合系统：实施一种以上的命名实体识别（NER）方法，以利用每种方法的优点。在CNER中，基于词典的系统通常与基于规则或机器学习的系统相结合，以提高性能。Zhang等[15]描述了一种高性能的复合CNER系统，该系统将基于规则的系统与基于机器学习的系统相结合，在BioCreative Ⅴ的CHEMDNER化学实体标注识别（CEMP）任务的21个参赛团队中，以87.18%的准确率、90.78%的召回率和88.94%的F值获得了第二名的成绩。

单独使用三种独立方法（基于词典、基于规则和基于统计）并不能达到最佳性能。基于词典的系统可以解决命名实体规范化的问题，但在识别新实体方面存在困难。对于专利中的化学实体识别，基于词典的系统通常召回率低、性能差；基于规则的系统可以弥补一些不足，通常与词典结合使用。然而，对于这两种方法来说，手动构建词典和设置规则都是耗时耗力的工作，需要依赖领域专家的知识，维护成本高昂。基于统计的系统，如机器学习或深度学习方法，可以识别新实体，也更易于维护和移植。与前两种方法相比，它们的性能也更好，已成为主流方法。不过，基于统计的系统需要足够大且有注释的语料库来训练模型，而模型的好坏直接取决于注释语料库的质量。对于专利化学实体识别而言，只有少量高质量的注释语料可供公众使用[16]。这三种方法的组合系统可以取长补短，有效提高CNER系统的性能。这就是为什么当今几乎所有新开发的高性能CNER系统都是基于机器学习或深度学习模型，并结合基于词典和规则的系统。

与化学文献相比，专利更为复杂，注释难度更大；因此，为专利开发CNER系统的难度也更大。因此，专门用于专利的CNER工具数量有限。ChemCurator是一款CNER工具，它结合了文本挖掘、结构处理和马库什技术，可识别和突出显示文档中的化学结构。ChemCurator可识别和突出显示各种文档中的化学信息，帮助查找相关数据，并可从本地文件或直接从Google Patents或IFI Claims中导入文档。

16.3.2.2 光学化学结构识别（OCSR）

光学化学结构识别（OCSR）旨在将化学结构图像转化为计算机可读的表示形式。光学化学结构识别方法可分为两类：基于规则的系统和基于统计的系统。

① 基于规则的系统：基于规则的系统试图模仿人类的感知模型，在光学化学结构识别中，人类的感知模型可以检测字符和形状，理解线条连接，并根据给定的分析构建公式。大多数基于规则的系统都遵循一个重构模型，该模型可识别原子和键线、图像矢量化以及连接表或图形。OCSR的识别过程可归纳如下：a.识别图片中节点（化学元素符号）的位置和类型以及连接线（化学键）的位置和类型；b.重建连接表，也可称为分子图；c.将重建的连接表转换为计算机可读格式（SMILES、InChI等）。1992年，第一个OCSR工具Kekulé发布[17]，Kekulé使用用户提供的扫描图像并将其矢量化。Kekulé使用基于规则的方法生成连接表，并有一个图形用户界面来检查和编辑结果。2009年，首个开源OCSR工具OSRA发布[18]。

② 基于统计的系统：基于统计的系统分为基于机器学习的系统和基于深度学习的系统。基于机器学习的系统，如ChemOCR[19]需要人工设计特征和训练模型，而基于深度学习的系统，如Chemgrapher[20]，可以自动提取特征并完成映射。与CNER不同，深度学习模型比机器学习模型更适合OSCR领域；因此，目前几乎所有主流方法和工具都是基于深度学习的系统。

基于规则的系统被用来主导OCSR，但它们有其局限性：a.化学规则多种多样，无法保证规则集的全面性；b.基于规则的系统对复杂、模糊、低质量图像的识别能力较差；c.基于规则的系统对噪声更敏感，极易误导识别结果。机器学习和深度学习已经取代了基于规则的系统，并取得了更高的性能。但是，这种系统依赖于训练数据，模型的结果取决于训练数据，因此仍然存在缺陷：a.对分辨率比较敏感，如果用高分辨率图像进行训练，模型对低分辨率图像的识别效果不佳；b.对超原子和复杂元素的识别比较困难。

16.3.2.3　化学信息专利数据挖掘面临的挑战

① CNER 和 OCSR 两种方法难以结合：化学专利包含两类化学信息，即文本和图像，但识别这两类信息涉及两个不同的信息挖掘领域。因此，更需要一种能够挖掘和关联两种类型化学信息的方法或工具。2020年发布的化学示意图解析器（ChemSchematicResolver）[21]，将文本挖掘与 OCSR 结合起来，从印刷文献中检索所有可能的信息。自动数据库生成和管理领域的一个主要问题是 OCSR 工具挖掘的信息与相应名称之间缺乏链条。ChemSchematicResolver 是第一个解决这一问题的工具，它以无监督的方式实现了大规模的信息挖掘。

② 专利中的马库什结构识别困难：马库什结构中可变取代基的复杂性给其检索和识别带来了困难。同时，专利中马库什结构的绘制方式不规则、缺乏开放获取的数据集以及传统算法的低效率也限制了马库什结构识别相关研究的发展。Wang 等[22]开发了一种基于多模态学习的文本和图像化学信息重构系统，实现了快速高效的马库什结构识别及其可变取代基文本的信息重构任务，进而自动提取专利中的化学分子结构。该方法是目前唯一快速高效的马库什结构图像识别系统。

③ 缺乏开放和开源工具：大多数都没有在任何可用工具中实现，只是在几篇公开发表的研究论文中描述了研究者开发的一些算法或将其作为原型。这是该领域潜力的巨大损失。公开的工具通常是商业软件，没有解释其算法和性能。ChemSchematicResolver 是第一个将文本挖掘与 OCSR 结合在一起的工具，它是在 OSRA 公开源代码的基础上开发的。

④ 仅限于识别化合物：大多数工具都忽略了专利中的基本数据，如化合物的物理化学性质和实验活性。新合成化合物的实验数据会在专利中公开，具有相当的研究和战略价值。然而，现有的专利化学信息挖掘手段（命名体识别或结构图识别）无法实现化学实体与其相关数据的关联功能。获取相关数据仍然需要人工提取。

16.3.3　专利化学信息数据库

16.3.3.1　Scifinder

Scifinder 是一个功能强大的工具，可从专利文件中提供多种格式的化学结构。只需输入专利号，就可以根据商业可用性、反应作用等过滤相关结构，然后以 PDF、Excel、Rich Text 和 SDF 文件格式下载。

16.3.3.2　SureChEMBL

SureChEMBL[23]是一个公开的大规模资源，包含从专利文件的全文、图像和附件中提取的化合物。SureChEMBL 基于自动文本和图像挖掘流程每天从专利文件中提取数据，可访问以前无法获得的、开放的和及时注释的化合物-专利关联集，并具有针对化合物库和专利文件库的完善的组合结构和基于关键字的搜索功能。该数据库目前包含从1400万份专利文件中提取的1700万个化合物。

16.3.3.3 中科院PatentPak数据库

中科院PatentPak数据库提供来自全球46个主要专利局的约1800万项可检索的专利全文。CAS科学家对重要的化学成分进行了注释，并可查看注释专利，以快速识别最重要的信息。符合CAS REFERENCES选择标准的九个主要专利局的所有专利记录均可在发布后两天内在线查阅，并在发布之日起不到27天内由CAS科学家编制完整索引。

16.3.4 常用OCSR工具比较

近年来，一些基于深度学习的OCSR因其优异的性能和用户友好性得到了广泛应用，下面将列举四款流行的OCSR工具，分别是Stonemind、InDraw、KingDraw、Img2Chem。这四款软件均免费供用户使用，并提供截图识别功能。为了测试这四款软件的能力，收集了100个化学结构图。其中，InDraw的准确率最高，90%以上的化学结构图都被完整正确地识别出来；Img2Chem和Stonemind的准确率都在60%左右，而KingDraw只有45%。

InDraw在识别复杂分子结构方面的表现远远超过其他三款软件，而且可以直接将图像粘贴到识别框中，无须上传。只有InDraw和KingDraw有完整的化学结构编辑选项，而Stonemind和Img2Chem只有最基本的简单选项。Stonemind具有批量识别功能，可以直接提取整个文档中的所有化合物，但鉴于识别准确率较低，批量识别后可能需要花费大量精力修正识别结果。

16.4 从专利数据中挖掘生物信息

数据的来源、分析工具和方法的选择以及对于最终结果的呈现方式，这些都是分析专利中所包含的生物序列的重要环节。本章节将根据专利中生物序列分析的基本流程，对上述内容进行介绍、补充和拓展。

16.4.1 专利中的生物信息

自21世纪以来，公开的生物序列数量正在逐年飞速增长。目前，全球约有数以亿计的生物序列。根据有关数据统计显示[24]，仅GenBank数据库，收录其中的生物序列数量大约每18个月就会增长一倍。这些海量的序列中有相当一部分来自专利。而专利中这些庞大的生物序列，包含了多种天然或人为干预的生物学信息。特别是在生物医疗领域，这些相关专利的生物序列往往还传递着生物药物的特性、选择和修饰，基因工程或蛋白质工程，治疗的靶标等信息。但是，这些信息琐碎冗杂，埋藏在无尽的专利数据之中。比起应用于传统的专利格局分析的方法，面对专利中含有的生物序列信息的分析方法要少得多。因此，如何挖掘并利用专利中有用的生物序列信息是一个崭新的分析问题的视角。

16.4.2 生物序列专利挖掘方法

16.4.2.1 BLAST序列分析工具

BLAST是生物信息学中最常用的序列分析工具。其算法是由Altschul等[25, 26]于1990年提出的一种双序列局部比对算法，这种算法既能保证较高的准确性，又能保证较快的计算速度。BLAST可以将查询序列与数据库中的序列进行快速序列比对，找出与查询序列相似的目标序列。而这些相似的序列可能已经有相关基因注释储存在数据库中，根据这些信息可以推断查询序列可能的功能信息。

BLAST包含一系列程序，可以基于不同的序列比对目的进行选择。比较常见的程序包括MegaBLAST、BLASTn、BLASTp、BLASTx、tBLASTn和tBLASTx。这些程序可以有效地帮助用户进行核酸序列之间的比对、蛋白质序列之间的比对以及核酸序列与蛋白质序列之间的比对[27, 28, 29]。其中，BLASTn和BLASTp是BLAST中最为常见和基础的功能，可分别帮助用户进行核苷酸序列之间和蛋白质序列之间的比较。BLASTx（核酸序列vs.蛋白质数据库）、tBLASTn（蛋白质序列vs.核酸数据库）和tBLASTx（核酸序列vs.核酸数据库）都涉及了将核酸序列翻译成蛋白质序列，这一过程会产生六条可能的蛋白质序列，然后将它们逐一进行比对并产生结果。而tBLASTx是BLAST中速度最慢的一种比对方式，查询序列和比对序列会被分别翻译成蛋白质序列。换句话说，每个序列要比对36次。更具体的程序和功能可参见NCBI的《BLAST用户手册》，根据自己的具体需要选择程序[27, 28, 29]。一般来说，BLAST程序为了能够更快地得到结果，会在准确性上做出一定的妥协，这可能会遗漏那些相似度较低的序列。因此，如果对序列有这方面的需求，可以选择PSI-BLAST程序。

BLAST提供多种搜索方法[27, 28, 29]。最快捷的方法是在NCBI BLAST上进行线上检索。线上使用BLAST的方法非常简便，无须注册。同时，BLAST也提供独立应用程序，对于那些计算资源充足，能够熟练掌握BLAST技能的用户来说，可以选择该方式进行检索。而需要进行多次检索或编写检索脚本的用户可以选择BLAST+远程服务。其他搜索选项可参见NCBI的BLAST手册和视频教程[30]。

除了BLAST以外，EBI提供的FASTA工具和UCSC Genome Browser（由University of California Santa Cruz创建）提供的BLAT工具也是常用的序列比对工具。FASTA算法最早由Pearson和Lipman[31]于1988年提出，主要针对蛋白质序列DNA序列之间的比对，经过多年以来的发展，FASTA包括FASTA、FASTAX、FASTAY、SSEARCH、GGSEARCH和GLSEARCH一系列程序，可以实现在DNA序列之间、蛋白质序列之间以及DNA和蛋白质序列之间的全局或局部比对策略[32]。同样地，EBI也在其网站中提供了FASTA工具的使用指南。

BLAT工具由James Kent[33]于2002年推出，意为BLAST类似比对工具。BLAT在功能上确实与BLAST有许多相似之处，但BLAT主要针对脊椎动物基因组中mRNA、DNA以及蛋白质之间的序列比对。它不能像BLAST那样找到较远的同源关系延伸，但比BLAST的反应时间更短。BLAT还经常被研究人员用来查找序列在基因组中的位置或确定mRNA的外显子结构[33, 34]。

另外，还有一些序列比对工具如针对多序列比对的Clustal Omega、ClustalW/ClustalX，用于双序列比对的Needle（EMBOSS）等，让使用者可以根据自己的需要选择合适的比对工具。

16.4.2.2　生物序列分析

生物序列十分多样，携带着遗传信息，是生物调节生理活动、完成生命活动不可缺少的物质基础。随着时代的发展，人们对蛋白组学、基因组学等学科研究的进一步深入，生物药在临床应用中逐渐发展，专利数量也相应迎来快速增长，这些专利中包含的生物序列无疑是一个潜在的宝库[35]。然而，从这些海量的生物信息中提取出有意义的结论是一个重大的挑战，需要进一步讨论如何标准化和处理数据冗余的问题[36, 37]。

分析专利中生物序列的核心思路基于以下步骤[38, 39]：首先，选取多个数据库进行原始数据的检索。其次，将获得的专利中的生物序列分离提取。然后，统一格式，分析宏观上的发展变化规律，再利用分析工具进行序列比对，描述序列之间的共性与差异。最后，归纳总结其在宏观和微观上的发展变化，利用图表等可视化手段对结果进行呈现。其最终得到的结论可以为医药行业内的相关从业人士提供信息上的支持与帮助。

然而，不同国家地区的专利政策，审评标准，公开信息原则，序列数据的可及性、标准化以及庞大的数据冗杂一直是干扰数据分析难题[40, 41, 42]。在检索了Web of Science、Scopus和ScienceDirect三个数据库后发现，目前相关的文献研究主要集中在那些含有专利中生物序列数据库的介绍、对比或搭建上，对于真正专利中生物序列的分析案例并不多。尽管如此，我们依然找到了一个有关方面较为完善的研究进行介绍与讨论（见15.4.4节专利中抗体序列数据挖掘—案例介绍）。这个案例让人们看到了专利中生物序列分析的具体操作的可行性，具有很大的参考价值[38]。

16.4.2.3　蛋白质结构

专利中的生物信息不仅包括基本核苷酸和氨基酸序列，还包括其他生物信息，如结构基因组学等。蛋白质结构与结构基因组学相关，是推断蛋白质功能的重要信息，在药物研发中有着宝贵的应用价值[43]。如果能在生物序列分析的基础上进一步整合和分析蛋白质结构信息，那么可以合理推断，人们可以从分子工程学的角度来挖掘出一些工程信息。然而，该领域的专利分析研究较少，存在一定的问题和困难。因此，本节将主要讨论以下几个方面：三维蛋白质结构的可专利性、专利局达成的共识、难点和建议。

蛋白质复杂多样的分子结构一直是研究人员研究的重点内容之一。然而，蛋白质分子结构的科研成本十分高昂，很少有大型制药公司进行蛋白质结构研究或基于结构的药物开发，更倾向于依靠现有的结构信息和试验来发现能激活或抑制目标蛋白质的化合物[44]。因此，蛋白质分子结构具有巨大的商业价值潜力。然而，就目前而言，蛋白质的3D结构专利仍是学术界争论的话题。在2004年，欧洲专利局（European Patent Office，EPO）、日本专利局（Japan Patent Office，JPO）和美国专利商标局（United States Patent and Trademark Office，USPTO）的领导人参加了一次三方会议，对蛋白质三维结构相关的权利要求进行了讨论，并达成了一定程度的共识[45]。有研究人员归纳总结了三个专利局在蛋白质三维结构和与之相关的权利要求的可专利性方面的基本相同点[46]。总的来说，三个专利局的观点是：蛋白质的计算机模型、蛋白质原子坐标的数据阵列、以蛋白质原子坐标编码的计算机可读存储介质、包括化合物名称和结构在内的数据编码的数据库以及药典的权利要求都不具有专利资格或成为法定发明。理由是上述内容只是信息或抽象概念的展示,没有得到实际的应用[45, 46]。但值得注意的是,三个专利局都认为蛋白质的结晶形式和由部分具有信号活性的蛋白质组成的分离和纯化的多肽符合专利申请的所有要求。

此外,虽然仅蛋白质三维结构以及空间坐标不能直接申请专利保护,但仍可作为其他专利申请的必要信息[43, 46, 47]。比如关于In-silico筛选方法的专利申请,其创造性是对整个发明进行评估的,包括蛋白质三维结构坐标数据本身。欧洲专利局认为,如果蛋白质三维结构坐标数据具有创新性,那么该方法就满足了新颖性和创造性的要求,但这一立场与美国专利商标局和日本专利局有所差异[46]。还有观点认为[47],在适当的情况下,可以通过将数据集与特定物理结构或用途联系起来,间接保护蛋白质或蛋白质的部分三维结构。比如当三维结构数据集包含在计算机可读存储器中,或当三维结构被证明可确定其作为激动剂或拮抗剂的类似物时,蛋白质的三维结构就可以获得保护[47]。不过,蛋白质结构目前还没有直接获得专利保护,这对于公司的研究和开发是相对不利的。

然而,一项美国专利(专利号:US6329184)为任何具有特定坐标集的结晶形式提供了保护。该专利对哺乳动物蛋白质抗酒石酸磷酸酶(tar-resistant purple acid phosphatase,TRAP)的结晶形式提出了权利要求,其中带有坐标的结晶形式已在专利申请中进行了描述[48]。该权利要求不受晶体获得方式的限制,并为任何具有这些坐标的哺乳动物TRAP提供了保护。这说明在蛋白质三维结构方面,不同国家地区之间的专利保护的差异是巨大的,这个例子也可对未来相关专利申请带来一定启发[43]。

综上所述,尽管蛋白质结构信息的重要性毋庸置疑,但与之相关的授权专利却较为有限。不过越来越多的个人或机构正在努力推进这种信息的专利化。如果一项发明具有足够的新颖性,那么用专利来保护与其结构信息相关的发明会变得更加可行[43, 46, 49]。对于那些有意申请蛋白质三维结构专利保护的申请者来说,从三维结构坐标的特异性变化、结构分析以及功能与结构之间可能存在的对应关系入手,提供足够的成为合理药物设计目标的特定化合物的信息,并使结构信息在现实世界中可用,可以帮助该蛋白质结构在申请处于更有利的地位[49]。

与所有新技术一样,蛋白质三维结构的专利保护问题不是一蹴而就的,需要坚持不懈地努力,才能在法律和科学理论之间找到更加合适的平衡点。而获得这种保护是非常有必要的,因为蛋白质结构的信息非常宝贵,它可以帮助研究人员更好地理解蛋白质工程和药物设计的原理。此外,尽管各国在专利保护方面的举措和审查标准较为相似,但仍可以看出不同国家地区在专利审评细节上的不同。因此,任何对专利申请感兴趣的人都应了解这些差异,合理安排产品专利的布局。

16.4.3 专利生物信息数据库

生物信息学领域的数据库种类繁多,其分类方式也各有不同。可以按照数据提供者分为公共数据库和商业数据库,或者按照数据处理和存储内容分为一级数据库和二级数据库。此外,还可以依据数据类型的不同进行分类,如序列数据库、结构数据库、文献数据库等[50]。其中,核酸数据库和蛋白质数据库是序列分析的主要数据来源。此外,与蛋白质数据库相比,大型公共核酸数据库有着更多的国际组织合作,数据覆盖面更加广泛。因此,在专利序列分析中，选择公共核酸数据库或在此基础上进行氨基酸翻译是使数据覆盖面更加全面合理的方法之一。下文将主要介绍几个知名的公共核酸数据库及相关的国际合作。

16.4.3.1　国际核苷酸序列数据库协作（International Nucleotide Sequence Database Collaboration，INSDC）

国际核苷酸序列数据库合作组织（INSDC）[51]至今已有三十多年的历史，是收集和提供核苷酸序列数据和元数据的核心基础设施。该组织的成员包括NCBI的GenBank、EMBL欧洲生物信息研究所（EMBL-EBI）的欧洲核酸数据库（ENA）和日本DNA数据库（DDBJ）[51, 52]。核酸序列数据在合作成员之间实现了交流与共享，并且可以同步更新。除此之外，这些成员还会组织年度会议，以确保数据标准、格式和注释的质量，为生物信息领域做出了重大的贡献[51, 52]。

16.4.3.2　美国国家生物技术信息中心（National Center for Biotechnology Information，NCBI）

NCBI成立于1988年11月，是世界上最大的生物信息学数据库之一，为众多国家和地区的科研人员和组织机构提供信息资源，在基因组织、序列分析和结构预测等方面做出了重大的贡献。NCBI创建并维护了许多不同的生物数据库，包括GenBank、RefSeq和PubMed OMIM[53, 54]。

GenBank主要用于分析专利中的生物序列。NCBI于1992年10月开始负责GenBank数据库，并将美国专利商标局存储的专利序列纳入GenBank管理[55]。目前，GenBank已发展成为一个收纳所有公开DNA序列的注释集的基因序列数据库[56]，并与前面提到的其他INSDC成员数据库交换数据。此外，GenBank每两个月发布一个版本[54]。

16.4.3.3　EMBL欧洲生物信息研究所（EMBL's European Bioinformatics Institute，EMBL-EBI）

EMBL-EBI于1994年9月在英国成立，其数据涵盖包括核苷酸、小分子、蛋白质和蛋白质结构等一系列不同类型的数据资源，是世界上最全面的分子数据库[57]。EBI拥有强大的数据资源管理、维护、研究和开发团队，用以维护数据库，开发新算法，并专注于生命科学和序列分析等多个领域。EMBL-EBI建立并维护了一系列生物信息学数据库，包括ENA和UniProt等[58]。

ENA是该领域使用的主要数据库，该数据库与其他INSDC成员共享数据，为相关领域的从业人员提供世界核苷酸序列信息的全面记录，涵盖原始序列数据、序列信息和功能注释。

16.4.3.4　日本DNA数据库（DNA Data Bank of Japan，DDBJ）

DDBJ于1987年开始正式运营，同属于INSDC的成员。DDBJ拥有的科研团队专注于利用计算机推动和发展生命科学等领域，通过INSDC实现在全球范围内的数据共享，极大地丰富了可供人们使用的生物信息学数据资源[59]。它也包含了许多生物信息领域的数据库，如DDBJ、BioSample和BioProject。我们将在16.6.3.3节中介绍DDBJ数据库以及与其他

INSDC 成员共享的数据。

16.4.3.5　美国专利商标局（United States Patent and Trademark Office，USPTO）

USPTO 成立于 1802 年，是授予美国专利和注册商标的联邦机构，旨在促进对知识产权的尊重，并在全球范围内推动更有效的知识产权保护[60]。美国专利商标局还提供多种专利信息资源。而在分析专利序列时，主要会用到以下两个数据库：Publication Site for Issued and Published Sequences（PSIPS）和 Patent full-text Databases（PatFT）[61, 62]。PSIPS 包含 2001 年之后在美国申请的专利序列，而 PatFT 包含 1976 年之后在美国申请的专利全文和 1790—1975 年中在美国申请的部分专利全文。PSIPS 提供文件编号检索和日期范围检索，其搜索结果可选择下载特定的序列或全部序列。但是，该数据库不提供 FASTA 格式，如果要进行后续的序列分析，则需要先进行序列格式的统一。

16.4.3.6　世界知识产权组织（World Intellectual Property Organization，WIPO）

WIPO 成立于 1967 年，是一个自筹资金的联合国机构，共有 193 个成员国。其使命是领导建立一个良好的国际知识产权制度，使创新和创造能够造福于每个人，提供大量知识产权资源，包括 PATENTSCOPE 数据库和 Global Brand 数据库[63]。

16.4.3.7　其他数据库

除了上述众所周知的由政府主导的公共数据库外，适当结合商业数据库也是增加数据覆盖面的一种方法。Lens-PatSeq 可以提供对专利、学术文章和专利序列的检索和分析[64]。难能可贵的是，PatSeq 是具有专门为检索和分析专利序列功能的数据库，其大部分功能对访问者都免费开放。其专利序列数据主要有三个来源：①国家专利局（如 JPO 等）；②合作的第三方公共数据库（如 NCBI、EMBL-EBI、DDBJ 等）；③地区性或全球性的知识产权组织（如欧洲专利局等）[65]。此外，Lens-PatSeq、Derwent Geneseq™ 的 GENESEQ 数据库[66]、Aptean 的 GenomeQuest（GQ）[67]、CAS 提供的 CAS REGISTRY/CAplusSM[68]、EMBL-EBI 的 UniProt 数据库[69]等一系列数据库中也包含了大量生物序列，可以在后续的分析中作为参考。其中，Aptean 与 CAS 已达成合作[70]，即在 GQ 中同时也会提供 CAS 的生物序列内容，帮助有关科研人员简化数据收集的过程。

总而言之，由 DDBJ、EMBL-EBI 和 NCBI 组成的 INSDC 是目前世界上覆盖面最广的核苷酸数据组织。INSDC 的成员可有效区分专利中的核苷酸序列，并共同拥有唯一的序列标识 ACCESSION。USPTO、WIPO 或其他国家或地区知识产权局的数据库也是重要的数据来源。这些数据库在专利领域的生物序列分析中具有独特的优势，它们的生物序列与专利的公开号紧密联系在一起，在研究人员确定了专利数据的范围后，就能很好地确定生物序列数据，其他数据库如 Lens、Derwent 也是如此。这也是为什么在之前章节中介绍数据库时强调要能识别生物序列数据是否来自专利以及是否能与特定专利相关联的原因。因为专利领域的生物序列分析比单纯的生物序列分析更加需要注意细节。

16.4.4 专利中抗体序列数据挖掘—案例介绍

抗体是目前生物医疗领域中最成功的生物治疗药物,虽然其研发周期十分漫长,但每年仍有越来越多的抗体治疗药物走向临床或者市场[71]。

这些成功的抗体在上市前都经历了大量的工程修饰与改造,而为了保护这一过程中的关键序列选择和相关选择,需要在专利文件中披露相关信息,这在一定程度上揭示了抗体工程的选择。然而,专利的目的是提供法律保护的依据,而不是解释学术问题,因此,专利能否有效传达相关领域的学术知识还有待探讨。Krawczyk等[38]重点研究了含有抗体序列的专利文件,量化其中有多少用于医疗目的,以及它们在多大程度上反映了治疗方法。这有助于他们评估专利数据对治疗性抗体工程的作用,以及是否可以用作开展抗体设计相关工作的参考。其研究数据来源包括USPTO[60]、WIPO[63]、DDBJ[59]和EMBL-EBI[57]中相关的专利。之所以选择这些数据库的原因是:首先,人们倾向于在世界知识产权组织专利合作条约(Patent Cooperation Treaty,PCT)体系和最大的医药市场(美国)寻求专利保护;其次,欧洲、日本和韩国的数据库可通过DDBJ和EBI获得。这项研究的作者认为,他们所选择的数据源合理地覆盖了全球抗体序列专利。

Krawczyk等于2020年1月30日从上述四个数据库中提取了原始序列数据,使用自定义的Python脚本将所有数据格式统一为FASTA格式,并用IgBlast扫描数据,确定了抗体序列部分并将其翻译成氨基酸。之后,他们用ANARCI分析原始氨基酸序列,以确定抗体的可变区链。在分析过程中,Krawczyk等使用Open Patent Service API v. 3.2识别了专利族,下载了每个专利族的基本信息,在命名实体识别(NER)的支持下进行了人工目标注释,最终以图表的形式展示了他们的分析结果。

Krawczyk等发现,在所有序列专利中,抗体的占比很高,并且相关专利文件的数量每年都在增加,这些含有抗体的专利大多以临床治疗为目的。此外,从列出抗体序列的专利中获得的靶标合理地反映了目前可用的治疗性抗体的靶标,这表明研究包含抗体序列的专利文件可以及早了解治疗性抗体领域的靶标和相关研究活动。此外,他们还发现,在专利文件中的抗体序列中,使用双特异性种系基因的主要是人类和小鼠种系基因,这与治疗性抗体种系基因选择的情况相吻合。而排在第三位的种系基因是羊驼,这暗示了单域抗体领域的发展,尤其是目前首个单域抗体药物Caplacizumab(Cablivi®)获得批准,这些大量的专利文件意味着未来会有更多的单域抗体出现。此外,在分析过程中,Krawczyk等还从治疗性抗体特性的工程角度进行了些许尝试。研究发现,专利抗体序列的长度会因为并不遵循自然分布而往往比较长,并且这些治疗性抗体的CDR-H3长度分布与专利抗体不同,这表明专利文件中包含了一些工程信息。他们的这一观点为今后挖掘这些工程信息提供了基础。

2008年,另一项研究[72]分析了1995年至2007年专利申请中序列数量和专利申请组织类型的变化,不涉及具体的生物序列分析,只涉及生物序列数量、专利文件数量和专利受让人随时间的变化,其数据来源只有GENESEQ数据库[66]。尽管如此,仍然可以从这项研究中发现某些变化趋势,即早年的序列申请要求更宽泛,审查标准更低,随着时间推移,序列专利申请的要求则变得更加具体,范围也更加狭窄。在含有生物序列的专利数量达到顶峰时,大量专利由生物技术公司持有,这些公司围绕核心产品或具有潜力的产品申请了一系列专利以保护产品的核心竞争力,并且这些专利包含的生物序列数量远远多于其他专利。

16.5　药剂学专利数据挖掘

药剂学是一门集药物、辅料、制造、技术于一体的系统工程。药物制剂通过提高药物吸收和生物利用度、减少毒副作用、增强药物稳定性和患者用药依从性来影响药物疗效,是实现从药物活性成分发展为临床使用药品的不可或缺的一门学科[73]。药物制剂专利包括剂型和赋形剂、药物递送系统、给药途径和药物制造等。

专利分析在药剂学研究中发挥着至关重要的作用。首先,专利分析有助于识别新颖的制药技术,例如,新型药物递送系统。这些信息可以显著提高药物制剂设计的效率,为目标领域的知识产权模式提供宝贵的见解。其次,专利格局分析能够揭示潜在的竞争者与合作者关系,有助于准确识别研发产品的市场定位,利于成果转化、技术转让和投资决策。此外,专利分析还可用于识别潜在的专利侵权行为,可有效避免法律诉讼的风险。因此,药剂学中的专利数据是值得挖掘和研究的。

16.5.1　药剂学专利分析

随着基因工程和精准医学的发展,药物递送系统(DDS)已成为药剂学研究的热点之一。DDS涉及多种技术,包括纳米、脂质体、控释等技术。DDS对于开发新型核酸生物制剂(如RNA药物和疫苗)起到十分关键的作用,DDS专利保护对于候选药物变得至关重要。基于纳米技术的药物递送系统已成为当前的研发趋势,纳米递送系统具有多种优势,例如生物利用度、渗透性和递送效率等[74]。DDS相关专利及新化学实体也层出不穷,例如,Nur Umairah Ali Hazis等[75]对纳米颗粒的主要类别进行了分类并总结了发展趋势。此外,还对剂型和相关赋形剂进行了专利分析[76]。另外,还有针对药物剂型和生产制备工艺的专利保护。例如,Karavasili C等对儿科口服剂型和相关设备进行了专利分析,总结了如迷你片剂和咀嚼剂型等新型赋形剂和方法[77]。代表性专利分析研究如表16-1所示。

表16-1　药物制剂代表性专利分析

专利题目	分类	公开年	DOI
Nanosponges-versatile platform as drug carrier	Drug carrier and delivery system	2023	10.2174/1872210516666220905092202
Nanoprecipitation technology to prepare carrier systems of interest in pharmaceutics: An overview of patenting	Drug carrier and delivery system	2022	10.1016/j.ijpharm.2021.121440
Pharmacokinetics of long-acting aqueous nano-/microsuspensions after intramuscular administration in different animal species and humans—A review	Dosage form and excipients	2022	10.1208/s12248-022-00771-5
Systematic patent review of nanoparticles in drug delivery and cancer therapy in the last decade	Drug carrier and delivery system	2021	10.2174/1872211314666210521105534
HP-β-CD for the formulation of IgG and Ig-based biotherapeutics	Dosage form and excipients	2021	10.1016/j.ijpharm.2021.120531

续表

专利题目	分类	公开年	DOI
Patent landscape of pediatric-friendly oral dosage forms and administration devices	Dosage form and excipients	2021	10.1080/13543776.2021.1893691
Prospection of chitosan and its derivatives in wound healing: Proof of patent analysis (2010—2020)	Dosage form and excipients	2021	10.1016/j.ijbiomac.2021.06.086
Application of liposomes in cancer therapy: An assessment of the advancement of technology through patent documents	Drug carrier and delivery system	2020	10.2174/1872210514666201223093321
A patent review on nanotechnology-based nose-to-brain drug delivery	Drug carrier and delivery system	2020	10.2174/1872210514666200508121050
Global research on artemisinin and its derivatives: Perspectives from patents	Natural product	2020	10.1016/j.phrs.2020.105048
Nanocarriers for the effective treatment of cervical cancer: Research advancements and patent analysis	Drug carrier and delivery system	2018	10.2174/1872211312666180403102019
Exploring sets of molecules from patents and relationships to other active compounds in chemical space networks	Chemical molecules	2017	10.1007/s10822-017-0061-2
Strategic patent analysis in plant biotechnology: terpenoid indole alkaloid metabolic engineering as a case study	Natural product	2014	10.1111/pbi.12134

16.5.2 药剂学专利数据挖掘

鉴于专利文献中存在大量非结构化数据，文本挖掘被广泛应用于专利数据处理。例如：i）通过集成文本挖掘和图像提取建立化合物空间网络，以研究生物活性化合物的相似性并进一步探索构效关系[78]；ii）基于文本挖掘算法的智能专利数据检索引擎和分析工具[79]。自然语言处理（NLP）是人工智能的一个分支，通过多种统计和人工智能模型将文本挖掘任务数字化。NLP已经用于生物医药专利数据挖掘，包括药物递送、药物相互作用探索和核心成分提取等。作为NLP的任务之一，命名实体识别（NER）涉及科学文献中化学和生物医学名称的识别和提取。主要的NER挑战包括三个独立的任务：专利中化学实体标注识别（chemical entity mention recognition in patents，CEMP）；基因和蛋白质对象识别（gene and protein-related object recognition，GPRO）；生物信息注释。药物制剂专利包含大量的化学和生物信息，因此在数据分析中可采用NER作为数据预处理的步骤之一。

此外，基于机器学习和深度学习方法建立的NER数据挖掘可以用于药剂学专利分析。它结合了CEMP和GPRO等任务，融合了条件随机场（conditional random field，CRF）和结构化支持向量机等算法[80]。还可以利用如长短期记忆（long short term memory，LSTM）神经网络等深度学习算法来提高NER性能。例如，LSTM Voter是一个深度学习NER系统，基于具有CRF层和基于注意力的特征模型的双向LSTM标记器（2019）。LSTM神经网络是基于将生物医学NER建模为序列标记问题而建立的[81]。专利文本挖掘采用了类似的深度学习NER模型（2018）[82]。ChEMU 2020作为一种数据分析工具可用于化学NER和化学反应事件提取，有助于化学专利中的关键信息提取[83]。研究表明，双向LSTM方法在NER任务中表现最好，而卷积神经网络在事件提取任务中表现较好[84]。有研究应用深度学习模型来预测特定专利的前向引用和市场反应作为产品估值衡量标准[85]。目前，已有多个数据库专注于基于文本挖掘的药剂学专利信息提取。例如，CHEMTABLES是一个拥有大型数据集的数据库，其中包含来自制药专利的788个化学表。附注释的化学专利语料库可用于文本挖掘，该数据集经过标准化文本处理和分割，可应用于机器学习和深度学习模型的训练和测试[86]。

16.6　实际操作及相关问题

随着互联网和计算机技术的快速普及，各种专利信息数据库和在线工具在过去几十年中蓬勃发展。本节将说明之前提到的专利数据库的具体使用方法和详细操作步骤。相关数据库的信息在表16-2中列出。

表16-2　专利数据库及相关在线工具总结

数据库名称	分类	专利范围
PATENTSCOPE	Patent database/Chemical information	US，EP，WO/PCT
FreePatentsOnline	Patent database	US，EP，WO/PCT，JP
The Patent Lens	Patent database/Biolgcal information	patents from 94 authorities
Derwent Innovation Index	Patent database	patents from 59 authorities
IncoPat	Patent database	patents from 120 authorities
PatentInspiration	Patent database	Based on the DOCDB database from the EPO (European Patent Office)
Google patents	Patent database	US，EP，WO/PCT，CN，DE，CA
United States Patent and Trademark Office（USPTO）	Patent database/Chemical information/Biolgcal information	United States Patent
World Intellectual Property Organization（WIPO）	Patent database/Chemical information/Biolgcal information	Patent Cooperation Treaty（PCT）
Scifinder	Chemical information	Chemical structure in patents
SureChEMBL	Chemical information	Chemical structure in patents
CAS PatentPak	Chemical information	Chemical structure in patents
International Nucleotide Sequence Database Collaboration（INSDC）	Biolgcal information	Biosequence in patents
National Center for Biotechnology Information（NCBI）	Biolgcal information	Biosequence in patents

数据库名称	分类	专利范围
EMBL's European Bioinformatics Institute（EMBL-EBI）	Biologcal information	Biosequence in patents
DNA Data Bank of Japan （DDBJ）	Biologcal information	Biosequence in patents
GENESEQ	Biologcal information	Biosequence in patents
GenomeQuest	Biologcal information	Biosequence in patents
CAS REGISTRY	Biologcal information	Biosequence in patents

16.6.1 专利检索数据库

16.6.1.1 PATENTSCOPE数据库

① 打开PATENTSCOPE数据库，点击"Access the PATENTSCOPE database"（图16-2）。

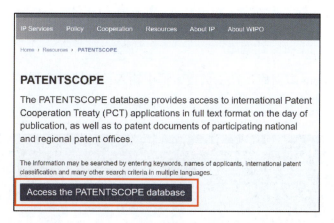

图16-2　PATENTSCOPE数据库操作界面

② PATENTSCOPE数据库提供不同类型的检索模式，包括"Simple Search"（图16-3）、"Advanced Search"、"Field Search"、"Cross-Language Extension"和"Compound Search（需登录后才能使用）"。将专利号输入"ID/Number"栏，即可检索到对应专利的内容（图16-4）。

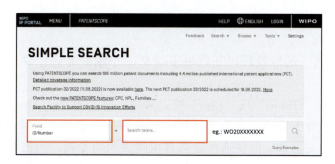

图16-3　PATENTSCOPE数据库操作界面（专利检索）

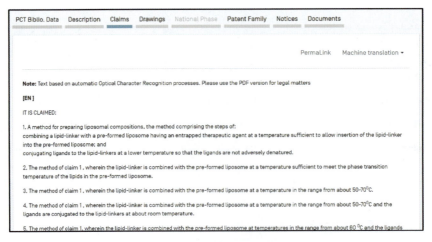

图16-4　PATENTSCOPE数据库操作界面（检索结果）

③ 专利中的生物序列在"Documents"部分中的"Sequence Listing"栏，可以提供浏览和检索功能。还可通过FTP批量下载数据[87, 88]。数据库包含从1999年至今的序列。然而，WIPO不提供FASTA格式；因此，如果需要进行生物序列分析，需要进行格式统一。

16.6.1.2　Patent Lens数据库

① 打开Patent Lens数据库，在主页搜索框中输入关键词、专利字段或专利号即可进行搜索（图16-5）。

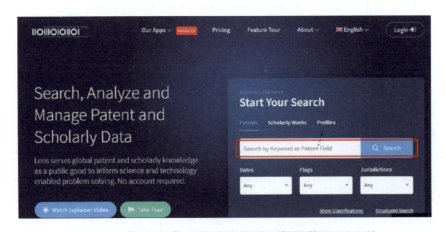

图16-5　Patent Lens数据库操作界面

② 点击专利标题下的标签可以获取更多信息，左侧的导航栏显示专利内容标签（图16-6）。

③ 专利可选择在"Table"或"List"模式呈现，并且可在"Analysis"中进行专利内容的可视化。对于包含生物序列的专利，每个序列都标有序列号、序列长度、类型、位置以及在PatSeq中的相关信息。可快速搜索具有相同序列的专利，也提供FASTA格式的序列下载。

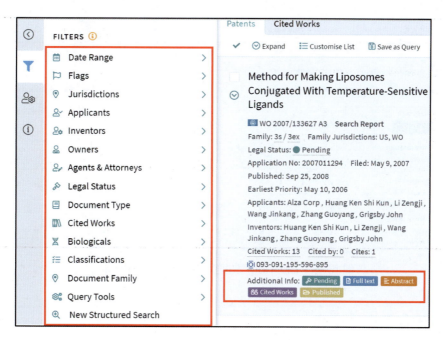

图16-6　Patent Lens数据库操作界面（导航栏）

16.6.2　化学信息数据库

Scifinder数据库提供专利相关的化学结构信息。

① 打开主页在搜索框中输入专利号，即可获得专利相关的化学结构（图16-7）。

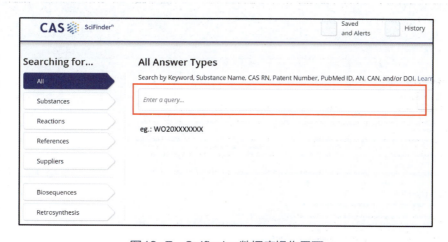

图16-7　Scifinder数据库操作界面

② 点击下载按钮并选择文件格式后即可下载。需要注意的是，如果化学结构超过500个，则仅下载前500个结构。如一个专利中的化学结构超过500个，则应分批下载才能获取该专利所包含的所有结构。图16-8为数据检索结果举例。

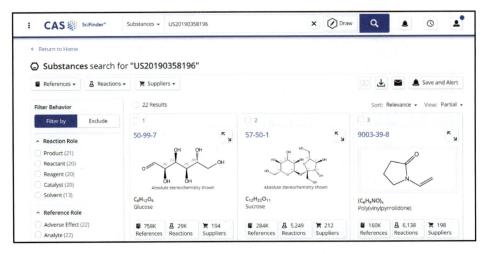

图16-8 Scifinder数据库操作界面（数据检索）

16.6.3 生物信息数据库

16.6.3.1 GenBank数据库

① 打开GenBank数据库并点击"Entrez Nucleotide"。生物序列位于"Entrez Nucleotide"部分，"BLAST"可用于序列比对。数据库可以提供单字段搜索、列表搜索等。详细规则可以在官网找到[89,90,91]。图16-9为该数据库的操作界面。

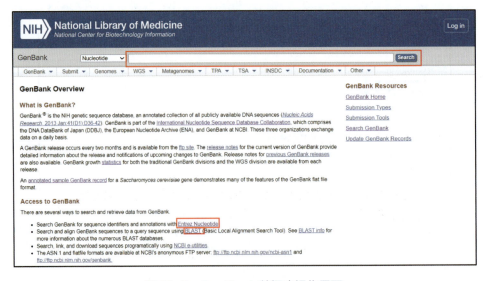

图16-9 GenBank数据库操作界面

② 打开GenBank样本记录（图16-10）。每个GenBank检索记录的数据格式都是固定的，每个记录都包含序列的简要描述，包括学名、物种分类、参考文献、序列特征和序列本身。其开头字段的完整含义在网站上有详细解释[92]。

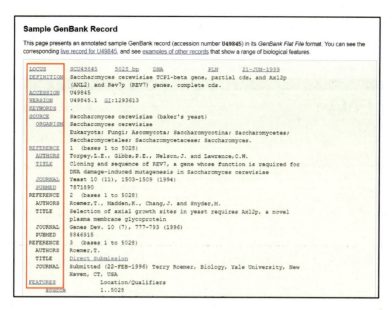

图16-10　GenBank数据库操作界面（数据记录）

③ 这里有几点需要注意："ACCESSION"是序列的唯一标识符，永远不会改变，而"VERSION"则包括入藏号后面跟"VERSION"。当顺序改变时，版本号将会增加。关键字包括描述序列的单词或短语，如果没有关键字，则仅包含句点。由于许多记录中不存在关键字，因此官方不建议使用关键字进行高级搜索。参考文献可以包含各种类型的出版物，包括期刊文章、书籍章节、书籍、论文、专著、会议记录和专利等。最先出版的出版物列在最前面。参考下的各个子字段位于"Entrez搜索"字段中。

④ 在搜索结果中，可以使用BLAST来搜索结果的序列匹配。对于序列部分，提供了FASTA格式，这是目前使用最广泛的序列格式。

16.6.3.2　欧洲核酸数据库（European Nucleotide Archive，ENA）

① 打开ENA。该数据库主要免费提供专利文本检索、高级检索、序列相似性检索等功能。还可以在搜索界面中搜索交叉引用并查看序列版本和历史记录。图16-11为该数据库操作界面。

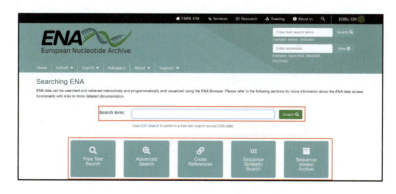

图16-11　ENA操作界面

② 在"Advanced Search"功能中，可根据五个基本要素扩大或缩小搜索范围（图16-12）。

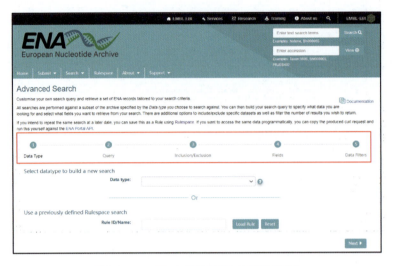

图16-12　ENA操作界面（高级搜索）

③ ENA中每条记录的数据格式是固定的，包含序列的简要描述，可以EMBL格式预览或下载，获得更详细的信息。虽然EMBL格式与GenBank不同，但涵盖的主要内容与NCBI类似。

④ 高级检索中的公开字段可以通过专利号进行检索，有利于专利中的序列分析。数据库提供序列FASTA格式，并可以在线预览[93]。

16.6.3.3　DNA Data Bank of Japan（DDBJ）数据库

① 打开数据库中"DDBJ Annotated/Assembled Sequences"，该数据库提供"ARSA"和"getentry"搜索（图16-13）。值得注意的是，DDBJ提供根据专利领域限制检索范围的方式。

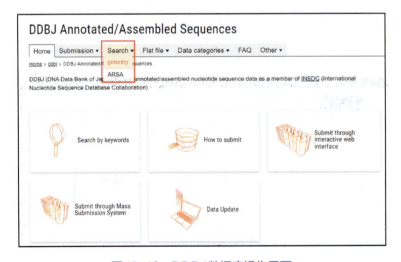

图16-13　DDBJ数据库操作界面

② DDBJ数据库"Getentry"选择框提供序列ID号的搜索，并可指定数据库类型和输出格式。还可以选择蛋白质数据库中的专利，获取该专利的氨基酸序列数据（图16-14）。

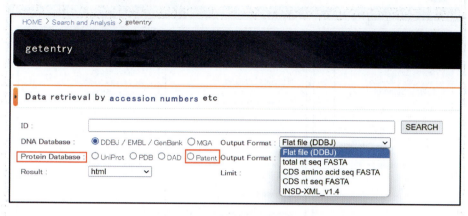

图16-14　DDBJ数据库操作界面（数据格式）

③ ARSA搜索有快速检索和高级检索可选，可以选择"Division"中的"PAT"和"Molecule Type"中的序列类型，如DNA、RNA、mRNA、rRNA等（图16-15），获取DDBJ/GenBank中PAT部分的数据。还可以在蛋白质数据库中获取专利中的氨基酸序列数据[94,95,96]。

④ 检索结果可以FlatFile、XML、FASTA格式在线预览，其中FlatFile格式与NCBI数据库格式相同，序列提供FASTA格式。

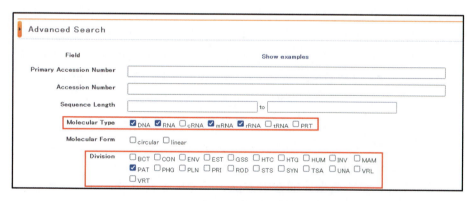

图16-15　DDBJ数据库操作界面（数据筛选）

16.6.3.4　Patent Full-text databases（PatFT）数据库

PatFT数据库提供多种检索功能，包括快速检索、高级检索、专利号检索、字段检索以及按专利号获取美国专利全页图片、获取专利全页图片等（图16-16）。需要注意的是，早期专利如1790年至1975年的专利只能按发布日期、专利号和当前分类（US、IPC或CPC）进行检索。

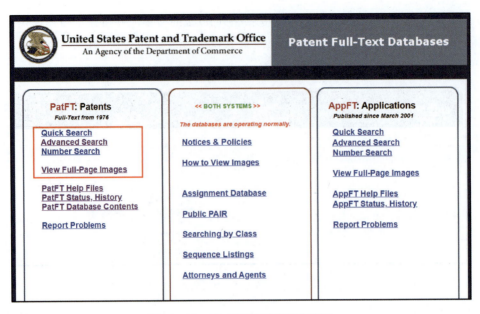

图16-16 PatFT数据库操作界面

16.6.4 现有专利数据库面临的挑战

16.6.4.1 数据缺失

在对专利数据进行分析之前，需要注意以下几点。首先，由于各个国家和地区的相关政策不同，并非所有关键信息（例如：专利中的生物序列）都得到充分披露。其次，尽管生物序列通常将某些格式视为主要序列格式，但并非所有数据库都提供统一格式。最后，没有一个数据库能够涵盖全球范围内已公开的所有数据。因此，与专利格局分析不同，专利中的生物信息和化学信息分析需要基于多个数据库以确保相对完整的数据覆盖范围[97,98]。

根据以往的研究结果[37,41,98,99]，数据缺失包括但不限于以下几点原因：

① 及时性：检索结果常常受到所选数据源的相对及时性的影响。

② 算法多样性：BLAST相似性检索可能会涵盖数量庞大的相似序列，使用者有可能选择不相关的序列而错过真正的目标序列。

③ 索引标准差异：每个数据库的索引方法、专利族定义以及处理专利族成员序号变更的方式各不相同。所有这些因素都会影响数据搜索的结果。

④ 真正的数据缺失。

16.6.4.2 数据库滞后

Cambia等在2011年的一项研究中发现[40]，在过去二十年中，专利序列数据在全球范围内向公众开放的程度仍然滞后。目前，还缺乏一个全球性的、完整的、透明的专利序列数据库。对包含专利生物序列的数据库的研究表明，商业数据库和公共数据库都有自己独特的序列数据，并没有彼此包含[40,41,99]。

16.6.4.3 数据范围差异

数据库之间的数据范围有差异，且会受到多种因素的影响[99]。例如，难以确定基础专利和授权专利之间的序列信息变化。EMBL-EBI和NCBI数据库不包含PSIPS中的序列表，USPTO审查的PCT申请的序列表一般不会出现在公共领域（同时出现在WIPO的除外）。另外，美国专利的序列，除非序列列表出现在PSIPS中，否则无法通过公众查询申请。

还有一点值得注意，数据库都有其自身的优缺点，研究人员需要评估数据缺失的潜在风险。而且，多个数据库一起检索必然会导致大量的数据冗余，需要分析人员明确同族专利的标准，及时排除冗余数据，以保证研究的顺利进行。

相关数据库的更多信息，还可参考 *Nucleic Acid Research* 杂志的数据库问题[100]。Database Issue收集了各种公共数据库，并每年进行扩充，为研究人员提供数据库的网址、更新情况、用途和主要内容，极大地便利了研究项目的开展。另外，还可使用数据库搜索工具，如Omictools等，来搜索所需的数据库。

16.6.5 生物医药专利分析流程

完整的生物医药研究专利分析应包括选题、数据检索、数据筛选、标准化、数据分析和讨论以及结论，应对照专利格局分析的标准完成分析项目。数据分析的方法具有开放性和多样性的特点，可以从实际的研究目的和数据类型等多方面出发，制定出有效且合理的数据分析方案。其工作流程如图16-17所示。

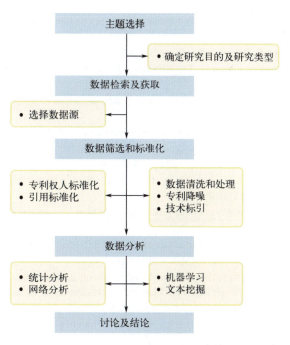

图16-17 生物医药专利分析流程

蓝色框表示专利分析的步骤，黄色框列举了分析步骤中的具体方法

16.7 总结

作为前沿技术的数据源，生物医药领域的专利申请呈现出快速增长的态势。目前，专利分析包含了手动数据挖掘和自动数据挖掘。专利相关数据库和在线工具的种类十分丰富。在专利分析中，已出现多种机器学习和深度学习算法进行化学信息学、生物信息学等数据挖掘，基于计算机技术的进步，未来这些算法开发将继续蓬勃发展。

然而，随着数据量的增加和数据处理要求的不断提高，专利数据分析也出现了更多的挑战。随着专利申请数量的快速增长，专利数据处理的负担将变得沉重，尤其是人工数据处理。涉及计算模型的自动数据处理可减轻人工负担，并且能够避免手动筛选产生的偏差。然而，自动方法也可能会引入错误，并且需要持续修正和维护。此外，专利数据挖掘还有其他挑战，例如NER的难度、现有的数据库数据重叠和缺失等问题。

尽管目前的专利分析方法存在局限性，但专利数据分析在未来的生物医药研究和开发中将变得越来越重要。基于专利分析，可以提供技术趋势，并且明确研究开发的边界，避免专利诉讼。总而言之，专利数据挖掘能够提升对目标领域多维度的了解，丰富理论基础的同时便于各方进行决策，对生物医药的新兴技术开发起到至关重要的作用。

参考文献

[1] Aggarwal S, Chandra A. Patentability challenges associated with emerging pharmaceutical technologies[J]. Pharm Pat Anal. 2021, 10(4): 195-207.

[2] Organization WIP. Guidelines for Preparing Patent Landscape Reports. 2015.

[3] Page M J, McKenzie J E, Bossuyt P M, et al. The PRISMA 2020 statement: an updated guideline for reporting systematic reviews[J]. BMJ. 2021, 372: n71.

[4] Smith J A, Arshad Z, Trippe A, et al. The reporting items for patent landscapes statement[J]. Nat Biotechnol, 2018, 36(11): 1043-1047.

[5] Chen Y, Xiong S H, Li F, et al. Delivery of therapeutic small interfering RNA: The current patent-based landscape[J]. Mol Ther Nucleic Acids, 2022, 29: 150-161.

[6] Eiblmaier J, Mazenc C, Geppert D, Isenko L, Saller H. Addition of chemical search capabilities to PATENTSCOPE: Turning a full-text search system into a chemistry database[M]. Washington: ABSTRACTS OF PAPERS OF THE AMERICAN CHEMICAL SOCIETY, 2017.

[7] Lynch D E, Hamilton D G. Croconaine dyes–the lesser known siblings of squaraines[J]. European Journal of Organic Chemistry, 2017, 2017(27): 3897-911.

[8] Senger S. Assessment of the significance of patent-derived information for the early identification of compound–target interaction hypotheses[J]. Journal of Cheminformatics, 2017, 9(1): 1-8.

[9] Jessop D M. Information extraction from chemical patents[M]. University of Cambridge, 2011.

[10] Fisanick W. The Chemical Abstract's Service generic chemical(Markush)structure storage and retrieval capability. 1. Basic concepts[J]. Journal of chemical information and computer sciences. 1990, 30(2): 145-54.

[11] Hettne K M, Stierum R H, Schuemie M J, et al. A dictionary to identify small molecules and drugs in free text[J]. Bioinformatics, 2009, 25(22): 2983-2991.

[12] Budi I, Bressan S. Association rules mining for name entity recognition. Proceedings of the Fourth International Conference on Web Information Systems Engineering 2003, WISE 2003, 2003: 325-328.

[13] Narayanaswamy M, Ravikumar K, Vijay-Shanker K. A biological named entity recognizer[J]. Pac Symp Biocomput, 2003: 427-438.

[14] Leaman R, Wei C H, Zou C, Lu Z. Mining chemical patents with an ensemble of open systems[J]. Database. 2016, 2016: baw065.

[15] Zhang Y, Xu J, Chen H, et al. Chemical named entity recognition in patents by domain knowledge and unsupervised feature learning[J]. Database, 2016, 2016: baw049.

[16] Krallinger M, Rabal O, Lourenço A, et al. Overview of the CHEMDNER patents task[J]. Proceedings of the fifth BioCreative challenge evaluation workshop, 2015.

[17] McDaniel J R, Balmuth J R. Kekule: OCR-optical chemical(structure)recognition[J]. Journal of chemical information and computer sciences, 1992, 32(4): 373-378.

[18] Filippov I V, Nicklaus M C. Optical structure recognition software to recover chemical information: OSRA, an open source solution[J]. J Chem Inf Model, 2009, 49(3): 740-743.

[19] Zimmermann M. Chemical Structure Reconstruction with chemoCR[C]. Proceedings of The Twentieth Text REtrieval Conference, TREC 2011, Gaithersburg, Maryland, USA, 2011.

[20] Oldenhof M, Arany A, Moreau Y, et al. ChemGrapher: optical graph recognition of chemical compounds by deep learning[J]. Journal of chemical information and modeling, 2020, 60(10): 4506-4517.

[21] Beard E J, Cole J M. ChemSchematicResolver: a toolkit to decode 2D chemical diagrams with labels and R-groups into annotated chemical named entities[J]. Journal of chemical information and modeling, 2020, 60(4): 2059-2072.

[22] Wang J, Shen Z, Liao Y, et al. Multi-modal chemical information reconstruction from images and texts for exploring the near-drug space[J]. Briefings in Bioinformatics, 2022, 23(6): bbac461.

[23] Papadatos G, Davies M, Dedman N, et al. SureChEMBL: a large-scale, chemically annotated patent document database[J]. Nucleic acids research, 2016, 44(D1): D1220-D1228.

[24] GenBank and WGS Statistics [Internet], 参见官方网址。

[25] Altschul S F, Madden T L, Schaffer A A, et al. Gapped BLAST and PSI-BLAST: a new generation of protein database search programs[J]. Nucleic Acids Research. 1997, 25(17): 3389-3402.

[26] Altschul S F, Gish W, Miller W, et al. Basic local alignment search tool[J]. Journal of Molecular Biology, 1990, 215(3): 403-410.

[27] Fassler J, Cooper P. BLAST® Help [Internet]. Bethesda(MD): National Center for Biotechnology Information(US), 2011.

[28] Madden T. The BLAST Sequence Analysis Tool. 2013. In: The NCBI Handbook [Internet] [Internet]. Bethesda(MD): National Center for Biotechnology Information(US).

[29] Wheeler D, Bhagwat M. BLAST QuickStart: example-driven web-based BLAST tutorial. Methods Mol Biol, 2007, 395: 149-176.

[30] BLAST Help Page(参见官方网址).

[31] Pearson W R, Lipman D J. Improved tools for biological sequence comparison[J]. Proc Natl Acad Sci U S A, 1988, 85(8): 2444-2448.

[32] Pearson W R. BLAST and FASTA similarity searching for multiple sequence alignment[J]. Methods Mol Biol, 2014, 1079: 75-101.

[33] Kent W J. BLAT : the BLAST-like alignment tool[J]. Genome Res, 2002, 12(4): 656-664.

[34] Bhagwat M, Young L, Robison R R. Using BLAT to find sequence similarity in closely related genomes[M]. Curr Protoc Bioinformatics, 2012.

[35] Li W Z, McWilliam H, de la Torre A R, et al. Non-redundant patent sequence databases with value-added annotations at two levels[J]. Nucleic Acids Research, 2010, 38: D52-D56.

[36] McDowall J. Prioritizing patent sequence search results using annotation-rich data[J]. World Patent Information, 2011, 33(3): 235-239.

[37] Dufresne G, Takacs L, Heus H C, et al. Patent searches for genetic sequences: How to retrieve relevant records from patented sequence databases[J]. Nature Biotechnology. 2002, 20(12): 1269-1271.

[38] Krawczyk K, Buchanan A, Marcatili P. Data mining patented antibody sequences[J]. Mabs. 2021, 13(1): 1892366.

[39] Alberts D, Yang C B, Fobare-DePonio D, et al. Introduction to patent searching. In: Current Challenges in Patent Information Retrieval[M]. Lupu M, Mayer K, Kando N, Trippe A J, editors. Berlin, Heidelberg: Springer Berlin Heidelberg, 2017: 3-45.

[40] Jefferson O A, Kollhofer D, Ehrich T H, et al. Transparency tools in gene patenting for informing policy and practice OPEN[J]. Nature Biotechnology, 2013, 31(12): 1086-1093.

[41] Jefferson O A, Köllhofer D, Ajjikuttira P, et al. Public disclosure of biological sequences in global patent practice[J]. World Patent Information, 2015, 43: 12-24.

[42] Stock M, Stock W G. Intellectual property information: A comparative analysis of main information providers[J]. Journal of the American Society for Information Science and Technology, 2006, 57(13): 1794-1803.

[43] Seide R K, Russo A A. Patenting 3D protein structures[J]. Expert Opinion on Therapeutic Patents, 2002, 12(2): 147-150.

[44] Chan K L, Fernandez D. Patent prosecution in structural proteomics[J]. Assay and Drug Development Technologies, 2004, 2(3): 313-319.

[45] Trilateral Project WM4, Comparative Studies in New Technologies. Report on Comparative Study on Protein 3-Dimensional Structure Related Claims. Vienna, Austria, 2002.

[46] Shimbo I, Nakajima R, Yokoyama S, et al. Patent protection for protein structure analysis[J]. Nature Biotechnology, 2004, 22(1): 109-113.

[47] Meyers T C, Turano T A, Greenhalgh D A, et al. Patent protection for protein structures and databases[J]. Nature Structural Biology, 2000, 7: 950-952.

[48] Uppenberg J. Crystalline form of activated tartrate-resistant and purple acid phosphatase. Google Patents, 2001.

[49] Vinarov S D. Patent protection for structural genomics-related inventions[J]. Journal of Structural and Functional Genomics, 2003, 4(2-3): 191-209.

[50] Krane D E, Raymer M L. Fundamental Concepts of Bioinformatics[M]. San Francisco: Benjamin Cummings, 2003.

[51] Arita M, Karsch-Mizrachi I, Cochrane G. The international nucleotide sequence database collaboration[J]. Nucleic Acids Research, 2021, 49(D1): D121-D124.

[52] Brunak S, Danchin A, Hattori M, et al. Nucleotide sequence database policies[J]. Science. 2002, 298(5597): 1333.

[53] Benson D A, Karsch-Mizrachi I, Lipman D J, et al. GenBank[J]. Nucleic Acids Research, 2006, 34: D16-D20.

[54] GenBank Overview(参见 GenBank 数据库官方网址).

[55] National Center for Biotechnology Information(参见 NCBI 数据库官方网址).

[56] Benson D A, Cavanaugh M, Clark K, et al. GenBank[J]. Nucleic Acids Research, 2013, 41(D1): D36-D42.

[57] About Us. In: EMBL's European Bioinformatics Institute(参见 EBI 数据库官方网址).

[58] Our Impact. In: EMBL's European Bioinformatics Institute(参见 EBI 数据库官方网址).

[59] DDBJ 数据库(参见 DDBJ 数据库官方网址).

[60] About Us | USPTO (参见 USPTO 数据库官方网址).

[61] The USPTO Publication Site for Issued and Published Sequences(PSIPS)(参见 USPTO 数据库官方网址).

[62] Patent Full-Text Databases(参见 USPTO 数据库官方网址).

[63] WIPO-World Intellectual Property Organization(参见 WIPO 官方网址).

[64] Search and Analyse Biological Sequences Disclosed in Patents.(参见 Lens 官方网址).

[65] PatSeq Data-The Lens .(参见 Lens 官方网址).

[66] Derwent SequenceBase Databases(参见 Clarivate 官方网址).

[67] Patent Sequence Search And Analysis(参见 GQ Life Sciences 官方网址).

[68] CAS REGISTRY(参见 CAS 官方网址).

[69] UniProt(参见 UniProt 官方网址).

[70] Aptean and CAS Collaborate to Offer CAS Biosequences Content in GenomeQuest(参见 CAS 官方网址).

[71] Kaplon H, Muralidharan M, Schneider Z, et al. Antibodies to watch in 2020[J]. Mabs. 2020, 12(1): 1703531.

[72] Cai R, Nirmala N R. Trends and impact of genome mining patents on target discovery[J]. Expert Opinion on Therapeutic Patents, 2008, 18(6): 563-568.

[73] Fang L. Pharmaceutics[M]. Beijing: People's Medical Publishing House；2021.

[74] Ravichandran R. Nanotechnology-based drug delivery systems[J]. NanoBiotechnology. 2009, 5(1): 17-33.

[75] Ali Hazis N U, Aneja N, Rajabalaya R, et al. Systematic patent review of nanoparticles in drug delivery and cancer therapy in the last decade[J]. Recent Adv Drug Deliv Formul, 2021, 15(1): 59-74.

[76] Nguyen V T T, Darville N, Vermeulen A. Pharmacokinetics of long-acting aqueous nano-/microsuspensions after intramuscular administration in different animal species and humans: A review[J]. AAPS J, 2022, 25(1): 4.

[77] Karavasili C, Gkaragkounis A, Fatouros D G. Patent landscape of pediatric-friendly oral dosage forms and administration devices[J]. Expert Opin Ther Pat, 2021, 31(7): 663-686.

[78] Kunimoto R, Bajorath J. Exploring sets of molecules from patents and relationships to other active compounds in chemical space networks[J]. J Comput Aided Mol Des, 2017, 31(9): 779-788.

[79] Ajay D, Gangwal R P, Sangamwar A T. IPAT: a freely accessible software tool for analyzing multiple patent documents with inbuilt landscape visualizer[J]. Pharm Pat Anal, 2015, 4(5): 377-386.

[80] Zhang Y, Xu J, Chen H, et al. Chemical named entity recognition in patents by domain knowledge and unsupervised feature

learning[J]. Database(Oxford). 2016, 2016: baw049.

[81] Hemati W, Mehler A. LSTMVoter: Chemical named entity recognition using a conglomerate of sequence labeling tools[J]. J Cheminform, 2019, 11(1): 3.

[82] Luo L, Yang Z, Yang P, et al. A neural network approach to chemical and gene/protein entity recognition in patents[J]. J Cheminform, 2018, 10(1): 65.

[83] He J, Nguyen D Q, Akhondi S A, et al. ChEMU 2020: Natural language processing methods are effective for information extraction from chemical patents[J]. Front Res Metr Anal, 2021, 6: 654438.

[84] Mahendran D, Gurdin G, Lewinski N, et al. Identifying chemical reactions and their associated attributes in patents[J]. Front Res Metr Anal, 2021, 6: 688353.

[85] Hsu P, Lee D, Tambe P. Deep Learning, Text, and Patent Valuation[J]. SSRN eLibrary, 2021.

[86] Akhondi S A, Klenner A G, Tyrchan C, et al. Annotated chemical patent corpus: A gold standard for text mining[J]. PLoS One, 2014, 9(9): e107477.

[87] PATENTSCOPE (参见WIPO官方网址).

[88] WIPO-Search International and National Patent Collections (参见WIPO官方网址).

[89] Schuler G D, Epstein J A, Ohkawa H, et al. Entrez: Molecular biology database and retrieval system[J]. Computer Methods for Macromolecular Sequence Analysis, 1996, 266: 141-162.

[90] Entrez Help [Internet]. Bethesda(MD): National Center for Biotechnology Information(US); 2006 Jan 20. (参见NCBI官方网址).

[91] Agarwala R, Barrett T, Beck J, et al. Database resources of the National Center for Biotechnology Information[J]. Nucleic Acids Research, 2018, 46(D1): D8-D13.

[92] Sample GenBank Record (参见NCBI官方网址).

[93] ENA Browser (参见ENA官方网址).

[94] Sequence Data Included in Patent Applications(参见DDBJ官方网址).

[95] DDBJ Sequence Search by Accession Numbers(参见DDBJ官方网址).

[96] About DDBJ Center(参见DDBJ官方网址).

[97] Xu G G, Webster A, Doran E. Patent sequence databases[J]. World Patent Information, 2002, 24(2): 95-101.

[98] Yoo H, Ramanathan C, Barcelon-Yang C. Intellectual property management of biosequence information from a patent searching perspective[J]. World Patent Information, 2005, 27(3): 203-211.

[99] Andree P J, Harper M F, Nauche S, et al. A comparative study of patent sequence databases[J]. World Patent Information, 2008, 30(4): 300-308.

[100] Rigden D J, Fernandez X M. The 2022 Nucleic Acids Research database issue and the online molecular biology database collection[J]. Nucleic Acids Research, 2022, 50(D1): D1-D10.

第17章

模型引导的药物研发（MIDD）监管要求与思考

王　维　　澳门大学，澳门，中国
王玉珠　　国家药品监督管理局药品审评中心，中国
欧阳德方　澳门大学，澳门，中国

17.1 MIDD发展的驱动力

传统药物开发主要依靠试错策略，通过大量的体外和体内测试验证和优化药物产品的疗效和安全性。然而，随着药物数据的急剧积累，自然的想法是将以前分散的数据或知识整合起来，以促进药物开发。因此，制药4.0时代不可避免地将要到来[1]。2004年，美国食品药品管理局（FDA）引入了创新药物研发计划（Innovative Path Program），旨在通过包括基于模型的药物研发（MBDD）方法在内的四项举措以提高创新药物的研发成功率。经过近二十年的发展，模拟技术现已变得至关重要，模型引导的药物研发（MIDD）[2]一词也越来越流行。

药物监管机构尤其是FDA释放出了一种向MIDD转变的关键驱动力。FDA认识到，无休止的试验并不一定能够提高产品质量，以及产品质量主要应由产品设计来决定[3]。因此，FDA在过去的十年里一直强调在药物开发中采用质量源于设计（QbD）的理念。

根据质量源于设计（QbD）理念，药物开发时应该考虑以下三点[3]：①确定关键质量属性（CQA），如影响药物性能的溶出曲线；②确定关键物料属性（CMA）（如颗粒大小）和关键工艺参数（CPP）（如研磨方法），以及CPP、CMA和CQA之间的关系；③制定CPP、CMA和CQA的规格或标准，以保证临床性能和质量控制制造策略；④认识到在制造过程中的可变性和持续改进。QbD策略有助于建立产品属性与临床性能之间清晰的关系，并建立关于这些属性的质量标准，据此研发者可以监控产品质量，提高工艺能力，提高生产效率，降低产品差异性，并为上市后（post-approval）生产工艺的改进提供合理化依据[4]。换言之，QbD策略强化了我们的"对制剂的理解"，基于这种理解，研发者和机构可以共同致力于优化过程，以给患者提供高质量的药品。

那么如何利用QbD策略呢？至少建模是一个很好的方法。生理药代动力学（PBPK）模型、群体药代动力学（Pop-PK）模型、药代动力学/药效动力学（PK/PD）或暴露-反应（E-R）模型等建模工具，是评估不同药物制剂生物等效性（BE）并设定临床相关性标准的重要方法[2]。PBPK模型通过基于机制的方式整合了与制剂和生理相关的参数，用于模拟药物暴露，从而可用于识别影响制剂性能的关键参数。Pop-PK模型考虑了个体间的变异，可用于进行虚拟生物等效性（VBE）模拟，从而指导生物等效性（BE）测试的研究设计。此外，Pop-PK模型可以利用稀疏采样的体内数据帮助确定对制剂差异敏感的PK指标。PK/PD或E-R模型是连接药物PK与治疗效果和安全性的桥梁，进一步发展出的定量系统药理学（QSP）模型还可通过药理机制模拟药物效应[5]。通过整合这些方法，可以从感兴趣的制剂中推断临床性能，从而促进药物制剂的开发和质量控制。

在临床药理学领域也可见到监管机构推动MIDD的努力。例如，欧洲药品管理局（EMA）最近发布了关于成人到儿科用药外推的科学指南[6]，该指南强调使用Pop-PK、PK/PD、PBPK等建模方法。如果成人和小儿疾病进展和治疗反应在某种程度上相似，推断是有希望的。外推法既满足了儿童的治疗需求，又尽可能减轻儿童参与临床试验的研究负担和伦理问题。类似的进步也出现在其他人群中，如孕妇和器官功能受损的患者，尽管应用程度还较低[7]。临床药理学中还有一个重要问题，药物相互作用（DDI），现已普遍涉及PBPK建模[8]。多种药物联合给药可能会改变单一药物的暴露，这通常由其他药物引起的代谢酶活性变化介导。PBPK模型通过模拟这种情况，可以为药物剂量调整提供指导，并支持药物处方信息的制定。

对于制药行业，应用建模来加速药物开发也备受热捧。在药物发现阶段，大数据工具、人工智能（AI）或机器学习（ML）等方法已被大量探索用于主导化合物筛选[9, 10]。在制剂开发阶段，包括AI、分子建模、PBPK、数学建模和计算流体动力学（CFD）建模在内的多种建模方法，对于选择制剂类型和理解制剂是很有用处的[11]。在生产阶段，过程分析技术（PAT）允许对生产流程进行连续监督和控制，从而实现"连续生产"，以确保药品质量[11]。因此，如今在提交给监管机构的文件中常常包含建模和模拟的内容，作为模型整合实证（MIE）。每年提交给FDA的包含三种建模方法信息的审评文件数量如图17-1所示。

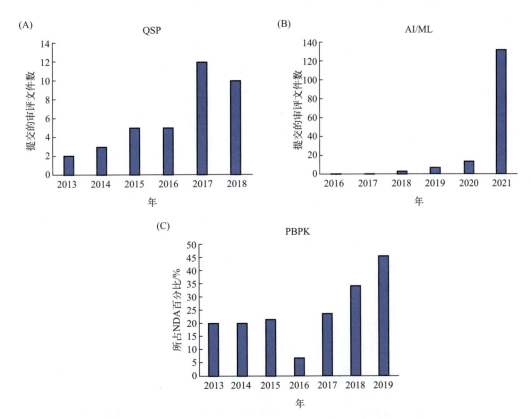

图17-1　向FDA提交的包含建模和模拟信息的年度报告。（A）包含QSP信息的IND和NDA申请（数据来自文献[12]）。（B）包含AI或机器学习信息的IND、NDA、ANDA和生物制品许可申请（BLA）申请（数据来自文献[13]）。（C）包括PBPK模拟的NDA的比例（数据来自文献[8]）

可见，MIDD的概念正在影响药物开发和监管的每一个部分。然而，作为一种新的方法，建模方法本身也需要规范化，以确保其被正确使用，并得出有效的结论。

17.2 建模方法的监管指南

迄今为止，监管机构已经发布了多种建模方法的指导原则，其中大多数涵盖了与PK相关的模型，例如E-R模型或PK/PD模型、Pop-PK模型和PBPK模型。这些模型与治疗的安全性和有效性密切相关，对监管决策产生影响。实施指导原则也反映了这样一个事实，即建模方法在现阶段得到了广泛应用。所有指导原则都包含了各机构当前关于良好建模实践的想法和建议，并不是实际的法律。通常，对于一种模型开发和验证的规则也适用于其他方法。

17.2.1 E-R模型或PK/PD模型

实际上，PK/PD模型在广义上是一种E-R模型，但是PK/PD模型更强调对药物暴露和反应的时间序列数据的分析[14]。2003年，FDA发布了关于E-R研究设计和分析的指导原则[15]。暴露-反应信息在评估药物的安全性和有效性方面起着核心作用。对此进行建模是为了将给药剂量对应的药物浓度度量（C_{max}、AUC、C_{ss}、浓度-时间曲线等）与临床效应的指标（临床终点、已建立的替代指标、相关生物标志物及其在时间上的变化）联系起来。通过这样，可以预测未测试剂量的反应，如果临床试验设计良好，可以估计诸如性别和体重等因素的影响。因此，E-R建模可以帮助优化剂量方案和个性化治疗。

在建立模型之前，开发人员应明确模型建立的目的，以及支持模型合理性所需的关于PK、PD和混杂因素的假设。然后，根据收集到的数据、药物作用机制、模型目的和假设，选择适当的模型结构或比较不同模型结构的性能，找到最佳模型。最终的模型应在拟合优度和模型简单性之间取得平衡。对于模型验证，将数据分为训练集和测试集是一种常见方法。最后，通过统计方法评估预测能力。E-R模型的预测能力非常重要，特别是在建模的目的是指导主要的疗效研究设计、应对安全性问题或为新的给药方案、新的用药人群和制剂变化提供依据时。

17.2.2 Pop-PK模型

由于人群中药物吸收、分布、代谢和排泄（ADME）参数的变异性，不同受试者对于相同剂量方案的体内药物暴露（如血浆浓度）是不同的。不幸的是，PK的这种个体间效应不太可能通过临床试验进行充分的调查，因为实际中存在的困难会影响从患者采集样本的数量和完整性。试验中常见血清药物浓度曲线无法覆盖完整的时间长度，从而导致数据稀疏。

Pop-PK模型提供了一种解决这些问题的途径[16]。Pop-PK模型将PK模型中单个个体对参数的贡献（如清除率、室体积）划分为人群典型值（人群中的共性）、协变量影响（如年龄、体重）和特定个体的随机效应（个体变异）。结合适当的统计算法，Pop-PK可以从包含不同人口和个体特征以及采样方案在内的训练数据中估计个体特异性参数和这些参数的个体间变异，从而使得对不同临床试验的汇总数据和稀疏数据进行分析成为可能。

FDA和EMA都发布了Pop-PK建模指南[17, 18]。Pop-PK模型的一个主要应用是预测不同特征的人群和个体在各种剂量方案下药物暴露情况，这是剂量优化和个体化治疗的重要证据。Pop-PK模型的另一个应用是指导临床试验的设计，例如应该包括多少受试者来估计协变量的效果。最后，Pop-PK模拟可以补充PK曲线中缺失的数据，并用于如PK/PD建模等后续工作。

Pop-PK模型的结果可以呈现在药物的说明书上，以描述其在不同人群和情况下的ADME。特定的人群可能是肝或肾功能障碍的患者，以及某个年龄、体重、性别或种族的小群体，尤其是儿科人群。合并用药是实践中常见的情况，Pop-PK模型也可以提供DDI的信息。在这些情况下，进行额外的E-R建模是很重要的，这样可以在考虑协变量时设定临床相关浓度界值，用以确定剂量是否需要调整。

若进行Pop-PK分析，首先要明确建模的目的，并审查手头所有的数据，评估样本量、协变量和数据质量等。详细描述建模所用的数据，尤其是排除数据的方法，对于评审机构来说非常重要，因为它是模型能力的基础。对于模型开发，应适当选择和论证模型结构和协变量分析方法。协变量-参数关系的制定应考虑数据的信息和其他机制或异速生长原理。建立模型后，应通过多种方法验证所宣称的用途的有效性（fit-for-purpose）。验证应该通过多种方法进行。良好拟合度（GOF）图可以首先用来显示整体拟合性能。此外，还应进行参数的收缩估计。高收缩降低了模型的信息性，在这种情况下，应使用基于模拟的诊断图。此外，还应估计和报告参数的不确定性。

17.2.3　PBPK模型

PBPK模型是一种基于机理的模型，强调利用生理或制剂相关属性以"自下而上"的方式预测药物PK。由于模型中的许多参数在现实中具有实际意义且可检测，因此PBPK建模显示出更高的模拟可解释性。

2018—2020年，FDA、EMA和日本监管机构发布了关于报告PBPK建模的指南[19-21]。此时，各机构已经收到越来越多的涉及PBPK模拟的提交材料，以解决临床药理学问题，如DDI、肝或肾功能障碍患者的以及儿童给药[7, 8]。与前面提到的指南类似，对建模目的、药物ADME特性、使用的数据、所做的假设以及模型开发过程的详细描述是模型具有高影响力的前提。

EMA指南[20]提供了一些关于PBPK模型验证的具体建议。一般而言，验证分为两个部分：PBPK平台的资格认证和特定药物模型的预测性能评估。平台资格认证意味着证明PBPK平台（如软件或程序）可以用于特定目的。为此，应使用具有相似ADME机制（如由相同酶代谢）的几种药物（指南中推荐的8至10种）的观察数据进行认证。然而，对资格认证的要求也随建模目的和模型影响力而有不同[7, 20]。指南中给出了不同影响力的一些示例以及资格认证要求。此外，平台资格认证还包含一个名为验证的部分，这是为了确保所使用的模型结构和方程是正确的。特定药物模型的预测性能评估意味着证明该模型对于声称目的的特定药物是有效的。该模型应尽可能多地捕获不同给药方案下的观察数据，例如不同的剂量水平、重复给药和不同的给药途径。基于虚拟人群的模拟结果应与观察结果进行比较。模拟和观察之间关于PK参数（例如C_{max}、AUC）的误差倍数是一般基准，以证明该模型是可接受的[22]。此外，对于关键参数或不确定参数，应进行敏感性分析以判断预测是否可靠。

PBPK模型在生物药剂学方面的应用是另一个主要的领域[23]，也被称为PBPK吸收模型或基于生理的生物药剂学模型（PBBM）。目前，FDA已发布的指南草案涵盖口服药物产品开发、生产工艺变更及控制等主题[24]。用于生物药剂学应用的PBPK模型是将口服产品的溶出结果与其他与吸收过程相关的参数相结合来预测PK。在这里，溶出结果是各种CMA和CPP与PK表现联系的桥梁，因为许多产品属性都会影响溶出性能。该方法应用十分广泛。例如，基于PK特征和吸收相关的参数，可以推导出体内溶出曲线，用于指导改善体外溶出试验方法，以开发用于产品质量控制的生物预测性溶出方案。更重要的是，PBPK模拟可以获得与临床相关的溶出接受范围，为其他制剂参数提供产品质量规范。通过VBE试验，可以确定制剂BE或非BE的溶出边界，该范围可作为设定接受标准和规范的依据。此举可能减轻批准前和批准后阶段中与制剂或生产工艺变化相关的体内研究负担。对影响较大的变化建议进行参数敏感性分析，这种方法还支持口服制剂的风险评估。

该指南还提供了有关生物药剂学应用模型在构建和验证方面的一些建议。对于模型结构，由于该应用侧重于药物吸收，因此吸收模型应该是基于生理的，而全身分布模型可以简化为非PBPK分布模型。对于模型验证，应使用来自多种剂型（具有可接受的或不可接受的生物利用度）的数据来提高模型置信度，并构建体内PK曲线和体外溶出曲线之间的等级关系，以表明该模型能够捕捉到溶出变化的影响。在进行VBE测试时，虚拟个体数量，个体内和个体间的变异性，以及试验方案（模拟方案）应模拟真实的BE试验。

17.2.4　计算流体动力学建模和其他建模技术

建模是医疗器械设计中的一种重要方法。2016年，FDA发布了指南文件，讨论了相关申请中计算建模部分应当具有的内容和格式，这与计算流体动力学、计算固体力学等方法有关[25]。

其实不同建模方法的指南有异曲同工之处。首先，要阐明建模的目的，以及应用背景。其次，需要描述代码的验证工作以确保程序的正确性。然后是控制方程和模拟设置。例如，CFD基于流体动力学方程对呼吸道药物沉积进行模拟，在呼吸道疾病吸入器的设计中尤其有用。因此需要提及这些控制方程、模拟装置和呼吸道的几何形状的设置以及呼吸道的离散化方法。最后，还需要提供模型验证的方法、数据以及结果。

17.3　关于MIDD的一些新思考

指导原则只能代表监管机构对MIDD的部分思考。这种药物开发的新范式才刚刚开始流行，因此许多概念需要不断升级。前沿的观点和最新的案例更多地会通过在线研讨会或会议的形式分享和讨论。这些活动的录像可以在FDA仿制药研究优先事项和项目网站和复杂仿制药研究中心（CRCG）活动网站以及FDA和CRCG在YouTube网站的频道上找到。一些相关视频也可以在FDA小企业和行业援助（SBIA）教育活动网站上找到。此外，某些重要研讨会或会议的总结会在活动结束后以文章的形式发布[26-28]。本章撰写的时间恰好是2022年10月27—28日举办的"利用建模方法支持仿制药产品开发的最佳实践"研讨会之后。

17.3.1　PBPK模拟用于体内试验的豁免

目前，PBPK已应用于几乎所有类型的制剂[29]。应用的主要方向是口服制剂。进行

PBPK的一个朴素目标是使用计算机模拟方法作为替代昂贵且耗时的体内研究方法，以提供令人信服且准确的关于药物PK的预测。然而，具有如此高影响力的模型需要严格的验证。哪种类型的PBPK模型可能被视为支持体内研究豁免的可信模型，这种经验对于预见监管机构对PBPK在药物开发中的机遇和挑战的态度非常有价值。

17.3.1.1 口服制剂中的应用

PBPK是一种重要的促进仿制药开发的计算辅助工具[2]。对于仿制药产品，新开发的产品必须与参比产品达到生物等效性。为减少不必要的体内研究，只有在产品符合某些特殊条件并有充分理由的情况下，才可以申请生物利用度（BA）或生物等效性（BE）测试的豁免。一般而言，对于口服药物，FDA指南[30, 31]指出，如果满足以下条件，BE测试可以豁免：①药物属于生物药剂学分类系统（BCS）Ⅰ类（高溶解度和高渗透性）或BCS Ⅲ类（高溶解度、低渗透性）；②药物产品是速释（IR）剂型；③对于BCS Ⅰ类药物，产品不具有影响吸收的辅料，而对于BCS Ⅲ类药物，产品的组成在质量上相同（Q1）且在数量上非常相似（Q2）。在这种情况下，PBPK模拟结果可以为生物利用度豁免申请提供更有力的证据。

上述要求尤其是对BCS Ⅲ类药物来说是比较保守的，因为人们担心不同的辅料对药物的吸收率和吸收程度的影响。然而，FDA的一项研究表明，只有25%的获得批准的BCS Ⅲ类仿制药达到上述Q1/Q2规则[32]。因此，应该有机会扩大BCS Ⅲ类药物用于生物利用度豁免的范围。关于该主题的PBPK建模研究在《仿制药使用者费用法案》（GDUFA）资助范围内。此外，PBPK建模也是研究辅料对药物吸收的影响的工具[33]。

对于BCS Ⅱ/Ⅳ类（低溶解度和高/低渗透性）药物和缓释（ER）制剂，PBPK是否可以在仿制药开发中支持其生物豁免，这方面的讨论还不太明确。这些制剂的PBPK建模可能更侧重于为关键属性设定规范，以确保不同制剂批次之间的生物等效性并免除体内生物等效性研究。从2008年到2018年，至少有24个提交给FDA的新药申请（其中71%是BCS Ⅱ或Ⅳ类药物）涉及PBPK模拟，其中许多申请用于设定溶出、粒径和粒径分布（PSD）[23]的规范。如前所述，这种应用有利于质量控制和批准后的制造工艺调整。对于缓释制剂，设定溶出规范或证明制造工艺调整通常还需要构建体内-体外相关性（IVIVC）。它将体外释放曲线映射到体内释放或吸收曲线[34]。IVIVC可以通过PBPK构建，与用传统方法构建IVIVC相比，PBPK方法考虑了更多的机制因素[23]。

在药物开发过程中，除了制剂的内在因素外，重要的外在因素也需进行调查。由于许多药物具有pH依赖的溶解性，其溶解和吸收对胃pH敏感，而胃pH可被抗酸药（ARA）轻易提高。通过整合pH依赖的溶解性，PBPK模型可预测在共用ARA情况下的PK。FDA发布的指南[35]已认可PBPK作为研究ARA引起的DDI的工具。另外一项FDA的研究使用了四个弱碱性药物，表明PBPK可以充分预测缺乏DDI效应的药物的PK，但只能定性预测具有阳性DDI效应的药物[36]。因此，PBPK至少可用于判断一种药物是否易受ARA影响。PBPK可以整合到常规ARA的DDI研究中，对于预测缺乏DDI的药物，可能可以免除体内ARA研究[37]。例如，帕纳博尼索坦，其中PBPK模拟被接受代替ARA的DDI研究[37]。然而，目前这种应用有一些限制，例如PBPK模型尚未对弱酸性药物和ER制剂进行充分的验证，并且该模型不能模仿真实世界中胃pH的动态变化行为。

食物是影响药物吸收的另一个常见的外在因素。食物作用评价较为复杂，与药物溶解性、脂溶性、吸收机制以及食物成分的吸收等因素有关。目前，PBPK被证明是预测食物对药物PK影响的一个很好的方法，比基于剂量数和BCS分类等其他估计方法具有更高的预测能力[38]。通过PBPK以预测30种药物的食物效应的研究表明，如果食物作用不是通过转运体介导的，则对于BCS Ⅰ和Ⅲ类药物可以实现高置信度的模拟；对于BCS Ⅱ和Ⅳ类药物，如果食物效应是由食物摄入引起的溶解度改变而导致的，也可以实现高置信度的模拟[39]。然而，由于食物影响的生理学是多方面的（例如pH、胆汁盐浓度、体液体积、传输时间等），因此这些药物只占所研究药物的50%。由于食物作用的复杂性，开发一种生物预测性溶出试验往往具有挑战性。此外，当考虑VBE试验时，建议对多种制剂进行模型验证，包括BE和非BE批次，但可能没有足够的数据来满足这一需求。这些因素可能导致目前PBPK对食物效应的模拟更多见于解决吸收相关问题，而在影响监管决策方面的应用（例如豁免体内研究）则较少提及[23]。

17.3.1.2 其他剂型中的应用

上述讨论仅围绕口服制剂。PBPK是否可以作为其他类型制剂的替代BE方法？是的。对于局部作用产品（LAP），作用部位的药物暴露测量通常很困难，并且比较临床终点的BE研究可能对制剂和剂量变化不敏感。PBPK是一种潜在的工具。2021年发表的一个典型的案例展示了PBPK模型如何支持FDA批准了一种仿制的皮肤用药双氯芬酸钠局部凝胶[40]。申请人开展了一项体内BE研究，以PK终点为依据，但没有开展双氯芬酸钠局部凝胶特定药品指导原则（PSG）中建议的体内临床终点比较研究，而是采用PBPK模型进行VBE测试作为替代。模型的开发和验证分为三个层次。在第一层中，使用双氯芬酸钠溶液和凝胶制剂的多种剂量水平和多个局部给药部位的PK数据来验证模型（特定产品验证）。在第二层中，使用具有各种活性药物成分（API）、剂型和剂量水平的各种局部制剂的数据进行验证（平台验证）。在第三层中，在测试和参考制剂之间进行VBE测试以支持BE。在模型开发和验证过程中，通过敏感性分析以确定风险评估的高影响因素。这个案例的成功归功于许多因素，包括出色的PBPK平台、审慎的模型开发与验证计划、全面的数据收集以及监管机构的帮助。

上述案例中提供的关于模型验证和确认的概念也适用于其他案例。然而，对于LAP，PBPK作为替代BE方法一般而言仅是有希望的，但具有挑战性。主要问题包括缺乏建立系统及局部间药物暴露关系的可靠方法，并且表征作用部位局部药物暴露的数据有限[41,42]。到目前为止，对于口服吸入产品，建议将PBPK模型与CFD建模结合使用，以更好地预测气道中药物的分布并增加模型说服力[41]。对于眼用制剂，PBPK模拟技术正在推进。最近，几种溶液产品的兔眼药物暴露已成功地用PBPK外推到人类[43]。然而，它仍需要一些时间才能被接受为豁免体内研究的高影响模型。

近年来，复杂的制剂如蛋白质药物、细胞治疗和核酸药物已受到广泛关注。虽然PBPK模型偶尔也参与这些制剂的开发，但目前对监管决策的影响有限。不过PK/PD模型和Pop-PK模型已被广泛应用于这些药物的评审，以支持不同人群的给药方案[44,45]。

17.3.2 通过PK相关的模拟以减轻BE研究的负担

如果需要进行体内研究，可以采用与PK相关的模型来优化研究设计。例如，建模可以帮助缩短研究时间并减少BE研究的受试者数量，如图17-2所示。

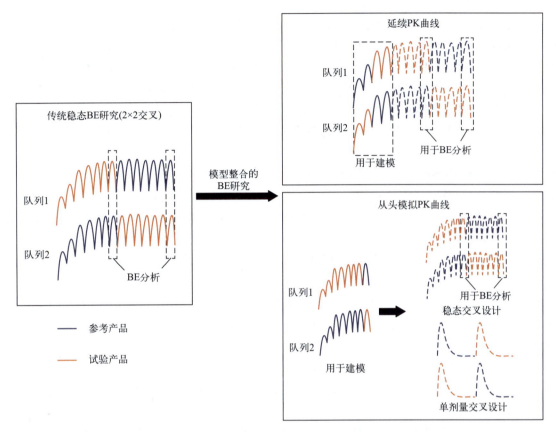

图17-2　传统的和模型整合的BE研究设计（实线表示从真实的体内PK研究中获得的PK曲线；虚线表示通过模型模拟的PK曲线）

交叉设计通常是BE研究的首选策略。在交叉研究中，每个受试者应接受一种治疗，再接受另一种治疗。然后，通过受试者内部比较两种治疗方法，因此这种设计减少了受试间变异的影响并提高了研究效力。然而，对于特殊制剂特别是长效注射剂（LAI），以常规方式进行理想的交叉研究可能不可行。对于这些制剂，BE通常需要在药物暴露达到稳态的条件下进行评估，而这需要很长时间才能达到，因为LAI的半衰期很长[46]。相反，模型整合的BE研究设计（图17-2）可以缩短体内研究阶段。患者在一个短的时间内以序贯方式多剂量地接受参考产品和试验产品，获得的PK数据可以用于建立两种制剂的Pop-PK和/或PBPK模型。之后，可以通过在受试者中延续PK曲线（in silico dosing MIE）以达到稳态的模拟，或是通过遵循稳态或单剂量设计从零开始建立模型（virtual BE MIE），以评估两种制剂之间的BE。

对于BE研究，一个关键问题是要招募多少受试者。较大的样本量有助于提高检验效能，得出强有力的结论，但也会增加研究成本。然而，通过在PK模型中改变虚拟受试者的数量并进行模拟，可以方便地估计适当且相对较少的受试者数量，以确保研究能力。用于建立初始PK模型的数据可能来自初步研究或文献资料。

17.3.3 机器学习及其统计方法的应用

机器学习（ML）或人工智能（AI）由于强大的分析多维大数据的能力，已经引起监管机构的关注。为促进AI在药品获益风险评估尤其在个体化给药中的应用，EMA和药品监管机构负责人组织（HMA）成立了大数据特别工作组[47]。特别工作组强调数据收集、数据处理和算法评估等框架，对于充分利用大数据技术非常重要。FDA最近发布了一份关于机器学习和人工智能在药物开发中潜在应用的讨论文件[48]，认可这项技术已被用于药物发现、非临床研究、临床研究、上市后安全监测和制药等多个阶段。FDA本身也进行了一些机器学习的应用。

2022年，Kineret被紧急授权用于治疗某些COVID-19患者。合适的患者的血浆可溶性尿激酶纤溶酶原激活剂受体（suPAR）应当≥ 6 ng·mL^{-1}。但是，检测suPAR不是一个市场化的方法，因此，研究者建立了一个机器学习模型通过其他一些可及的检测指标来预测suPAR水平，由此为这种药物进行患者优化[49]。这是机器学习应用在药物评估阶段的一个意义深远的事件。此外，一些研究人员试图使用机器学习模型进行临床数据分析，并发现它们很擅长识别协变量和治疗效应之间的关系[51, 52]。自然语言处理类的模型也有所尝试。例如，已有研究者开发了一个机器学习模型以自动识别药物标签中包含与食物效应相关的信息段落[50]。食物效应是仿制药开发中的一个重要问题，因此在PSG中突出了这一点。这种机器学习模型应该能提高信息检索任务的效率，从而促进PSG的发展。

应当注意的是，报告也指出尽管机器学习和人工智能应用取得了成功，但该方法中的一些局限性在未来应该得到改进，包括模型的数据质量、潜在的偏差、透明度、可解释性、概括性以及法律或伦理等问题[48]。

除了新型的ML模型外，多种统计模型也有开发应用，其中许多模型支持仿制药产品的批准。例如，稀疏主成分分析（Sparse-PCA）可被用来比较高效液相色谱-质谱法（LC-MS）谱图，并证明新开发的格拉替尼注射液和参比药品的成分相同[53]。基于EMD距离（Earth Mover's Distance）的模型证明，环孢素眼用乳剂的测试样品和参比药品的复杂粒度分布是等效的[54]。2020年，FDA批准了一种用于治疗或预防4岁及以上患者支气管痉挛的硫酸沙丁胺醇吸入气雾剂的仿制药，以应对COVID-19大流行。这种仿制药的批准部分归功于使用了新的基于似然的建模（M3模型），通过利用数据插补，分析包含大量截断值（检测限之外）的支气管挑战PD生物等效性研究数据[55]。

17.3.4 监管部门正努力促进MIDD的应用

新药和仿制药的开发中，都融入了MIDD方法。对于新药开发，MIDD一方面可以指导临床试验设计，另一方面可以深入分析临床数据，提取剂量、协变量和效应之间的关系，影响个体化给药方案和药品说明书的制定。为促进MIDD在新药开发中的应用，FDA从2018—2022的第六次处方药使用者费用法案（PDUFA Ⅵ）开始，启动了MIDD配对会议试点计划[56]。在该计划下，药物开发者可以与FDA讨论如何恰当地为特定药物使用MIDD方法，并在药物生命周期中分享他们的信息，旨在实现成功与协调的MIDD应用。同样，对于复杂的仿制药，在GDUFA的简化新药申请申报前（pre-ANDA）计划下，开发者也有机会在药物开发早期与FDA讨论。

预测模型的价值不应局限于某一具体案例，相反，它应该为未来案例提供洞察力。监管机构致力于制定有关模型重复使用的监管路径。适用于特定目的倡议（Fit-for-Purpose Initiative）提供了一个彻底评估根据声称目的提交的模型的监管流程[55]。如果用于类似目的，通过评估的模型可以用于各种药物开发项目。此外，该计划还提供了与 FDA 就 MIDD 的适当使用进行交流的机会。促进模型重用和共享的另一项行动是关于模型主文件（model master file，MMF）的讨论，这是已实施的药物主文件（drug master file）的类比。一般来说，MMF 预期将呈现验证模型所需的所有证据，包括建模目的、收集的数据以及模型验证方法和结果。如果实施，MMF 可以被多个申请交叉引用，以提高审查效率。

当前 MIDD 方法也面临许多挑战。为了改进仿制药开发中的 MIDD 应用，GDUFA 计划每年公布科研优先事项，并为资助了多项内部或外部的合作项目[55]，包括预测方法（PK 相关模型、CFD 模型、机器学习算法、生物预测溶出法等）、复杂 API 和制剂（悬浮制剂、脂质体药物、长效注射剂等）、各种给药途径（口服、眼用、皮肤、吸入、生殖道等）、MIDD 平台和监管工具的开发研究。

17.4 我国在定量药理学方面的进展

尽管基于数学的药物开发理念在 20 世纪 90 年代已经在中国学术界提出，但我国定量药理学的发展落后于其他发达国家。尽管一些大学领导人认识到定量药理学的潜力和重要性，但由于缺乏新药开发和出于可及性原因而侧重仿制药，定量药理学在过去 20 年中的增长受到了限制。

然而，随着 2015 年国务院《关于改革药品医疗器械审评审批制度的意见》的发布，情况开始改变。尽管在这方面缺乏经验，但更多的中国公司开始投资创新药物开发。这些公司获得了政府的鼓励。而且由于某些原因，投资新药成为这些公司不得不做出的选择。国家药品监督管理局（NMPA）看到了支持这些公司的迫切需求，需要发布包括 MIDD 方法在内的指南，以提高我国创新药物开发的效率和成功率。

近 2019 年末，中国药品审评中心（CDE）决定改进定量药理学指南，因为越来越多的创新药物在中国开发。2020 全年，CDE 启动与行业、学术界、政府及其内部工作组的讨论，就此事进行协商。2020 年 12 月 31 日，经过一年的协商，CDE 发布了"模型引导的药物研发技术指导原则"（MIDD 指南），正式向我国药品行业引入模型方法，鼓励我国公司在整个创新药物的发现和开发过程中使用定量药理学和模型模拟方法。这一指南被认为是我国定量药理学发展的一个重要里程碑。该指南由我国专家撰写，是世界上第一份此类指南。

在第一份 MIDD 模型指导原则发布后，过去三年我国定量药理学的发展快速推进。CDE 在不同的会议上介绍了 MIDD 指导原则。到目前为止，NMPA 已经发布了一些指导方针，包括为 MIDD 指导原则同一天发布的《群体药代动力学研究技术指导原则》，这被广泛认为是最常用的技术方法。这两项指导方针是我国首批模型相关指导方针，对于业界和监管机构来说都成为了一个里程碑。2022 年，CDE 已经启动关于定量药理学在儿科用药中应用的讨论，预计很快会发布新的指导意见。不同适应证的指导原则，例如肿瘤和抗生素，也已经发布。

定量药理学被应用于多个领域，包括药物相互作用研究和暴露-反应分析，这在评价临床药理学中的创新药物方面至关重要。模型与模拟方法以及暴露-反应研究已然成为探索和优化患者（包括肝肾功能损害患者）给药方案的核心方法。

随着创新药物开发和指导在我国不断增长，定量药理学专业在大学和企业中得到了认可。然而，由于定量药理学在我国的历史相对较短，受训学生和有经验的专家的短缺在一定程度上阻碍了其发展。鼓舞人心的是，越来越多的培训课程，包括免费的课程，开始介绍定量药理学和模型模拟。

17.5 总结

MIDD是一种新颖的药物开发方法。对如何恰当使用它达成共识对制药领域很重要。为此，监管机构的努力不可或缺。到目前为止，已经有几个指导文件讨论了一些建模方法的潜在应用和关注点。然而，应当注意MIDD本身正在快速发展，在谨慎的模型验证后，建模方法可能会用于更广泛的目的。尽管还没有一致的框架和标准来验证各种模型应用，但一般的验证规则可能存在。监管审查的模型应包含模型的明确目的、模型开发和验证的数据，以及关于模型结构和参数的每一个细节，以便审查者重新构建模型。对于模型验证，模型应尽可能再现尽可能多剂量和API的数据，并且非常重要的是要证明模型表现对关键参数变化有正确的敏感性。开发和验证完善的模型有望在未来被再次用于其他药物应用。

MIDD方法在药物开发中显示出巨大的潜力。尽管该技术和对它的理解仍需改进，监管机构对它的态度是开放和审慎的。因此，这个领域的未来看上去是很光明的。

参考文献

[1] Steinwandter V, Borchert D, Herwig C. Data science tools and applications on the way to Pharma 4.0[J]. Drug Discov Today, 2019, 24: 1795-805.

[2] Zhao L, Kim M J, Zhang L, Lionberger R. Generating model integrated evidence for generic drug development and assessment[J]. Clin Pharmacol Ther, 2019, 105: 338-349.

[3] Yu L X, Amidon G, Khan M A, et al. Understanding pharmaceutical quality by design[J]. AAPS J, 2014, 16: 771-783.

[4] The U.S. Food and Drug Administration. Guidance for industry: CMC postapproval manufacturing changes to be documented in annual reports, 2014.

[5] Derbalah A, Al-Sallami H, Hasegawa C, et al. A framework for simplification of quantitative systems pharmacology models in clinical pharmacology[J]. Brit J Clinical Pharma, 2022, 88: 1430-1440.

[6] The European Medicines Agency. ICH guideline E11A on pediatric extrapolation-Scientific guideline, 2022.

[7] Shebley M, Sandhu P, Emami Riedmaier A, et al. Physiologically based pharmacokinetic model qualification and reporting procedures for regulatory submissions: A consortium perspective[J]. Clinical Pharmacology and Therapeutics, 2018, 104: 88-110.

[8] Zhang X, Yang Y, Grimstein M, et al. Application of PBPK modeling and simulation for regulatory decision making and its impact on US prescribing information: An update on the 2018-2019 submissions to the US FDA's office of clinical pharmacology[J]. J Clin Pharmacol, 2020, 60(Suppl 1): S160-178.

[9] Vamathevan J, Clark D, Czodrowski P, et al. Applications of machine learning in drug discovery and development[J]. Nat Rev Drug Discov, 2019, 18: 463-477.

[10] Mak K K, Pichika M R. Artificial intelligence in drug development: present status and future prospects[J]. Drug Discov Today, 2019, 24: 773-780.

[11] Wang W, Ye Z, Gao H, Ouyang D. Computational pharmaceutics: A new paradigm of drug delivery[J]. J Control Release, 2021, 338: 119-136.

[12] Zineh I. Quantitative systems pharmacology: A regulatory perspective on translation[J]. CPT Pharmacometrics Syst Pharmacol, 2019, 8: 336-339.

[13] Liu Q, Huang R, Hsieh J, et al. Landscape analysis of the application of artificial intelligence and machine learning in regulatory submissions for drug development from 2016 to 2021[J]. Clinical Pharmacology & Therapeutics, 2023, 113: 771-774.

[14] Overgaard R, Ingwersen S, Tornøe C. Establishing good practices for exposure-response analysis of clinical endpoints in drug development[J]. CPT Pharmacometrics Syst Pharmacol, 2015, 4: 565-575.

[15] The U.S. Food and Drug Administration. Guidance for Industry: Exposure-Response Relationships — Study Design, Data Analysis, and Regulatory Applications, 2003.

[16] Owen J S, Fiedler-Kelly J. Introduction to population pharmacokinetic/pharmacodynamic analysis with nonlinear mixed effects models[M]. Hoboken, New Jersey: Wiley, 2014.

[17] The European Medicines Agency. Guideline on Reporting the Results of Population Pharmacokinetic Analyses, 2007.

[18] The U.S. Food and Drug Administration. Guidance for Industry: Population Pharmacokinetics, 2022.

[19] The U.S. Food and Drug Administration. Physiologically Based Pharmacokinetic Analyses — Format and Content Guidance for Industry, 2018.

[20] The European Medicines Agency. Guideline on the Reporting of Physiologically Based Pharmacokinetic(PBPK)Modelling and Simulation, 2018.

[21] Japan MHLW. Guidelines for analysis reports involving physiologically based pharmacokinetic models, 2020.

[22] Kuemmel C, Yang Y, Zhang X, et al. Consideration of a credibility assessment framework in model-informed drug development: potential application to physiologically-based pharmacokinetic modeling and simulation[J]. CPT: Pharmacometrics & Systems Pharmacology, 2020, 9: 21-28.

[23] Wu F, Shah H, Li M, et al. Biopharmaceutics applications of physiologically based pharmacokinetic absorption modeling and simulation in regulatory submissions to the U.S. Food and Drug Administration for new drugs[J]. AAPS J, 2021, 23: 31.

[24] The U.S. Food and Drug Administration. The Use of Physiologically Based Pharmacokinetic Analyses-Biopharmaceutics Applications for Oral Drug Product Development, Manufacturing Changes, and Controls-Draft Guidance for Industry. The U.S. Food and Drug Administration, 2020.

[25] The U.S. Food and Drug Administration. Reporting of Computational Modeling Studies in Medical Device Submissions, 2016.

[26] Suarez-Sharp S, Cohen M, Kesisoglou F, et al. Applications of clinically relevant dissolution testing: Workshop summary report[J]. AAPS J, 2018, 20: 93.

[27] Mitra A, Suarez-Sharp S, Pepin X J H, et al. Applications of physiologically based biopharmaceutics modeling(pbbm)to support drug product quality: A workshop summary report[J]. J Pharm Sci, 2021, 110: 594-609.

[28] Parrott N, Suarez-Sharp S, Kesisoglou F, et al. Best practices in the development and validation of physiologically based biopharmaceutics modeling: A workshop summary report[J]. J Pharm Sci, 2021, 110: 584-593.

[29] Wang W, Ouyang D. Opportunities and challenges of physiologically based pharmacokinetic modeling in drug delivery[J]. Drug Discov Today, 2022, (8): 27.

[30] The U.S. Food and Drug Administration. Guidance for Industry: Waiver of In Vivo Bioavailability and Bioequivalence Studies for Immediate-Release Solid Oral Dosage Forms Based on a Biopharmaceutics Classification System, 2017.

[31] The U.S. Food and Drug Administration. M9 Biopharmaceutics Classification System-Based Biowaivers, 2021.

[32] Zhang Y. Biopharmaceutics Classification System Class 3 Waiver. Advancing Innovative Science in Generic Drug Development Workshop, 2020.

[33] Chow E C, Talattof A, Tsakalozou E, et al. Using physiologically based pharmacokinetic (pbpk) modeling to evaluate the impact of pharmaceutical excipients on oral drug absorption: Sensitivity analyses[J]. AAPS J, 2016, 18: 1500-1511.

[34] Guidance for Industry: Extended Release Oral Dosage Forms: Development, Evaluation, and Application of In Vitro/In Vivo Correlations, 1997.

[35] The U.S. Food and Drug Administration. Evaluation of Gastric pH-Dependent Drug Interactions With Acid-Reducing Agents: Study Design, Data Analysis, and Clinical Implications Guidance for Industry-Draft Guidance for Industry. The U.S. Food and Drug Administration, 2020.

[36] Dong Z, Li J, Wu F, et al. Application of physiologically-based pharmacokinetic modeling to predict gastric pH-dependent drug-drug interactions for weak base drugs[J]. CPT Pharmacometrics Syst Pharmacol, 2020, 9: 456-465.

[37] Lin W, Chen Y, Unadkat J D, et al. Applications, challenges, and outlook for PBPK modeling and simulation: A regulatory, industrial and academic perspective[J]. Pharm Res-Dordr, 2022, 39: 1701-1731.

[38] Fink C, Sun D, Wagner K, et al. Evaluating the role of solubility in oral absorption of poorly water-soluble drugs using physiologically-based pharmacokinetic modeling[J]. Clin Pharmacol Ther, 2020; 107: 650-661.

[39] Riedmaier A E, DeMent K, Huckle J, et al. Use of physiologically based pharmacokinetic (PBPK) modeling for predicting drug-food interactions: An industry perspective[J]. AAPS J, 2020, 22: 123.

[40] Tsakalozou E, Babiskin A, Zhao L. Physiologically-based pharmacokinetic modeling to support bioequivalence and approval of generic products: A case for diclofenac sodium topical gel 1%[J]. CPT Pharmacometrics Syst Pharmacol, 2021, 10: 399-411.

[41] Walenga R L, Babiskin A H, Zhao L. In silico methods for development of generic drug-device combination orally inhaled drug products[J]. CPT Pharmacometrics Syst Pharmacol, 2019, 8: 359-370.

[42] Zhao L, Seo P, Lionberger R. Current scientific considerations to verify physiologically-based pharmacokinetic models and their implications for locally acting products[J]. CPT Pharmacometrics Syst Pharmacol, 2019, 8: 347-351.

[43] Le Merdy M, Alqaraghuli F, Tan M L, et al. Clinical ocular exposure extrapolation for ophthalmic solutions using PBPK modeling and simulation[J]. Pharm Res, 2022, 40(2): 431-447.

[44] Belov A, Schultz K, Forshee R, et al. Opportunities and challenges for applying model-informed drug development approaches to gene therapies[J]. CPT: Pharmacometrics & Systems Pharmacology, 2021, 10: 286-290.

[45] Fairman K, Li M, Ning B, et al. Physiologically based pharmacokinetic(PBPK)modeling of RNAi therapeutics: Opportunities and challenges[J]. Biochem Pharmacol, 2021; 189: 114468.

[46] Sharan S, Fang L, Lukacova V, et al. Model-informed drug development for long-acting injectable products: Summary of American College of Clinical Pharmacology Symposium[J]. Clin Pharm Drug Dev, 2021, 10: 220-228.

[47] Hines P A, Herold R, Pinheiro L, et al. Artificial intelligence in European medicines regulation[J]. Nat Rev Drug Discov, 2023, 22(2): 81-82.

[48] The U.S. Food and Drug Administration. Artificial Intelligence and Machine Learning (AI/ML) for Drug Development, FDA, 2023.

[49] The U.S. Food and Drug Administration. Emergency Use Authorization (EUA) for Kineret (Anakinra), n.d.

[50] Shi Y, Ren P, Zhang Y, et al. Information extraction from FDA drug labeling to enhance product-specific guidance assessment using natural language processing[J]. Front Res Metr Anal, 2021, 6: 670006.

[51] Gong X, Hu M, Zhao L. Big data toolsets to pharmacometrics: Application of machine learning for time-to-event analysis[J]. Clin Transl Sci, 2018, 11: 305-311.

[52] Gong X, Hu M, Basu M, et al. Heterogeneous treatment effect analysis based on machine-learning methodology[J]. CPT Pharmacometrics Syst Pharmacol, 2021, 10: 1433-1443.

[53] Rogstad S, Pang E, Sommers C, et al. Modern analytics for synthetically derived complex drug substances: NMR, AFFF-MALS, and MS tests for glatiramer acetate[J]. Anal Bioanal Chem, 2015, 407: 8647-8659.

[54] Hu M, Jiang X, Absar M, et al. Equivalence testing of complex particle size distribution profiles based on earth mover's distance[J]. AAPS J, 2018, 20: 62.

[55] Madabushi R, Seo P, Zhao L, et al. Review: Role of model-informed drug development approaches in the lifecycle of drug development and regulatory decision-making[J]. Pharm Res-Dordr, 2022, 39: 1669-1680.

[56] Madabushi R, Benjamin J M, Grewal R, et al. The US Food and Drug Administration's model-informed drug development paired meeting pilot program: early experience and impact[J]. Clin Pharmacol Ther, 2019, 106: 74-78.